Introduction to
Healthcare
Informatics

Second Edition

Sue Biedermann, MSHP, RHIA, FAHIMA
Diane Dolezel, EdD, RHIA, CHDA

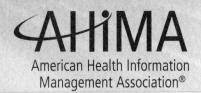

AHIMA
American Health Information
Management Association®

ISBN: 978-1-58426-528-3
AHIMA Product No.: AB120015

AHIMA Staff:
Chelsea Brotherton, MA, Assistant Editor
Ashley Latta, Production Development Editor
Elizabeth Ranno, Vice President of Product and Planning
Caitlin Wilson, Project Editor
Pamela Woolf, Director of Publications

Cover image: ©teekid, iStockPhoto

For more information, including updates, about AHIMA Press publications, visit http://www.ahima.org/education/press.

American Health Information Management Association
233 North Michigan Avenue, 21st Floor
Chicago, Illinois 60601-5809
ahima.org

Table of Contents

Detailed Contents

Chapter 5

Chapter 6

Chapter 7

Chapter 8

Chapter 9

Chapter 10

Chapter 11

Chapter 12

Chapter 13

Chapter 14

Chapter 15

Online Resources

About the Authors

Lead Authors

Sue Biedermann, MSHP, RHIA, FAHIMA, is associate professor emeritus and the former chair of the HIM Department at Texas State University. She has served the Texas Health Information Management Association in various appointed and elected positions including president. At the national level, she has been an accreditation site visitor for more than 15 years with additional past service including the Professional Conduct Committee, Nominating Committee, AOE Strategy Task Force, and project manager for the Professional Resource Task Force. Ms. Biedermann completed the AHIMA Research Institute and was most recently funded by the Texas Higher Education Coordinating Board for a project preparing for HIT students to advance to bachelor's level education. She has been author or coauthor on a number of publications and reports and presents frequently at state and national meetings. During her tenure as a faculty member, she has received the College of Health Professions Faculty Excellence Award and was selected as an Alpha Chi Favorite Professor.

Diane Dolezel, EdD, RHIA, CHDA, is an assistant professor in the HIM Department at Texas State University where she teaches informatics, analytics, and data use; healthcare research and data analysis; and quality management to graduate and undergraduate students. At the university, she serves on the faculty student research forum. Dr. Dolezel has published several peer-reviewed research articles on usability of web-based PHRs, data migration for EHRs, metadata, data analysis relational databases, and other informatics topics. She is a frequent speaker at national and regional AHIMA, HIMSS, and TSAHP conferences on electronically stored information, relational databases, and informatics topics. She worked in the information technology field for many years as a senior developer and consultant with significant experience in database programming and systems integration. She has served on the AHIMA Foundation Council for Academic Excellence, Faculty Development Workgroup and was awarded an AHIMA Merit Scholarship as a graduate student.

Contributing Authors

Juliana J. Brixey, PhD, MPH, MSN, RN, is currently an associate professor at the University of Texas Health Science Center at Houston. She holds a joint appointment with the School of Biomedical Informatics and School of Nursing. Her faculty position entails teaching biomedical and nursing informatics courses. Brixey is also director for the UT Health Center for Interprofessional Collaboration. She previously held the position of operations manager for Outreach and Education for the Gulf Coast Regional Extension Center.

Kelly McLendon, RHIA, CHPS, was awarded the 2015 AHIMA Innovation Award. The Innovation Award honors those individuals who are focused on moving Healthcare Informatics/Health Information Management into the future of the healthcare and wellness industry. It honors individuals who have promoted important advances in areas related to HIM practice, quality data, standards development, patient safety, systems development, and any domain where visionary thinking has made a difference.

Kelly has been a HIM (medical records) practitioner for over 36 years. Most recently he founded CompliancePro Solutions, a company that has brought the state-of-the-art HIPAA privacy compliance product PrivacyPro™ to the healthcare marketplace. He routinely works with a large network of healthcare providers and vendor business associates. He volunteers his time and expertise to professional associations, such as AHIMA, including serving on their Privacy and Security Practice Council.

Kelly is considered an innovator and subject matter expert in HIPAA Privacy and Security, Legal Health Records and is a computer system functional designer. Kelly's career includes many contributions to the migration of HIM into the electronic environment, an effort that has taken decades to achieve. He is a well-known speaker and author and has published a book on the topic of legal health records. He has been recognized with the 2003 AHIMA Visionary Award, the 2008 FAHIMA Distinguished Member, as well as numerous literary awards.

Joanne D. Valerius, PhD, MPH, RHIA, is the director of Health Information Management Graduate Programs at the Oregon Health and Science University in Portland, Oregon. Ms. Valerius's interests center on human resource development in healthcare settings and the impact of the electronic health record. Her focus is on a holistic approach to the workplace and how diversity impacts the workplace. Ms. Valerius is a published writer, as well as a national and international speaker. Currently, she serves on the Functioning and Disability Reference Group (FDRG) committee of the WHO for the International Health Information Management Association. She is an educational professional with 40-plus years of experience in HIM; and 20-plus years as a diversity consultant.

Susan White, PhD, RHIA, CHDA, is the administrator of Analytics at the James Cancer Hospital at the Ohio State University Wexner Medical Center and an associate professor of Clinical Health and Rehabilitation Sciences in the Health Information Management and Systems (HIMS) Division at the Ohio State University. Dr. White is responsible for the Cancer Program Analytics Department as well as driving the design and implementation of alternative payment models for cancer. In her academic role, she teaches classes in statistics, data analytics, healthcare finance, and computer applications. She has written numerous articles and presented to national audiences regarding the benchmarking of healthcare facilities and appropriate use of claims data. Dr. White has also published articles covering outcomes assessment and risk adjustment using healthcare financial and clinical data analysis, hospital benchmarking, and claims data mining. She is the author of AHIMA's *Healthcare Financial Management for Health Information and Informatics* and *A Practical Approach to Analyzing Healthcare Data.* Dr. White received her PhD in Statistics from the Ohio State University. She is a member of AHIMA, the American Statistical Association, and the Healthcare Financial Management Association. Prior to joining OSU, Dr. White was a vice president for Research and Development for both Cleverley and Associates and CHIPS/Ingenix. She has 20 years of experience in the practice of healthcare financial and revenue cycle consulting.

Foreword

Congratulations!

Health information professionals are moving into the field of informatics at warp speed. There are countless articles and quotes saying that this is one of the fasted growing careers. The US Department of Labor Statistics projects that employment in health informatics and related fields will grow nearly 17 percent from 2014 to 2024, much faster than average for all professions (BLS 2015).

Informatics involves people, processes, and technologies to produce and use trusted data for better decision making. The difference in our roles of the past, compared to our jobs of today, is that we now share and communicate information via technology rather than through paper records. This allows us to continue providing health information when and where it is needed but through electronic health records and other technology solutions.

The mission of the American Health Information Management Association (AHIMA) is to transform healthcare by leading health information management, informatics, and information governance. We believe that informatics will enable us to improve health through trusted information. Our goal is to gain recognition as the professional association of choice and present a widely accepted definition of informatics recognized by the healthcare industry.

Sue Biedermann, MSHP, RHIA, FAHIMA and Diane Dolezel, EdD, RHIA, CHDA, wrote and edited this text to inform health information professionals about the major roles associated with the field of informatics. Along with industry experts, they provide a roadmap to understand the foundations of this emerging field and the different competencies needed to succeed.

By reading this book, you will begin the journey of leading the healthcare industry into a world where decision making is better and more informed. *Introduction to Healthcare Informatics* helps the reader to understand the evolution of informatics and covers key issues from standards to clinical decision support. The editors and authors have provided information about computer science, technology, the provision of care, education, and research aspects of medicine.

Information management and informatics has never been more important. Only through trusted information will providers be able to continue driving down costs and improving the quality of care. Become part of the evolution to a better, more informed healthcare environment by reading this book and learning about the emerging field of health informatics.

Lynne Thomas Gordon, MBA, RHIA, CAE, FACHE, FAHIMA
Chief Executive Officer
American Health Information Management Association

REFERENCE

US Department of Labor Bureau of Labor Statistics. 2015 (December 8). Press Release: EMPLOYMENT PROJECTIONS—2014-24. https://www.bls.gov/news.release /pdf/ecopro.pdf

Acknowledgments

I would like to acknowledge the significant contributions of Dr. Susan Fenton in the planning and writing of the first edition of this text and of Diane Dolezel who joined me in this revision. My thanks and appreciation extends to the chapter authors for sharing their expertise with us for inclusion in the text. Recognition should also be given to the many HIM and other related professionals who are making a difference in healthcare with their influence in the healthcare informatics evolution. Last, but not least, thank you to my husband, Jim, and daughter, Amy, for your continued love and support.

Sue Biedermann

I want to acknowledge the contributions of Dr. Susan Fenton in the writing of the first edition of this text. I also want to acknowledge the work of Sue Biedermann who guided my efforts in the writing of the second edition of this text. Professionally, I continue to be inspired by Jackie Moczygemba who supports my efforts and provides an excellent role model for this dynamic field.

Diane Dolezel

Both authors wish to thank Ashley Latta and the AHIMA Press staff who supported us during the process of writing this book. We hope our fellow faculty and students find this book to be of benefit.

AHIMA Press would like to thank the authors who contributed to previous editions of this textbook:

- ⊙ Christopher G. Chute, MD
- ⊙ Susan H. Fenton, PhD, RHIA, FAHIMA
- ⊙ Desla Mancilla, DHA, RHIA
- ⊙ Jackie Moczygemba, MBA, RHIA, CCS, FAHIMA
- ⊙ Kim Murphy-Abdouch, MPH, RHIA, FACHE

AHIMA Press would also like to thank Susan H. Fenton, PhD, RHIA, FAHIMA, and Julie Swavely, MHA, RHIA, for their review and feedback of this publication.

Chapter

1

Foundations of Healthcare Informatics

Learning Objectives

- Examine the evolution of the field of health informatics
- Interpret the health informatics core competencies
- Apply the terms related to health informatics
- Compare the methods associated with health informatics
- Determine the need for current policies and procedures to support electronic health records and use of data
- Articulate ethical issues associated with health informatics
- Contrast the major roles associated with the field of health informatics

KEY TERMS

ASC X12 Accreditation Standards Committee

AMA Transactions and Code Set Standards

American Society for Testing and Materials (ASTM) on Computerized System Standards for HIT

Biomedical informatics

Chief clinical information officer (CCIO)

Chief information officer (CIO)

Chief knowledge officer (CKO)

Chief medical information officer (CMIO)

Clinical decision support

Clinical informatics

Computer-aided diagnosis (CAD)

Computerized provider order entry (CPOE)

Consolidated Health Informatics (CHI)

Consumer informatics

Data mining

Decision analysis

Digital Imaging Communication in Medicine (DICOM)

e-Health

Fast Healthcare Interoperability Resources Specification (FHIR)

Genetic Information Nondiscrimination Act of 2008 (GINA)
Genomics
Health informatics
Health information technology (HIT or health IT)
Health Insurance Portability and Accountability Act (HIPAA)
Health Level 7 (HL7)
Human Gene Nomenclature (HUGN)
Informaticist
Informatics
International Classification of Functioning and Disability (ICF)
Internet of Things (IoT)
Interoperability
Logical Observation Identifiers Names and Codes (LOINC)
Meaningful use of information
Medical informatics

Medical scribe
National Council for Prescription Drug Program (NCPDP)
National Drug File–Reference Terminology (NDF–RT)
Nursing informatics
Personal health record (PHR)
Physician Consortium for Performance Improvement (PCPI), American Medical Association
Population Health
Probability
Protected health information (PHI)
Public health informatics
RxNORM
Systematized Nomenclature of Medicine Clinical Terms (SNOMED CT)
Telehealth
Telemedicine
Translational medicine

The transformation in patient health records and their use with the move from paper-based patient records to electronic health record systems is a testament to the effects of advances in technology. These health informatics technologies facilitate the delivery of health information for use in clinical decision making, telehealth, predictive modeling, and population health studies. Moreover, new professional roles are emerging as a result of the increased focus on patient information utilization.

⊙ Definitions, Policies, Methods, and Ethics

Informatics is defined as "a field of study that focuses on the use of technology to improve access to and utilization of information" (AHIMA 2014, 78). **Health informatics** is "a science concerned with the cognitive, information processing and communication tasks of healthcare practice, education, and research, including the information science and technology to support these tasks" (AHIMA 2014, 68). The health informatics field continues to change with the development of newer and more advanced technology and applications. **Health information technology (HIT or health IT)** includes the technical aspects of processing health data and records including classification and coding, abstracting, registry development, and storage as stated at HealthIT.gov and includes electronic health records (EHRs), personal health records (PHRs), e-prescribing, health information exchange (HIE), and interoperability (HealthIT 2016a). The health informatics domain includes computer and data science, technology, and the provision of care, education, research aspects of medicine and the usability of information and information systems. Despite consistencies among informatics and healthcare professionals on the basic components comprising health informatics, the frame of reference continues to change as new health informatics applications emerge across the healthcare disciplines. These referential changes have generated varying definitions of health informatics, and currently no single consistently accepted definition exists. The first chapter of this book provides an introduction to health informatics by briefly reviewing its history, relevant definitions, and associated methods and roles.

Figure 1.1 presents the interrelationships of the aspects of health informatics, which includes clinical, financial and administrative data, and technology. The technology component provides the means for the acquisition, compiling, analysis, transmission, and storage of the clinical data. Clinical data includes all that is amassed in the treatment of the patient and is driven by the needs of the users and the availability to support the provision of care. The financial and administrative data are related to the need for quality healthcare provided in a cost-effective and secure manner. Health informatics is the overlapping area in the middle where all three components come together to produce new knowledge to be used in healthcare delivery. Indeed, advances in technology, including the utilization of the electronic health record, have been the major catalysts for the rapid advancement of health informatics.

New terms often emerge and the uses of these terms evolve as new technologies and fields are developed. It is important to understand the terminology that defines a concept or activity to truly be able to comprehend it. Many new health informatics terms are explored in this section, which covers the history of health informatics, core competencies, specific health informatics applications, methods for creating systems, and ethics.

Figure 1.1.   Relationship aspects of health informatics

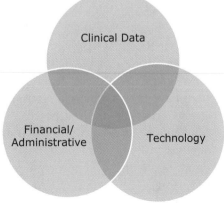

History of Health Informatics

Health informatics is a relatively new discipline that has received substantial attention primarily from healthcare providers and others who rely on reliable and substantial information to support decision making in both the provision of care and management and administrative endeavors. Much federal legislation has been enacted to promote the utilization of technology in healthcare and the **meaningful use of certified EHR technology. Meaningful use of information** is using systems with certified software to enhance the use of data contained in and obtained from health records. This requires meeting measurements such as the recording of patient information as structured data to exchanging information that provides summaries of care provided (HealthIT 2016b). The goals for the use of this data are to improve quality, safety, and efficiency; reduce health disparities; improve the engagement of patients and families; improve care coordination; and support population and public health while maintaining privacy and security. The objectives and measures for meeting the meaningful use program requirements as outlined by the Centers for Medicare and Medicaid Services (CMS) are:

- ⊙ Providers are required to attest to a single set of objectives and measures that replace the core and menu structures of previous stages. Core and menu structures required meeting all 15 core requirements and 5 of 10 menu requirements.

- ⊙ For eligible professionals (EPs), there are 10 objectives, and for eligible hospitals and critical access hospitals (CAHs), there are 9 objectives to meet. All providers must attest to objectives and measures using EHR technology certified to the 2014 edition. All providers may attest to objectives and measures using EHR technology certified to the 2015 edition, or a combination of the two (CMS 2016a).

As of October 2015, more than 479,000 healthcare providers received payment for participating in the Medicare and Medicaid EHR Incentive Programs (CMS 2016a). This meaningful use of information continues to be very important. Through the EHR Incentive Programs' requirements for 2015 through 2017 (Modified Stage 2) and Stage 3, CMS will focus on advanced use of certified EHR technology to support health information exchange and interoperability, advanced quality measurement, and maximizing clinical effectiveness and efficiencies. The EHR reporting period for eligible professionals, eligible hospitals, and CAHs begins and ends based on the calendar year (CMS 2016a; 42 CFR 412 and 495).

The significant increase in awareness of the field of health informatics has led to the belief that it is a new field, but the term health informatics was coined a number of years ago. There have been numerous references in the literature to the use of computers in the provision of healthcare, information processing, and a reference to data management in medicine, as well as the use of the terms "computer technology" together with "medicine" and "healthcare." Some healthcare institutions were just beginning to use systems with patient care applications during this time (Saba et al. 1994). Transaction or process oriented systems used in healthcare in the earlier times were primarily for the financial and accounting functions (Sewell and Thede 2012). A report, "Benefits of Health Informatics for Patients," published by the University of Illinois at Chicago related that, in the 1950s, "healthcare experts realized the need to integrate health records of patients along with the use of computers and that originally, this process was called medical computing" (UIC 2016). As the capabilities of computer technology continued to evolve with more applications and opportunities for utilization to support the provision of healthcare, there was a pressing need for a recognizable name for the new domain. However, difficulties arose due to the diversity of science, technology, engineering, and healthcare that were the key components of the domain. The US government was instrumental in supporting and developing the medical informatics movement through the initial funding for academic medical centers. The academic medical centers had considerably more patients than most other hospitals, with more diverse and complicated medical cases where the utilization of information in diagnostics and treatment was vital, plus the prohibitive cost for many facilities of the large mainframe computers that were required in the 1960s. Reports from the early 1970s indicated that **medical informatics** was used "to cover both the information and data parts as well as the controlling and automatic nature of data processing itself" (Anderson and Jay 1987).

In the ensuing years additional working definitions were considered. Definitions included terms such as computer science, information science, engineering, and technology related to the fields of health and medicine and includes practice, education, and research. For example, in the computer science realm, **computer-aided diagnosis (CAD)** was introduced, which uses computers and information science for provision of care designed to improve the outcomes of the practice of medicine. CAD incorporates computer images with aspects of artificial intelligence to detect and identify potential disease factors. Furthermore, disease information such as symptoms, duration, medical history, and diagnostic information from numerous cases can be stored in CAD systems. This allows similar patient information to be compared to the stored data using computer algorithms and a list of probable diagnoses can be generated for the physician to consider (Dior et al. 1999).

As health informatics continued to develop, the need for standards and models became apparent. Definitions of standards appropriate for the health informatics movement include such phrases as, "A scientifically based statement of expected behavior against which structures, processes, and outcomes can be measured" or "A model or example established by authority, custom, or general consent or a rule established by an authority as a measure of quantity, weight, extent, value, or quality" (AHIMA 2014, 137). When health informatics is incorporated in the delivery of healthcare, the need for models or examples for quality measurements is vital to assure valid outcomes are obtained.

The following is a list of current standards specific to health data and health informatics:

- **PCPI (Physician Consortium for Performance Improvement, American Medical Association [AMA])** develops, evaluates, uses, and disseminates best practices based on evidence-based measures.

- ⊙ **AMA Transactions and Code Set Standards**, for compliance with HIPAA, provides standards for the electronic exchange of protected health information (AMA 2016).

- ⊙ **ASTM (American Society for Testing and Materials) on Computerized System Standards for HIT** provides procedures for the development, implementation, utilization, and maintenance of health information systems. Specifies data dictionary definitions to support other standards programs.

- ⊙ **Health Level 7 (HL7)** "is a not-for-profit, standards-developing organization dedicated to providing a comprehensive framework and related standards for the exchange, integration, sharing, and retrieval of electronic health information that supports clinical practice and the management, delivery, and evaluation of health services" (HL7 2013; AHIMA 2014, 69). These standards have been identified as the default messaging standard for meeting three of the meaningful use public health standards (CDC 2015). Meaningful use will be covered in a later chapter but is related to assuring that patient health information can be transmitted and used appropriately.

- ⊙ **FHIR (Fast Healthcare Interoperability Resources) Specification** "is a standard for exchanging healthcare information electronically" (HL7 2015). It provides a new specification for data exchange related to new approaches for accomplishing this. This specification can be used exclusively, although it can be used with existing data exchange standards.

- ⊙ The **Value Set Authority Center (VSAC)** "is a central repository for the official versions of value sets that support the electronic Clinical Quality Measures. The National Library of Medicine (NLM) maintains the NLM Value Set Authority Center and provides downloadable access to the value sets and the Data Element Catalog" (HealthIT 2016c).

- ⊙ **Systematized Nomenclature of Medicine Clinical Terms (SNOMED CT)**, by the College of American Pathologists, is a processable collection of medical terminology covering most areas of clinical information such as lab results, nonlab interventions and procedures, anatomy, diagnosis and problems, and nursing.

- ⊙ **Logical Observation Identifiers Names and Codes (LOINC)** is a standardization of electronic exchange of laboratory test orders and drug label section headers.

- ⊙ The **Health Insurance Portability and Accountability Act (HIPAA)** addresses standards for transactions and code sets for electronic exchange of health-related information to perform billing or administrative functions and for terminologies related to medications including the Food and Drug Administration's names and codes for ingredients, manufactured dosage forms, drug products, and medication packages.

- ⊙ **RxNORM** (normalized names for clinical drugs), by the National Library of Medicine, for describing clinical drugs

- ⊙ **National Drug File–Reference Terminology (NDF–RT)**, by the Veterans Administration, for specific drug classifications
- ⊙ The **Human Gene Nomenclature (HUGN)** for exchanging information regarding the role of genes in biomedical research in the federal health sector

Additional resources have been developed to support the electronic exchange of clinical information across the federal government. Designed to build on the previously mentioned standards, these are used to support the implementation of new information technology systems.

Resources to support the electronic exchange of data include:

- ⊙ **Digital Imaging Communication in Medicine (DICOM)**, which enables the exchange of multimedia information
- ⊙ **RxNORM** for the exchange of medication allergy information
- ⊙ **HL7, International Classification of Functioning and Disability (ICF)**, and related **Consolidated Health Informatics (CHI)** endorsed vocabularies for the exchange of Clinical Assessments and Disability and Functional Status. The ICF includes a list of body functions and structure and a list of domains of activity and participation. The CHI initiative is a collaborative effort of the federal government to adopt standards.
- ⊙ **NCPDP (National Council for Prescription Drug Program)** provides standardization for communication between pharmacies and payers.
- ⊙ **ASC X12 Accreditation Standards Committee** was created by ANSI (American Standards Institute) for developing and maintaining EDI (electronic data exchange) and CICA (Context Inspired Component Architecture) to help resolve incompatibility in data exchange for business processes.

Although computers are easily used in many nonhealthcare industries to compile, manage, and utilize large quantities of information, applications related to the provision of healthcare present unique technological challenges. The primary challenge is that the majority of providing healthcare is based on subjective information and thus is hard to define because terms such as pain, feelings, and perceptions are used to describe the condition of the patient. A second challenge is that the sheer amount of information generated for individual patients and aggregated patient groups pushes the boundaries of the computer systems and those who work with them. Consequently, designing systems that will enhance the delivery of healthcare, contribute to the quality of care, and facilitate cost-effective means of healthcare delivery requires proficiency in computer science and information systems as well as familiarity with how the delivery of healthcare is carried out. When considering the information generated in the provision of care, the who, what, where, when, why, and how must be taken into consideration. Then, just as important, but even more challenging to understand, is where the information is needed and how it is used, how it is transmitted, and the form and format required for the transmissions while continuing to protect the confidentiality of the patient's information throughout the process.

Technology professionals are knowledgeable in computer science and computer information systems. Healthcare providers are knowledgeable in the aspects of care that they provide and are familiar with the health information that they generate and use. The various other providers and staff members who use health information are familiar with what they need to carry out their responsibilities. Health information management (HIM) professionals are experts in understanding the regulations for patient records, recognizing who is responsible for documenting in the record, and knowing the majority of the uses of the patient information because access is controlled and facilitated through the HIM department. Healthcare informatics brings together all of these aspects to enhance patient care through the use of technology. The following statement from the American Medical Informatics Association (AMIA) summarizes all that health informatics encompasses:

> The science of informatics drives innovation that is defining future approaches to information and knowledge management in biomedical research, clinical care, and public health. Informatics researchers develop, introduce, and evaluate new biomedically motivated methods in areas as diverse as data mining (deriving new knowledge from large databases), natural language or text processing, cognitive science, human interface design, decision support, databases, and algorithms for analyzing large amounts of data generated in public health, clinical research, or genomics/ proteomics. The science of informatics is inherently interdisciplinary, drawing on (and contributing to) a large number of other component fields, including computer science, decision science, information science, management science, cognitive science, and organizational theory (AMIA 2016).

Health informatics will provide the tools to enable the production of the right information to the right people in the right format at the right time. The evolving science of health informatics will provide for the continued development of the supporting, necessary systems.

Check Your Understanding 1.1

Match the following terms with the appropriate phrase.

    a. Health Level 7
    b. SNOMED CT
    c. LOINC
    d. AMA Transactions and Code Sets
    e. DICOM

    1. _____ Processable collection of medical terminology covering most areas of clinical information such as lab results, nonlab interventions and procedures, anatomy, diagnoses, problems, and nursing

2. _____ International standards developing organization for data exchange

3. _____ A standardization of electronic exchange of laboratory test orders and drug label section headers

4. _____ Enables the exchange of multimedia information

5. _____ Provides standards for the electronic exchange of protected health information to be HIPAA compliant

Answer the following questions.

6. Increases the use of data obtained from health records by using EHR systems with certified software:
   a. Standards
   b. Meaningful use
   c. Clinical data
   d. Informatics

7. Healthcare informatics is comprised of:
   a. Clinical data only
   b. Healthcare-related technology and clinical data
   c. Financial and administrative data
   d. Clinical, financial, and administrative data and technology

8. What provides tools to control processes in healthcare, acquire medical knowledge, and communicate information between all people and organizations involved with healthcare?
   a. EHR
   b. HIPAA
   c. Meaningful use of information
   d. Health informatics

Core Competencies

Within the past 20 years, the movement to utilize information systems in healthcare has experienced varying degrees of success for a variety of reasons. The lack of a trained informatics workforce throughout all levels in an organization from the highest levels in administration and technological positions to those less skilled data entry and scanning employees has been an issue. The lack of an adequate workforce has not impeded the creation of new positions with new skills from developing as the capabilities and regulations continue to move forward. The new positions are directly related to the use of the EHR, increased utilization of data, and increased regulatory requirements as borne out by data from the US Bureau of Labor Statistics (BLS) and advertisements for open positions across the country. The BLS projections for medical and health services managers is projected to increase by 17 percent through the year 2024 and 15 percent for computer systems managers for this same time period (Bureau of Labor Statistics 2016).

In the past, training for these evolving positions was typically developed by individual healthcare entities to meet their immediate needs as they arise or the training has been vendor specific to support the acquisition of their specific product. The increased reliance on computer technology and the increasingly more sophisticated software and systems require the continued development of job training methods as well as formal educational programs. In recent years, more universities have modified degree programs in nursing and other direct patient care degrees to include informatics as a required domain. Health information, health administration, and other nonpatient care programs related to healthcare have also changed their degree programs to include this content. New and developing programs at the baccalaureate, master's, and doctoral level are increasing as well to meet the needs of the workforce in acquiring the new knowledge and skills in the increased and potential use of the healthcare data that is now available in an exponentially expanding manner along with the escalating demand for the information that can now be acquired through the electronic health records and statistical software.

The reasons for lack of workforce development to support health informatics are complex and include many contributing factors. With the rapid evolution of information systems and advancement within systems and procedures already developed for use in other industries, it would seem that deployment in the healthcare environment would be occurring at a more rapid pace. The diversity and magnitude of the healthcare workforce is huge. Nearly all healthcare workers will be required to interact with the computerized information systems in some manner. In addition to learning new technical skills, the workforce must also become familiar with a new lexicon of terms and acronyms that have emerged as systems arise. The terminology in question is related to HIM, medical or clinical informatics, and health informatics. This is compounded by the plethora of applications utilized within one system within a facility. Another contributing factor is the varying degree of implementation of information systems across the full spectrum of healthcare facilities.

For all of these reasons, attention must be given to technical training programs and formal educational programs from the associate degree to the doctoral levels. The need for a skilled workforce at all levels was addressed by the federal government with the funding made available through the American Recovery and Reinvestment Act of 2009 (ARRA) for the creation of many programs. These programs included certificate programs at the associate's, baccalaureate, and master's degree levels and as continuing education course offerings. These funds were limited and for a defined period of time. These programs were also envisioned before training needs were clearly understood, so many areas were not addressed. A number of the programs were focused primarily on assessing user needs, making a purchase decision, and implementing the systems. Data analytics is now a key function in the health informatics field whereby data are turned into useful information. Skills needed to support these positions include an understanding of issues and challenges related to data collection, assessing the data for correctness and reliability, using statistical software to abstract information from the data, and presenting the information in the most effective format, especially for decision making.

Electronic Health Records Core Competencies

In 2008, the Joint Work Force Task Force of AMIA and the American Health Information Management Association (AHIMA) published the report *Health Information Management and Informatics Core Competencies for Individuals Working with Electronic Health Records.* The Electronic Health Record Core Competency domains identified by this task force are

  I. Information literacy and skills

 II. Health informatics skill using the EHR

III. Privacy and confidentiality of health information

IV. Health information/data technical security

 V. Basic computer literacy skills (AHIMA and AMIA 2008, 8)

Core competencies for each of the domains were identified and a matrix tool was developed to provide guidance for the competencies needed by a variety of disciplines. For example, all healthcare workers need an awareness of privacy and security regulations for keeping patient information confidential. However, the privacy officer, often an HIM professional, will require an in-depth understanding of the HIPAA Privacy Rule.

Domain II specifically addresses the health informatics skill set, but many competencies from the other domains are applicable to informatics-related roles directly or indirectly depending on the role. The model presented by this group was intended to be used to encourage the development of models of health information and informatics education and training programs and to serve as a resource for policy makers when considering funding for such programs. For health informatics skills using the EHR and PHR, needed skill sets and knowledge are the following:

1. Create and update documents within the EHR and the PHR

2. Locate and retrieve information in the EHR for various purposes

3. Perform data entry of narrative information

4. Locate and retrieve information from a variety of electronic sources

5. Differentiate between primary and secondary health data sources and databases

6. Know the architecture and data standards of health information systems

7. Identify classification and systematic health-related terminologies for coding and information retrieval

8. Know the policies and procedures related to populating and using the healthcare content within primary and secondary health data sources and databases

9. Apply appropriate documentation management principles to ensure data quality and integrity

10. Use software applications to generate reports

11. Know and apply appropriate methods to ensure the authenticity of health data entries in electronic information systems

12. Use electronic tools and applications for scheduling patients (AHIMA and AMIA 2008, 9)

Accreditation

Many discipline-specific accrediting entities have started updating their curriculum requirements to address informatics and what should be covered in their educational programs to appropriately prepare their students. The Commission on Accreditation for Health Informatics and Information Management Education (CAHIIM) accredits associate's and baccalaureate degree programs in health information, and approves master's degree programs in health informatics and health information management. CAHIIM Domain III of the curriculum requirements is focused on informatics for the associate's and baccalaureate educational programs. The CAHIIM Domain III and Subdomains are as follows:

> Domain III. Informatics, Analytics and Data Use
> > Subdomains
> > > A. Health Information Technologies
> > > B. Information Management Strategic Planning
> > > C. Analytics and Decision Support
> > > D. Health Care Statistics
> > > E. Research Methods
> > > F. Consumer Informatics
> > > G. Health Information Exchange
> > > H. Information Integrity and Data Quality

Accreditation is a reflection that an educational program has met a standard of quality that is important both to the institution and to the general public. What is most important though is the process that is required to develop the curriculum and the educational program to meet the accreditation requirements and the employment demands for the community of interest. This effort is guided by the domains of knowledge required for specific content areas as shown in Domain III. One can better understand what is encompassed in the content area and what is required to be adequately prepared for potential positions by reviewing the subdomain statements. As can be seen from the subdomains shown above, the informatics, data use, and analytics area is diverse with the need to have general knowledge and experience in all of these content areas but allows for one to specialize or develop proficiency in a specific area such as analytics and decision support for jobs as a data analyst, informaticist researcher, and data integrity analyst (AHIMA 2016).

Definitions and Terms

HIT-related terms and definitions have continued to emerge due to the advancements in technology and the methods of delivery of care and the need for governmental leaders, policy makers, and healthcare providers to have a more standardized terminology. The terms "health information technology" and "health informatics" are still not clearly defined or understood. Health information technology is a broad term often used to identify the computers and programs used in the maintenance of health records. Federal legislation such as the Affordable Care Act, HITECH Act, HIPAA, and the EHR Incentive Programs brought the term "health information technology" (health IT or HIT) to the forefront in healthcare (Hersh 2009).

Figure 1.2 provides an example of transforming data into informatics using temperature to determine which medications are prescribed for fevers over a six-month period. Figure 1.1 illustrated the basic concepts that comprise health informatics, the clinical, the technology, and the financial and management aspects. In figure 1.2, the temperature, 40 C/104 F is the clinical data, the technology is the EHR and pharmacy systems, and the financial and management aspects could be related to which medication seemed to be the most effective in treating the elevated temperature. The financial and management implications could be determined by analyzing the patient's return to normal temperature in a timely manner, length of hospital stay, comparison of outcomes with drugs of varying costs and then comparing these outcomes to other patients and medications. The results of the comparisons could then be used in the treatment of future patients and for considering the most cost-efficient manner for treating patients with similar conditions.

Designing new solutions is the goal of informatics. In healthcare this includes augmenting biomedical science and improving the quality of care and health in a cost-effective manner. Biomedical informatics is the term that reflects the broad

Figure 1.2.   Example of transforming data into informatics

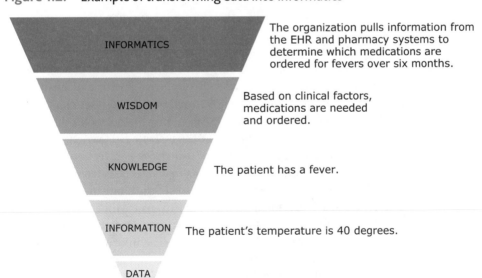

INFORMATICS — The organization pulls information from the EHR and pharmacy systems to determine which medications are ordered for fevers over six months.

WISDOM — Based on clinical factors, medications are needed and ordered.

KNOWLEDGE — The patient has a fever.

INFORMATION — The patient's temperature is 40 degrees.

DATA — 40 degrees Celsius

Source: Wiedemann 2014

definition for the underlying science across functional domains. The names of these functional domains provide more specificity than biomedical informatics. The five application focus areas emphasized by AMIA, the leading professional association for informaticians, are defined here (AMIA 2016).

Biomedical Informatics

Biomedical informatics has multiple definitions and can be considered from several perspectives. Publications from the Stanford School of Medicine allude to the fact that modern science has given us tools for scientific research but produces a preponderance of data that is impossible to analyze with traditional methods (Altman and Klein 2007). However, the biological data are key to learning the causes of disease and developing new treatment modalities. A clear definition or statement of the meaning of biomedical informatics is important to provide a perspective from which to consider the topic. One example of such a definition is presented here.

> Biomedical informatics, by definition, incorporates a core set of methodologies that are applicable for managing data, information, and knowledge across the **translational medicine** continuum, for the purpose of improving health through bench biology to clinical care and research to public health (Sarkar 2010, 22).

Translational Bioinformatics is "the development of storage, analytic, and interpretive methods to optimize the transformation of increasingly voluminous biomedical data, and genomic data, into proactive, predictive, preventive, and participatory health" (AMIA 2016). It is taking the new knowledge gained from basic advances in research to transform the delivery of medical care provided to patients and improving community health by developing new procedures and modes of treatment.

Clinical Research Informatics is a subdiscipline within biomedical informatics. It is the use of informatics to facilitate the acquisition and management of new health- and disease-related knowledge with the intent to improve health and healthcare. This new knowledge is obtained through clinical trials and use of clinical data in secondary research. An example of clinical research informatics would be a study of wireless monitoring of pulmonary function at the bedside (BUMC 2012).

Clinical informatics is applying informatics principles and technology in the delivery of healthcare services. Clinical informatics may also be referred to applied clinical informatics or operational informatics. It is part of the biomedical continuum, as outlined above. It is focused on information systems to ensure they support patient care that is safe, efficient, effective, timely, patient-centered, and equitable (Detmer et al. 2009, 167–168). A more specific definition for clinical informatics would infer that it is the scientific study of patient care, clinical research, and medical education and the effective use of information to support these activities, establish standards, and set policy. The goal of clinical informatics is to provide healthcare practitioners with timely, accurate data to support the delivery of care efficiently to improve quality of care in a cost-effective manner. The users of clinical information systems include all providers of care and may include consumers as well.

Case Study: Improving Provider Performance

This case study outlines how a medical staff used EHRs to obtain data on provider performance to improve the healthcare provided to the patient. The key aspects of the study are provided in table 1.1.

This case study is an example of using the technology (the EHR) to improve the success and utilization of information, which are the key components of the definition of health informatics. The EHR system was enhanced to automatically generate a list of patients with high LDL who were also due for a cholesterol check. Without the system created list, a staff member would be required to manually generate a list and remember to monitor it for the test to be performed at next visit. With the automatically generated list, the affected patients are readily identified and scheduled for the cholesterol testing at their next visit.

Table 1.1. Leveraging Health IT to improve provider performance

Background	This study was done at an 11 hospital Accountable Care Organization (ACO) with a large rural population, many of whom are on Medicare and Medicaid. The physician ACO's Performance Improvement Coordinator led the project.
Problems/ Challenges	• The need for providers to improve quality of healthcare and be more cost efficient • There are 11 different hospitals with different leadership and differing standards among them, which makes standardization, monitoring, and training more difficult
Goal	• Use existing IT • Improve physician performance to assure patients at risk for high LDL cholesterol level were targeted by physicians to have cholesterol checks performed when due • Improve quality of care of the patients as a result of this close monitoring and checking of their cholesterol level
Approach	• Establish a collegial organizational culture among the hospital leaders • Obtain agreement on uniform set of provider performance standards • Secure buy-in
Data	• Developed a tool for the EHR system that allowed providers to generate lists of patients with high LDL who were due for a cholesterol check. Providers could use these lists to target health interventions for the checks and subsequent treatment • Monitored performance measures to monitor health status

Source: Adapted from HealthIT.gov. Health IT Success Stories 2013

Other Types of Healthcare Informatics

Consumer informatics is consistent with other kinds of healthcare informatics in that it is the intersection of health, computers, and information management. In this case, the focus is on the interest of the consumer. A goal of consumer informatics is to support and inform consumers to facilitate the management and participation in their own care. Activities within this subset of health informatics may include evaluating the information needs of the consumers and developing means of providing accessible and meaningful information to the patient or family consumer of the healthcare. Another important aspect of consumer informatics is utilization of consumer input and preferences in the development of information systems to maximize their perspective and promote usability. The gamut of information to be made available to the consumer includes that for prevention, wellness, and treatment options.

Consumer informatics should be distinguished from patient education information, which is more commonly considered to be the instructions provided by a healthcare provider to instruct and communicate specific information for a specific treatment option. Examples of patient education include the instructions provided by the healthcare provider for activity restrictions, special diets to be followed, signs and symptoms to monitor, wound care, and the drug information that is provided to the patient with new prescriptions. Consumer informatics could include things such as interactive health communication. An example of this is where a consumer can access a website to seek information on a specific symptom or condition and possibly even be able to submit questions to be answered. Physicians who offer a patient portal (a secure site for access to their personal health information) provide a method for patient engagement with their own care through enhanced patient–provider communication, means of reviewing their health information and add to it in some instances, and support care between visits, which all help to improve patient outcomes (HealthIT 2016). Other functionality may also be available to the patients such as scheduling, sharing health data, means to communicate with the provider, disease specific information, and links to other sites. Patients can use their patient information gained through the portal in addition to data from other providers and diagnostic reports to develop their own **personal health record (PHR)**, another example of consumer informatics. A PHR is "an electronic or paper health record maintained and updated by an individual for himself or herself, a tool that individuals can use to collect, track, and share past and current information about their health or the health of someone in their care" (AHIMA 2014, 114). E-mail exchanges between a provider of care and a patient and mobile device applications (apps) such as those for monitoring blood sugar and blood pressure readings, educating about exercise and diet, and informing about the meanings of lab values, signs and symptoms of conditions, and the specific disease also fall in the category of consumer informatics. Unobtrusive sensing and wearable technologies are especially important informatics tools for early prediction and treatment of major diseases. These devices provide information seamlessly and pervasively with sensors that can be integrated into clothing and in the living environment (Zhang et al. 2010).

Also aiding consumer informatics is the **Internet of Things (IoT),** "the network of physical objects that contain embedded technology to communicate and sense or interact with their internal states or the external environment" (Gartner 2016). The information applications are a part of the equipment or appliance being used and are integrated into the home/work environment. An example of an IoT object is a medicine bottle cap that uses light, sound, and text in communication with other devices. The cap sends reminders to the consumer to take medication and sends refill requests to the pharmacy by pushing a button on the cap, both of which aid in the management of prescribed medications (Nuvem Consulting 2014). New consumer informatics applications continue to proliferate with the advances in technology and impetus to support and improve patient care.

Public health informatics is the systematic application of information and utilization of computer technology to support public health initiatives as related to research, education, and delivery of public health services (CDC 2005). Public health is

> an organized effort by society, primarily through its public institutions, to improve, promote, protect and restore the health of the population through collective action. It includes services such as health situation analysis, health surveillance, health promotion, prevention, infectious disease control, environmental protection and sanitation, disaster and health emergency preparedness and response, and occupational health, among others (WHO 2016).

Discussions of public health commonly include topics such as disease prevention, health promotion, increasing life expectancy, and threats or health perils, along with terms such as population analysis, biostatistics, and monitoring of diseases, all of which require large amounts of information. The focus of public health is not on the individual patient but rather large groups of individuals and communities. A large amount of redacted aggregate data are collected and analyzed. The data are on all members of the population under study to include the healthy as well as those suffering from illness and other health conditions. With the increased use of technological advances to aggregate and analyze public health data, public health data will be a key component with health exchange initiatives (HealthIT 2013). This information can also play a greater role in the treatment of conditions such as cancer with the potential for IT-supported surveillance and care.

Population health has become a frequently used term regarding "the health outcomes of a group of individuals, including the distribution of such outcomes within the group," and that "the field of population health includes health outcomes, patterns of health determinants, and policies and interventions that link these two" (Kindig and Stoddard 2003). A definition of population health from the health information management perspective is "the capture and reporting of healthcare data that are used for public health purposes. It allows the healthcare providers to report infection diseases, immunizations, cancer, and other reportable conditions to public health officials" (AHIMA 2014, 116). **Population Health Management (PHM)** can be defined as "the discipline of managing the clinical and financial risk of a defined group of individuals" (Cassidy 2013). The intent of PHM is to improve the overall general health and well-being of defined groups such as tobacco users or patients with diabetes, that will in turn reduce the need for costly medical interventions.

Other terms are used to define informatics such as **nursing informatics**. This is not a separate type of informatics but is specific to one specialized group of providers of care. Nursing informatics would fall into one of the categories of Translational Bioinformatics, Clinical Research Informatics, or Clinical Informatics depending on the emphasis of the activity. The term **health informatics** is commonly used in reference to applied research with the application of informatics for both the clinical and public health domains. The term medical informatics is used less and less due to the growth and what all bioinformatics encompasses.

Genomics is a biological science in which the structure and function along with the evolution and mapping of genomes is the focus and provides a wealth of data for informatics activities. Genomic mapping, or the creation of a genetic map, is where the DNA fragments are assigned to chromosomes. Studies of genomic maps can identify major risk factors for certain illnesses at the individual level and can also assess a person's risk of inherited diseases. In 1990, the US Human Genome Project was started in the United States. The project, coordinated by the US Department of Energy and the National Institutes of Health, was originally planned to take 15 years. The project was completed after only 13 years due to the acceleration of the project because of technological advances moving forward at an unexpected rate. While the focus of the project was to identify an estimated 20,000 to 25,000 genes and the sequences of three billion pairs that comprise human DNA, the storing of the associated information in databases and designing improved data analysis tools were also established goals of the project (National Human Genome Research Institute 2013). The final goals of the project were to make the use of the technology available in the private sector and to address the ethical, legal, and social issues that were anticipated to arise from the project.

The Human Genome Project provided a significant impact on the kinds and amount of health information maintained and was part of the motivation for the emergence of health informatics. The term health informatics is currently used more in reference to applied research and application of informatics principles in the clinical and public health domains. The term **genomic informatics** is specific to the use of genome sequence data along with computer capabilities and statistical methods to obtain biological information. The consequences of the advances in genomic informatics are the ability to study the precursors, markers, and presentations of disease over time. The issue that discrimination might occur due to knowledge of genetic information does present an ethical challenge, which led to the **Genetic Information Nondiscrimination Act of 2008 (GINA)**. This law provides the legal standard to be followed for the collection, use, and disclosure of genetic information. In general, Title I of GINA prohibits health plans from discriminating against covered individuals based on genetic information (National Human Genome Research Institute 2013). The law further clarifies that genetic data are health information. As health information it is then considered **protected health information (PHI)**, which according to the HIPAA Privacy Rule is that which could be used to identify the patient and therefore must be protected.

Telemedicine is the remote delivery of healthcare services over the telecommunications network. Although used interchangeably, use of the term **telehealth** tends to include both medical and nonclinical elements of care to include education, monitoring, and administration to facilitate the prevention or treatment of medical conditions. In either case, it is the use of technology that allows the service to be provided when the patient and the healthcare provider are remote from each other, which has caused a paradigm shift in the provision of healthcare. The technology for telehealth and telemedicine range from e-mail and videoconferencing to the use of imaging and monitoring devices with results recorded and transmitted to the provider and to the transmission of health information for the use of diagnosis and treatment. The application of informatics in telemedicine relies on the strength of the patient-specific data combined with statistical and epidemiological data to facilitate decision making and quality of care. The use of informatics in telemedicine ultimately will enhance standardization of care and the provision of leading-edge expertise that might not otherwise be available in remote or low-population areas or to home-bound patients.

E-health is using the Internet and other technologies to improve information and health services; a combination of public health, business, and medical informatics (Eysenbach 2001). E-health can include anything related to computers and medicine and has sometimes been referred to as Internet medicine by the business-related entities. However, academicians desired a more scientific inclusive definition:

> In a broader sense, the term characterizes not only a technical development, but also a state-of-mind, a way of thinking, an attitude, and a commitment for networked, global thinking, to improve health care locally, regionally, and worldwide by using information and communication technology (Eysenbach 2001).

Simply stated, e-health is the use of the Internet and other electronic media to provide access to health-related information including that for specific medical conditions and services as well as for information related to lifestyle information and services. The scope of e-health is quite broad. It includes clinical information systems such as radiology information systems; telemedicine and home care including remote patient monitoring; integrated health information networks and distribution systems as used for EHR systems for e-referrals; and secondary usage nonclinical systems like health portals and biostatistics programs for outcome analysis. The increased utilization of e-health services is the result of a number of factors that have made it possible, and it has become a popular option for many service providers. Consumerism and patient expectations are a key factor in the increased use of e-health resources with the desire to have immediate and more information and to become more engaged in their care and self-management of medical conditions. E-health sites are becoming more sophisticated, linking much information together in one place on an easily navigable site. Some healthcare providers are encouraging the use of e-health via their own sites where patients are directed to a number of services including disease and treatment information, links to sites such as governmental sites that allow access to needed forms and information, scheduling, and payment options, and for some a portal to a PHR. These kinds of sites not only support the needs of the patient but also aid in staffing issues for the provider.

Check Your Understanding 1.2

Answer the following questions.

1. To facilitate decision making and quality of care, the application of informatics in telemedicine relies on:
   a. The strength of the patient-specific data combined with epidemiological data and statistical methods
   b. Technology
   c. Epidemiological data
   d. Willingness of the patient to participate

2. Which of the following is the use of genetic sequence data along with computer capabilities and statistical methods to obtain biological information?
   a. Genomic informatics
   b. Biomedical informatics
   c. Clinical informatics
   d. Public health information

3. The discipline of managing the clinical and financial risk of a defined group of individuals is the meaning of:
   a. Population health
   b. Informatics
   c. Population health management
   d. E-health

4. The Internet of Things is:
   a. Population health management
   b. Network of physical objects with embedded technology
   c. Telehealth
   d. Data resource document

5. Assign numbers 1 through 5 to indicate the order in which these items would fall in the process of the transformation of data to informatics:
   _____ knowledge
   _____ data
   _____ informatics
   _____ information
   _____ wisdom

Policies

A facility must continuously ensure that effective policies are in place to address the new ways of maintaining patient information and the expanded use of the data available in an electronic system. All policies related to the patient health record must be reviewed to determine whether changes need to be made once the record is electronic rather than in the paper format. Hybrid record systems must be reviewed to determine the needed policy changes for this interim step to a fully functioning EHR. Key policies relating to privacy and security, compliance with HIPAA, and the assurance that the needed information is available to support the federal meaningful use requirements are of prime importance. An example of a new policy that might need to be developed relates to systems that utilize alerts such as **computerized provider order entry (CPOE)**. CPOE systems are applications that allow providers to write orders for medications or other treatments and transmit them electronically. A policy would need to address the requirements for alert monitoring to guide the provider in the appropriate way to respond to alerts. Policies that might need to be changed are those that relate to privacy and security and HIPAA compliance. A facility should already have policies in place to address these, but a review will need to be done to see how these functions have changed in the electronic environment. Examples of this would include how access to the system is granted to employees and what specific information can be accessed by each employee. Another related policy would be one that outlines sanctions for employees inappropriately accessing information relating to patients not under their care.

The responsibility for assuring that policies related to the data used in informatics functions now falls under the auspices of Information Governance (IG). AHIMA defines IG as "the accountability framework and decision rights to achieve enterprise information management (EIM). IG is the responsibility of executive leadership for developing and driving the IG strategy throughout the organization. IG encompasses both data governance (DG) and information technology governance (ITG)" (AHIMA 2014, 78). An IG program is expected to be the means of governing the information for a healthcare facility.

Methods

Technical aspects of creating systems include programming HIT systems to recognize the language of healthcare. One key application requiring this ability is **clinical decision support**, which uses codified information from a patient record and aids in diagnosis and treatment. The multiple ways that medical information can be stated presents significant challenges in creating these systems. The work of **informaticists** is to define the way information is represented in HIT systems. This can be done by interpreting the data, codifying it, and identifying relationships between the data. An example of the outcome of the work of a health informaticist is a system for CPOE. Error prevention software is typically included in CPOE systems where prompt alerts are made in cases when there is the possibility of drug interaction, allergy, or overdose. To assure the correctness of orders prior to processing and administering it, other pertinent information may be a part of a CPOE system (AHIMA 2014, 33). Incorporated into such a system would be the relevant drug information including the different names the drug could be identified by, the typical dosage protocol, contraindications for taking the drug, symptoms of untoward events such as allergies, and interactions with other drugs. This drug data would be codified, which reduces words to codes of numbers and letters. Once the codes are assigned, the relationships are identified. There are a multitude of relationships that would need to be identified to reflect the potential interactions that could occur between the data elements. For example, the generic name for a common anticoagulant drug is Warfarin, the alternate (brand) names also used to identify the drug are Coumadin and Jantoven. The standard dosage, common side effects, and the names of other drugs that are contraindicated need to be identified. An example of how this CPOE system could then contribute to improved patient care is a scenario where the standard dosage is keyed in incorrectly, such as 25 milligrams versus 75 milligrams. In this instance in most CPOE systems, the physician would receive an immediate prompt questioning this order as entered. Available for the physician to review would be manufacturer information that indicates the normal drug dosage with a request for the physician to confirm the correct dosage to be prescribed. A defined vocabulary to identify clinical conditions is imperative in creating the system. The difficulty of defining a vocabulary in healthcare is exacerbated by multiple terms meaning the same thing as in the terms laceration and cut, compounded by all the words that can then be used to further describe such a term. Coding systems that use specific clinical terminologies provide a means for providing specific definitions with more standardized terms. The implementation of ICD-10-CM/PCS provided an expanded lexicon for enhanced standard terminology and SNOMED is commonly used for informatics purposes.

With health informatics consideration must also be given to the development of standards for software to be used in the EHR and the exchange of data. Compatibility and **interoperability**, allowing different "health information systems to work together within and across organizational boundaries in order to advance the effective delivery of healthcare for individuals and communities" (HIMSS 2013, 75), are a key focus in health informatics. Vendors have a vested interest in the establishment of standards to assure their products are compatible and competitive with the multiple applications required to build an EHR system.

Using the information to make decisions relies on the technology, the defined vocabulary, and the standards. These are tools to achieve the ultimate goal of having usable, meaningful information to facilitate the decision-making process. Informatics processes utilized to support this include **probability** and making predictions. Probability in informatics is to use patient-related data to determine the likelihood of various occurrences in the disease process and modes of treatment. Informaticists must apply probability modes numerous times when developing systems to assist with making treatment decisions, often while utilizing incomplete, minimal, or even conflicting information. The various methods of decision analysis may be incorporated to identify the course to be taken in treatment or in making administrative decisions and setting policies. **Decision analysis** is "a systematic approach to decision making under conditions of imperfect knowledge; it is a practical application of probability theory that is used to calculate the optimal strategy from among a series of alternative strategies" (Studdert et al. 2012). The results of this process are often expressed graphically in the form of a decision tree. With the wealth of data that can be transformed into information, opportunities exist to create new knowledge through numerous statistical applications and activities such as **data mining**, which involves searching, analyzing, and summarizing large data sets from different perspectives to identify trends and other useful information.

Check Your Understanding 1.3

Answer the following questions.

1. True or false: There is no need to review and rewrite policies when a record goes from paper to electronic.

2. Using patient data to determine the likelihood of occurrences in the disease process and modes of treatment is an example of
   a. Reliability
   b. Probability
   c. Standardization
   d. Decision analysis

3. Interoperability can best be described as
   a. A certified system
   b. Where multiple users can be accessing and using a system at the same time
   c. When there is complete standardization of data that can be accessed in a system
   d. Where there is the ability to exchange and use data between systems

4. Data mining is
   a. Searching, analyzing, and summarizing large data sets from different perspectives to identify trends and other useful information
   b. A statistical analysis software program
   c. Abstracting and categorizing large amounts of information
   d. Building flags into systems to automatically identify certain data elements

5. Under conditions of imperfect knowledge, a practical application of probability theory that is used to calculate the optimal strategy from among a series of alternative strategies is
   a. Strategizing
   b. Alternative analysis
   c. Decision analysis
   d. Data mining

6. The advantage(s) of utilizing clinical terminologies is(are):
   a. Providing specific definitions
   b. More standardized terms
   c. Both a and b
   d. A consistent vocabulary

Ethics

Ethics involves the standards of moral practice, values, and a code of conduct. Ethical issues with EHRs and health informatics are inherently due to the nature of the information involved, the confidential patient information. The goal of health informatics is to convert the patient-related data into information that can be used to make treatment decisions and to compile information that can be used to enhance the care of large populations of patients. This information is valuable for administration and policy making. To support this activity, the information must be compiled, shared, transmitted, and reviewed by a variety of entities. As more patient data are generated and used across the spectrum of healthcare, the potential for ethical challenges arise. Probability and predictability of the incidence of a medical condition or potential survival with a meaningful life could influence who receives healthcare and to what extent the services are provided.

The hybrid state of patient health records where part of an individual patient record is generated and maintained in paper format and part is generated and maintained electronically, can lead to the potential for medical care errors due to system issues with incomplete, incorrect, or unavailable information. The difficulty in keeping the patient information secure and confidential is a continuing problem whether the records are electronic, paper, or hybrid (AHIMA 2005). Quality issues exist as well with occurrences such as poor quality of images transmitted via an electronic system, medical errors when protocols are inadequate to support quality care, and lack of staff or inability to use the system appropriately.

Ethical issues could arise as a consequence of making an incorrect self-diagnosis. With regard to telemedicine, there is also the reliance on the technology and the inherent problems of availability and quality of the information and the electronic transmission and storage of information. For aggregate data reported on large groups of patients, the selective use and distribution of the analysis of the information, privacy concerns, and unscrupulous use of data for commercial gain are all of concern from an ethical standpoint. Ethical issues are not new in the provision of healthcare. It must be recognized that for all of the positive outcomes that technological advances can bring, such as the amount of and enhancement of patient data with the ability to transmit and share it, the potential for ethical issues still exists and such issues are arguably more complex than with the paper record.

Check Your Understanding 1.4

Answer the following questions.

1. The term used to identify a patient record that is maintained partly in hard copy and partly in an EHR system is:
   a. Patient health record
   b. Electronic health record
   c. Hybrid record
   d. There is no accepted term for this occurrence

2. Informatics creates new potential uses for patient health information. Which of the following is not an area of concern for using this kind of information?
   a. Ability to aggregate data for decision making
   b. Increased concern for protecting the privacy of the information
   c. Limited opportunities to use the information
   d. Lack of data

3. Ethics encompasses:
   a. Code of conduct
   b. Laws
   c. A set of actions to be followed in any situation
   d. Previously handled situations

Indicate whether each of the following is true or false.

4. The utilization of informatics does not change the potential ethical concerns.

5. Ethical issues are more prevalent with EHRs rather than the paper health record.

⊙ Roles

The field of health informatics and subsequent positions differ from one facility to another and can vary significantly in terms of responsibilities. Individuals who play key roles in health informatics include HIM professionals, physicians, and other care providers, computer and information specialists, data specialists, and administrators. Each role contributes to the success of the health informatics initiatives with their specific area of expertise but the diversity of the roles illustrates the breadth of knowledge and skills necessary to meet the goals and realize the potential of informatics in the healthcare environment. An introduction to several of the primary roles and how professionals in a variety of existing roles will play an important part in the informatics movement utilizing their knowledge and skills from their perspective is shown below. The existing roles will inherently continue to evolve and new roles will be identified to meet the needs of health informatics and as advances continue to be made.

Health Information Management Professional

The foundation of the HIM profession has always been to ensure the integrity of patient information through its life cycle while maintaining patient confidentiality. As the regulations, laws, technology, and payment methods have changed over the years, the HIM professional domain of knowledge and skills has also changed. Advances and utilization of technology within the past few years have resulted in a fundamental change in the functions and roles of all levels of HIM professionals. In the first years of EHR deployment, the focus of many positions was on the acquisition and implementation of systems, so more were related to the technology itself. Data analysis has now emerged as a key focus area. The wealth of data that can be generated with the many ways that it can be compiled and analyzed continues to become more critical. As improved systems are deployed more and more information becomes available and new uses for the data continue to be identified. The selection, acquisition, and

Table 1.2. Job titles for AHIMA career map section on informatics and data analytics

Level	Job title	Related jobs
Master	Chief Clinical Information Officer	Professor Consultant
	Director of Clinical Informatics	Program Director Consultant
Advanced	Research and Developmental Scientist–Emerging	Chief Learning Officer Professor Program Director
	Project Management	Director of Clinical Informatics Business Analyst
	Mapping Specialist	Coding Trainer Coding Manager Consultant Director of Clinical Informatics
	Data Integrity Analyst	Consultant Data Quality Manager
	Informatics Researcher	Clinical Information Coordinator
Mid	**Clinical Informatics Coordinator**	Director Clinical Informatics Information Researcher
	Data Analyst	Informaticist Researcher Data Integrity Analyst
	Content Analyst	Informaticist Researcher Data Architect

Source: AHIMA 2016

implementation of systems require the ongoing input of HIM professionals. HIM roles that support this process include those related to project management, work redesign, and privacy concerns. HIM professionals transitioning in these roles will require the acquisition of IT knowledge and leadership capabilities. Numerous other new roles continue to emerge to include those associated with data analysis, research activities, information exchange, the PHR, and consumer health informatics to name a few.

A career map with job titles and information about HIM careers in informatics and data analytics can be found at the AHIMA website (AHIMA 2016). The AHIMA Career Map is a web-based tool for students and health information professionals to identify and map various career paths. The map is representative of positions that reflect the scope of the field including some of the emerging positions. The job titles and level for the positions from the Informatics/Data Analysis category of the Career Map are shown in table 1.2. The jobs will be covered more in chapter 16 with skills needed.

The bolded job titles in table 1.2 are shown to be a transitional path: the clinical informatics coordinator to the information researcher position and a promotional path to the director of clinical informatics position. Job descriptions and additional information about these positions can be linked to from the AHIMA Career Map. General skills required for most positions are critical thinking, detail orientation, and excellent verbal and written communication skills. Common skills related to the informatics positions specifically, but dependent on the individual jobs, are mapping, knowledge of EHR applications, knowledge and experience in health IT to use and plan for health information, managerial ability, technical and professional skills of systems and procedure analysis, proficiency with analytical tools, and use of presentation software.

CIO, CMIO, and the C-Suite

The chief administrative positions related to health informatics may vary from facility to facility and may not even be present in some facilities as a named position. In this instance the related responsibilities are shared by many throughout the organization, mostly to carry out the tasks within their domain and area of expertise. Over the past few years the scope of information technology within a facility has increased significantly and permeates every aspect of the delivery of healthcare. The following statement indicates the prevalence of health informatics tasks throughout healthcare organizations:

> Whether it involves sending laboratory test results and appointment reminders to patients on their smart phones, giving nurses earlier warnings that a patient's vital signs are trending in a dangerous direction, or developing the paradigm-changing clinical and financial systems needed to put an accountable care organization into place, health information technology's (HIT) presence is pervasive. And it has become integral to virtually every process and operation within the healthcare field, from clinical decision making to materials management (Birk 2011).

Administrative positions in health informatics may include the **chief information officer (CIO)**, **chief clinical information officer (CCIO)**, and the **chief medical information officer (CMIO)**. The CIO is the senior manager responsible for the overall management of information resources in an organization (AHIMA 2014, 25). The CMIO is typically a physician with medical informatics training who provides physician leadership and direction in the deployment of clinical applications in healthcare organizations (AHIMA 2012, 73). The CCIO usually provides leadership for nurses, physicians, and other clinicians for using information systems for the delivery of care, education, and research. Additionally, health information managers are filling the role of **chief knowledge officer (CKO)**, the person who oversees the entire knowledge acquisition, storage, and dissemination process and identifies subject matter experts to help capture and organize the organization's knowledge assets (AHIMA 2014, 25). Although job descriptions for CIOs would vary significantly for those holding this position from one facility to another, the required knowledge and skills for the position would include technical skills, but just as important would be the need for strategic planning and thinking, leadership, and the ability to predict and prepare for the future.

The CMIO provides that vital link between the medical aspect of care and the information technology or systems departments within the healthcare facility. The individual who holds this title may either be a physician who has a particular interest or knowledge of the use of technology or an individual with a technology background specifically in health informatics, utilizing information in medical treatment and research. Common requirements for a CMIO position would include the ability to integrate systems to support the delivery of healthcare, the ability to evaluate and analyze the outcomes of using technology on patient care, and the more administrative-related tasks of planning, setting standards, project management, and being an advocate of the use of technology with the members of the medical staff.

The CKO is someone who has a broader view of the effective use of the information in ways that contribute to the knowledge of workers and the organization. An effective CKO can help utilize improved technology and expanded data assets to efficiently convert data into knowledge and strategically meet an organization's needs in regard to cost reductions, clinical outcomes, pay-for-performance, competitive advantage, and best practices (Cassidy 2011).

Physician

The role the physician plays in the adoption and utilization of the EHR is key to capturing the information needed to support informatics-related activity. Their role is to work with technology and healthcare professionals to provide the physicians' perspective of firsthand knowledge of patient care. They are key to determining information and knowledge needs, to refining clinical processes and potential clinical support systems, and to participating in continual improvement of the clinical information systems. One of the programs of the American Recovery and Reinvestment Action (ARRA) of 2009 was to promote the adoption and use of EHRs. In this law, the Health Information Technology for Economic and Clinical Health (HITECH) Act refers to the HIT components of the stimulus package that was a part of the ARRA bill. The ultimate purpose of HITECH is for quality and efficiency of healthcare, not just for the components that comprise HIT:

> One of HITECH's most important features is its clarity of purpose. Congress apparently sees HIT—computers, software, Internet

connection, telemedicine—not as an end in itself but as a means of improving the quality of health care, the health of populations, and the efficiency of healthcare systems (Blumenthal 2009).

Information Technology Specialists

The role of information technology specialist cannot be well defined based on job title or role alone. This generalist title can be interpreted or designed to meet the specific needs of a facility or defined based on a specific perspective or frame of reference. Within the scope of this job title or domain would be the knowledge and ability to use computers for the collection, maintenance, and use of patient health information. Aspects of using hardware and software would be important as would the ability to utilize the data that could be obtained from the systems that maintain patient care data, along with the skills to then use that data to enhance the quality and efficiency of healthcare. Using a job description posted on the National Institutes of Health (NIH) website as a guide, table 1.3 illustrates a job description indicative of the current role of the information technology specialist.

Table 1.3.   Sample job description for health information technology specialist

Job Title	Health Information Technology Specialist
Job Description	Health Information Technology (HIT) Specialists are experts in the development, implementation, management, and support of systems and networks. HIT specialists plan and carry out complex assignments and develop new methods and approaches in a wide variety of IT specialties.
Job Specialties	Bioinformatics Systems analysis Customer support Information security Applications software Data management Internet applications Network services Operating systems Systems administration
Job Sequirements	Knowledge of IT principles, concepts and methods Systems testing and evaluation principles, methods, and tools IT security principles and methods COTS (Commercial Off-the-Shelf) products (nondevelopmental items such as computer software and hardware systems) Internet technologies Emerging technologies

Source: NIH 2012.

Scribes

The term scribe alludes to one who authors or writes. A **medical scribe**, many times a medical student, nurse practitioner, or physician's assistant, assists the physician with the required documentation in the patient's medical record. The benefits to direct patient care are twofold with improved productivity of the physician in terms of time and ability to focus more directly on the patient and the ability of the scribe to support the treatment by providing the physician with needed information. This could include updates on diagnostic information and other information from the patient's record to enhance the encounter with the patient by providing timely and comprehensive information. With the increased use of the EHR, scribes are instrumental in incorporating the documentation into the EHR system thus again freeing up the physician's time and ensuring that required fields and other documentation requirements are met including legibility with handwritten notes. A more comprehensive record will enhance the aggregate use of data in research and meaningful use activities and in making administrative decisions.

The Centers for Medicare and Medicaid Services (CMS) regulations allow for the use of scribes, with the stipulation that the physician is clearly the one providing the service, with the scribe serving to record the spoken words of the practitioner (CMS 2016b). Notation must be made attesting to the involvement of the scribe with the practitioner authenticating the information with signature upon completion of the report. Improved patient care may be one of the benefits when scribes are utilized. Other benefits documented in various studies include the increased productivity of physicians in seeing a greater number of patients, increased physician morale with the significant burden for documentation lifted, improved compliance with core measures, and enhanced reimbursement with improved capture of the data elements to support the billing function. Limitations in the use of scribes include the acceptance of providers to utilize them appropriately and the cost to the organization.

Companies that provide scribe services to hospitals and practitioners are reporting an escalation in demand for their services due in part to the increased use of the EHR. It is their opinion that physicians feel that documenting in the EHR takes time away from engaging with their patients plus the increased time just to document. These time constraints are coupled with the increased need for quality documentation to support initiatives such as meaningful use, ICD-10, and value-based purchasing.

Chapter 1 Review Exercises

Answer the following questions.

1. The benefits of using scribes include:
    a. Relieving the physician from the responsibility for completing documentation in the record
    b. Providing medical students the opportunity to learn to document
    c. Providing entries that are legible and easier to read
    d. Freeing up physician time and providing comprehensive documentation

2. The primary role of the CMIO is to:
   a. Be a physician
   b. Provide a vital link between the medical aspect of care and the information/systems departments
   c. Ensure that all necessary perspectives are represented when health information technology is implemented
   d. Design the EHR system

3. With the advances in genomic information, the probability and predictability of medical conditions can be determined in many instances. What potential ethical issues arise out of this?
   a. It could influence who receives healthcare.
   b. It can lead to medical errors due to incomplete information.
   c. It would require documentation for such a patient to be filed separate from the rest of the record.
   d. Whether or not to tell the patient about the information.

4. The person charged with the primary functions of strategic planning, leadership, and ability to predict future technology needs would be the
   a. Facility administrator
   b. CIO
   c. CMIO
   d. Informaticist

5. Someone who has a broader view of the effective use of the information in ways that contribute to the knowledge of workers and the organization:
   a. CIO
   b. Director of HIM
   c. CKO
   d. Project director

6. The role of the informaticist is:
   a. Defining the way information is presented in the system
   b. Designing the technical aspects of a system
   c. Making decisions based on information acquired
   d. Developing the EHR software to be used

7. The strength of a CAD system is:
   a. The ability to generate a treatment plan for the patient.
   b. That x-rays are the primary sources documents.
   c. That it can use only the patient's data to predict the diagnosis.
   d. That patient information can be compared to stored data of similar patients for consideration by the physician to arrive at a diagnosis.

Discussion.

8. What are common skills and knowledge that would be needed across the various roles of those involved with health informatics?

9. Why are computer applications in healthcare such a challenge?

10. From this introduction to informatics, what impact has the evolution of the field had on healthcare?

REFERENCES

42 CFR 412 and 495: Medicare and Medicaid Programs; Electronic Health Record Incentive Program—Stage 3 and Modifications to Meaningful Use in 2015 through 2017; Final Rule 2015.

AHIMA. 2016. Health Information Careers. http://hicareers.com/CareerMap/.

AHIMA. 2014. *Pocket Glossary for Health Information Management and Technology*, 4th ed. Chicago: AHIMA Press.

AHIMA. 2012. *Pocket Glossary for Health Information Management and Technology*, 3rd ed. Chicago: AHIMA Press.

AHIMA. 2005. e-HIM Work Group on Maintaining the Legal EHR. Update: Maintaining a legally sound health record—Paper and electronic. *Journal of AHIMA* 76(1): 64A-L.

AHIMA and AMIA. 2008. Joint Work Force Task Force, Health Information Management and Informatics Core Competencies for Individuals Working with Electronic Health Records.

Altman, R., and Klein, T. 2007. Biomedical informatics training program at Stanford University in the 21st century. *Journal of Biomedical Informatics* 40(1):55–58.

American Medical Association. 2016. *Transaction and Code Set Standards.* http://www.ama-assn.org/ama/pub/physician-resources/solutions-managing-your-practice/coding-billing-insurance/hipaahealth-insurance-portability-accountability-act/transaction-code-set-standards.page.

AMIA. Informatics Core: Science of Informatics. 2016. https://www.amia.org/about-amia/science-informatics.

Anderson, J., and S. Jay, eds. 1987. *Use and Impact of Computers in Clinical Medicine, Invited Volume in the Computers and Medicine Series.* New York: Springer-Verlag Publishing.

Birk, S. 2011. The evolving CIO: From IT manager to key healthcare delivery strategist. *Healthcare Executive* May/June, 20–27.

Blumenthal, D. 2009. Perspective: Stimulating the adoption of health information technology. *New England Journal of Medicine* 360:1477–1479.

BUMC. 2012. New Service: Using Technology and Informatics in Clinical Research. http://www.bumc.bu.edu/ocr/clinical-research-informatics-and-technology-consultation-service/.

Bureau of Labor Statistics, U.S. Department of Labor, Occupational Outlook Handbook, 2016-17 Edition, Administrative Services Managers. http://www.bls.gov/ooh/management/administrative-services-managers.htm.

Cassidy, B.S. 2011. Teaching the future: An educational response to the AHIMA core model. *Journal of AHIMA* 82(1):34–38.

Centers for Disease Control and Prevention. 2005. National Center for Public Health Informatics (CPE). http://www.cdc.gov/maso/pdf/NCPHIfs.pdf.

Centers for Medicare and Medicaid Services. 2016a. Medicare and Medicaid EHR Incentive Program Basics. https://www.cms.gov/Regulations-and-Guidance/Legislation/EHRIncentivePrograms/2016ProgramRequirements.html.

Centers for Medicare and Medicaid Services. 2016b. Ensuring Proper Use of Electronic Health Record Features and Capabilities. https://www.cms.gov/Medicare-Medicaid -Coordination/Fraud-Prevention/Medicaid-Integrity-Education/Downloads/ehr -decision-table.pdf. Detmer, D.E., J.R. Lumpkin, and J.J. Williamson. 2009. Defining the medical subspecialty of clinical informatics. *Journal of the American Medical Informatics Association* 16(1):167–168.

Dior, K., MacMahon, H., Katsuragawa, Nishikawa, R., Jiang, Y. 1999, August. Computer-aided diagnosis in radiology: potential and pitfalls. *European Journal of Radiology* 31(2).

Eysenbach, G. 2001. What Is e-Health? *Journal of Med Internet Research.* 3(2):e20. Published online June 18, 2001. doi: 10.2196/jmir.3.2.e20.

Gartner. 2016. *IT Glossary.* http://www.gartner.com/it-glossary/internet-of-things/.

HealthIT. 2013 How can electronic health records improve public and population health? https://www.healthit.gov/providers-professionals/faqs/how-can-electronic-health -records-improve-public-and-population-health-.

HealthIT. 2016. Basics of health IT. https://www.healthit.gov/patients-families/health -it-terms.

HealthIT. 2016a. What does "interoperability" mean and why is it important? https:// www.healthit.gov/providers-professionals/faqs/what-does-interoperability-mean -and-why-it-important.

HealthIT. 2016b. Meaningful use regulations. https://www.healthit.gov/policy -researchers-implementers/meaningful-use-regulations.

HealthIT. 2016c. Value Set Authority Center (VSAC). e-CQI Resource Center. https:// ecqi.healthit.gov/ecqm-tools/tool-library/value-set-authority-center-vsac.

Hersh, W. 2009. A stimulus to define informatics and health information technology. *BMC Medical Informatics and Decision Making* 9(24). doi:10.1186/1472-6947-9-24.

HIMSS. 2013. *HIMSS Dictionary of Healthcare Information Technology Terms, Acronyms and Organizations.* 3rd ed. Chicago, IL: HIMSS Publishing.

Kindig, D., and G. Stoddard. 2003. What is population health? *American Journal of Public Health* 93(3):380–383.

National Human Genome Research Institute. 2013. http://www.genome.gov.

National Institutes of Health. 2012. NIH: Jobs@NIH-Job Descriptions-Information Technology Specialist. Administrative careers at NIH. https://www.jobs.nih.gov /vacancies/administrative.htm.

Nuvem Consulting. 2014. Top 5 Internet of Things Examples. http://blog .nuvemconsulting.com/top-5-internet-of-things-examples/.

Saba, V. K., J. E. Johnson, and R. L. Simpson. 1994. *Computers in Nursing Management.* American Nursing Publishers.

Sarkar, I. 2010. Biomedical informatics and translational medicine. *Journal of Translational Medicine* 8(22).

Sewell, J., and L. Thede. 2012. *Informatics and Nursing: Opportunities and Challenges* 4th ed. Philadelphia: Lippincott, Williams and Wilkins.

Studdert, V.P., C.C. Gay, and D.C. Blood. 2012. Saunders Comprehensive Veterinary Dictionary, 4th Edition. "Decision making process." Retrieved January 18 2017 from http://medical-dictionary.thefreedictionary.com/Decision+making+process.

Wiedemann, L.A. 2014. Informatics harnesses healthcare's wild, rich data. *Journal of AHIMA* 85(1):68–69.

World Health Organization. 2016. Health Systems Strengthening Glossary. http://www .who.int/healthsystems/hss_glossary/en/index8.html#17.

Zhang, Y., X. Yang, X. Han, and R. Xia. 2010. The research of data management technology in telemedicine diagnosis system based on multimedia. 2010 International Conference on Computer Application and System Modeling (ICCASM 2010).

ADDITIONAL RESOURCES

AHIMA Work Group. 2014. Defining the basics of health informatics for HIM professionals. *Journal of AHIMA* 85(9):60–66.

Arya, R., D. Salovich, P. Ohman-Stricklan, and M. Merlin. 2010. Impact of scribes on performance indicators in the emergency department. *Academy of Emergency Medicine* 17(5):490–494.

Betts, H., and G. Wright. 2009. Observations on Sustainable and Ubiquitous Healthcare Informatics from Florence Nightingale. *Connecting Health and Humans.* Edited by K. Saranto et al. Amsterdam: IOS Press.

Birnbaum, C.L. 2015. Evolving practice of health informatics. *Journal of AHIMA* 86(5):8.

Brandt, M. 2000. Health informatics standards: A user's guide. *Journal of AHIMA* 71(4):39–43.

Brittain, J., and A. Norris. 2008. Delivery of health informatics education and training. *Health Libraries Review* 17(3):117–128.

Butler, M. 2015 Reformatting healthcare through standards: AHIMA building a standards strategy to improve interoperability and healthcare. *Journal of AHIMA* 86(11):18–21.

Campbell, R. 2005. Getting to the good information: PHRs and consumer health informatics. *Journal of AHIMA* 76(10):46–49.

Carter-Templeton, H., R. Patterson, and C. Russell. 2009. An Analysis of Published Nursing Informatics Competencies. *Connecting Health and Humans.* Edited by K. Saranto et al. Amsterdam: IOS Press.

Cassidy, B. 2013. The next HIM frontier: Population health information management presents a new opportunity for HIM. *Journal of AHIMA* 84:40–46.

Cassidy, B. 2011. Stepping into new e-HIM roles: The e-HIM transition changes HIM roles and responsibilities. *Journal of AHIMA* 83(9):10.

Centers for Disease Control and Prevention. 2015. Introduction to Health Level Seven (HL7), Version 2.5 www.cdc.gov/EHRmeaningfuluse/Docs/Introduction_to _HL7_03022011_Anderson_CLEARED.pptx.

Cesnik, B. and M. Kidd. 2010. History of health informatics: A global perspective. *Studies in Health Technology Information* 151:3–8.

Collen, M. 1986. Origins of medical informatics. *Medical Informatics* (Special Issue). 145:778–785.

Dolan, M., J. Wolter, C. Nielsen, and J. Burrington-Brown. 2009. Consumer health informatics: Is there a role for HIM professionals? *Perspectives in Health Information Management.*

Embi, P., S. Kaufman, and R. Payne. 2009. Biomedical informatics and outcomes research: Enabling knowledge-driven healthcare. NIH Public Access. December 8; 120(23):2393. doi:10.1161/CIRCULATION AHA. 108.795526.

Expanded scribe role boosts staff morale and templates help organize care. *ED Management.* July 2009; 21(7):75–77.

Eysenbach, G. 2000. Consumer health informatics. *British Medical Journal* 320(7251):1713–1716.

Forgey, D., and J. Vickrey. 2005. Informatics: How an emerging field of study benefits HIM. *Journal of AHIMA* 76(6):46–49.

Fox, L. 2004, October. Health record paradigm shift: Consumer health informatics. IFHRO Congress and AHIMA Convention Proceedings.

Georgiou, A. 2002. Data, information and knowledge: The health informatics model and its role in evidence-based medicine. *Journal of Evaluation in Clinical Practice* 8(2):127–130.

HealthIT 2013. Health IT Success Stories. 2013. https://www.healthit.gov/providers -professionals/dr-bragg-leverages-health-it-improve-provider-performance.

Health Level Seven. 2013. About HL7. http://www.hl7.org/about/index.cfm?ref=nav.

Health Level Seven. 2015. Introducing HL7 FHIR. http://www.hl7.org/implement /standards/fhir/summary.html.

Health Level Seven International. 2016. Introduction to HL7. http://www.hl7.org /implement/standards/index.cfm.

Ellis, B., R. Hedges, and P. Lane. 2014. Information governance: Why should I care? *Journal of AHIMA.* http://journal.ahima.org/2014/12/17/information-governance -why-should-i-care/.

Houston, T., B. Chang, S. Brown, and R. Kukafka. 2001. Consumer health informatics: A consensus description and commentary from the American Medical Informatics Association members. AMIA, Inc.

Hovenga, E. 2010. National Standards in Health Informatics. *Health Informatics.* Edited by E. J. S. Hovenga et al. Amsterdam: IOS Press.

Imhoff, M., A. Webb, and A. Goldschmidt. 2001. Health informatics. *Intensive Care Medicine* 27:179–186.

Jesse, W. 2011. Healthcare IT is more than EHRs. *MGMA* Connexion, 5–6.

Joint Work Force Task Force. 2008. *Health Information Management and Informatics Core Competencies for Individuals Working with Electronic Health Records.* AHIMA and AMIA.

Kampov-Polevoi, J., and B. Hemminger. 2011. A curricula-based comparison of biomedical and health informatics programs in the USA. *Journal of American Medical Informatics Association* 18:195–202.

Lau, F. 2004. Toward a conceptual knowledge management framework in health. *Perspectives in Health Information Management* 1:8.

Layman, E. 2009. Research and policy model for health informatics and information management. *Perspectives in Health Information Management* 6.

Macpherson, B. 2010. The role of a health information manager in creating data fit for purpose. *Health Information Management Journal* 39(3):58–59.

Martin-Sanchez, F., V. Maojo, and G. Lopez-Campos. 2002. Integrating genomics into health information systems. *Methods in Informatics Medicine* 41:25–30.

McKinney, M. 2010. Most wired CMIOs steadily on the rise. *Hospital and Health Networks* 84(3):41–42.

Murphy, G., and M. Brandt. 2001. Health informatics standards and information transfer: Exploring the HIM role (AHIMA Practice Brief). *Journal of AHIMA* 72(1):68A–D.

Murphy, J. 2011. The nursing informatics workforce: Who are they and what do they do? *Nursing Economics* 3(29).

National Institutes of Health. National Human Genome Research Institute. 2015. All about the Human Genome Project. https://www.genome.gov/10001772/all-about -the--human-genome-project-hgp/.

Norris, A. 2002. Current trends and challenges in health informatics. *Health Informatics Journal* 8:205.

Oachs, P., and A. Watters. 2016. *Health Information Management: Concepts, Principles, and Practices.* Chicago: AHIMA.

Osborne, K., L. Spellman, and D. Warner. 2014. Setting the norm: HIM increasingly involved in developing and using standards. *Journal of AHIMA* 85(6):52–53.

Public Health Informatics Institute. 2016. *Defining Public Health Informatics.* http://www .phii.org/defining-public-health-informatics.

Russo, M. 1998. Consumer health informatics: The medical librarian's role. *Journal of AHIMA* 69(8):38–40.

Scribes. 2009. ER please docs, save $600,000. *ED Management* 21(10):117–118.

Sethi, P., and K. Theodos. 2009. Translational bioinformatics and healthcare informatics: Computational and ethical challenges. *Perspectives in Health Information Management* 6, Fall.

Shiraishi, J., Li, Q., and Doi, K. 2011. Computer-aided diagnosis and artificial intelligence in clinical imaging. *Seminars NuclearMedicine* Nov.

Smith, S., L. Drake, J. Harris, K. Watson, and P. Pohlner. 2011. Clinical informatics: A workforce priority for 21st century healthcare. *Australian Health Review* 35:130–135.

Tegen, A. and J. O'Connell. 2012. Rounding with scribes: Employing scribes in a pediatric inpatient setting. *Journal of AHIMA* 83(1):34–38.

University of Illinois at Chicago (UIC). Downloaded 2016. Benefits of Health Informatics for Patients. UIC Publisher. http://healthinformatics.uic.edu/resources/articles/benefits-of-health-informatics-for-patients/.

US Department of Energy Genome Programs. Human Genome Project Information. http://genomics.energy.gov.

Yasnoff, W., P. O'Carroll, D. Koo, R. Linkins, and E. Kilbourne. 2000. Public health informatics: Improving and transforming public health in the information age. *Journal of Public Health Management Practice* 6(6):67–75.

Zeng, X., R. Reynolds, and M. Sharp. 2009. Redefining the roles of health information management professionals in health information technology. *Perspectives in Health Information Management* 6, Summer.

Chapter

2

Ethics

Learning Objectives

- Define ethics
- Use basic ethical terms and concepts
- Explain the importance of ethical issues related to technology
- Analyze ethical issues related to health informatics
- Apply the AHIMA Code of Ethics to ethical scenarios
- Apply the steps of the ethical decision-making process to a given scenario
- Develop policies and procedures for ethics related to informatics

KEY TERMS

Autonomy
Beneficence
Code of Ethics
Confidentiality
Ethics
Ethical decision making
Hacker ethics
Justice
Morals

Nonmaleficence
Privacy
Secondary release of information
Security
Sentinel event
Social media
Values
Whistle-blower

Decisions of an ethical nature must be made on a daily basis in providing quality healthcare services across an organization and with individuals carrying out their professional responsibilities. Determining the course of action in these situations becomes more difficult with the added dimension of cultural and religious beliefs, values, and experiences of all those involved with or affected by the decision. One definition of medical ethics is "moral principles that govern the practice of medicine" (Oxford 2016). Healthcare informatics with the increased use of technology and health information for supporting the delivery of healthcare services has changed and introduced new situations resulting in the potential for new ethical situations to arise. Related to health informatics, there is now more patient information available and used, along with increased rights of the patient for privacy, autonomy, and to be an active participant in decision making regarding their care and in the management of their information, and the higher perceptions of parity pertaining to access to their information and care among many other types of situations (HIMSS 2016). There are many laws, regulations, and standards for protecting patient information related to privacy, security, unauthorized disclosure, use, and maintenance from creation to planned destruction. **Privacy** is the patient's right to control the disclosure of their protected health information (AHIMA 2014) while **security** is the means to control access and protect the information from disclosure, accidental or intentional, to unauthorized individuals and to protect from alteration, destruction, and loss (AHIMA 2014). Ethical situations and dilemmas surface when there is a conflict between one of the formal means of protection with what is perceived as the right thing to do in a given situation. An example of this is deciding how much and what information to give a terminally ill patient. The patient has the right to their information and to be engaged in the decision-making process regarding their healthcare. Those close to the patient and even some of the providers of care may think it is more humane to withhold such information.

The pervasive use of these new informatics technologies and activities, such as electronic health records (EHRs), personal health records (PHRs), health information exchanges (HIEs), and data analytics, creates a complex ethical landscape that must be navigated carefully to avoid misuse, loss of protected health information (PHI), or unintentional destruction of PHI. Healthcare informatics can result in increased accessibility to patient information, but it is imperative that the integrity and quality of the data in the patients' health records be maintained. To navigate this shifting landscape, HIM professionals must balance the benefits provided by the functionality of the informatics systems that facilitate sharing of patients' healthcare data from internal and external sources on multiple platforms in multiple locations with the need to protect patients' privacy and respect their autonomy (Layman 2008).

⊙ Defining Ethics

The word ethics is derived from the Greek word ethos, which refers to letting your conscience guide you when deciding on the right or wrong action to take in a given situation (McWay 2014). **Ethics** is defined as "a field of study that deals with moral principles, theories, and values; in healthcare, a formal decision-making process for dealing with the competing perspectives and obligations of the people who have an interest in a common problem" (AHIMA 2014, 56). Humans constantly process data about the daily activities occurring in their surroundings into information used for making a multitude of ethical decisions. **Ethical decision making** is a process where everyone must contemplate others' perspectives, even if they disagree on the issue (AHIMA 2014, 56).

Ethical decisions have varying levels of difficulty. In general, the decision-making process must be internalized and ethical principles debated to reach equitable conclusions about the right and wrong actions for a given situation. Sometimes the decisions are relatively easy because the correct behaviors are dictated by outside forces. An example of easy ethical decision making would be that anyone driving an automobile must obey the rules of the road or face the undesirable consequences of getting a traffic ticket. Most drivers realize that driving ethics is an example of common courtesy that has been translated into a set of laws designed to make the highways safer for everyone and that they represent the acceptable choices, but it can be tempting to break the speed limit or run a red light in order to get to your destination faster. An example of a more difficult situation would be the decision-making process for whether or not to include outliers in a data analysis project. There are no laws or specific requirements for including or excluding the outliers and their presence can be attributed to several different things such as errors in data collection or the presence of an extreme figure. These things, along with determining the influence of the outlier, require further analysis to determine whether the outlier is to be left in or removed (Murphy and Lau 2008). It would be simple to either keep it or remove it but then the integrity of the statistical analysis may be in jeopardy and the use of the analysis would be less useful. Thus, most ethical answers are not nearly as apparent in all situations and the decision making can be a difficult process.

Values and Morals

The ethical choices made by individuals are based on their morals and values. **Morals** are the principles of right conduct that an individual adopts (McWay 2014). Morals are grounded in the teachings of family, friends, religion, and other influential persons or groups such as significant teachers or workplace mentors. Morals may be conceptualized as the principles that people follow when deciding on what ethical actions they will take. **Values** are what ethics and morals are based on; the beliefs or standards on which judgment is based (McWay 2014). For example, if a childhood background included a hard working parent, kind teacher, honest and loyal friend, or a strong religious framework then these will likely be the values drawn upon when making moral decisions as an adult.

An individual's moral compass, one's capacity to assess right from wrong and perform accordingly, is strongly influenced by the groups they belong to, the ethics of their workplace, and where they live. Individuals tend to norm to the groups' standards by bending their personal moral philosophy toward the group's moral philosophy in order to be accepted, which may have undesirable effects in the long run. For example, a coworker clocking in for another coworker when they are late for work, or falsifying their favorite doctor's delinquent record list to gain favor.

Several widely used ethical concepts especially relevant to health informatics are autonomy, beneficence, nonmaleficence, and justice, which are discussed here (Budinger and Budinger 2006).

Autonomy

Autonomy refers to the freedom of an individual to choose their own actions. Autonomy is "a core ethical principle centered on the individual's right to self-determination that includes respect for the individual; in clinical applications, the patient's right to determine what does or does not happen to him or her in terms of healthcare" (AHIMA 2014, 14). Autonomy would be exercised when obtaining informed consent from the patient for surgery. For the conditions of autonomy to be met, the preoperative patient would be given enough information about the surgery and its consequences, be able to understand that information, and cognitively reason to decide to sign the consent form for the surgery (Layman 2008). A related concept is **confidentiality,** protection against unauthorized access or unintended disclosure of the patient's written or verbal information (45 CFR 164.304 2013), which health information and health informatics professionals must protect. This could be done by restricting access to the protected health information to those who do not have the proper authorization or right to access the information. Technically, confidentiality could involve the use of passwords and biometric user authentication for log-ons and having updated policies and procedures that are consistent with HIPAA Privacy and Security regulations.

Beneficence

Beneficence is doing good for others. Beneficence, an act of goodness or kindness, implies that informatics professionals have a duty to assist patients toward positive outcomes (Layman 2008). This principle is embodied in the Hippocratic Oath that physicians' take upon graduation, which requires them to treat patients in a manner that maximizes the patients' positive health outcomes (McWay 2014). In the field of HIM, this could include verifying that the patient's information is being accessed only by the patient and others who will use this information for treatment, payment, or healthcare operations purposes that benefit the patient and those who have been authorized access. Beneficence is also being practiced when using available data to support clinical decision making and the provisioning of quality healthcare (Cellucci et al. 2011). The increased use of self-monitoring devices for diabetics, telehealth psychiatric consultations for remote areas, and the ability to print out discharge instructions are all beneficial to the patient (Layman 2008).

Nonmaleficence

Nonmaleficence is doing no harm to others. Nonmaleficence, protecting from wrongdoing, requires preventing access to the patient's data that could harm the patient (AHIMA 2014, 103). For example, testing to ensure that electronic data are transmitted accurately between the laboratory computer and the electronic health record (EHR). Nonmaleficence would include preventing harm to the patients by retesting clinical decision support algorithms after the system upgrades or security patches. Additionally, backup procedures must be in place to ensure business continuity in the event the system goes down, and antivirus programs must be kept up to date in order to prevent potentially harmful destruction of clinical data and ensure that recovery can be effected when needed.

Justice

Justice is treating all people fairly. Justice is displayed by treating everyone fairly and equally at all times. Equal treatment can be demonstrated by maintaining everyone's PHI in a confidential and secure environment that is HIPAA compliant (International Medical Informatics Association 2016). Another example of treating patients in a fair and equal manner is providing digital access via cell phones to facilitate a low-income patient's access to the Internet and consequently portals and information. The application of justice is important in the ethical decision-making process, which will be discussed in greater detail later in this chapter.

Legal Influence

At a minimum, members of society must abide by the legal rules set forth by that society. Thus, the laws of the land influence our ethical choices. In particular, the laws are the foundation for the development of the principles surrounding the ethical use of health information and technology in healthcare. When a circumstance is found to be in violation of the law or other regulation, it is not likely to be an ethical situation. The laws briefly mentioned here are covered in more detail in chapters 12, 13, and 14.

HIPAA

The Health Insurance Portability and Accountability Act of 1996 (HIPAA) is federal legislation enacted in 1996, which, in part, assures privacy and security of health information (AHIMA 2014, 69). HIPAA is complex and comprehensive covering many different facets of both patient health information and the use of technology for creating, maintaining, accessing, disclosing, storing, using, and transmitting it. Consideration must also be given to the type of technology used with increased use of such things as mobile devices and Internet computing.

HITECH

The Health Information and Technology for Economic and Clinical Health Act (HITECH), a part of the American Recovery and Reinvestment Act of 2009 (ARRA), is legislation designed to support the adoption of technology that will result in the meaningful use of patient health information (AHIMA 2014, 68). Privacy, security, and the electronic exchange of data are key components in the act to reach the meaningful use goal. The electronic exchange of healthcare data involves the electronic transfer among various entities.

GINA

Title II of the Genetic Information Nondiscrimination Act of 2008 (GINA), a federal law that took effect in 2009, was enacted to prohibit discrimination based on genetic information for health coverage and employment (HHS 2009). For GINA, due to the nature of the information obtained in genetic testing, genetic information was defined as information about an individual's genetic tests, their family's genetic tests, or their family medical history. Different from most other medical tests, identifying a genetic marker in one person also identifies it for some family members as well.

HIPAA Omnibus Rule

The HIPAA Omnibus Rule was enacted in 2013 to strengthen privacy and security protections that were established in the initial HIPAA (HHS 2009). The Omnibus Rule primarily addresses the privacy protections, new rights for individuals related to their health information and provides the government with increased ability for enforcement. All of the changes are consistent with the other laws, HITECH and GINA, that have been enacted since HIPAA first went into effect and with the increasing digital world.

Even when there are laws or rules in place to govern a situation, ethical issues may still arise when the law is not explicit in a given circumstance. The nature of health information and the increased use of health information technology can foster the development of ethical situations where existing laws may be in conflict with personal values. Examples of these instances include where some are in favor of sharing protected health information when a communicable disease is involved or with sharing genetic information to alert other family members of their risk for potential conditions. With the increased use of technology throughout the healthcare enterprise there are many more employees who have access to health information via the electronic system but may not have the right or need to know the PHI.

Ethical Standards of Practices

Ethical dilemmas occur when there are differing perspectives among the individuals involved in the situation including the patient, patient's family, and friends to the countless healthcare professionals who treat and provide services from all facets of supporting the delivery of healthcare. A **code of ethics** is "a statement of ethical principles regarding business practices and professional behavior" (AHIMA 2014, 30). Professional associations and societies support a sound ethical framework that members are obligated to follow. A common statement in many of the healthcare code of ethics includes one referring to protecting patient privacy and respecting the patient. One professional code of ethics directly associated with healthcare informatics is that of the American Medical Informatics Association (AMIA) whose members are engaged in transforming healthcare through science, educational opportunities and biomedical and health informatics practice (AMIA 2016). Figure 2.1 shows AMIA's Code of Professional and Ethical Conduct with the full document available at the AMIA website.

Figure 2.1.   Principles of Professional and Ethical Conduct for AMIA Members

A member of AMIA has the professional duty to uphold the following principles of, and guidelines for, ethical conduct.

    I. Key ethical guidelines regarding <u>patients, guardians and their authorized representatives</u> (called here collectively "patients").

        A. Given that patients have the right to know about the existence and use of electronic records containing their personal healthcare information AMIA members involved in patient care should:

            1. Not mislead patients about the collection, use, or communication of their health information;

            2. Enable and—as appropriate, within reason and the scope of their position and in accord with independent ethical and legal standards—facilitate patients' rights to access, review, and correct their electronic health information. Further, they should:

        B. Advocate and work as appropriate to ensure that health and biomedical information is acquired, stored, analyzed and communicated in a safe, reliable, secure and confidential manner, consistent with applicable laws, local policies, and accepted informatics processing standards.

        C. Never knowingly disclose biomedical data in violation of legal requirements or accepted local confidentiality practices, or in ways that are inconsistent with the explanation of data disclosure and use previously given to the patient. Even if an action does not involve disclosure, one should not use patient data in ways inconsistent with the stated purposes, goals, or intentions of the organization responsible for these data—except as appropriate for approved research, public health or reporting as required under the law.

    II. Key ethical guidelines regarding <u>colleagues</u>. AMIA members should:

        A. Endeavor, as appropriate, to support and foster colleagues' and/or team-members' work in a timely, respectful, and conscientious way to support their roles in healthcare and/or research and education;

        B. Advise colleagues and others, as appropriate, about actual or potential information or systems issues (including system flaws, bugs, etc.) that affect patient safety or could hinder colleagues' ability to discharge responsibilities to patients, other colleagues, involved institutions, or other stakeholders;

        C. If a leader:

            1. Be familiar with these guidelines and their applicability to your practice, unit or organization;

            2. Communicate as appropriate about these ethical guidelines to those you lead;

            3. Strive to promote familiarity with, and use of, these ethical guidelines.

III. Key ethical guidelines regarding <u>institutions, employers, business partners and clients</u> (called here collectively "employers"). AMIA members should:

   A. Understand their duties and obligations to current and former employers and fulfill them to the best of their abilities within the bounds of ethical and legal norms.

   B. Understand and appreciate that employers have legal and ethical rights and obligations, including those related to intellectual property. Understand and respect the obligations of their employers, and comply with local policies and procedures to the extent that they do not violate ethical and legal norms.

   C. Inform the employer and act in accordance with ethico-legal mandates and patient rights when employer actions, policies or procedures would violate ethical or legal obligations or agreements made with patients. AMIA's Ethics Committee might be a resource in such cases.

IV. Key ethical guidelines regarding <u>society</u> and regarding <u>research</u>. AMIA members involved in research should:

   A. Be mindful and respectful of the social or public-health implications of their work, ensuring that the greatest good for society is balanced by ethical obligations to individual patients. Seek the advice of institutional ethics committees, AMIA's Ethics Committee or appropriate institutional review boards, as necessary.

   B. Strive as appropriate in the context of one's position to foster the generation of knowledge and biomedical advances through appropriate support for ethical and institutionally approved research efforts.

   C. Know and abide by the applicable governmental regulations and local policies that define ethical research in their professional environment.

V. <u>General professional and ethical guidelines</u>. AMIA members should:

   A. Maintain competence as informatics professionals;

     1. Recognize technical and ethical limitations and seek consultation when needed;

     2. Obtain applicable continuing education;

     3. Contribute to the education and mentoring of students and others, as appropriate for job function.

   B. Strive to encourage the adoption of informatics approaches supported by adequate evidence to improve health and healthcare; and to encourage and support efforts to improve the amount and quality of such evidence.

   C. Be mindful that their work and actions reflect on the profession and on AMIA.

Source: Goodman, Kenneth W; Adams, Samantha, AMIA's Code of Professional and Ethical Conduct, *Journal of the American Medical Informatics Association*, 2013, 20(1), by permission of Oxford University Press.

Because AMIA's Code of Professional and Ethical Conduct is specifically for an organization of informatics professionals in healthcare it stands to reason that their entire code is focused on the informatics aspect. There are other code of ethics for healthcare professionals with the focus primarily on their discipline or area of practice but most of these codes still include statements about privacy and/or use of patient information. For example, AHIMA credentialed health information professionals are guided by the AHIMA Code of Ethics, AHIMA Standards of Ethical Coding, and Ethical Standards for Clinical Documentation Improvement Specialists (AHIMA 2008, 2011). Specific principles in the AHIMA Code of Ethics, which address patient information and informatics include:

> I. Advocate, uphold and defend the individual's right to privacy and the doctrine of confidentiality in the use and disclosure of information

> III. Preserve, protect and secure personal health information in any form or medium and hold in the highest regards health information and other information of a confidential nature obtained in an official capacity, taking into account the applicable status and regulations

> X. Facilitate interdisciplinary collaboration in situations supporting health information practice (AHIMA 2011).

As can be seen with these statements, patient and other confidential information in any form must be protected and the concern for the individual is of utmost importance.

Policies and Procedures for Ethics Related to Informatics

To operationalize the laws and other regulations, consistent codes of ethics such as AHIMA Code of Ethics, AMIA's Code of Professional and Ethical Conduct, or another code of ethics, policies, and procedures must be developed that protect the privacy, security, and confidentiality of PHI and serve as a deterrent to unethical workplace practices. These policies and procedures must facilitate personal freedom as it relates to technology use (autonomy), ensure technology is used for good (beneficence), and prevent technology from causing harm to others (nonmaleficence) (Anderson 2004). This requires balancing the need to give access against the need to secure the information systems. The following example shows the number and types of informatics policies and procedures that are used to create an ethical healthcare workplace by explaining the process of getting a new hire's technical work environment set up, which illustrates the minimum necessary policies and procedures to ethically use healthcare informatics.

A new employee, John, has been hired for the HIM department. To begin, after completing the new hire paperwork and passing the required background check, he is assigned a job title and a job role, and a department in the Human Resources database system. When John arrives for his first day at work, he is unable to enter the building until he goes to the security office, presents identification, and has a plastic identification badge issued. Security personnel call his department, and someone comes to escort him to the HIM department where he is required to test his badge by swiping it on the electronic badge reader in the HIM department's door.

After being shown to his cubical, John finds that he does not have a computer system on his desk. At this point, the HIM department manager follows the procedure for ordering a new computer for the new employee with the company's approved computer configuration. The manager knows that this standardization is needed to more easily maintain the facility's systems (Abdelhak et al. 2011). The IT department places the order specifying an up-to-date system. When the new employee's computer arrives at the facility, the type and characteristics of the machine are recorded to be used for later maintenance and inventory tracking. Next, the new computer is assigned an internal asset code, which is etched into a plastic plaque and attached to the machine as part of the security procedure to uniquely identify the machine, to prevent theft of the machine, and to allow asset tracking. The facility will use a "standard build" that is a set of specific software (for example, Microsoft Word, Outlook e-mail and a web browser), which will be installed on all new machines and specific tests will be run to ensure that the machine is working according to specifications (Denić et al. 2014).

When the machine is ready, it is taken to the department and placed on John's desk. Unfortunately, he finds that he cannot log on to the machine until he goes to his boss and gets his log-on and temporary password, which is a standard security procedure. Using his network ID and password, John logs on the network and is then able to access his Windows system, but his e-mail and web browser are giving errors related to not having an Internet connection. Due to the number of healthcare breaches occurring over the Internet, his boss must complete a second form stating that he needs the Internet access to perform his work activities (Butler 2015; HHS 2014). After receiving Internet access and having a network connection physically set up on his computer, John's manager tells him to go ahead and complete the mandatory online HIPAA training on privacy and security, and to take the other mandatory classes on facility security, ethics, and the use of emergency codes. He is also given the HIM department policy and procedure book to read and must sign a form stating that he has read it. John learns that use of employer-owned property for personal use is prohibited. He will e-mail his friends after work.

While completing this training, he has some technical issue with his e-mail and calls support who follows security procedures by directing him to read the asset tracking code from the machine and to tell them his network ID. While using his computer, he notices that some websites he tries to access are blocked because they do not have valid security certificates and he observes that virus tracking software and routine backups are running on the machine (Abdelhak et al. 2011). John has completed all these preliminary steps and is ready to get started on his work assignments. His manager tells him that he will be using three pieces of software at work, which are an electronic health record, a chart tracking system, and a system that tracks record deficiencies. Each of these systems require further training and each system has its own procedure for security access and for logging on with different user names and passwords. John learns that his access levels for these systems will be determined by his assigned role at work, which is called role-based access, and that this security feature helps IT manage and track system usage.

In the lunchroom, John ends up sitting at a table with Jane, the IT employee who set up his new machine. Jane tells him that he should feel confident that IT is using technology for the benefit of all employees and patients. Specifically, the IT department stores the servers in a restricted area that requires biometric access, they perform regular backups of servers, and their maintenance schedule includes regular updates to all system hardware and software as well as an annual disaster recovery drill. They also have offsite storage of their backups, and uninterruptable power systems to provide power if the system goes down. In addition, they monitor the audit logs on all servers to determine who has accessed the systems and what they have done.

Jane notices that John has brought a personal electronic notebook to work and is using a cell phone to read his work e-mail at meetings. She tells him that there is a policy requiring him to report any personal device usage at work to his boss and that he will have to come into the IT department to have his devices physically checked or he will not be able to continue bringing the devices to work (HIMSS 2011; Imgraben et al. 2014; Tan and Aguilar 2013; Thomas 2007). She also mentions that he needs to be encrypting all his work e-mail to protect the PHI. At this point Jane has to leave to return to a workshop on implementing secure patient-centered protected health information, which is part of her department's mandatory professional development training designed to keep all employees up to date on the latest technology. As John walks back to his desk, he is tired but highly impressed by the numerous policies and procedures in place to protect the employee's and patient's data that form the ethical framework of this hypothetical workplace.

This example shows the number and types of policies and procedures required for protected health information for a facility to be compliant with the laws for privacy and security. Professionals working in this environment are personally obligated to conduct themselves with ethical behavior and managers are accountable for assuring that the employees have the tools in the form of the policies and procedures and a culture that respects ethical behavior to promote ethical decision making.

The Ethics Committee

Traditional functions of a healthcare ethics committee are to provide consultation when ethical issues arise, generate and revise policies and procedures for clinical ethics, and facilitate entity educational activities for employees (Pearlman 2013). The committee membership may vary based on the emphasis and function of the committee; that is, a clinical ethics committee will likely be comprised of mainly physicians while a more comprehensive hospital ethics committee will have a more diverse membership from across the facility. More facilities are expanding the functions of their ethics committees to cover issues related to both clinical and organizational ethics situations. In addition to the patient and provision of care-related goals of the traditional clinical ethics committee, the current trend is expanding the ethics committee goals to include:

- ⊙ "Integrating ethics throughout the health care institution from the bedside to the boardroom,
- ⊙ Ensuring that systems and processes contribute to/do not interfere with ethical practices, and
- ⊙ Promoting ethical leadership behaviors, such as explaining the values that underlie decisions, stressing the importance of ethics, and promoting transparency in decision making" (Pearlman 2013).

The inclusion of goals addressing ethical situations across the organization's personnel, their systems, and their processes is significant. These items also suggest that the leadership in an organization must strive for an institutional culture that values ethical decision making and demonstrates ethical behavior.

Check Your Understanding 2.1

Answer the following questions.

1. What is a field of study that deals with principles, theories, and values related to our moral choices?
   a. Ethics
   b. Values
   c. Morals
   d. Economics

2. What is the freedom of an individual to choose their own actions?
   a. Autonomy
   b. Beneficence
   c. Nonmaleficence
   d. Justice

3. Treating all people fairly is referred to as
   a. Autonomy
   b. Beneficence
   c. Nonmaleficence
   d. Justice

4. Which is an example of beneficence?
   a. Verify patient's identity during ROI
   b. Let your friend use your password
   c. Locking your computer when you go to lunch
   d. Getting an informed-consent form signed

Indicate whether each of the following is true or false.

5. Nonmaleficence would include retesting clinical decisions support systems after a security patch was applied.

6. HIPAA includes penalties for failing to secure mobile devices.

7. GINA does not address discrimination based on genetic history specifically.

8. There are no requirements for a hospital to have an ethics committee.

⊙ Potential Ethical Issues in Healthcare

Numerous ethical dilemmas arise during the provisioning of healthcare. For example, how can healthcare professionals use health information ethically? How can they protect the privacy and security of the patients' data while simultaneously providing access to patients and providers via electronic health records, personal health records, and mobile devices? Additional ethical concerns surround data sharing though the internal processes of release of information, the secondary release of information, and the external collaborations inherent in the health data exchange systems. **Secondary release of information,** or redisclosure, is releasing the health information that was originally obtained per a request from an external facility (AHIMA 2009). A growing body of research on health literacy raises concerns about what patients really take away from their perusals of public websites, or from the handouts they are given at their doctor's office. Finally, the use of social networks is pervasive and this creates a gray area for employers because information from work shared via social networks can do irreparable harm in minutes, and it is hard to retract all copies.

Provisioning of Care

Facilities have a responsibility to establish a corporate culture that rewards ethical behavior and applies sanctions to unethical activities (Lefkowitz 2006). When the provision of healthcare meant that the doctor and the patient were in the same room, there was a strong connection between the healthcare provider and the patient. Similarly, the healthcare providers' daily ethical decision making was influenced by the everyday interactions with coworkers, managers, and the top leadership of the facility. Although technology has provided many beneficial advances in healthcare utilizing robotic surgery, telehealth, patient portals, and remote management of patients' chronic diseases via smart devices, unfortunately, it has also created the potential for new and different kinds of ethical dilemmas. Indeed, many of the healthcare workers will never set foot inside the facility, but they will manage the patients' data (through cloud computing or remote data storage center) or the patient's care from a distance (for example, telehealth).

In the past, workers commuted to work, entered the healthcare facility, and were exposed to the corporate ethical culture of their company's top management, they interacted face to face with patients and staff, attended department meetings in person, and had a chance to observe firsthand the demeanor of their department heads as they conducted business. Consequently, a facility with strong ethical leaders and a culture that fostered autonomy, beneficence, equality, charity, and justice provided a strong moral compass for their employees to follow. In this era of globalization and virtual private networks there are more and more health employees telecommuting from home, from other states, or even from other countries, as is common in the field of teleradiology. One researcher argues that the old concept of employee's wanting to be seen as good corporate citizens has gone by the wayside as virtual healthcare workers and electronic medical record systems become the norm (Lefkowitz 2006). Consequently, while the ethical behavior practiced by top management still strongly influences their employees' ethical behavior, the effectiveness of this positive influence is diffused when the face to face element between employer and employee is lacking.

Ethical Use of Health Information

Using health information ethically means honoring the ethical concepts of autonomy, beneficence, nonmaleficence, and justice. In the workplace, health informatics professionals must deal with complex ethical issues in accordance with the standards of practice clearly outlined in the AHIMA Code of Ethics. Unfortunately, everyday workplace ethical dilemmas are multifaceted and usually do not have clear-cut answers. Although it is ethically and morally correct to report overcoding for the purpose of higher reimbursement, the reality is that the **whistle-blower**, one who reports a wrongdoing, may be asked to seek other employment, which is a misuse of justice (Crawford 2011). Similarly, failing to report delinquent records in order to stay below the required Joint Commission delinquency rate is dishonest, but reporting the oversight to your manager may cause you harm if the manager is the one who is generating the delinquency reports. There are also situations where the person behaving unethically is not aware of the rules governing the situation, which is why healthcare facilities require employees to remain up to date by completing annual professional development classes on relevant rules and regulations for their jobs. Indeed, the principles of ethics and risk management are interrelated because the facility is responsible for maintaining current policies and procedures and documenting that employees have received training on those policies and procedures.

The use of EHRs has introduced functionality for entering information into a patient's record where the information may not be as precise or as specific to an individual patient as intended while still being technically correct. One example of this is the copy and paste functionality, which includes copying material from one document such as a previous hospital stay and pasting into a patient's EHR or copying from one part of a record to another without deleting from the original location (AHIMA 2014, 17). This is a shortcut for documenting but can have consequences primarily related to the integrity of the record. When blocks of information are copied and pasted, there could be parts of it that are inaccurate for the current encounter and the possibility of contradictions with other information in the record could occur easily. There are also some situations that could result in legal issues such as the pasted information having a higher reimbursement than what the patient actually was being treated for and this would then be considered fraud. An example of this is a patient with two hospitalizations just months apart but both for respiratory conditions. On the first visit the patient was treated for a bacterial pneumonia and on the second visit was treated for bronchitis. Both conditions had many of the same symptoms, tests, and treatments but in the end they were different conditions. Copying and pasting from the first visit for the second visit, without deleting symptoms, diagnostics, and treatments that were only done in the pneumonia visit could inadvertently trigger the reimbursement rate for payment for pneumonia rather than bronchitis. Knowingly providing documentation that may not be current or specific to a given situation is not in the best interest of the healthcare of the patient. Even when fraud is not an issue, once it is recognized that the copy and paste has been done the credibility of the record is in question.

Autonomy and confidentiality of patient information can be hard to preserve in this digital era where camera phones are used to transmit photographs of patients to their doctors and hospitals have surveillance cameras in the halls (van der Rijt and Hoffman 2015). Similarly, administering beneficence in the context of making choices for health information technologies that benefit patients has become a balancing act. There are evidence-based long-term benefits from funding multiyear high-dollar electronic record system implementations, such as a reduction in medical record errors, more complete and more specific documentation for billing, and a facilitated release of information cycle. However, a study by the Joint Commission on sentinel events associated with the implementation of computerized provider order entry (CPOE) reflect that health IT has been a contributing factor in medical errors. A **sentinel event** is "an unexpected occurrence involving death or serious physical or psychological injury or risk" (AHIMA 2014, 134). Findings of the Joint Commission review of 3,375 sentinel events occurring between January 1, 2010, and June 30, 2013, indicate the following:

- 120 identified health IT as a contributing factor
- 15 different types of events associated with the most common events (1) medication errors, (2) wrong-site surgery (wrong side/site wrong procedure performed or on wrong patient), and (3) delays in treatment
- Multiple contributing factors to any one sentinel event with 305 health IT–related factors identified across the 120 health IT–related sentinel events with most common:
  - Human-computer interface, 33 percent
  - Workflow and communication, 24 percent
  - Clinical content, 23 percent
- There were 120 sentinel events; however, 147 were related to medical devices. More than one health IT device may have been involved in a sentinel event.
  - 66 percent of the sentinel events involved EHRs or some component of the EHR (includes CPOE, pharmacy, and clinical documentation systems [for example, progress notes], e-MARs, and clinical decision support) (HHS 2015).

The Joint Commission study illustrates that there are associated risks when incorporating health IT, although the majority of these cases caused only minor health issues or delayed appropriate treatment. Another study that reported much more dire results attributed to CPOE system implementation, completed in 2005, brought attention to the issue. The study findings reported:

> Of 1,942 children admitted for specialized care during the study period, 75 died, a 3.86% mortality rate. Further analysis revealed the mortality rate to be 2.80% (39 of 1,394) before CPOE and 6.57% (36 of 548) after CPOE was implemented. This finding was an unexpected increase in mortality coincident with CPOE implementation. The study recognized that CPOE technology has the capability to reduce human error but the unexpected finding indicates continued evaluation of the mortality effects and medication error rates especially for children dependent on time-sensitive therapies (Han et al. 2005).

The Han report brings attention to the serious nature of outcomes, mortality, that can occur when there are errors made in using the CPOE systems, which is in conflict with what has been touted as a benefit to using CPOE. Moreover, malpractice claims related to EHR risks have resulted from system issues such as poor system design (10 percent), system or technology failure (9 percent), alert or alarm issues (7 percent), electronic data routing failure (6 percent), lack of space for documentation (4 percent), or fragmented EHRs (3 percent). User factors have also caused risk issues, with the top three reported issues being incorrectly entered information (16 percent), problems with hybrid health records or EHR conversion (15 percent), and issues with preloading information (13 percent) (Crysts 2016, 15).

All of these studies could be considered a violation of ethical principles when considering the rights of patients, expectation of sound medical, patient-centered outcomes, and ensuring effective systems and practices to support the delivery of care and patient privacy.

Protected Health Information

The ethical concept of autonomy, also called freedom of choice, is closely related to the legal concept of privacy. Privacy in healthcare is considered to be the right of patients to control disclosure of their PHI (AHIMA 2014, 119). Historically, there was a limited concept of patient privacy, other than that related to the patient's medical record, and it was not unusual to see the patients' name on the door of their room and also on a chalkboard in the hall by the nurses' station so that visitors and staff could more easily locate a patient. For many years, nursing stations had a bulletin board that listed the patient's name, room number, and physician, and the procedures they were having (for example, upper GI or gallbladder surgery) so that staff could keep track of who had gone to surgery or radiology and who still needed to be transported. When the patient was transported to x-ray, the paper chart was placed beside the patient on the stretcher, which meant that the chart was somewhat accessible to anyone walking by who wanted to take a look at their information.

In the digital era, most PHI is collected, transmitted, and stored electronically, thus there is no one "door" that can be locked to control access to the data. For example, while the architecture of the Internet facilitates the remote monitoring of a Sudden Infant Death Syndrome baby and the subsequent data transmission to cloud storage for later download to the provider's smartphone, it also makes it almost impossible to guarantee that the patient's private data are safe from unauthorized disclosure (Levine 2015).

Genetics

Compared to most protected health information, additional ethical questions arise with genetic information due to the nature of the information that is obtained with the testing (NSW Health 2016). Genetic data is different because it engenders the concept of shared ownership of genetic information, due to its familial nature. Moreover, genetic testing is not always definitive because it identifies the presence of present or potential conditions but cannot determine when the condition may present itself or the severity of the condition if it does present. This uncertainty about future conditions complicates current ethical decision making. How the information is used also causes ethical dilemmas, such as when the genetic information is used for employment screening, for obtaining insurance, and for making reproductive decisions. Genetics information is valuable with the potential to significantly improve health outcomes utilizing preventive measures and personalized treatment based on genetic test results. However, caution must be exercised with the information as illustrated in the following case study.

Case Study: Genetic Predictive Testing

Huntington's disease (HD) is a neurological progressive degenerative disease with no cure. Onset is usually between 30 to 50 years of age with symptoms of declining movement, cognition, and general ability to function with respiratory conditions commonly the cause of death. It is an inherited disease. A child of a person who has the disease has a 50 percent chance of inheriting the faulty gene. Individuals over the age of 18 who have an affected parent or relative can obtain genetic predictive testing. The results of the test will reliably reveal whether they will develop the disease at some point in their life.

The situation: Mr. C is a 25-year-old male. His grandfather died from Huntington's disease 10 years ago, which means that his mother has a 50 percent chance of developing HD. She was genetically tested and does have the faulty gene, which indicated that she will certainly develop HD at some time and now Mr. C. is at a 50 percent risk of developing HD.

Mr. C. is an air traffic controller and he does not want to have the test. He likes his job and feels that he can carry out his duties appropriately for years whether he carries the faulty gene or not. His employer is not aware of the family medical history of HD.

(Continued)

The ethical questions at this point are:

- Whether or not to have the predictive testing, which is a "to know or not to know" dilemma.

- Do employers have the right to know family medical history especially where public safety could be an issue? At what point do they have the right to this information, while the individual is still healthy, later when symptoms to start to appear, never?

- Whose information is this, the mother's, Mr. C's, both? And, who can make the decision to release it?

- What if in this situation Mr. C. wanted the testing but his mother refused? His results may reveal the genetic status of the mother (if Mr. C has it, he must have inherited it from his mother).

- Consideration and implications for Mr. C's reproductive choices. Does he tell the potential mother of his children and at what point in the relationship? If a child is conceived, should prenatal testing be done and what choices must be made? (NSW Health 2016).

This case study illustrates an ethical dilemma with a number of implications and decisions to be made by several individuals. There are no right or wrong actions with much left to personal choice. For this reason, genetic counseling is a common part of the genetic testing process. This case also illustrates the importance of protecting the PHI.

Electronic Health Records

Electronic health records (EHRs) are "an electronic record of health-related information on an individual that is created and managed by clinicians and staff across two or more healthcare organizations" (AHIMA 2014, 53). The use of EHRs has made PHI documentation by physicians more legible and accessible, which can benefit patients by contributing to the reduction in medical errors, providing data integrity, and facilitating communication among interdisciplinary healthcare teams (Cheshire 2014). EHRs enable e-prescribing and computerized order entry, they provide alerts for physicians, and they are accessible from multiple locations (Cheshire 2014). Conversely, the confidentiality of the patient's e-PHI is harder to protect due to the increased accessibility and many feel that the patient–provider connections may suffer (Clark 2014; Cochran et al. 2015).

Today PHI is stored electronically and the virtual storage media makes it easier to steal. First, e-PHI can be accessed remotely using mobile devices, web-based PHRs and patient portals, which greatly reduces the danger of being observed during the theft. Second, the thief is pilfering data from a computer thus their sense of connectedness to stealing an actual person's healthcare data is diminished.

Healthcare entities who do attempt to persecute malicious users, soon realize that these unauthorized users believe they are not subject to the laws of society (Cross 2006). Researchers have coined the term **hacker ethics** to refer to the hackers' beliefs that restrictions on data are objectionable and that technology is a tool that should be used to perform hands-on actions that make nonhackers' private data publicly accessible while protecting the hacker's personal privacy (Kirkpatrick 2002). The size of this problem cannot be underestimated, hackers are not just a local issue involving one disgruntled IT employee in his garage. Hackers form global groups to share system vulnerabilities and system access codes on their websites. HIM personnel should conduct a security audit to assess vulnerabilities. As a final note, there are some hackers called white hat hackers who use their abilities to help companies detect their vulnerabilities (Vaas 2007). Essentially a white hat hacker breaks or hacks into protected systems and networks to assess the security and identify vulnerabilities.

To reduce security vulnerabilities, measures like antivirus software, role-based access levels, passwords, data encryption, audit trails, and server security are needed to protect PHI against hackers (HIMSS 2011). The facility should develop a security profile to be used when selecting vendors. New computers should have a standard security configuration. Computer system inventories must be kept up to date so that the location and security measures in use on each system can be tracked, this will also assist in the timely replacement of older systems. Policies and procedures must address the level of system access to give the patient's family and visitors through wireless connections (HIMSS 2011). An example of how the EHR system facilitated the unauthorized access to a patient's information is

> a nurse practitioner who has privileges at a multi-hospital health care system and who is part of the system's organized health care arrangement which allows access to all patient records across the system impermissibly accessed the medical records of her ex-husband. Following a determination by the OCR, the covered entity: terminated the nurse practitioner's access to its electronic records system; reported the nurse practitioner's conduct to the appropriate licensing authority; and provided the nurse practitioner with remedial Privacy Rule training (HHS 2016).

This example illustrates the importance of strong policies and procedures, appropriate access levels granted, and the employees' education. In this particular situation, a review of the practice of granting access to all patient records across the systems should be conducted to determine if that is necessary and policies and procedures to address whatever access is provided should be updated.

Personal Health Records

The CMS federal incentive Stage 2 Meaningful Use program promotes the meaningful use of EHRs and recommends patient engagement through access to their personal health information (PHI) through a patient portal or by obtaining a copy of their personal records from their provider (HHS, Centers for Medicare and Medicaid 2012). A **personal health record (PHR)** is a paper or electronic record maintained by the patient for the purpose of collecting and sharing their data (AHIMA 2014, 114). There are two types of PHRs. A stand-alone personal health record is patient generated from their own records with information stored on a personal computer or the Internet. These have the capability to accept information from external sources.

Patients have control of what to include and may include such things as diet or exercise logs. They also control who to share the information with. A tethered or connected PHR is linked to a specific organization's EHR system. Patients have access via a portal (HealthIT 2016). PHRs provide patients with more autonomy by providing greater access to their health data and greater ownership of that data. In PHR portals, patients can view health information about diseases, examine their diagnostic results, e-mail providers, or schedule appointments (Tang et al. 2006).

A PHR can be hosted on a vendor's website where the patient logs on and enters the information (stand-alone) or it can be integrated into the hospitals' system such that part of the data is entered automatically by the hospital's systems and part of the data is entered by the patient (Househ et al. 2014). The patient portal functionality of an EHR is controlled by the healthcare organization. The patient has read-only access to view only the designated sections. E-mail and appointment scheduling may also be available, similar to the PHR portal.

There are two major barriers to increasing PHR usage. First, the absence of a standard design for PHR systems or a standard PHR data set for data transmission has led to a lack of interoperability among PHRs and other healthcare systems (Studeny and Coustasse 2014). Second, patients are concerned about the privacy of their PHR data.

The following are examples of PHR software systems:

- ⊙ Microsoft's HealthVault
- ⊙ Department of Veteran Affairs' MyHealtheVet
- ⊙ Health Companion

Additionally, Blue Cross Blue Shield and several other health plans offer PHRs to their enrollees, as do some major companies (Kaelber et al. 2008).

One technical challenge with PHRs is ensuring the privacy and security of PHI in the PHR systems due to the lack of standard designs and data sets. Moreover, because so much computer code has to be generated to move PHR data between these disparate healthcare systems, and because there is no standard design or standard transmission data set, there are concerns about data accuracy. Physicians are especially cautious about the legality of making medical decisions based in part on data recorded by the patient in their PHR (Studeny and Coustasse 2014).

Ethical challenges include the concerns for maintaining complete and current information and determining what is the level of responsibility for maintaining the PHR. Although physicians have a concern for using patient-generated data, patients have a similar concern about the information populated for them in their PHR. Concerns include whether the test results and medication records are up to date, if all their reports are there, and if there is a possibility of information for another patient ending up in their record.

Release of Information

Release of information (ROI) refers to the process of disclosing PHI from health records (AHIMA 2014, 128). ROI process requires corresponding policies and procedures designed to restrict access to the patient's information to those individuals who are authorized by the patient to receive the information to be in compliance with existing laws. An organization is bound to use systems and processes that assure that improper disclosure is prevented. The following is an example in which a health plan had a computer flaw that resulted in mailing EOBs (Explanation of Benefits) to the wrong person and the corrective action taken:

> A HMO sent an EOB by mail to a complainant's unauthorized family member. An investigation by the OCR identified a flaw in the health plan's computer system that put the PHI of approximately 2,000 families at risk of disclosure in violation of HIPAA Security Rule. The corrective action required the insurer to correct the flaw in its computer system, review all transactions for a six month period and to correct all corrupted patient information (HHS n.d.)

With an organization's responsibility to use systems that assure only proper disclosures are made, it is imperative that system testing be done periodically to make sure they are working as intended. Correcting corrupted information can be costly both in terms of time and money.

Health Information Exchange

To receive incentive money from the HITECH act, a facility must demonstrate use of electronic records for data sharing. This can be accomplished with a **health information exchange** (HIE), which expedites data sharing between healthcare systems located in different facilities (Vest and Gamm 2010). HIEs can contain massive amounts of data with the potential for meaningful biomedical and public health research. The concepts of beneficence, to do good, and nonmaleficence, to do no harm, are in conflict in this instance. The research would benefit the health of individuals and the populace but to do no harm would require both that the data in the exchange be protected from unauthorized use and that consent be given from each individual in the exchange for the specific use of their data and for researchers who will require access to the systems. HIE systems at this time do not have the capacity to be research compatible and adding this capacity would be very costly and legally challenging (Mercuri 2010).

Social Networking

Social networking refers to social communications conducted using Internet-based **social media** tools such as e-mail, text messaging, Facebook, Twitter, LinkedIn, and YouTube. Social media use is becoming pervasive in our society. In 2016 there were 320 million Twitter users and 1,590 million active Facebook users (Chaffey 2016). The use of social media at work for communications among healthcare professionals is increasing because it can provide instantaneous communications irrespective of the geographic locations of the two providers. Clinicians are texting and e-mailing each other to discuss cases (Kolowitz et al. 2014). Nurses are using social media at work to research the side effects of medicines and the symptoms of diseases. Patients are texting and e-mailing their doctors. The Mayo Clinic is active in their use of YouTube, Facebook, and blogs, and in 2016 they reported they had more than 1.36 million Twitter followers (Twitter.com/MayoClinic2016). The goal of the Mayo social media network is to improve global health by engaging patients using social media to share health information.

Social media use in healthcare has many benefits. The sender and receiver of social media information can quickly and easily locate each other, which saves time and reduces frustration. Collaboration is easier with social media because everyone can be online at the same time. With patients, social media has been shown to improve the health literacy skills of older adults, by increasing their cognitive functions through increased Internet use and their engagement in social activities (Kobayashi et al. 2015), and to provide much needed healthy living information for rural adolescent mothers (Logsdon et al. 2015). Local health departments are using Twitter and Facebook to disseminate health information on topics that include child safety, health, and smoking cessation (Harris et al. 2013). For example, a local health clinic uses Facebook to post daily information on healthy behaviors.

A few examples of ethical dilemmas in social networking include a family member who shared health information on an individual on their Facebook page, nursing students posting pictures of patients they come in contact with as a part of their educational training, and others posting pictures of individuals seen at a particular healthcare facility, such as a person leaving a planned parenthood clinic or substance abuse clinic. In many of these instances, this would not be against the law but would be unethical and likely against institutional policy. The following is an example of a situation where using a social networking site could be in conflict with institutional policy, which is based on the Privacy Law, but the patient's permission has been given:

> Scenario: You are an HIM professional employed at a cancer clinic, and also a member of a private group hosted on a social networking site. Mary is not a member of the social networking group, but she is a friendly acquaintance of all the group members. Mary is a cancer survivor. She has attended many parties and community events with various members of the group. At these events, she has been very open about her cancer, her treatment, and her prognosis. It has been several months since the group members have seen Mary. One day Mary comes into the cancer clinic for a follow-up appointment while you are working. She encourages you to let "the gang" know that she is doing well. The easiest way for you to convey this great update is via the group's private site. What would you do?
>
> Option 1: Go ahead and post the happy update to the group page; after all, Mary said it was okay.
>
> Option 2: Do not put yourself at risk by using the social networking site at all. Instead, tell just a few of Mary's friends—the ones you are certain she would want you to tell.
>
> Option 3: Explain to Mary that because you are learning this information about her in your capacity as an employee, it is important that any information sharing come from her—and not from you. You use this opportunity to talk to Mary about your organization's commitment to patient privacy.

Option 3 is the best ethical choice. Key points in this situation are that the information was obtained while you were in an employee role, which means that the facility policy that is based on the Privacy Law governs your actions and makes it the legal thing to do even though she has given you the permission to post the information (AHIMA Professional Ethics Committee 2013).

Health Literacy

In order for patients to give informed consent for the use of the healthcare data, they must have the details of the consent form explained to them and they must understand those details. One factor that affects their ability to understand these details is health literacy, which is the ability to obtain, process, and understand basic health information (Center for Health Care Strategies 2011, 13). Health literacy levels have been shown to be lower for individuals for whom English was a second language and among those living in poverty (Center for Health Care Strategies 2011, 13; HHS 2010). The patient with low health literacy lacks the skills to interpret medical documents and numbers, which impacts their clinical health outcomes and increases healthcare costs (Chen et al. 2013).

The Department of Health and Human Services developed an action plan to study health literacy in order to guarantee that all US citizens have been provided with accurate, understandable healthcare information (HHS 2010). The plan was written to:

- ⊙ "Provide access to accurate and actionable health information
- ⊙ Deliver person-centered health information and services
- ⊙ Support lifelong learning and skills for good health

The seven goals of the plan are:

1. Develop and disseminate accurate, accessible, actionable health and safety information
2. Promote changes in the healthcare system that improve the health information, communication, informed decision making, and access to health services
3. Incorporate accurate, standards-based, and developmentally appropriate health and science information and curricula in child care and education through the university level
4. Support and expand local efforts to provide adult education, English language instruction, and culturally and linguistically appropriate health information services in the community
5. Build partnerships, develop guidance, and change politics
6. Increase basic research and the development, implementation, and evaluation of practices and interventions to improve health literacy
7. Increase dissemination and use of evidence-based health literacy practices and interventions" (HHS 2010, 6)

Specific actions include clear labeling of food and drugs, use of the Internet and social media for disseminating health information, use of consumers to evaluate healthcare materials, conducting ongoing health literacy training at work and in schools, and providing patient-centered care (HHS 2010). Additionally, mandatory continuing education in health literacy for health professionals was one suggestion.

Check Your Understanding 2.2

Answer the following questions.

1. Which of the following is an issue with the electronic provisioning of healthcare?
   a. Loss of connection between patient and physician
   b. Faster access to patient data
   c. Legibility of documentation
   d. Appropriate authorization required for accessing system

2. The concept of autonomy in healthcare is most closely related to the concept of
   a. Security
   b. Privacy
   c. Trust
   d. Responsiveness

3. Which of the following is an HIT factor that can contribute to errors in care:
   a. Lack of technology skills
   b. Workflow and communication
   c. Limited access to clinical information
   d. Time to access needed documentation

4. Type(s) of personal health records are:
   a. Stand-alone
   b. Tethered
   c. Patient portal
   d. a and b

Indicate whether each of the following is true or false.

5. Autonomy and confidentiality of patient information can be hard to preserve in this digital era.

6. Preventing harm to the patient would not include checking for valid authorization before releasing PHI.

7. It is important for the organizational leaders to create a strong ethical corporate culture.

8. According to HIPAA, a patient's PHI can be sold or disclosed without the patient's written consent.

9. Health literacy is an issue with informed consent because the patient may not understand the details of the consent form.

10. The literacy level of a patient should not be of concern if they are provided with all of the key pertinent information.

◉ Ethical Decision Making

Handling ethical issues correctly falls into the realm of risk management. Conflicts resulting from differing ethical viewpoints can disrupt the workflow, cause upheaval between coworkers and result in harm to patients and to staff morale. A plan for ethical decision making should be put in place and employees should be given examples of correct and incorrect use of the process. Steps to manage ethical situations should include assessing all situations for their ethical subcontexts, identifying the underlying ethical issues, evaluating the situation including the perspectives of all involved in the situation, and deciding on a course of action. After the event, ongoing monitoring should be implemented to prevent future occurrences of similar situations.

Assessing Potential

This chapter has discussed many nuances of ethical issues related to technology that could form the basis for a risk assessment of potential ethical hotspots related to health informatics. Policies, procedures, hardware, software, and education surrounding the use of PHI, PHRs, HIEs, mobile devices, social media outlets and release of information technology must be assessed for their potential to cause harm to the patient.

Identifying

The PHRs, HIEs, mobile devices, servers, personal computers, and other computing systems should be cataloged and the level of risk potential for these systems should be rated. The potential of the human resources for generating unethical behavior should be added to this list. Several instruments are available for ethics screenings of employees. For example, Oncology and ICU nurses at Mayo Clinic attended an ethics workshop where they were trained to use an ethics screening tool that was developed by nurses to identify early warning signs of ethical conflict (Pavlish et al. 2015). Participants then evaluated the tool for three months. Results indicated the tool was beneficial in early identification and the researchers recommend it be administered as part of the admission assessment.

Evaluating

Each item on the potential risk list should be evaluated step by step to determine when, where, and how the risk might occur. The cost and benefits of each risk should be evaluated. For example, while mobile application use is correlated with higher risks of data breaches, the use of mobile devices for looking up drug interactions or treatment modalities can provide better patient outcomes due to the fact that online references are updated more frequently than paper-based medical references (Bullock 2014). The completed risk evaluation should be documented and put in a repository that is accessible to e-HIM project managers as it will serve to assist them in their project planning with regard to costs, resources, and timelines.

Deciding on a Course of Action

For each item on the list of risks, several potential courses of action should be outlined. Using the weightings for each path of action, a cost–benefit analysis should be conducted to determine the critical path and decide on which of many paths is the most optimal one. These decisions may expose a need for creating or modifying the organizations policies and procedures. Once determined, the course of action should be carried out and the results documented.

Preventing Future Occurrences

Ongoing vigilant prevention is essential for the success of any risk management initiative. Indicators should be put in place and the necessary data collected for reporting on the previously identified risk situations. Mandatory annual training on ethics should be conducted for all employees. Top management should attend workshops and retreats designed to emphasize their role in creating an ethical work culture and rewarding ethical behavior.

Educational programs and practice in working through ethical situations can take many forms and can be adapted for different groups and different situations. One example of a tool to use in working through the ethical decision-making process is a matrix as shown in figure 2.2.

As can be seen in this tool, ethical decision making is a process to be worked through with many aspects to consider. Solving ethical situations is not a quick decision to be made. Working through the steps of this process, the first thing to determine is the question. What is the question in a situation where a potential

Figure 2.2.   Ethical decision-making matrix

Steps	Information	
1. What is the question?		
2. What is my "gut" reaction?		
3. What are the facts?	Known	To be gathered
4. What are the values? Stakeholders:	Patient: HIM Professional(s): Healthcare professional(s): Administrators: Society: Others as appropriate:	
5. What are my options?		
6. What should I do?		
7. What justifies my choice?	Justified	Not justified
8. How can I prevent this problem?		

Source: Harman, L.B. and F. Cornelius, *Ethical Health Informatics: Challenges and Opportunities*, 2017, Jones & Bartlett Learning, Burlington, MA. www.jblearning.com. Reprinted with permission.

employer has been given genetic information that suggests the likelihood of a potential job applicant getting a disease that could be costly for the employer's health plan and could cause missed work if the employee were to actually develop the condition? Is the problem that the employer's livelihood and the financial well-being of his family could be jeopardized? Or is the problem that using this information in making an employment decision is considered discrimination? Next is the "gut reaction," which is setting aside consequence and personal feelings about the course of action to be taken. This should then be followed up with gathering pertinent information. In the employment issue, this could be finding out exactly what the law says about using genetic information in the hiring decision and working with HR to assure the screening and hiring process follows procedures (Harman and Cornelius 2017).

The next step is to evaluate the values of all those involved in the particular situation. In the previous employment example, the values of the potential employee, the hiring supervisor, the organization, and others are in conflict much of the time. From all of this, options can be identified followed by choosing what should be done. This should then be followed by articulating the justification for action to be taken based on the steps in the ethical decision making. To avoid similar situations in the future, this final step is important for determining what could have been done to avoid the situation. This may result in rewriting policies and procedures, more training, or other similar activities. Although every situation will be different, using this process should lead to better decision making.

Chapter 2 Review Exercises

Match the term with its description.
- a. Electronic record maintained by the patient for collecting and sharing their health data
- b. Principles of right conduct that an individual adopts
- c. What ethics and morals are based on
- d. An individual's capacity to understand health information
- e. Doing good for others

1. _____ PHR
2. _____ Values
3. _____ Morals
4. _____ Health literacy
5. _____ Beneficence

Indicate whether the following statements are true or false.

6. Autonomy would be used when obtaining informed consent.

7. Verifying that the patient's medical record is being accessed only by authorized users is an example of beneficence.

8. Nonmaleficence includes making sure that the wrong lab results are not put on a patient's chart.

9. An example of the ethical use of justice would be letting a friend see her aunt's chart.

10. The AHIMA Code of Ethics should serve as an ethical guideline at all times.

Discussion.

11. As the HIM manager, what would be the best response to a complaint that one of your employees was posting information about a patient on Facebook?

12. How would you apply the AHIMA Code of Ethics to a report that a medical coder has consistently been overcoding medical records to increase reimbursement?

13. Apply the steps of ethical decision making to a case where a physician is accepting money from a vendor to recommend the vendor's new EHR system.

REFERENCES

Abdelhak, M., S. Grostick, and M.A. Hanken. 2011. *Health Information: Management of a Strategic Resource.* 4th ed. St. Louis, MO: Saunders.

AHIMA. 2014. *Pocket Glossary of Health Information Management and Technology.* 4th ed. Chicago, IL: AHIMA Press.

AHIMA. 2009. Redisclosure of PatientHealth Information (2009 Update). *Journal of AHIMA* 80(2):51–54.

AHIMA. 2011. AHIMA Code of Ethics. http://bok.ahima.org/doc?oid=105098#.WHkUkVMrJaQ.

AHIMA. 2008. AHIMA Standards for Ethical Coding. http://bok.ahima.org/doc?oid=106344#.WHkU4lMrJaQ.

AHIMA Professional Ethics Committee. 2013. Reality check 2013: Ethical issues in HIM. *Journal of AHIMA*: web extra. http://journal.ahima.org/2013/10/01/reality-check-2013-ethical-issues-in-him/.

AMIA. 2016. Ethical, legal, and social issues. https://www.amia.org/programs/working-groups/ethical-legal-social-issues.

Anderson, J.G. 2004. The role of ethics in information technology decisions: A case-based approach to biomedical informatics education. *International Journal of Medical Informatics* 73(2):145–150. doi: 10.1016/j.ijmedinf.2003.11.015.

Budinger, T.F., and M.D. Budinger. 2006. *Ethics of Emerging Technologies: Scientific Facts and Moral Challenges.* Hoboken, NJ: Wiley.

Bullock, A. 2014. Does technology help doctors to access, use and share knowledge? *Medical Education* 48(1):28–33. doi: 10.1111/medu.12378.

Butler, M. 2015. Cracking encryption: Despite benefits, technology still not widely used to combat multi-million dollar breaches. *Journal of AHIMA* 86(4):18–23.

Cellucci, L.W., E.J. Layman, E.M. Campbell, and Z. Xiamong. 2011. Integrating healthcare ethical issues into IS education. *Journal of Information Systems Education* 22(3):215–224.

Center for Health Care Strategies. 2011. Health literacy interventions and outcomes: An updated systematic review. AHRQ.

Chaffey, D. 2016. Global Social Media Research Summary 2016. http://www.smartinsights .com/social-media-marketing/social-media-strategy/new-global-social-media-research/.

Chen, J.-Z., H.-C. Hsu, H.-J. Tung, and L.-Y. Pan. 2013. Effects of health literacy to self-efficacy and preventive care utilization among older adults. *Geriatrics & Gerontology International* 13(1):70–76. doi: 10.1111/j.1447-0594.2012.00862.x.

Cheshire, W.P. 2014. Can electronic medical records make physicians more ethical? *Grey Matters* 30(3):135–141.

Clark, J.R. 2014. Making your mark. *Air Medical Journal* 33(5):194–196. doi:http://dx.doi .org/10.1016/j.amj.2014.06.007.

Cochran, G.L., L. Lander, M. Morien, D.E. Lomelin, C. Reker, and D.G. Klepser. 2015. Consumer opinions of health information exchange, e-prescribing, and personal health records. *Perspectives in Health Information Management* (Fall):1–12.

Crawford, M. 2011. Everyday ethics. *Journal of AHIMA* 82(4):30–33.

Cross, T. 2006. Academic freedom and the hacker ethic. *Communications of the ACM* 49(6):37–40. doi: 10.1145/1132469.1132498.

Crysts, A. 2016. Preventing malpractice lawsuits due to EHR errors. *Medical Economics* 93(9):13–17.

Denić, N., V. Moračanin, M. Milić, and Z. Nešić. 2014. Risk management in information system projects. *Upravljanja rizicima projekta informacijskih sustava* 21(6):1239–1242.

Department of Health and Human Services. 2015. Breaches affecting 500 or more individuals. https://www.hhs.gov/hipaa/for-professionals/breach-notification/index.html.

Department of Health and Human Services. 2014. Annual report to Congress on breaches of unsecured protected health information for calendar years 2011 and 2012.

Department of Health and Human Services. 2010. National action plan to improve health literacy. Washington, DC. https://health.gov/communication/initiatives/health -literacy-action-plan.asp.

Department of Health and Human Services. 2009. The Genetic Information Nondiscrimination Act of 2008. Information for researchers and health care professionals. https://www.genome.gov/pages/policyethics/geneticdiscrimination /ginainfodoc.pdf.

Department of Health and Human Services. 2016. Large Health System Restricts Provider's Use of Patient Record. http://www.hhs.gov/hipaa/for-professionals /compliance-enforcement/examples/all-cases/index.html.

Department of Health and Human Services. 2016. Health Information Privacy. All case examples. http://www.hhs.gov/hipaa/for-professionals/compliance-enforcement /examples/all-cases/index.html#case15.

Department of Health and Human Services, Centers for Medicare and Medicaid. 2012. Medicare and Medicaid programs: Electronic health record incentive program— Stage 2. *Federal Register* 77 42 CFR Parts 412,413, and 495 (171):53967–54162.

Goodman, K.W., S. Adams, E.S. Berner, P.J. Embi, R. Hsiung, J. Hurdle, D.A. Jones, C.U. Lehmann, S. Maulden, C. Petersen, E. Terrazas, P.Winkelstein. 2013. AMIA's Code of Professional and Ethical Conduct. *J Am Med Inform Asso:* 20 (1):141-143.

Han, Y, J. Carcillo, S. Venkataraman, R. Clark, R. Watson, T. Nguyen, H. Bayir, and R. Orr. 2005. Unexpected increased mortality after implementation of a commercially sold computerized physician order entry system. *Pediatrics* December 116(6):1506–1512.

Harman, L.B., and F. Cornelius. 2017. *Ethical Health Informatics.* Burlington, MA: Jones and Bartlett.

Harris, J.K., N.L. Mueller, and D. Snider. 2013. Social media adoption in local health departments nationwide. *American Journal of Public Health* 103(9):1700–1707. doi: 10.2105/AJPH.2012.301166.

HealthIT. 2016. Are there different types of personal health records (PHRs)? https://www.healthit.gov/providers-professionals/faqs/are-there-different-types-personal-health-records-phrs.

HIMSS. 2016. Ethical Issues in the Use of Health Information. http://www.himss.org/ethical-issues-use-health-it.

HIMSS. 2011. Security of mobile computing devices in the healthcare environment. http://www.himss.org/security-mobile-computing-devices-healthcare-environment.

HIPAA. 1996. Health Insurance Portability and Accountability Act of 1996. Public Law 104-191.

Househ, M.S., E.M. Borycki, W.M. Rohrer, and A.W. Kushniruk. 2014. Developing a framework for meaningful use of personal health records (PHRs). *Health Policy and Technology* 3(4):272–280. doi: 10.1016/j.hlpt.2014.08.009.

Imgraben, J., A. Engelbrecht, and K.-K. R. Choo. 2014. Always connected, but are smart mobile users getting more security savvy? A survey of smart mobile device users. Rochester, NY: Social Science Research Network.

International Medical Informatics Association. 2016. The IMIA Code of Ethics for Health Information Professionals. http://www.imia-medinfo.org/new2/pubdocs/Ethics_Eng.pdf.

Kaelber, D.C., A.K. Jha, D. Johnston, B. Middleton, and D.W. Bates. 2008. A research agenda for personal health records (PHRs). *Journal of the American Medical Informatics Association* 15(6):729–736. doi: 10.1197/jamia.M2547.

Kirkpatrick, G. 2002. The hacker ethic and the spirit of the Information Age. *Max Weber Studies* 2(2):163.

Kobayashi, L.C., J. Wardle, and C. von Wagner. 2015. Internet use, social engagement and health literacy decline during ageing in a longitudinal cohort of older English adults. *Journal of Epidemiology & Community Health* 69(3):278–283.

Kolowitz, B., G. Lauro, J. Venturella, V. Georgiev, M. Barone, C. Deible, and R. Shrestha. 2014. Clinical social networking—A new revolution in provider communication and delivery of clinical information across providers of care? *Journal of Digital Imaging* 27(2):192–199.

Layman, E.J. 2008. Ethical issues and the electronic health record. *The Health Care Manager* 27(2):165–176.

Lefkowitz, J. 2006. The constancy of ethics amidst the changing world of work. *Human Resource Management Review* 16(2):245–268.

Levine, B.A. 2015. Digital OB/GYN: Gadgets for Health Tracking. *Conteporary OB/GYN.* http://contemporaryobgyn.modernmedicine.com/contemporary-obgyn/news/digital -obgyn-gadgets-health-tracking.

Logsdon, M.C., M. Mittelberg, and J. Myers. 2015. Use of social media and Internet to obtain health information by rural adolescent mothers. *Applied Nursing Research* 28(1):55–56.

McWay, D.C. 2014. *Legal and Ethical Aspects of Health Information Management.* 4th ed. Clifton Park, NY: Cengage Learning.

Mercuri, J. 2010. The ethics of electronic health records. *Clinical Correlations, The NYU Langone Online Journal of Medicine.* http://www.clinicalcorrelations.org/?p=2211.

Murphy, T., and A. Lau. 2008. Dealing with outliers, *Datapoits, ASTM.* http://www.astm .org/SNEWS/ND_2008/datapoints_nd08.html.

NSW Health. 2016. Fact Sheet 19/Ethical Issues in Human Genetics and Genomics. *Health Centre for Genetics Education.* http://www.genetics.edu.au/Publications-and -Resources/Genetics-Fact-Sheets/FactSheetELSI.

Oxford Dictionaries. 2016. https://en.oxforddictionaries.com/.

Pavlish, C.L., J. Henriksen Hellyer, K. Brown-Saltzman, A.G. Miers, and K. Squire. 2015. Screening situations for risk of ethical conflicts: A pilot study. *American Journal of Critical Care* 24(3):248–257. doi: 10.4037/ajcc2015418. https://depts.washington .edu/bioethx/topics/ethics.html.

Pearlman, R. 2013. *Ethis Committees, Programs and Consultation.* Ethics in Medicine, University of Washington School of Medicine.

Studeny, J., and A. Coustasse. 2014. Personal health records: Is rapid adoption hindering interoperability? *Perspectives in Health Information Management* 11 (Summer).

Strategies for Overcoming Barriers to Adoption. *Journal of the American Medical Informatics Association.* 13(2): 121. doi:10.1197/jamia.M2025.

Tan, M., and K.S. Aguilar. 2013. An investigation of students' perception of Bluetooth security. *Information Management and Computer Security* 20(5):364–381. doi: 10.1108/09685221211286539.

Tang, P., J. Ash, D. Bates, J. Overhage, and D. Sands. 2006. Personal Health Records: Definitions, Benefits, and

Thomas, G. 2007. Secure mobile device use in healthcare guidance from HIPAA and ISO17799. *Information Systems Management* 24(4):333–342. doi: 10.1080/10580530701586060.

Twitter.com/MayoClinic. 2016. https://twitter.com/MayoClinic.

Vaas, L. 2007. Inside the mind of a hacker. *eWeek* 24(24):38–46.

van der Rijt, R., and S. Hoffman. 2015. Ethical considerations of clinical photography in an area of emerging technology and smartphones. *Journal of Medical Ethics* 40:211–212. doi: 10.1136/medethics-2013-101479.

Vest, J.R., and L.D. Gamm. 2010. Health information exchange: Persistent challenges and new strategies. *Journal of the American Medical Informatics Association* 17(3):288–294.

ADDITIONAL RESOURCES

AMA. 2016. AMA Code of Medical Ethics.

Archer, N., U. Fevrier-Thomas, C. Lokker, K.A. McKibbon, and S.E. Straus. 2011. Personal health records: A scoping review. *Journal of the American Medical Informatics Association* 18(4):515–522. doi: 10.1136/amiajnl-2011-000105.

Aulisia, M. 2016. Why Did Hospital Ethics Committees Emerge in the U.S.? *AMA Journal of Ethics* 18(5):546–553.

Bagley, J.E., D.D. DiGiacinto, and K. Hargraves. 2014. Imaging professionals' views of social media and its implications. *Radiologic Technology* 85(4):377–389.

Bates, M., C. Black, F. Blair, L. Davis, S. Ingram, D. Lane, A. McElderry, B. Peagler, J. Pickett, C. Plettenberg, and S. Hart-Hester. 2014. Perceptions of health information management educational and practice experiences. *Perspectives in Health Information Management* 11 (Summer):2–12.

Bønes, E., P. Hasvold, E. Henriksen, and T. Strandenæs. 2007. Risk analysis of information security in a mobile instant messaging and presence system for healthcare. *International Journal of Medical Informatics* 76(9):677–687. doi: 10.1016/j.ijmedinf.2006.06.002.

Buelow, J.R., P. Mahan, and A.W. Garrity. 2010. Ethical dilemmas as percieved by healthcare students with teaching implications. *Journal of Teaching and Learning* 7(2):85–92.

Darr, K. 2002. *Ethics in Health Services Management.* 5th ed. Baltimore, MD: Health Professions Press.

Department of Health and Human Services. 2006. HIPAA security guidance.

Department of Health and Human Services, ONC, HealthIT. 2015. Investigations of Health-IT related deaths, serious injuries or unsafe conditions. Final report. The Joint Commission. https://www.healthit.gov/sites/default/files/safer/pdfs/Investigations_HealthIT_related_SE_Report_033015.pdf.

Eddy, N. 2014. Mobile devices still unsecured in the workplace. *eWeek.* http://www.eweek.com/mobile/mobile-devices-still-unsecured-in-the-workplace.html.

HIMSS. 2015. Cloud computing toolkit: Cloud privacy and security 101.

Kurzman, P.A. 2012. Workplace Ethics: Issues for Human Service Professionals in the New Millennium, In *Encyclopedia of Applied Ethics* (Second Edition), edited by Ruth

Chadwick, Academic Press: San Diego, Pages 559-564, http://www.sciencedirect .com/science/article/pii/B9780123739322000879Lau, L.K., B. Caracciolo, S. Roddenberry, A. Scroggins. 2011. College students' perceptions of ethics. *Journal of Academic and Business Ethics* 5:1–13.

Markel Foundation 2011. PHR Adoption on the Rise. http://markle-stage.svr04.com /publications/1440-phr-adoption-rise.

Putrillo, R.B., and R.F. Doherty. 2010. *Ethical Dimensions in the Health Professions.* 5th ed. St. Louis, MO: Saunders.

Samuel, H.W., and O.R. Zaiane. 2014. A repository of codes of ethics and technical standards in health informatics. *Online J Public Health Inform* 6(2):e189. doi: 10.5210 /ojphi.v6i2.5484.

Sittig, D.F., and H. Singh. 2013. A red-flag-based approach to risk management of EHR-related safety concerns. *Journal of Healthcare Risk Management: The Journal of the American Society for Healthcare Risk Management* 33(2):21–26. doi: 10.1002 /jhrm.21123.

US Congress. 2009. Health Information Technology for Economic and Clinical Health (HITECH) Act. Code of Federal Regulations.

US Department of Labor Family and Medical Leave Act (1993). Family and Medical Leave Act. https://www.dol.gov/whd/fmla/.

US Equal Employment Opportunity Commission. 2009. Genetic Information Nondiscrimination Act of 2008.

US Food and Drug Administration. 2016, June. *Mobile Medical Devices.* http://www.fda .gov/MedicalDevices.

Chapter

3

Electronic Health Records

Learning Objectives

- Relate the evolution in the development of the electronic health record
- Analyze the issues surrounding the deployment and implementation of the electronic health record
- Contrast the differences in electronic health record systems
- Articulate the aspects of the CMS EHR Incentive Program
- Summarize the advantages and disadvantages of the electronic health record
- Evaluate the current status and documented outcomes of EHR utilization
- Articulate the role of the patient health record
- Explain the outcomes of EHR utilization

KEY TERMS

American Recovery and Reinvestment Act (ARRA)
Certified Electronic Health Record Technology (CEHRT)
Clinical decision support
Clinical decision support system (CDSS)
Clinical documentation
Computer-based patient record (CPR)
Computerized provider (physician) order entry (CPOE)

Continuity of care document (CCD)
Electronic health record (EHR)
Electronic medication administration record (EMAR)
Episode of care
E-prescribing
Evidence-based medicine
Health and Medicine Division (HMD)
Health information exchange (HIE)
Health information system (HIS)
Health information technology (HIT)

Health Information Technology for
   Economic and Clinical Health
   (HITECH) Act
Healthcare Information and Management
   Systems Society (HIMSS)
Integration
Interface
Interoperability

Laboratory information system (LIS)
Meaningful use
Office of the National Coordinator
   for Health Information
   Technology (ONC)
Picture archiving and communication
   system (PACS)
Regional Extension Center (REC)

The evolution of the field of informatics cannot be fully understood or appreciated without consideration of the introduction and advancement of information systems in healthcare and the continued emphasis on the implementation of the **electronic health record (EHR)** along with the subsequent analysis and use of the health information. The EHR is "an electronic record of health-related information on an individual that conforms to nationally recognized interoperability standards and that can be created, managed, and consulted by authorized clinicians and staff across more than one organization" (AHIMA 2014, 53). **Interoperability** is "the capability of different information systems and software applications to communicate and exchange data" (AHIMA 2014, 82). Interoperability standards "allow different health information systems to work together within and across organizational boundaries in order to advance the effective delivery of healthcare for individuals and communities" (HIMSS 2005). The interoperability is the key component for an EHR system to provide the seamless sharing of patient information.

Paper medical records and EHRs contain the same patient information, including the notes of the physicians, nurses, therapists, and all healthcare professionals who provided direct care to the patient. Also recorded in the patient records, whether paper or electronic, are consent for treatment and other consent forms; lab, imaging, and other diagnostic reports; reports of procedures; and medication records; all of which provide complete documentation of the medical care provided to a patient. Paper records provide a record of the **episode of care**, which is the specific instance of a condition or illness with a defined time frame of care in which the patient is treated. An episode of care can apply to ambulatory encounters at a physician's office, outpatient clinic, ambulatory surgery center, or stand-alone laboratory and imaging facilities. It can also be an inpatient stay where the patient is admitted to a hospital or other healthcare facility for comprehensive care with multiple services provided within one setting. The limitation of the paper record is that a paper record is initiated when the patient arrives at a physician's office or when the patient is admitted to a hospital and it ends when the patient leaves the physician's office or is discharged from the hospital. Thus, the documentation is for just that one episode of care, which is a well-defined, time-limited encounter. A second limitation is that access to the information in paper form is limited to its location or to being copied and distributed to others via delivery, fax, or mail.

Similar to the paper record, the patient information for the EHR is initially collected for an individual episode of care. However, once the information is maintained electronically the information from all episodes of care can be accessed at one time, from many different locations, and in different formats than the original record. With the EHR, the individual data elements in the record become searchable across visits. For example, a patient's medication history for one month could be accessed without reviewing each individual record of care to compile the information for the entire month. Other benefits of the EHR are the ability of multiple authorized individuals to access it at the same time as opposed to a paper record, which can only be accessed by one person at a time. EHRs also provide alerts and reminders about preventive services and provide information to support diagnostic and therapeutic decision making. EHRs are a key factor in the exchange of data, which is the sharing of data between systems and organizations. To better understand the EHR systems of today, it is important to review the history of the evolution of the use of technology for maintenance of patient health information.

⊙ History

EHRs have evolved over time, beginning in the late 1960s with advances in technology introducing keyboards instead of punch cards as a medium for data entry and terminal hardware devices used to display data instead of printouts. For the most part, EHRs were stand-alone, software based, and did not accept input from other clinical systems like the lab or radiology. These systems were not interoperable, which means that they ran on specialized software at one facility and were not accessible outside the facility. Early adopters of these systems included Latter Day Saints Hospital utilizing Logical Processing System; El Camino Hospital incorporating CPOE and ability for multiple, simultaneous users; and Massachusetts General Hospital with the utilization of vocabulary mapping (Tripathi 2012). Utilization of early EHRs involved collecting information for decision support. The development of software applications evolved with the development and the adoption of **health information systems (HISs)**. A health information system can be defined as a "set of components and procedures organized with the objective of generating information which improve health care management decisions at all levels of the health system" (Lippeveld et al. 2012).

With the anticipated potential of electronic systems for maintaining and utilizing patient information, there were multiple driving forces supporting the continued development and implementation of such systems. Physicians supported the movement for two reasons: due to concern for care of their patients as medical care increased in complexity and because there was a growing need for critical patient information to be available in a timely manner. Healthcare administration supported HIS implementation with early systems developed to support billing and financial services. The transactional nature of the hospital's billing and financial services allowed the development of systems similar to those used in banking and by other early adopters of information technology (IT) to support business processes.

The availability of smaller computers in the 1970s enabled the development of early **clinical information systems (CISs)** to support individual clinical departments such as pharmacy, radiology, and laboratory. These clinical information systems were designed to facilitate the management of the activities of the clinical departments and to provide electronic charge capture and results reporting (McCullough 2008). Each department's CIS functioned as a stand-alone system within the department but could also be connected with other systems using an interface. **Interfaces** are hardware or software that enable disparate CIS and HIS software systems to communicate with each other. For example, interfaces eliminated the need to enter patient demographic information multiple times into separate laboratory, radiology, or pharmacy systems. Interfaces also enabled users to have a single sign-on to access information from any of the stand-alone clinical information systems that facilitated access to data, but interfaces were expensive and time consuming to develop. Once implemented, interfaces consumed considerable resources of time and manpower to maintain and update. An update to one system required testing of the interface and modification if needed. Information on how the interface was written had to be documented, maintained, and updated. Incorporating new or changing existing interfaces increased the challenges in troubleshooting problems to determine which system or interface was the cause.

A significant milestone in the development of these early systems in the early 1970s was the implementation of a **computerized provider (physician) order entry (CPOE)** system such as the one mentioned at El Camino Hospital. The CPOE system allowed providers the ability to directly enter medication, other orders, and medical instructions electronically. The utilization of CPOE systems reduces medical errors that may result from handwritten orders. CPOE systems are now "electronic prescribing systems that allow physicians to write and transmit them electronically" (AHIMA 2014, 33). CPOE systems currently in use commonly contain software with alerts for possible allergies, dosing errors, and other contraindications to the order as entered. CPOE applications coupled with decision support applications are an important tool to reduce medical errors, improve healthcare quality, and provide efficient care.

One of the first comprehensive electronic health record (EHR) systems was developed in the 1970s by the Regenstrief Institute in Indianapolis, Indiana. Samuel Regenstrief was an industrial production expert who founded the Regenstrief Institute in 1968 to promote the use of computer automation and industrial efficiency techniques in healthcare delivery. One of the earliest benefits of the Regenstrief EMR was improved access to patient information wherever and whenever clinical decisions were being made, independent of where the data were originally acquired. The Regenstrief Medical Record System (RMRS) has advanced over time and now functions as a citywide EHR system, allowing emergency room physicians to view a single virtual record for all patient care previously provided at any of 18 participating hospitals. Ambulances in Indianapolis also have laptops that can access the EHR in real time to provide up-to-date clinical information for diagnosis, treatment, and referral decisions about the patient (Regenstrief Institute 2012).

In addition to providing access to patient data for clinical decision support for the treatment of the patient, the RMRS also provides a rich source of data for health services research. **Clinical decision support (CDS)** is "the process in which individual data elements are represented in the computer by a special code to be used in making comparisons, trending results, and supplying clinical reminders and alerts" (AHIMA 2014, 27). RMRS has a database of "over 14.7 million distinct patients and 4.7 billion clinical results and observations" (Regenstrief Institute 2016). These data are useful for research to support implementation of evidence-based practices. **Evidence-based medicine** is defined as "healthcare services based on clinical methods that have been thoroughly tested through controlled, peer-reviewed biomedical studies" (AHIMA 2014, 56).

Major milestones in the evolution of the EHR in the 1980s included the implementation by the Veterans Health Administration (VHA) of an electronic health record system that is still in use today. Prior to the 1980s, the VHA was using comprehensive patient scheduling software programs but no clinical systems were in use. As the VHA system evolved through the 1970s and the 1980s, the numerous agencies and organizations involved in developing their scheduling systems encouraged them to implement an expansion that included systems that supported clinical functions. The first of these programs was the Decentralized Hospital Computer Program (DHCP), which was implemented in 1981. The name of the system was eventually changed when new groups, such as dentists, were added because the practice of these new groups was not reflected in the name of the system. Other changes occurred as different organizations became involved or new applications were added. In 1994, the system was renamed VistA (Veterans Health Information System and Technology Architecture) and adopted. Vista is still in use today as an enterprise-wide open source information system with approximately 160 integrated modules comprising the integrated system for clinical care, financial functions, and infrastructure (US Department of Veterans Affairs 2015).

The 1990s saw the first Windows-based software for electronic health records. Software for **e-prescribing** enjoyed significant advances during this time. In recent years e-prescribing was included as a requirement of the federal government's EHR Meaningful Use Incentive Program, which provides financial incentives for providers and for implementing health information technology (CMS 2016). With e-prescribing, practitioners can use electronic devices to write and submit prescription orders directly to a participating pharmacy rather than faxing the orders or providing the patient with a written prescription that must then be taken to the pharmacy. E-prescribing systems incorporate reference software for practitioners' use as they consider the options of medications to be ordered.

The **Health and Medicine Division (HMD)**, formerly Institute of Medicine (IOM) of the National Academies of Sciences, has been a major force in the development of the EHR. The HMD is "an independent, nonprofit organization that works outside of government to provide unbiased and authoritative advice to decision makers and the public" (National Academies 2016). Originally, the IOM presented a blueprint for the **computer-based patient record (CPR)** in 1991. The report defined the CPR as "an electronic patient record that provides complete and accurate data, alerts, reminders, clinical decision support, links to medical knowledge, and other aids" (IOM 1997). The IOM proposed the adoption of CPR as the standard for all records related to patient care, and recommended the establishment of a public or private organization to focus on a national agenda and provide support for CPR research, development, and demonstration. They also proposed the promulgation of national standards for data and security, and laws and regulations to facilitate implementation of CPRs. A follow-up report in 1997 reported that the healthcare industry was lagging behind other industries in automating their data and called for the establishment of CPRs as the standard within 10 years (IOM 1997). In 2007 the IOM lauded the US Department of Health and Human Services for the momentum generated with the 2004 creation of the position of National Coordinator for Health IT. The **Office of the National Coordinator for Health Information Technology (ONC)** was legislated in 2009 in the HITECH Act. The ONC is "the principal federal entity charged with coordination of nationwide efforts to implement and use the most advanced health information technology and the electronic exchange of health information" (AHIMA 2014, 107).

As a result of the gradual adoption of IT over time in the complex business of healthcare, health IT is not a single product, but rather a collection of hardware and software working within the healthcare organization or the healthcare delivery system. Although there were published standards for the content of the paper medical record as defined by the Medicare Conditions of Participation and accrediting bodies such as the Joint Commission, the complex nature of healthcare and the lack of standardization for EHRs have impeded the development and implementation of these systems when compared to information systems development in business and financial arenas. Although data in the business and financial arenas are generally standardized and structured, in 2012 approximately 60 percent of healthcare documentation contained unstructured narrative text (Health Story Project 2012). This number continues to grow as an August 2015 report indicated that approximately 80 percent of healthcare data was unstructured based on a consensus of the industry (Smithwick 2015). Structured data are binary, computer-readable data, whereas unstructured data are nonbinary, human-readable information. For example, history and physical examinations, discharge summaries, nursing observations, physician progress notes, and consultation reports are generally written or dictated and transcribed. In this unstructured narrative form, there are many ways to say the same thing, multiple terms that can have the same meanings, and acronyms may represent multiple different phrases. For instance, the medical term jaundice is synonymous with icterus. The acronym CVA is frequently used to refer to a cerebrovascular accident but is just as commonly used to refer to costovertebral angle. The lack of continued development and/or utilization of the EHR due to the sheer amount of unstructured data is one issue with the structured versus nonstructured data situation. Another concern is that of the providers who many times have a distrust of the structured data because it is computer generated more for purposes of transmission rather than patient care. Unstructured data tends to be more descriptive and provides better communication for patient care (Hersh

2015). This is not an easy situation to resolve with the amount of unstructured data and the difficulty of converting this kind of information to a structured format but much of it is very useful information that could be utilized more if it were in a structured format.

In 2001, the IOM noted that for most individuals "health information is typically dispersed in a collection of paper records which are not easy to retrieve, making it nearly impossible to manage illnesses, especially chronic conditions which require frequent monitoring and ongoing patient support" (IOM 2001, 15). The IOM called for a system in which knowledge is shared and information flows freely, where clinicians and patients communicate effectively and share information. The IOM emphasized the need for a commitment to the development of a national information infrastructure, with the expectation that such commitment could lead to the elimination of most handwritten clinical data by the end of the decade.

Despite the development of EHRs over three decades, research indicating improved quality of care, and the suggestions of the IOM, it was not until President George W. Bush noted in his 2004 State of the Union address "By computerizing health records, we can avoid dangerous medical mistakes, reduce costs, and improve care" that the issue of EHR came to the forefront for the American people and significant federal investment in health IT was initiated (Bush 2004). President Bush created the ONC in 2004. The ONC's function is that of principal advisor to the Secretary of the Department of Health and Human Services on the development, application, and the use of HIT.

Between 2005 and 2009, there was a gradual adoption of EHRs and the ONC developed and promulgated standards for health IT, but it was not until 2009 that the **American Recovery and Reinvestment Act (ARRA)** of 2009 provided a significant impetus to HIT through the allocation of over $20 billion in funds to promote HIT. ARRA was an economic stimulus bill created to help the United States recover from the downturn of the economy with a total amount of $787 billion allocated to the recovery (GPO 2009).

The **Health Information Technology for Economic and Clinical Health (HITECH) Act**, one part of ARRA, designated funding to modernize the healthcare system by promoting and expanding the adoption of HIT. HITECH provided $20 billion in Medicare and Medicaid incentive payments to physicians and hospitals for meaningful use of EHRs and $2.6 billion to support ONC initiatives (HealthIT 2013). **Meaningful use** "is using certified electronic health record (EHR) technology to: (1) improve quality, safety, efficiency, and reduce health disparities, (2) engage patients and family, (3) improve care coordination, and population and public health, and (4) maintain privacy and security of patient health information" (HealthIT 2015). Eventual outcomes of the meaningful use initiatives should be improved clinical outcomes and health of populations as a whole, improved efficiency and transparency in the provision of care, and considerably more data that can be used for research.

The HITECH funding and the ONC's coordinated nationwide effort to implement and standardize health IT resulted in a surge in health IT implementation with primary care providers signing up with Regional Extension Centers (RECs) to participate in Medicare and Medicaid EHR Incentive Programs. **Regional Extension Centers** provide support and serve as resources for healthcare providers for EHR implementation and use (HealthIT 2015). A 2015 REC report on outcomes reflected the following:

- ⊙ 157,000 providers enrolled with an REC with 146,000 live on an EHR (actual setting and patients in real time) and more than 116,000 demonstrating meaningful use

- ⊙ 46 percent of PCPs nationally enrolled and 54 percent of rural PCPs enrolled

- ⊙ 93 percent of REC-enrolled providers live on an EHR compared to 73 percent of general provider population live on an EHR (HealthIT 2015)

These data indicate that while a significant number of primary care practitioners are utilizing EHRs and, more importantly, using the data in a meaningful way, there are still many more who are not. One of the goals of the RECs is to support the deployment and use of EHRs, and the data indicate their efforts appear to be effective with REC enrollees, who have a 20 percent higher rate of implementing an EHR.

RECs were established by the ONC to assist primary care providers in quickly becoming adept and meaningful users of EHRs. RECs provide training and support services to assist doctors and other providers in adopting EHRs, share information and guidance to help with EHR implementation, and give technical assistance as needed. ONC reported that by the end of 2014 there was at least a basic EHR system in 76 percent of the hospitals and 97 percent had a certified EHR technology (ONC 2015). The ONC's 2014 report to Congress on adoption and exchange of health information indicated that the exchange of health information has increased in 60 percent of hospitals with 14 percent of physicians reporting (ONC 2014). Participating in HIE by both hospitals and physicians is hindered by technology, policy concerns, and the concern for maintaining privacy and security. Follow up reflects that when the exchange does occur, there is improvement in healthcare and lower costs in the provision of care (ONC 2014).

With mounting evidence supporting the premise that health IT can improve quality, safety, and cost effectiveness of care, it could be expected that the adoption rate would be high. While the adoption of EHRs started out slowly, there has been a significant increase in the number of nongovernmental hospitals that have adopted EHRs from 2008 to 2015. See table 3.1 for data illustrating this growth in the number of facilities implementing EHRs. As the table shows, almost all of the nongovernmental hospitals have an EHR (HealthIT 2015).

A summary completed by the Agency for Healthcare Research and Quality (AHRQ) in 2006 compiled published findings of 20 previous reports and studies. The summary findings indicated that cost was one of the most commonly identified barriers to implementing the EHR (HHS, AHRQ 2006). More recent studies include one reported in Health Affairs (Fleming et al. 2011) that identified the direct costs but also factored in the indirect costs of time. A 2012 report published by Health IT identified that the costs include those for the hardware, software, implementation assistance (tech support, legal input, consultant expertise plus other associated

Table 3.1. Percent of hospitals with an EHR

Hospital EHR adoption	Percent of hospitals with an EHR							
	2008	2009	2010	2011	2012	2013	2014	2015
All hospitals with a basic EHR*	9%	12%	16%	28%	44%	59%	76%	84%
All small hospitals with a basic EHR*	6%	8%	11%	22%	39%	53%	70%	81%
All rural hospitals with a basic EHR*	6%	8%	11%	22%	36%	53%	70%	80%
All critical access hospitals with a basic EHR*	4%	7%	10%	20%	35%	54%	68%	80%
All hospitals with a certified EHR	–	–	–	72%	85%	94%	97%	96%

*Basic EHR with clinician notes
2014 estimate was 96.9 and 2015 estimate was 96.0; the difference is not statistically significant
Source: HealthIT 2015

expenses), training and ongoing network and maintenance fees (HealthIT 2012). These two studies indicate that the cost factor continues to be a deterrent for some, primarily for physicians in small group practices. Much of the growth in adoption of EHRs can be attributed to the incentive program supporting the purchasing of systems to facilitate the meeting of meaningful use requirements for reporting and to the monetary penalties for not having an EHR.

Check Your Understanding 3.1

Match the term with the appropriate description.
  a. Clinical decision support
  b. E-prescribing
  c. Evidence-based medicine
  d. Regional Extension Centers
  e. Meaningful Use

1. _____ Using certified EHR information as a measure of quantity and quality of care

2. _____ Provides support to providers in the use of electronic health records

3. _____ Facilitates transmission of medication orders from a physician to a pharmacist

4. _____ Using information to make comparisons, trending results, and supplying clinical reminders and alerts to aid in diagnosing

5. _____ Relies on clinical expertise and the best research-based clinical evidence

Answer the following questions.

6. The primary goal of meaningful use is to:
   a. Have more physicians using computers
   b. Improve clinical outcomes
   c. Facilitate billing
   d. Gather data for statistical purposes

7. One of the first significant historical milestones in the development of systems is:
   a. Interoperability
   b. Clinical decision support
   c. CPOE
   d. Computer-based record

⊙ Components

The electronic health record is not just software or a single computer system but is composed of multiple integrated applications. An integrated system is one that has been designed to bring together multiple information systems, and allows them to communicate in a timely and effective manner and work together as one system. There may be variations among systems regarding which ancillary services are included. There may be differences in the ways the interfaces provide access to the ancillary systems, but all EHRs are designed to create an electronic record to bring together information from disparate systems that are in compliance with standards for the purpose of supporting quality of care, administrative functions, and research. Current 2015 Certification Electronic Health Information Technology (CEHRT) criteria provides assurances to those purchasing and using EHR systems that "a system meets the technological capability, functionality, and security requirements adopted by HHS" in addition to being secure and interoperable (HealthIT 2015). The CEHRT 2015 standards and specifications for implementation stipulates the minimum requirements related to the ability to support meaningful use for those required to do so (HealthIT 2015). A comprehensive EHR system is quite complex and supports more than the data needed for meaningful use purposes. The systems are also used for capturing diagnostic and treatment information such as medications, lab, x-ray, and other clinical information in addition to the administrative uses. Refer to figure 3.1, which depicts how all of the healthcare data is integrated from various systems for a record on a single patient.

The element that is identified as administrative in nature includes those data that accurately identify the patient, such as the name and other demographics, and the registration, admissions, discharge, and transfer information, including such things as chief complaint and patient disposition. A vital administrative consideration is the unique patient identifier, which is at the core of an EHR because it is the means by which all information from the various components is linked to the patient. For confidentiality and security purposes the patient identifier is unique to the organization and not known outside the organization.

Figure 3.1. Electronic health record—concept overview

The EHR represents the integration of healthcare data from a participating collection of Systems for a single patient.

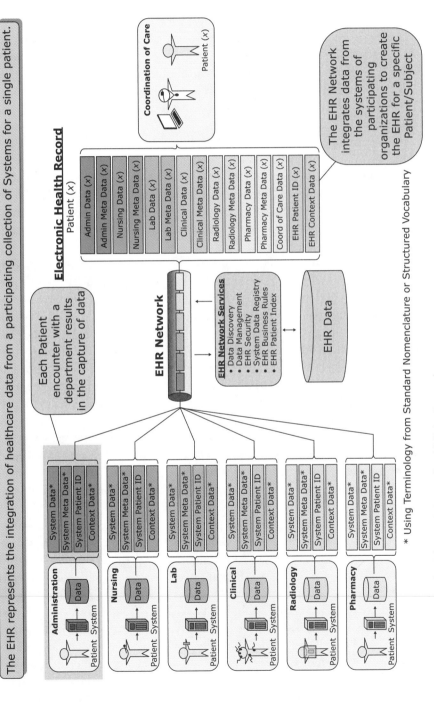

Source: Used with permission from The MITRE Corporation. All Rights Reserved.

In the majority of EHR systems, the laboratory systems remain as stand-alone systems that interface with the EHR and with numerous laboratory instruments that process the lab specimens. A **laboratory information system (LIS)** is a system for the integration of laboratory information related to the processing and storage of medical tests (physician orders for the tests and reports of results) that interfaces with the EHR to provide this information for inclusion in individual patient records. **Integration** involves ensuring that all aspects of an information system communicate appropriately and function as a uniform system (AHIMA 2014, 80). Other LIS functionality includes scheduling, billing, and other information specific to the needs of the lab but not made a part of the EHR nor available to those with EHR access privileges.

Radiology information systems (RIS) bring together patient radiology data with images. As seen with laboratory systems, RIS systems many times include patient tracking, scheduling, and reporting of results. Many systems are used with **picture archiving and communication systems (PACS)**. PACS provide storage of electronic images and reports. Although many hospitals have some sort of electronic system to support radiology, it does not mean that the system is necessarily integrated with the EHR.

Clinical documentation is "any manual or electronic notation (or recording) made by a physician, or other healthcare clinician, that is associated with a patient's medical condition and treatment" (AHIMA 2014, 27). Structured or discrete data that are entered using a controlled vocabulary rather than narrative is referred to as structured data entry (AHIMA 2014, 140). This would include patient assessments and clinical reports such as flow sheets and medication administration records. Conversely, clinical documentation entered into the patient record as text is narrative data and is not as easily automated due to the unstructured nature of the information. Examples of unstructured, narrative clinical information would include notes written by the physicians and other practitioners who treat the patient, dictated and transcribed reports, and legal forms such as consents and advanced directives. Information from medical devices may also be integrated into the information flow such as vital sign readings or intravenous pump dosages and flow rates that can be sent directly to the patient record from the device where the data originated.

Within the framework of the components of the EHR systems, a number of other factors must be considered in a discussion of the electronic health record. Many of these topics are related to regulations whereas others are identified as core functions and uses of the EHR that have been developed over time with the implementation and advancement of the systems. First HITECH funding for the EHR incentive program required eligible providers to implement an EHR that was certified for **meaningful use**. Three general types of payers established eligibility for providers. These are (1) Medicare Fee for Service, (2) Medicare Advantage (MA), and (3) Medicaid. Eligible hospitals include acute care, critical access, and children's hospitals. Eligible providers included non-hospital-based physicians with reimbursement from Medicare FFS or with a contractual affiliation with a qualifying MA program (CMS 20016). Meaningful use (MU) was defined earlier in the chapter and focuses on using information to improve the quality and efficiency of care and the safety of the patients and reduce health inequalities (HealthIT 2015). Key to success of this initiative is the EHR and certified software to be able to access, compile, and analyze data to provide the information needed to make the changes necessary to meet these goals. MU criteria and how to achieve the meaningful use of electronic health records was designed to be implemented in three stages. The meaningful use criteria for Stages 1, 2, and 3 are presented in table 3.2. When a provider meets this level of meaningful use of their EHR system, an improvement in outcomes should result. There has been an increase in EHR adoption since ARRA was enacted in 2009 and the majority of hospitals have attested to Stage 1 of meaningful use. Meeting Stage 2 has been more difficult with over 60 percent of hospitals and approximately 90 percent of physicians unable to attest to Stage 2 compliance (ONC 2016). The challenges stem from EHR implementation, lack of adequate interoperability, and issues outside the provider's control such as information exchange recipients who are not involved with the meaningful use initiatives. The time frame for attesting compliance for the different stages depends on when a provider initially starts and then achieves Stage 1 compliance. Table 3.3 shows when each stage must be met, determined by the year a provider first became compliant.

Table 3.2.   Meaningful use criteria and how to attain meaningful use of EHRs

Stage 1: Meaningful use criteria focus on:	Stage 2: Meaningful use criteria focus on:	Stage 3: Meaningful use criteria focus on:
Electronically capturing health information in a standardized format	More rigorous health information exchange (HIE)	Improving quality, safety, and efficiency, leading to improved health outcomes
Using that information to track key clinical conditions	Increased requirements for e-prescribing and incorporating lab results	Decision support for national high-priority conditions
Communicating that information for care coordination processes	Electronic transmission of patient care summaries across multiple settings	Patient access to self-management tools
Initiating the reporting of clinical quality measures and public health information	More patient-controlled data	Access to comprehensive patient data through patient-centered HIE
Using information to engage patients and their families in their care		Improving population health

Source: HealthIT 2015

Table 3.3.   Stage of meaningful use criteria by first year

First Year Demonstrating Meaningful Use	Stage of Meaningful Use				
	2015	2016	2017	2018	2019 and Future Years
2011	Modified Stage 2	Modified Stage 2	Modified Stage 2 or Stage 3	Stage 3	Stage 3
2012	Modified Stage 2	Modified Stage 2	Modified Stage 2 or Stage 3	Stage 3	Stage 3
2013	Modified Stage 2	Modified Stage 2	Modified Stage 2 or Stage 3	Stage 3	Stage 3
2014	Modified Stage 2	Modified Stage 2	Modified Stage 2 or Stage 3	Stage 3	Stage 3
2015	Modified Stage 2	Modified Stage 2	Modified Stage 2 or Stage 3	Stage 3	Stage 3
2016	NA	Modified Stage 2	Modified Stage 2 or Stage 3	Stage 3	Stage 3
2017	NA	NA	Modified Stage 2 or Stage 3	Stage 3	Stage 3
2018	NA	NA	NA	Stage 3	Stage 3
2019 and Future Years	NA	NA	NA	NA	Stage 3

Source: CMS 2016

To receive the MU incentive payments specific thresholds must be met to reflect that the eligible provider is meaningfully using their information. Figures 3.2 and 3.3 are indicative of the progress being made with meaningful use, predominantly with Stage I. Figure 3.2 illustrates the number of hospitals, listed by type of facility, that have achieved MU. Figure 3.2 also indicates those facilities that have received the adopt/implement/upgrade payment, the number registered for MU, or are not participating. For example, in the data reflected, about 71 percent of children's hospitals have attested to meaningful use, 7 percent have received the adopt/ implement/upgrade payment, and 6 percent are not participating. Figure 3.3 reflects the percentage of primary care providers by credentials who have enrolled in a REC and are live on an EHR and demonstrating that they are meaningfully using the patient information. From this illustration, it can be seen that chiropractors have the highest rate of REC enrollment and all of those enrolled are meaningfully using the information. All of the other categories have a high rate of REC enrollment and a significant number of these facilities have achieved meaningful use.

Figure 3.2. Hospital progress to meaningful use by size, practice setting, and geographic area

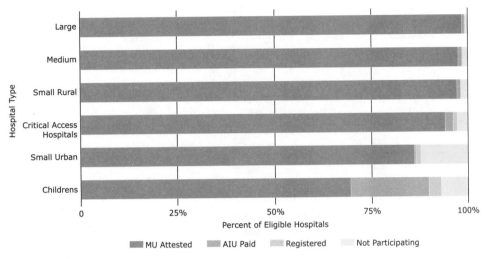

Source: ONC HIT 2016

Figure 3.3. Percent of REC-enrolled primary care providers by credentials live on an EHR and demonstrating meaningful use

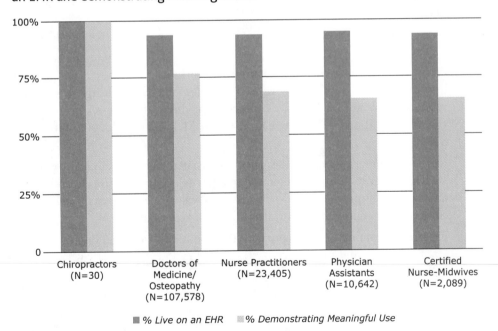

Source: ONC HIT 2016

Table 3.4.   Primary and secondary uses of an EHR system

Primary uses	Secondary uses
Patient care delivery	Education
Patient care management	Regulation
Patient care support processes	Research
Financial and other administrative processes	Public health policy and homeland security
Patient self-management	Policy support

Source: IOM 2003 (adapted from IOM 1997)

In 2003 a committee of the IOM identified potential primary and secondary uses of an EHR system as outlined in table 3.4. Primary uses are the direct recording of care on individual patients and the secondary uses involve aggregating patient data to improve the delivery of healthcare.

In addition to identifying the primary and secondary uses of information, the IOM outlined eight core functions that EHR systems should be capable of performing. These functions are designed to promote greater safety, quality, and efficiency in healthcare delivery. The eight functionalities with a brief description include:

1. Health information and data—information for care providers to make clinical decisions

2. Results management—management strategy using feedback for development to achieve goals

3. Order entry/management—"can improve workflow processes by eliminating lost orders and ambiguities caused by illegible handwriting, generating related orders automatically, monitoring for duplicate orders, and reducing the time to fill orders" (Lepage et al. 1992; Mekhjian et al. 2002; Sittig and Stead 1994)

4. Decision support—system designed to assist in making clinical decisions such as prescribing drugs, detection of adverse events and disease outbreaks, and computer prompts for such areas as vaccinations, breast cancer and colorectal screening, and cardiovascular risk reduction

5. Electronic communication/connectivity—communication among healthcare team members and other care partners (for example, laboratory, radiology, pharmacy) and with patients

6. Patient support—patient access to their health record and educational materials to engage the patient more in their healthcare and to participate in the clinical control of chronic illnesses

7. Administrative processes and reporting—to increase the efficiency of healthcare organizations and provide better, timelier service to patients with electronic scheduling billing, and inventory

8. Reporting and population health management—reduce the significant data collection burden at the provider level with the associated costs and increase the accuracy of the data reported with a standardized terminology and in a machine-readable format (IOM 2003)

Ambulatory and inpatient EHRs have evolved differently over time and the specific components or functions also vary between ambulatory and inpatient EHRs. Ambulatory care is provided in a variety of locations by individual or groups of healthcare providers. Settings for ambulatory care may include physician offices, outpatient clinics, ambulatory surgery centers, urgent care clinics, retail clinics, and stand-alone laboratory and imaging facilities. In the ambulatory setting the patient generally moves themselves from setting to setting when receiving services from multiple providers. Inpatient care is generally provided in the hospital setting with many levels of providers and services concentrated within one setting. See table 3.5 for an example of the different clinical functions that might be present in an EHR.

Table 3.5.   Examples of clinical functions in an EHR

Health information and data
  Patient demographic information
  Patient problem list
  Patient medication lists
  Clinical notes
  Minimum data set
  Notes including medical history and
  follow-up notes
	Electronic communications and
	connectivity
	  Electronic health information
	  exchange (eHIE)
	  Access to shared patient histories
	  Continuity of Care Document (CCD)

Results management
  Viewing lab results
  Viewing imaging results
  Electronic images are returned
	Patient support
	  Patient portal to EHR
	  E-mail communication with
	  clinicians

Order entry management
  Computerized orders for prescription
  Computerized orders for labs
  Computerized orders for radiology
  Orders sent electronically for prescriptions
  Orders sent electronically for labs
  Orders sent electronically for radiology
	Administrative processes
	  Scheduling/appointments
	  Billing
	  Inventory

Decision support
  Warnings of drug interactions or
  contraindications are returned
  Out of range lab levels are highlighted
  Reminders for guideline-based interventions
  and screenings
  Access to online clinical guidelines
	Reporting and population health
	management
	  Disease reports
	  Disease registries
	  Quality measured and improvement
	  reports
	  Patient safety
	  Immunization information exchange

Source: IOM 2003

Check Your Understanding 3.2

Match the term with the appropriate description.

   a. Clinical documentation
   b. Integrated applications
   c. Laboratory information systems (LIS)
   d. Picture archiving and communication system (PACS)
   e. Radiology information system (RIS)

1. _____ That which brings together multiple systems

2. _____ Related to processing and storage of medical tests

3. _____ Having to do with scheduling, tracking, and results reporting of radiology images and data

4. _____ Storage means for reports and electronic images

5. _____ Notation or recording made by clinician, can be paper or electronic

Answer the following questions.

6. The ultimate goal of meaningful use is to:
   a. Engage patients
   b. Improve health outcomes and health of populations
   c. Provide data for aggregate data analysis
   d. Provide monetary support to physicians for obtaining EHR systems

7. Which of the following is a primary use of an EHR system?
   a. Patient care delivery
   b. Research
   c. Patient self-management
   d. Financial processes

⊙ Inpatient EHR

As described earlier in this chapter, inpatient EHRs have evolved over time, beginning with business- and financial-based hospital information systems, followed by clinical information systems, and evolving to EHRs. Inpatient EHRs are generally comprised of integrated, interoperable multiple applications. In contrast, most ambulatory EHRs have been developed as complete systems that include practice management and clinical applications. An inpatient EHR's components may include financial and administrative applications, clinical systems, CPOE, **electronic medication administration records (EMARs)** (use of technology and bar coding to track medications from when ordered to when given to the patient), clinical data repositories, clinical decision support, document imaging, and PACS.

Inpatient EHRs certified for meaningful use purposes may be classified as complete or modular. Complete systems are those that meet all of the MU criteria tested for CEHRT certification. Certified modular systems meet one or more of the MU criteria so would require multiple modular systems working together

Figure 3.4.   Source systems feeding data into the inpatient EHR

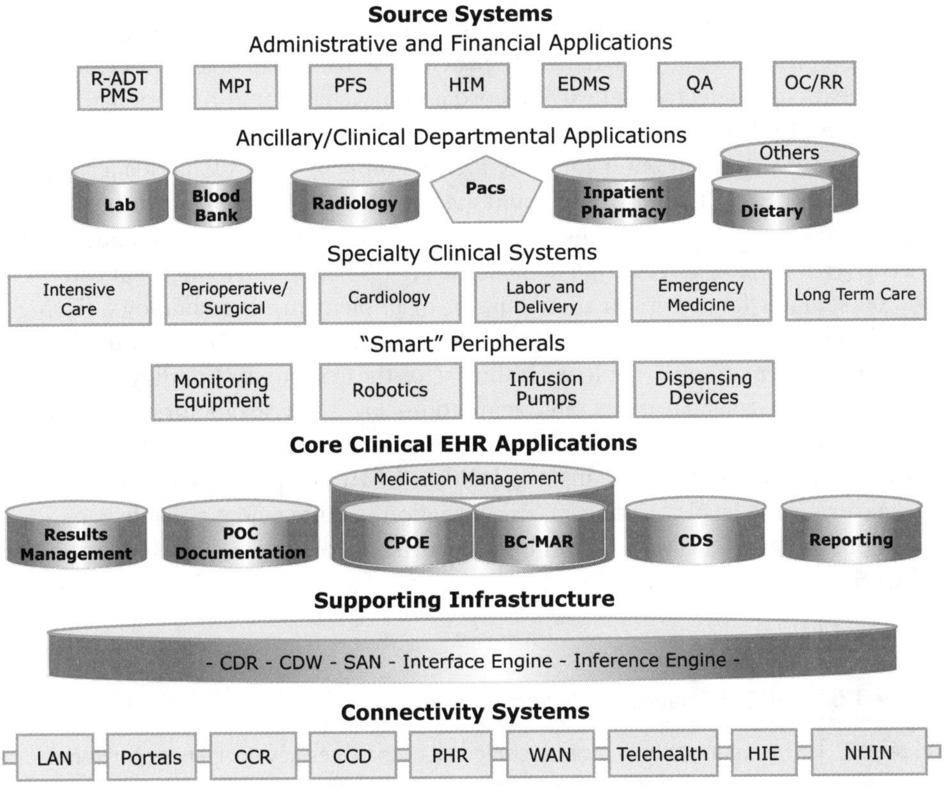

Source: Copyright © 2012, Margret\A Consulting, LLC. Reprinted with permission.

to attest compliance with Stage 1. Modular systems are used by 33 percent of hospitals but only by 6 percent of eligible practitioners (ONC 2014). Figure 3.4 illustrates all of the source systems potentially feeding into the EHR. There are administrative and financial systems in the EHR system that include R-ADT for registration/admission discharge, transfer; MPI, the master patient index; and PFS practitioner/physician fee schedule. The ancillary/clinical and specialty clinical applications provide data when they are utilized for an individual patient. For example, if a patient had an x-ray, the radiology system would transmit the report to become a part of the EHR. For patients who were in ICU, that system would provide reports specific to the time there. The "smart" peripherals are the devices that can submit reports directly from the device to the EHR, such as an EKG equipment monitoring a patient's heart function transmits reports that become a part of the record. With all of this patient information in the patient record it will then be used to carry out the core clinical applications to treat and document the care given to the patient. Examples of this are the point-of-care recommendations (POC), computerized physician order entry (CPOE) for medications, diagnostic tests and other things that must be ordered for the patient, and clinical decision support (CDS) information for provider to use for reference. The other parts of the system are those required for making the system function.

The **Health Information and Management Systems Society (HIMSS)** EHR Adoption Model (EMRAM[SM]) provides a framework for describing the components of an electronic health record and measuring and reporting the stage of adoption by healthcare organizations (see table 3.6). HIMSS is a cause-based not-for-profit organization exclusively focused on providing global leadership for the optimal use of IT and management systems for the betterment of healthcare. The HIMSS mission is to lead healthcare transformation through the effective use of HIT (HIMSS 2016). Table 3.6 depicts the HIMSS adoption model that can serve as a benchmark for others in their pursuit of implementing technology (HIMSS 2016). Electronic health record systems have increased in numbers and the level of use of the information available with the use of these systems. Funding initiatives, reimbursement considerations, and regulations are the reasons for the increased deployment of EHRs. The extent to which systems have adopted the potential system components varies. Using the HIMSS EMR Adoption Model as the basis of measuring the level of adoption, this variation is quite evident. Table 3.7 shows the adoption level of EMRs through 2015 based on the seven stages identified by HIMSS.

Table 3.6.   HIMSS Analytics Adoption Model

Stage 0	The organization has not installed all of the three key ancillary department systems (laboratory, pharmacy, and radiology).
Stage 1	All three major key ancillary clinical systems are installed.
Stage 2	Major ancillary clinical systems feed data to a clinical data repository (CDR) that provides physician access for reviewing all orders and results. The CDR contains a controlled medical vocabulary, and the clinical decision support/ rules engine (CDS) for rudimentary conflict checking. Information from document imaging systems may be linked to the CDR at this stage. The hospital may be health information exchange (HIE) capable at this stage and can share whatever information it has in the CDR with other patient care stakeholders.
Stage 3	Nursing/clinical documentation (for example, vital signs, flow sheets, nursing notes, eMAR) is required and is implemented and integrated with the CDR for at least one inpatient service in the hospital; care plan charting is scored with extra points. The Electronic Medication Administration Record application (eMAR) is implemented. The first level of clinical decision support is implemented to conduct error checking with order entry (that is, drug–drug, drug–food, drug–lab conflict checking normally found in the pharmacy information system). Medical image access from picture archive and communication systems (PACS) is available for access by physicians outside the Radiology department via the organization's intranet.

Stage 4	Computerized Practitioner Order Entry (CPOE) for use by any clinician licensed to create orders is added to the nursing and CDR environment along with the second level of clinical decision support capabilities related to evidence-based medicine protocols. If one inpatient service area has implemented CPOE with physicians entering orders and completed the previous stages, then this stage has been achieved.
Stage 5	A full complement of radiology PACS systems provides medical images to physicians via an intranet and displaces all film-based images. Cardiology PACS and document imaging are scored with extra points.
Stage 6	Full physician documentation with structured templates and discrete data is implemented for at least one inpatient care service area for progress notes, consult notes, discharge summaries or problem list & diagnosis list maintenance. Level three of clinical decision support provides guidance for all clinician activities related to protocols and outcomes in the form of variance and compliance alerts. The closed loop medication administration with bar coded unit dose medications environment is fully implemented. The eMAR and bar coding or other auto identification technology, such as radio frequency identification (RFID), are implemented and integrated with CPOE and pharmacy to maximize point of care patient safety processes for medication administration. The "five rights" of medication administration are verified at the bedside with scanning of the bar code on the unit does medication and the patient ID.
Stage 7	The hospital no longer uses paper charts to deliver and manage patient care and has a mixture of discrete data, document images, and medical images within its EMR environment. Data warehousing is being used to analyze patterns of clinical data to improve quality of care, patient safety, and care delivery efficiency. Clinical information can be readily shared via standardized electronic transactions (i.e., CCD) with all entities that are authorized to treat the patient, or a health information exchange (i.e., other non-associated hospitals, ambulatory clinics, sub-acute environments, employers, payers and patients in a data sharing environment). The hospital demonstrates summary data continuity for all hospital services (e.g., inpatient, outpatient, ED, and with any owned or managed ambulatory clinics). Blood products and human milk are included in the closed-loop medication administration process.

Source: Adapted from HIMSS 2016. Used with permission from HIMSS.

Table 3.7.   Adoption level of EMRs through 2016

Stage	Cumulative capabilities
Stage 7	Complete EMR; CCD, Data analytics to improve care
Stage 6	Physician documentation (templates), full CDSS. Closed loop medication administration

(Continued)

Table 3.7.   Adoption level of EMRs through 2016 (*Continued*)

Stage	Cumulative capabilities
Stage 5	Full R-PACS
Stage 4	CPOE, clinical decision support (clinical protocols)
Stage 3	Clinical documentation, CDSS (error checking)
Stage 2	CDR, controlled medical vocabulary, CDS, may have document imaging; HIE capable
Stage 1	Ancillaries—Lab, Radiology, Pharmacy—All installed
Stage 0	All three ancillaries not installed

Source: Data from HIMSS Analytics® Database ©2015. Used with permission from HIMSS.

Case Study: Stage 7 Organization Brief Outline

The clinical staff of a network of 50 primary clinics, dental clinics, pharmacies, wellness centers, and HIV care/case management were trained in a short time frame for Stage 7 to be successfully implemented. This implementation failed. It was learned that the governance needed to be revamped to include a standardized workflow across the enterprise, communication was needed that embraced change, training methodology needed to be reexamined, the entire staff needed to be retrained, and people needed to be removed from their personal comfort zones so each could bring a different perspective.

The results of the implementation showed that the level of confidence in staff increased across the organization and staff became less fearful of change. Satisfaction increased with staff and patients and their ability to leverage educational resources. As a result, the staff achieved Stage 6 five months following implementing the new system and one year later achieved Stage 7.

From this implementation, the study demonstrated that many may not be comfortable communicating their lack of understanding of new technology and the need for training. Also, not everyone is suited to teach and explain complex technologies and processes.

The participants in this case study were clinicians whose primary focus is on the treatment of their patients. Policies and procedures with tools were always readily available and familiar to meet their data needs from development to acquisition to using the data. Important initial aspects of training included developing an understanding of workflow, process, and technology. It also became important to see the technology as a tool used in the process but keeping the focus on the information, not the technology. Stage 7 requirements introduce new requirements for utilizing an EHR in addition to increased use and analysis and use of the data required. It was important for the physicians to be engaged in the process of training and be familiar with it so they would be more likely to accept ownership and be proponents for meeting this level.

⊙ Ambulatory EHR

EHRs in the ambulatory setting are similar to those seen in the inpatient environment. Major differences between these two kinds of EHRs are that the ambulatory record is longitudinal rather than episodic, has fewer practitioners documenting in the record, may not have in-house diagnostics (lab, x-ray, and such) so requires a link to this information, and has more referrals made to outside practitioners than seen in the hospital. Ambulatory EHRs include:

- ⊙ Problem lists
- ⊙ Medication lists
- ⊙ History and physical examinations
- ⊙ Immunization records
- ⊙ Patient progress and visit notes
- ⊙ Clinical templates
- ⊙ Electronic prescribing
- ⊙ Medication management
- ⊙ Health maintenance
- ⊙ Disease management
- ⊙ Outcomes reporting
- ⊙ Clinical decision support
- ⊙ Lab order entry
- ⊙ Results reporting

Ambulatory EHRs may be characterized as complete or modular systems just as seen in the in-patient environment. By 2014, 83 percent of physicians had an EHR in their practice, 74 percent were using certified EHR systems, and 51 percent were using all of the basic EHR functionalities (ONC 2015). Health IT reports that as of the end of 2015, meaningful use has been exhibited by 56 percent of office-based physicians participating in the CMS EHR incentive pay program with 16 percent of nurse practitioners and less than 2 percent of physician assistants doing so and an over percentage of 48 percent for physicians, nurse practitioners, and physician assistants (ONC 2016). In 2016 the EHR Incentive Program for physician and individual providers was discontinued as a separate program. The use of EHRs will be combined with quality measures and other items in payment and penalty consideration.

The rates of adoption of ambulatory EHRs through the end of 2015 based on the HIMSS adoption model are shown in table 3.8. This reflects that more than 50 percent of the eligible ambulatory practitioners are at Stage 2 or below (HIMSS 2016). Table 3.8 shows the adoption level of ambulatory EHRs through quarter four of 2015.

Table 3.8.   Adoption level of ambulatory EHRs through Q4 2015

Stage	2015 Q4
7	7.89%
6	12.21%
5	6.81%
4	1.32%
3	11.19%
2	22.17%
1	35.6%
0	2.77%

Source: Data from HIMSS Analytics® Database ©2016. Used with permission from HIMSS.

⊙ Long-Term Care EHR

EHR systems in long-term care (LTC) facilities provide the same benefits as do those for acute care and will allow these facilities to participate in the exchange of data. Most LTC facilities have submitted the federally required Minimum Data Set (MDS) electronically for some time (AHIMA 2014). Other electronic functionality is limited in this environment primarily due to lack of financial and technical support. Future changes for LTC would most likely be processing changes rather than functionality changes. Specifically, processing changes in chart processing (assembly, auditing), moving and thinning of records and release of information (electronic exchange and documentation of disclosures), and reports/screen design could optimize processing time and output and provide more storage space and greater access to information. Practical LTC activities that would be enhanced with an EHR include care coordination with access to information that is already available, facilitating communication with all of the providers associated with the patient and for quality improvement to protect this high-risk group with prevention of additional conditions and earlier interventions when they do occur. Forces that are behind the desire for the EHR in LTC include quality of care, consumerism, and provision of care in a more efficient and effective way.

⊙ Behavioral Healthcare EHR

Behavioral healthcare can be provided in the ambulatory or inpatient settings. **Behavioral healthcare** is a "broad array of psychiatric services provided in acute, long-term, and ambulatory care settings; includes treatment of mental disorders, chemical dependency, mental retardation, and developmental disabilities, as well as cognitive rehabilitation services" (AHIMA 2014, 16).

⊙ Enterprise EHR

Health records, whether in paper or electronic format, provide documentation of an episode of care. The EHR provides a health record with information from a variety of healthcare organizations where the patient has been seen. EHRs provide the means for the focus to be more on the patient's health over time rather than the condition present at a specific time. They also provide the ease of access to a broader group of practitioners treating the patient as well as access to the patient, which affords the opportunity for them to be more engaged in their own healthcare. **Enterprise integration** under HITECH means the electronic linkage of healthcare providers, health plans, the government, and other interested parties, to enable the electronic exchange and use of health information among all the components in the healthcare infrastructure in accordance with applicable law (AHIMA 2014, 55). This integration is what provides the means by which the information can be shared. The information exchange requires interoperability systems and policies defined for supporting the exchange while protecting the privacy and security of the information. Utilizing information across the enterprise allows for better and faster access to information, which in turn improves care and cost efficiency.

Chapter 3 Review Exercises

Answer the following questions.

1. A key factor that allowed EHR systems to evolve to the current state:
   a. Interoperability
   b. HIPAA
   c. More systems to choose from
   d. Willingness of physicians to participate

2. A significant amount of investment of funds to support stand-alone deployment and utilization of EHRs was provided by:
   a. HIPAA
   b. ONC
   c. HITECH
   d. Meaningful Use

3. The process where individual data elements are represented by special code so they can be used for comparisons, trends, reminders, and results is:
   a. Clinical information systems
   b. Clinical decision support
   c. EHR
   d. CPOE

4. A disadvantage of unstructured data?
   a. Easily compiled into reports
   b. Typically more descriptive
   c. Constitutes only a small part of the patient record
   d. The large amount of this type of data that is available

5. The purpose of meaningful use is:
   a. Improves healthcare quality, safety, and efficiency
   b. Provides documentation standards
   c. Aids in coding and billing.
   d. Supports the exchange of data across healthcare entities

6. A comprehensive EHR system is important to:
   a. Assure the meaningful use of information
   b. Meet administrative needs
   c. Exchange healthcare data
   d. Provide appropriate information to enhance patient care

7. Which of the following are challenges in hospitals' ability to attest to Stage 2 meaningful use?
   a. Cost, lack of interoperability, and physician resistance to use the technology
   b. Lack of systems for hospitals and physician offices to be able to implement
   c. Inability to generate appropriate data
   d. Unwillingness of patients to participate

8. The program that currently certifies EHR systems that meet meaningful use:
   a. CCHIT
   b. CEHRT
   c. ONC
   d. Multiple organizations are approved to do this.

Discussion.

9. What are some of the advantages of having the EHR?

10. Why are unstructured data more difficult to work with in the deployment of EHRs?

REFERENCES

AHIMA. 2014. *Pocket Glossary for Health Information Management and Technology*, 4th ed. Chicago: AHIMA Press.

Amatayakul, M.K. 2013. Electronic Health Records: Conceptual Framework. Chapter 5 in *Health Information Management: Concepts Principles and Practice*. 4th ed. Edited by LaTour, K.M., S. Eichenwald Maki, and P. Oachs. Chicago: AHIMA.

Bush, G. 2004. The 2004 State of the Union Address: Complete transcript of President Bush's speech to Congress and the nation. http://whitehouse.georgewbush.org /news/2004/012004-SOTU.asp.

Centers for Medicare and Medicaid Services (CMS). 2016. Electronic Health Records Incentive Programs. https://www.cms.gov/Regulations-and-Guidance/Legislation /EHRIncentivePrograms/index.html?redirect=/ehrincentiveprograms.

Department of Health and Human Services, Agency for Healthcare Research and Quality (AHRQ). 2006. Barriers to HIT Implementation. https://healthit.ahrq.gov /health-it-tools-and-resources/health-it-costs-and-benefits-database/barriers-hit -implementation.

Fleming, N.S., S.D. Culler, R. McCorkle, E.R. Becker, and D.J. Ballard. 2011. The financial and nonfinancial costs of implementing electronic health records in primary care practices. *Health Affairs* 30(3):481–489. http://content.healthaffairs.org/content /30/3/481.full.

GPO. American Recovery and Reinvestment Act of 2009. H.R. 1 Bill. https://www.gpo .gov/fdsys/pkg/BILLS-111hr1enr/pdf/BILLS-111hr1enr.pdf.

Health Story Project. 2012. https://healthstoriesproject.com/.

HealthIT. 2015. Meaningful use definitions and objectives. https://www.healthit.gov /providers-professionals/meaningful-use-definition-objectives.

HealthIT. 2013. EHR incentives and certification. https://www.healthit.gov/providers -professionals/ehr-incentive-programs.

HealthIT. 2012. How Much Is This Going to Cost Me? https://www.healthit.gov /providers-professionals/faqs/how-much-going-cost-me.

Hersh, B. 2015. The Conundrum of Structured vs. Unstructured Data. http:// informaticsprofessor.blogspot.com/2015/02/the-conundrum-of-structured-vs.html.

HIMSS. 2016. U.S. EMR Adoption Model Trends. https://app.himssanalytics.org /stagesGraph.asp.

HIMSS. 2005. Interoperability definition and background. http://www.himss.org/himss -interoperability-definition-and-background.

HIMSS Analytics. 2015. ARcare Stage 7 Case Study. https://www.himssanalytics.org /case-study/arcare-stage-7-case-study.

Institute of Medicine (IOM), Committee on Data Standards for Patient Safety. 2003. Key Capabilities of an Electronic Health Record System. Washington, DC: National Academy Press.

Institute of Medicine (IOM), Committee on Improving the Patient Record. 1997. *The Computer-Based Patient Record: An Essential Technology for Health Care.* rev. ed. Washington, DC: National Academy Press.

Institute of Medicine (IOM), Committee on Quality of Health Care in America. 2001. *Crossing the Quality Chasm: A New Health System for the 21st Century.* Washington, DC: National Academy Press.

Lepage, E.F., R.M. Gardner, R.M. Laub, and O.K. Golubjatnikov. 1992. Improving blood transfusion practice: role of a computerized hospital information system. *Transfusion (Paris)* 32(3):253–259.

Lippeveld, T., R. Sauerborn, and C. Bodart. 2012. Section 3, Module 7. Health Information Systems from *Health Systems Approach: A How-to Manual.* Arlington: Management Sciences for Health.

McCullough, J. 2008. Adoption of hospital information systems. *Health Economics* 17: 649–664.

Mekhjian, H.S., R.R. Kumar, L. Kuehn, T.D. Bentley, P. Teater, A. Thomas, B. Payne, and A. Ahmad. 2002. Immediate Benefits Realized Following Implementation of Physician Order Entry at an Academic Medical Center. *Journal of the American Medical Informatics Association* 9(5):529–539.

National Academies. 2016. About the IOM. http://www.nationalacademies.org/hmd/.

Office of the National Coordinator for Health Information Technology (ONC). 2016. Hospital progress to meaningful use by size, type, and urban/rural location. Health IT Quick-Stat #5. dashboard.healthit.gov/quickstats/pages/FIG-Hospital-Progress-to-Meaningful-Use-by-size-practice-setting-area-type.php.

ONC. 2015. Data Brief No. 28. Any, Certified, and Basic: Quantifying Physician EHR Adoption.

ONC. 2014 Report to Congress. Update on the adoption of health information solution technology and related efforts to facilitate the electronic use and exchange of health information.

Regenstrief Institute. 2012, 2014, and 2016. http://www.regenstrief.org.

Sittig, D.F., and W.W. Stead. 1994. Computer-based physician order entry: The state of the art. *Journal of American Medical Informatics Association* 1(2):108–123.

Smithwick, J. 2015. *Unlocking the Value of Unstructured Patient Data.* Becker's Health IT and CIO Review. http://www.beckershospitalreview.com/healthcare-information-technology/unlocking-the-value-of-unstructured-patient-data.html.

Tripathi, M. 2012. EHR evolution: Policy and legislation forces changing the EHR. *Journal of AHIMA* 83(10):24–29.

US Department of Veterans Affairs. 2015. E-Health. http://www.ehealth.va.gov/vista.asp.

ADDITIONAL RESOURCES

AHIMA. 2014 Update. AHIMA Longitudinal Coordination of Care Practice Council E-HIM Strategy Team. *Electronic Health Record Adoption in Long Term Care.* AHIMA Practice Brief.

American Recovery and Reinvestment Act of 2009. Public Law 111–115.

CDC. 2012. National perceptions of EHR adoption: Barriers, impacts, and federal policies. http://www.cdc.gov/nchs/ppt/nchs2012/SS-03_JAMOOM.pdf.

Charles, D., Gabriel, M., and Searcy T. 2015, April. Adoption of Electronic Health Record Systems among U.S. Non-Federal Acute Care Hospitals: 2008–2014. ONC Data Brief, no. 23. Office of the National Coordinator for Health Information Technology: Washington, DC.

Department of Health and Human Services. 2012. Press Release: More doctors adopting EHRs to improve patient care and safety. https://content.govdelivery.com/accounts/USHHS/bulletins/61c93a.

Dick, R.S., and E.B. Steen. 1991. *The Computer-Based Patient Record: An Essential Technology for Healthcare.* Washington, DC: National Academy Press.

HIMSS. 2004. Top Line: President Bush calls for EHRs for most Americans in 10 years; Creates new NHII coordinator. *Health IT News.* http://www.healthcareitnews.com /news/president-bush-continues-ehr-push-sets-national-goals.

Jha, A., C. DesRoches, E. Campbell, K. Donelan, S. Rao, T. Ferris, A. Shields, S. Rosenbaum, and D. Blumenthal. 2009. Use of electronic health records in U.S. hospitals. *The New England Journal of Medicine* 360:1628–1638.

Sackett, D. 1996. Evidence based medicine: What it is and what it isn't. *British Medical Journal* 312:71–72. https://www.ncbi.nlm.nih.gov/pubmed/8555924.

Chapter 4

Information Infrastructure

Learning Objectives

- Articulate the goals of a distributed system
- Construct examples of different types of distributed systems
- List the differences between two- and three-tiered network architectures
- Relate the purpose of middleware
- Apply the concepts of collaborative computing
- Compare design models of distributed systems
- Articulate the development process of a distributed system
- Apply the basic principles of cloud computing
- Describe the five basic characteristics of a cloud computing system
- Relate examples of the three major cloud computing service models

KEY TERMS

Architectural models
Audit log
Broad network access
Centralized
Client-server
Clinical data repository (CDR)
Cloud computing
Community cloud
Concurrent processes
Cost of ownership

Database management system (DBMS)
Decentralized
Dependability
Distributed system
Electronic document management system (EDMS)
Ergonomics
Extended or Enhanced Entity Relationship (EER)
Fault tolerant

103

File server	Private cloud
Firewall	Random access memory (RAM)
Future-proofing	Rapid elasticity
Hard disk	Read only memory (ROM)
Hybrid cloud	Resource pooling
Hypertext markup language (HTML)	Resource sharing
Information infrastructure	Scalability
Infrastructure as a service (IaaS)	Security
Local area network (LAN)	Software
Measured service	Software as a service (SaaS)
Middleware	Terminal emulation software
Mobile computing	Terminal-to-host
Mobility	Three-tiered architecture
On-demand self-service	Topology
Open System Interconnection	Transparency
Model (OSI)	Two-tiered model
Openness	Unified Modeling Language (UML)
Physical models	Virtual private network (VPN)
Platform as a service (PaaS)	Wide area network (WAN)
Public cloud	Wireless network

Healthcare information professionals are increasingly finding a need for **information infrastructure**, specifically processing, tools, and technologies to support the creation, use, transport, and storage of information (Pironti 2006). This infrastructure will allow them to work faster, more efficiently, and more economically when managing healthcare data and information. There is also an increasing need to share expensive resources and to collaborate with others via networked systems and the applications that run in these environments. This can be accomplished by the use of collaborative computing. In the best of all possible scenarios, this would occur seamlessly without the user having to know any of the details, such as the location or types of the machines or applications functioning in the networked health information (HI) system environment, which is the idea behind **cloud computing**. Cloud computing "is the dynamic delivery of information technology resources and capabilities as a service over the Internet" (Sarna 2010, 2). Effectively using technology infrastructure involves selecting the correct hardware, software, computer language, and database system for the job. After selecting the hardware, the network, physical, and storage architectures are constructed, databases are designed and loaded with data, interfaces are built, and system testing commences.

    This chapter introduces the topic of the hardware, software, and networks used in distributed systems and their development relative to the healthcare informatics industry. The uses of technology are explored with particular reference to the role of these systems in facilitating collaborative computer communication as well as their design and development. Cloud and mobile computing are examined. The advantages and disadvantages of these systems are highlighted. Next, assessing systems for regulatory compliance, recommending device selection, and developing and evaluating systems is explored. Finally, evaluating information systems with systems testing and interface management as it relates to these networked distributed systems is addressed.

⊙ Using Technology

Increasingly health information data are stored in archival systems like clinical data repositories or electronic document management systems (EDMS). Informaticists wishing to interact with these systems must first understand the basic concepts of computer hardware, software, and networks, then master the distributed architectural models. A **clinical data repository (CDR)** stores structured and unstructured clinical data in a database (Amatayakul 2013, 18). Structured data are generated when the user selects data from a predefined selection of data on a webpage dropdown, radio button, or check box. Data typed into a textbox on a webpage are unstructured because they are not input according to a predefined selection list. Unstructured data, like scanned documents, are harder to index for database searches and cannot be separated into individual components like the structured data. CDRs can store data in the form of digitized x-ray images, audio recordings, and video. As documentation requirements and regulations increase in number and complexity, so does the need for generating, storing, and retrieving the clinical data for regulatory and diagnostic usage. **Electronic document management systems (EDMSs)** are utilized to manage the plethora of electronically stored images and documents (Reynolds and Sharp 2016, 136). These useful systems provide workflow management, digital signature authentication, and laser disk output.

Computer Concepts

Information infrastructure references the hardware, software, and networks that comprise a computer system. System software includes the machines' operating system and any application software installed on the system, such as a database management system. In networked systems, one or more machines are connected by physical or wireless networks to form distributed networked systems that can exchange data. For example, a distributed cloud computing system allows seamless connectivity to a remote archival storage area that may contain data or applications for the users.

Hardware

Computer hardware is the physical part of the computer system that includes the monitor, keyboard, mouse, printer, and scanner (Sayles and Trawick 2014, 5). Inside the computer, central processing unit (CPU) hardware mimics the human brain as it directs the electrical circuits in the computer to perform math, make logical comparisons, and store calculation results in long-term random access memory (RAM) (Sayles and Trawick 2010, 5).

Computers differ in terms of size and computing power. Smaller less powerful computers used by individuals for activities such as e-mailing or searching the Internet are called personal computers (PCs), while larger more powerful mainframe computers with special hardware and software that allow multiple individuals to connect at one time in order to use the machines' hardware or software are referred to as servers. Servers dedicated for special usage are referenced by their intended usage. A network server handles network requests, database and application servers handle requests for database information and application access, respectively. The current trend is toward smaller portable systems like notebooks, tablets, smart phones, or personal device assistants (PDAs) that can be used at the bedside (Amatayakul 2013, 292).

Hardware input peripherals commonly found attached to the outside of a PC include the mouse, keyboard, touch screen, microphone, bar code reader, and web camera. Output peripherals such as printers, speakers, digital cameras, and network cards provide the user with the ability to print documents, take pictures, connect to other computers, and listen to music.

Computer systems have several types of memory. When a software application is in use or when the computer starts up, temporary memory called **random access memory (RAM)** is utilized to perform the needed tasks. Information stored in RAM memory is not saved when the application is closed or the computer is turned off. In contrast, **read only memory (ROM)** is programmed into a computer chip. It is permanent memory that can be read from but not changed by any applications' or users' actions. If a computer application is running slowly, the CPU may elect to use its own temporary cache memory to supplement the RAM memory used by the application. The permanent memory of a computer that stores application software, files created by the user, and the operating system is called the **hard disk** (Amatayakul 2013, 297).

Software

Software is a program that directs the hardware in the computer (AHIMA 2014, 137). Software inside the computer primarily falls into two categories: operating systems and application software. The type of operating system platform installed on a computer determines applications the computer can run and the functions it can perform (Amatayakul 2013). Examples of operating systems include Microsoft Windows, Linux, and Apple Mac OS X. When a MS Word file is opened, the operating system directs the computer to read data from a Microsoft Word file, display the data on the screen, send the data to the printer, and store the file on a USB key.

Conversely, application software performs specific tasks that include word processing (for example, Microsoft Word), graphics display, statistics, spreadsheet calculations (for example, Microsoft Excel), and database processing. Application software programming languages provide the set of instructions for performing the application software tasks. **Hypertext markup language (HTML)** is "a standardized computer language that allows the electronic transfer of information and communications among many different information systems" (AHIMA 2014, 75).

Architectural Models

Distributed information systems are difficult to develop due to their complex and decentralized nature (Kart et al. 2007), basic safety (and security) requirements (Lamport 2001), as well as the need to achieve consistently high performance across a wide range of deployment settings (Mao et al. 2008). Healthcare, along with many other industries, faces these challenges, so a broad array of information modeling methods has been developed. These methods are often termed information **architectural models** as they provide a framework or structure for the flow of data and information within systems. This section will provide a brief review of different modeling approaches including Enterprise Knowledge Development (EKD), Service-Oriented Architecture (SOA), and Business Process Simulation (BPS). Each of these has its own methods, techniques, and tools, which are used to analyze, plan, design, and possibly change businesses (Stirna and Persson 2008, 85).

Before exploring the different approaches and frameworks, it is important to understand that there are "languages" associated with information modeling. The most common are the **Unified Modeling Language (UML)**, and **Extended Entity Relationship (EER)** (Halpin et al. 2008, 18). UML is a data-modeling notation for object-oriented database design (AHIMA 2014, 148). With the use of various tools utilizing UML an organization can "specify, visualize, and document models of software systems, including their structure and design" (Object Modeling Group Inc. 2005). The Extended Entity Relationship system is an enhanced entity relationship design tool that has additional symbols for object-oriented modeling. The EER has been the subject of much research and is now widely used in various forms (Alkoshman 2015). It uses graphical and textual languages to model and query information, as well as a procedural language for designing conceptual models.

Enterprise Knowledge Development (EKD)

Enterprise Knowledge Development is focused on managing technology, information, and knowledge across an organization (Zhao et al. 2012). EKD helps organizations to better utilize scarce resources, manage acquisition of knowledge, update existing knowledge stores, and develop EKD sources. Because knowledge is related to productivity, EKD facilitates are getting the most economical and efficient use out of knowledge resources across the enterprise, which makes the company more competitive (Zhao et al. 2012).

Service-Oriented Architecture (SOA)

Service-Oriented Architecture is a distributed computing system framework that is used to integrate existing software components (Kuan-Li and Chin-Yu 2014). It is defined as "a logical way of designing software in modular and flexible components, called services, that are often provided over the Internet or intranet" (Amatayakul 2013, 654). Specifically, interoperable web-based SOA architecture that meets web service standards is referred to as web services architecture (Amatayakul 2013, 300). SOA has a discovery system that searches the Internet for existing services that can be used by existing systems (Rodriguez et al. 2016).

By reusing services, SOA can help minimize software development costs and reduce the time to develop new services. In fact, legacy systems can continue to provide their services within the structure of an SOA architected system until the replacement system is fully implemented. SOA also helps organizations provide more robust systems because these systems can recover faster from system errors due to the built-in service software redundancies (Kuan-Li and Chin-Yu 2014). Another benefit is that SOA facilitates interoperability for disparate software systems by providing standardized interfaces and adaptable deployment of a system's services (Kuan-Li and Chin-Yu 2014).

Business Process Simulation (BPS)

The final information systems development process to be explored is BPS. BPS is defined as

> designing a model of a real system and conducting experiments with this model for the purpose either of understanding the behavior of the system or of evaluating various strategies (within the limits imposed by a criterion or set of criteria) for the operation of the system (Elliman et al. 2008, 242).

BPS can help information system developers understand current system operations, identify bottlenecks, evaluate various alternatives, and assess quantitative results on all of the above (Elliman et al. 2008, 251). BPS requires the active involvement of technical experts as well as business users to ensure the simulations created are accurate.

Check Your Understanding 4.1

Answer the following questions.

1. What is the term for the physical part of a computer system that includes the monitor, keyboard, and mouse?
   a. Hardware
   b. Software
   c. Operating System
   d. Computer language

2. What is temporary memory used by a laptop to perform application software tasks?
   a. ROM
   b. Hard disk
   c. RAM
   d. CPU

3. What is permanent memory that stores the applications installed by a user, such as Microsoft Word?
   a. ROM
   b. Hard disk
   c. RAM
   d. CPU

4. Architectural models are used for information systems to
   a. Provide a framework or structure for the flow of data and information within systems
   b. Determine the hardware necessary for the system
   c. Help technicians isolate problems in the system
   d. Assess quantitative results of evaluation data

5. Which of the following is not a goal of Service-Oriented Architecture?
   a. Build information systems that enable business to reuse existing assets effectively
   b. Support changes that will occur in the business and its needs
   c. Create new assets
   d. Ensure services are delivered effectively

⊙ Assess Systems for Regulatory Requirements

A primary consideration when selecting a system for use in healthcare informatics is whether or not the systems meets the current regulatory requirements. There is no single regulatory body that determines all the health informatics regulatory requirements for all systems. For example, the Office of the National Coordinator for Health Information Technology monitors HIT certification (Amatayakul 2013, 6). The Health Information Technology for Economic and Clinical Health (HITECH) provides guidance for electronic health record (EHR) certification (Amatayakul 2013, 69). The Food and Drug Administration (FDA) regulates electronic signatures, bar coding, and medical devices.

Assessing the system capabilities should begin in the design and development stage by carefully comparing the systems' regulations to the functional specifications of the hardware, software, and networks prior to procurement. In particular, security capabilities of potential hardware and networks must be scrutinized to assure that the system will provide the highest levels of security when implemented. The pervasive nature of mobile computing in today's healthcare systems is a special security concern. Other topics that require special attention are electronic signatures, data corrections, and audit log maintenance.

Design and Development

A fully functioning information infrastructure for healthcare systems requires careful, considered, and informed design and development. Many factors must be considered beginning with user needs, the physical environment, the technology available, industry regulations, internal constraints, and any external threats. There are usually two different types of models, physical and architectural (logical), that are used to fully describe the information infrastructure for an organization.

Physical Models

Physical models capture the hardware composition of a system in terms of the computer and other devices. The physical infrastructure generally refers to the computers (workstations, servers, and so on) and connection media used for a network. The model is a pictorial representation of the arrangement of the different pieces and connection points (Wager et al. 2009, 206–207). A network consists of two or more computers linked by a communication line. There are many types of computers, including servers and user interface devices such as personal computers, laptops, tablet computers, and smart phones, among others. The communication media used in a network includes cabled and noncabled media such as microwaves and radio waves, more commonly known as Wi-Fi, short for wireless fidelity.

The selection of servers, along with their configuration and capabilities, is very technical and usually the responsibility of the chief technology officer (CTO), chief information officer (CIO), or director of information systems. Generally, these same people are responsible for either the selection of user interface devices (computers, tablets, smart phones, and such) or setting standards for the user interface devices that may be purchased by others in the organization. Hopefully, these decisions will be made based upon the needs of the organization and users of the system. For example, an inadequate number of computers in an emergency room could lead to extreme user frustration or even a failure to document all of the care delivered.

The cabled communication media chosen for the physical infrastructure and model are categorized according to their varying transmission speeds. Coaxial cable is typically used only for cable television, with twisted pair and fiber-optic preferred for other uses. Twisted pair can transmit a variety of speeds, though usually only over short distances. Fiber-optic can be used to transmit over longer distances; however, it is more expensive (Wager et al. 2009, 208).

Noncabled communication media are usually termed wireless. When a network is created using noncabled communication methods to connect the computers and other resources it is known as a **wireless network**. They take the form of microwaves, including those used for satellite transmissions; other radio waves including the Institute of Electrical and Electronics Engineers (IEEE) 802.11(a-n) standards used for Wi-Fi local area networks; cellular telephone technology; and the Bluetooth standard (Wager et al. 2009, 209). These wireless standards all have different specifications for speed of transmission, as well as supported distance between the sending device and receiving device.

There are additional devices that enable networked communication. Generally, these consist of hubs, bridges, routers, gateways, and switches. Much like a transportation hub such as a major rail station, a network hub brings together the data from a network. A bridge can be used to connect networks using the same communication protocol, while the more sophisticated router can play a role in directing the network traffic. Gateways connect networks using different communication protocols, while switches route data to their destination and may also be a gateway or router.

Physical models are described in terms of a **topology**. The topology is the network's physical layout. Types of cabled network topologies include point-to-point, star, bus, tree, or ring. The advantages and disadvantages are summarized in table 4.1. The last topology in the table is a mesh topology, which is largely

Table 4.1. Network topologies pros and cons

Network Topology	Advantages	Disadvantages
Point-to-point	• Speed	• Limited to two devices
Star	• Easy installation and device connection • Can connect and remove devices without disruption • Problems are easily identified	• Requires more cable than bus topology • Failure of a hub, switch, or concentrator disables nodes • More expensive than bus topology
Bus	• Easy device connection • Uses less cable than other topologies	• One break disables network • Terminators required at both ends of the backbone • Problems are hard to identify
Tree	• Point-to-point wiring for certain segments • Vendor neutral	• Length of a segment is limited by type of cable used • If backbone breaks an entire segment fails • More difficult to configure and wire
Ring	• Can support better performance than a star topology • Provides for orderly data transmission	• High performance under low loads • Expensive to implement • Any fault can cause network failure
Mesh	• Extensive redundancy with multiple connections • "Self-configuring" when new nodes are added • "Self-healing" to continue operations even when some nodes fail • More nodes increase speed	• Still in development, with no standards • Wireless is inherently unreliable • They are not completely seamless; moving nodes may result in failure

Source: Adapted in part from Florida Center for Instructional Technology 2013

confined to wireless networks, due to the exorbitant costs if a mesh network were to be attempted with cable.

The physical model and distribution systems of a network are very important. Although they do not determine the entire functionality, they can limit what can be done with a given system. It is important to involve users as well as technical experts to ensure the choices made support the organizational needs.

Mobile Computing

Mobile computing is quickly emerging as a technology infrastructure challenge for healthcare organizations (Kim and Glassman, 2013; Oscar 2013). Mobile computing is defined as providing healthcare with mobile devices, which include smart phones, tablets, PDAs, and other portable wireless devices (Harvey and Harvey 2014). Mobile devices of today have as much, if not more, computing power as desktop computers of the past. They offer practically unlimited access for busy clinicians and staff. However, they come with a separate set of concerns, which must be managed to maintain effective, efficient, and secure operations.

Initial issues to be addressed include the type and ownership of the devices. Whether the system is compatible with Apple's iOS or Google's Android operating system is a technical, infrastructure decision, which may be constrained by the EHR or other systems already installed. Related to the decision of which platforms or operating systems to support is the ownership of the device. This decision can be very difficult, especially when users are vocal and do not always understand the complexity of the situation. The technical requirements for each platform come with their own challenges and organizations must be able to manage all of them effectively, while complying with myriad regulations. Users will often want to use their personal devices, often called "bring your own device" (BYOD). This is certainly easier for the user; however, using a personal device for accessing protected health information (PHI) requires the device to meet very specific encryption standards. The healthcare organization is responsible for ensuring that any access to individually identifiable HI via any method is legal and secure.

Securing healthcare data on mobile devices is especially challenging. According to a recent Department of Health and Human Services report, the majority of all healthcare data breaches affecting over 500 users involved mobile devices (HHS 2015). Facilities must have policies and procedures in place to regulate mobile device use. Data encryption should be used for devices and e-mail, and computer logs should be monitored regularly to determine who is accessing PHI (HIMSS 2011). Physical security for laptops and other mobile devices is essential to prevent theft (HHS 2014).

Lawmakers have increased HIPAA monetary penalties for not securing smart phone, e-mail, laptop, and tablet data and now require a separate risk management plan for mobile devices (HHS 2006). Yet the healthcare industry does not currently agree on a standard for mobile device security, thus healthcare facilities must create their own standards (Thomas 2007). National Institute of Standards and Technology (NIST) suggests educating users on security measures such as the creation of strong passwords and use of e-mail encryption (Scarfone et al. 2007). At a minimum, the facility must address virus protection, backups, firewalls, encryption, disaster recovery, annual security training, as well as regular security audits, updates, and ongoing monitoring of mobile devices. As with all tools, this functionality comes with a price. It is ultimately up to senior management to establish the level of acceptable risk versus the cost to protect the organization and its information assets.

Another decision point is the access to be supported. The organization must decide whether to only allow application access, such as with the EHR, or whether to include more expanded communication methods such as e-mail or text messaging, which are more difficult to manage. Additionally, the organization must determine whether to support mobile access for all employees or to limit it to physicians or some other combination of user types. Organizations must be cautious when authorizing access because increased mobile access will increase the mobile support needs. As with the platform and device ownership decisions, the access decision must be carefully considered. Theft of mobile devices is increasing and facilities must include scheduled checks on the physical locations of their mobile devices in their risk management plans.

Mobile computing is becoming pervasive in healthcare. Development and growth in this market is exponential with the advent of radio frequency identification (RFID) for tracking assets and patients, real-time locator systems (RTLS), and portable wireless devices such as glucose monitors and blood pressure monitors. Other devices in use that must be protected include internal monitors (that is, pacemakers), portable Holter heart monitors, and wearables (that is, exercise monitors). Health informatics professionals must work with vendors to stay current regarding the security features of these devices. Healthcare organizations and health informatics professionals will have to engage in lifelong learning to provide their users, including patients, with the very latest technological tools in a protected environment.

Electronic Signatures

An ongoing security concern is providing strong electronic signatures for electronic health records. The process of electronically signing a record, called e-signing, is a complex workflow involving the initial access of the user to the systems, and the authentication of the user through strong passwords or PINs (AHIMA e-HIM Workgroup: Best Practices for Electronic Signature and Attestation 2009). The system must carefully check that the authenticated user has the necessary permissions to sign off on the record. Complications arise when multiple users must sign off on one record, such as an operation performed by multiple physicians or a doctor who is supervising residents and cosigning their entries. Physician groups often allow other doctors in the group to round on the groups' patients and sign off orders. Absences of the person originating the entry creates a need for allowing alternate signers. Facilities must also generate security policies to address electronic record amendments and deletions, and all versions on the record must be retained for legal reasons and a reference must be added to identify the original uncorrected document (McWay 2016, 165). Risk management teams must be heavily invested in monitoring this process due to the potential for damaging data integrity, which generates legal liabilities for the hospital.

Audit Logs

One tool used by security teams to monitor user activity is an **audit log**, also called an audit trail, which records the user's log-on information as well the activities they performed in the systems (Sandefer 2016, 379). Audit logs are maintained by many clinical applications, like databases, and by electronic document management systems. For example, when the user logs on to a CDR, the CDR logging component begins writing information to a file about the machine and software the user employed for access, the method of authentication (for example, PIN, user's ID), the date and time of systems access, the files or applications the user accessed, the actions they performed, and when the user logged off the system. Audit logs are searchable and they are part of a systems backup. Risk management and security teams routinely monitor log files, and there are preset flags that trigger special attention to a users' activities. Audit files may be subpoenaed and examined to determine if fraudulent activities occurred.

◎ Device Selection Recommendations

Healthcare devices are selected using multiple criteria such as cost, intended usage, user requirements, system features, and interoperability. In general, the usability of information systems increases if the user is comfortable with the systems. Consideration should be given to workflow and ergonomics when selecting healthcare devices. **Ergonomics** are natural laws that govern work (LeBlanc 2016, 726). Ergonomic work environments are designed to increase the workers' comfort as they go about the daily activities. An initial ergonomic analysis is used to examine the workers' assigned tasks as well as the physical work environment. Human factors are considered regarding how much workers sit or stand, perform repetitive activities, bend, or lift heavy objects. Management should encourage workers who spend long hours at their computer to stretch, move, and walk around periodically. A variety of computer and office equipment is available to address the human factors correlated with injuries, fatigue, and stress. Ergonomic keyboards, foot pads, and computer display screens can increase worker comfort and reduce eyestrain. A track ball mouse helps to reduce carpal tunnel syndrome, electronic staplers reduce the number of repetitive motions for administrative workers, ergonomic chairs with specially designed backrests reduce back strain and encourage correct posture. Computer screens should reduce glare, be comfortably positioned and large enough to see the applications and documents easily, and have a high screen resolution. Employees with preexisting conditions requiring special office environments should be encouraged to discuss their needs.

Point-of-care (POC) systems include EHRs, picture archiving systems, laboratory information systems, and patient monitoring systems (Ventola 2014). When selecting mobile devices for POC use, consideration must be given to the system uses and the system functionalities. End users should be surveyed to determine what applications and functionalities they need on the POC system, and a set of device selection criteria should be established and used for vendor selection. The presence of features like voice messaging, e-mail, text, conferencing, search tools, reporting, cloud-based storage, online references, and user-defined alerts should be evaluated. Security requirement for security features like encrypting and the ability to wipe the device remotely in case of threat should be documented and communicated to the vendor selection committee (Ventola 2014). It is also important to determine what applications and software are desired on the mobile systems in order to ensure the vendors providing the mobile device will support the mobile software. Interoperability of this system with existing systems must be tested prior to purchasing the device.

Computers on wheels (COWs) are mobile notebook computers on rolling carts that are used by clinical personnel (AHIMA 2014, 33). COWs can provide an easy way for an informatics professional to move around the patient care area to check paper charts for completeness, which can be recorded using the COW's laptop. Other uses of COWs could include checking inventory, nursing medication administration, chart audits, and other point-of-care uses. COWs use wireless technology to transmit and receive data as they are moved around buildings, which means that PHI security must be addressed prior to system selection with the system's vendor. Regarding COW device selection, the screen size, battery life, cart size, and ergonomics must be considered (PC Connection 2016). A larger screen provides the user with more area for viewing applications, but it adds to the weight of the device. Screens on these devices should have password protected screen savers that lock after a timeout, and they should have a screen protector that prevents viewing the screen by anyone not directly in front of the screen. A bigger cart allows a larger notebook or a laptop, but may not fit into the physical spaces as needed (for example, between patient beds) (Andersen et al. 2009). Mobile carts and bedside terminals used for point-of-care patient activities should be adjustable to accommodate a variety of users of different heights, and they should have ergonomic keyboards and displays. When using COWs, it is important that the notebook on the COW have the longest battery life possible as this will help avoid workflow interruptions while using a charging station to recharge the batteries. Dockable notebooks that are plugged into a physical dock on the chart are more portable but must be secured to reduce the threat of theft. This can be accomplished by attaching the notebook to the COW using a special computer cable that requires a key to unlock.

Healthcare-associated infections (HAIs) are infections acquired in a healthcare setting that are associated with the use of indwelling medical devices (for example, central venous lines), surgical procedures, and environmental contamination (ODPP 2015). Although many HAIs are preventable, there are still 1 million HAIs reported in the US healthcare system each year, which indicates that HAIs pose a significant threat to patient safety (ODPP 2015). The Centers for Disease Control and Prevention (CDC) aims to eliminate HAIs in US hospitals in order to improve patient outcomes by reducing the number of HIA-associated deaths and diseases (CDC 2014). A CDC report indicates that this goal has not been achieved, although the HAI infection levels have been reduced in many areas (CDC 2014). Some example of HAI reductions are: central line–associated infections decreased 35 percent, catheter-associated urinary tract infections decreased 10 percent, and methicillin-resistant *Staphylococcus aureus* (MRSA) infections decreased 71 percent (CDC 2015). In response to the HAI threat, healthcare facilities are using medical devices treated with antimicrobial agents designed to reduce infections (Saint et al. 2013). However, a survey of infection prevention personnel at US hospitals indicated that antimicrobial device use varied by clinical area with antimicrobial urinary catheters being used in 45 percent of hospitals, and antimicrobial central venous catheters being used 33 percent of the time (Sanjay et al. 2013). These results are important for informatics professionals who should apply this knowledge to selecting and maintaining medical devices used for point-of-care tools. The FDA regulates medical devices, and they provide a guideline for antimicrobials (FDA 2007).

Check Your Understanding 4.2

Answer the following questions.

1. What is a noncabled method for computer communications using microwaves or radio waves called?
   a. Wireless
   b. Fiber optic
   c. Twisted pair
   d. Coaxial

2. This network design is more expensive than a hub; however, it is easier to install. It is what type of network?
   a. Star
   b. Mesh
   c. Tree
   d. Bus

3. What is a private network that uses a public network (usually the Internet) to connect remote sites or users together privately?
   a. Extranet
   b. FTP
   c. VPN
   d. SFTP

4. What is the information distribution system that is the most widely employed in information systems?
   a. Internet
   b. Client-server
   c. Peer-to-peer
   d. Network

5. Decisions regarding mobile computing should be made
   a. After new technology emerges
   b. After IT personnel tests the product
   c. When users demand it
   d. Following a thorough risk analysis

6. According to the DHHS, the majority of all healthcare data breaches affecting over 500 users involved which devices?
   a. Servers
   b. Desktops
   c. Printers
   d. Mobile devices

7. According to HIPAA, what are facilities required to have for mobile devices?
   a. Adequate power supply
   b. Correct network architecture
   c. A separate risk management plan
   d. A policy forbidding Bring Your Own Devices

8. Which of the following would decrease the usability of a new Clinical Data Repository?
   a. Develop workflow reports as they relate to the CDR
   b. Review reports of other users of the same system
   c. Survey users regarding what they want in the new system
   d. Exclude users from systems testing activities

9. What is the term for the natural laws that govern work?
   a. Ethics
   b. Ergonomics
   c. Economics
   d. Procedures
   e. Processes

10. Which is the main goal of creating ergonomic office environments?
    a. Provide an up-to-date work place
    b. Color coordinate the office furniture
    c. Spend money leftover in the annual budget
    d. Increase users' comfort as they perform their daily activities
    e. Ergonomics

⊙ Development of Systems

Computer systems have evolved from large mainframe computers that took up an entire room and were used mainly by scientists and government agencies to the small, compact, wireless handheld tablets found in most homes today. Similarly, the technologies have progressed from huge vacuum tubes to microchips that are scant millimeters long. The evolution of networks and availability of Internet technologies have been a driving force for increasing consumer use of computers.

Communication Technologies

Data in interconnected systems are communicated across local and wide area networks using a set of rules called communication protocols, like the IEEE protocols, that regulate the flow of data between computers with respect to data packet composition, authentication, and session management (PC Magazine 2015). A **wide area network (WAN)** is a computer network that connects devices across a large geographic area (AHIMA 2014, 434). A **local area network (LAN)** is a network that connects various devices together via communications within a small geographic area such as a single organization (Abdelhak et al. 2012, 270). For example, the Internet is a WAN. Data traveling across the Internet are transmitted through networks connected by Ethernet cables or by light pulse in the case of fiber-optic systems. Locally, PCs with wireless network interface cards, present in most of today's systems, can wirelessly transmit data.

Figure 4.1. Firewall

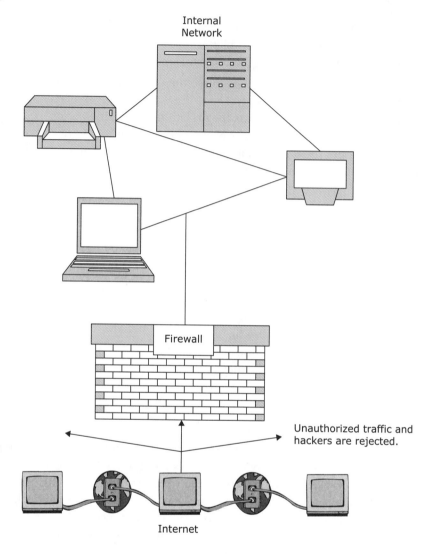

Regarding secure data transmission, **firewalls** and **virtual private networks (VPNs)** are software components that are integral parts of network communication security (Amatayakul 2013, 300–301). A firewall monitors and controls all communication into and out of an intranet. It is implemented by a set of processes that act as a gateway to a network, applying the organizational security policy. Firewalls in healthcare organizations usually keep hackers and other external threats from the Internet outside of the internal network; however, firewalls can also keep sensitive data such as individually identifiable patient HI from leaving the organization. Firewalls can help protect PHI from viruses attached to documents or from hackers trying to get identifying information to sell (for example, SSNs or insurance numbers) (Microsoft Corp. 2016). See figure 4.1 for an illustration of a firewall.

Sometimes there is a need to communicate across wide networks, which includes sending data via the Internet. Virtual private networks (VPNs) extend the firewall protection boundary beyond the local intranet by the use of cryptographically protected secure channels at the Internet Protocol (IP) level. A VPN is a private network that uses a public network (usually the Internet) to connect remote sites or users together privately (Amatayakul 2013, 659).

Networks are often described in terms of the methods they use to distribute information. The most common distribution methods are **terminal-to-host**, **file server**, and **client-server**. With terminal-to-host, the application and any data stay on a host computer with the user connecting either via a "dumb" terminal or using **terminal emulation software** on a personal computer to connect as if the user is on a dumb terminal. Sometimes this arrangement is also termed a thin client, with most of the actual processing taking place on a central computer (Wager et al. 2009, 210). A file server system runs entirely on the end user's workstation and transfers entire files, while the client-server method has multiple servers dedicated to different functions with workstations running the application and retrieving data from a server as needed. Client-server is the most used method, whereby some information and applications will sit on a local client; however, information or data can be pulled from a server (Wager et al. 2009, 210). A common example of client-server is the use of e-mail, such as Microsoft Outlook, where Outlook runs on the local computer but pulls e-mail and other information from a server. MS Office can also be used as a cloud-based application, which is convenient for mobile users.

Internet Technologies

The Internet is a complex compendium of networked technologies. Several communications standards are used for data transmission. Foremost, the International Standards Organization's protocol called the **Open System Interconnection Model (OSI),** which is a well-established standard set of protocols used by most industries (ISO 2016). This seven-layer model, shown in figure 4.2, presents an overview of the protocol layers that a typical data packet traverses beginning with the electronic signal that starts the source data transmission, and ending with the application layer in the destination application on a PC or server that receives the transmitted data packet and translates it into meaningful data for display. The target application could be e-mail on a PC or a table in a clinical database on an EDMS server. The upper layers 4–7 (application, presentation, session, transport) define standards more specific to the target application, and lower layer protocols can be generalized to most networked systems. For example, the network layer sends the data across the LAN or WAN, and the Presentation Layer handles decrypting the data and unpacking the data packet so that the target application can process it for the user.

The prevalent Internet protocol set utilized for implementing the OSI model is the Transmission Control/Internet Protocol (TCP/IP) that was developed by the Department of Defense (Microsoft Corp. 2015b). This four-layer model consists of application, transport, Internet, and network interface protocols. Starting at the lowest level, data travels from a PC to the Ethernet through optical fiber cables

Figure 4.2.   Open system interconnection model

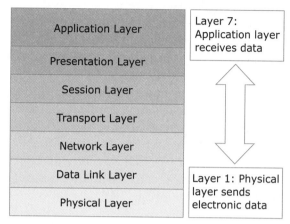

Source: Adapted from Wager et al. 2009

Figure 4.3.   Four-layer TCP/IP model

Application Layer
Transport Layer
Internet Layer
Network Interface Layer

(network interface layer). It is grouped into data packets having start and end addresses (Internet layer) then pushed into a TCP session (transport layer). The TCP session pushes the data to a remote PC where the user accesses the data in the e-mail and opens the attachment to read the original report (application layer). A key reason that TCP/IP can find the destination server and send the requesting server a transmission success or error message is the fact that every machine on the Internet has a unique numerical address called the IP address. Figure 4.3 displays the four-layer TCP/IP model containing application, transport, Internet, and network interface layers.

Within a TCP/IP session, file transfer protocol (FTP) can be used on a dedicated FTP server to poll the network for data packet requests. When a request is received, the data are transmitted from the requesting client to the destination server where it can be downloaded. Typically, FTP facilitates data downloads from websites, but a user can start a local FTP session and type in commands to upload, download, copy, and move files. FTP data are transmitted unencrypted or modified, called clear text, so it is essential that security protocols be in use for FTP sessions (Microsoft Corp. 2015a).

A web server that delivers webpages to the user utilizes hypertext transfer protocol (http) and XML messaging. The http protocols are used to move the data from the web server across the Internet to the IP address that is mapped to the client's web browser. In fact, the URL for a webpage, which starts with "http," actually maps to a numerical Internet address and that is what TCP/IP uses to find the data destination. As an illustration, the IP address for www.google.com is 74.125.239.98. The data sent to web servers is contained in XML messages, which are a set of system independent tags widely used that are read by the web server's services to generate the client's webpage display.

Check Your Understanding 4.3

Answer the following questions.

1. Which network design connects various devices in one hospital building so that they can communicate?
   a. WAN
   b. VPN
   c. LAN
   d. Firewall

2. Which network design connects various computers across one state so that they can communicate?
   a. WAN
   b. VPN
   c. LAN
   d. Firewall

3. Which device monitors and controls all data transmission in and out of Valley General Hospital?
   a. WAN
   b. VPN
   c. LAN
   d. Firewall

4. Which of these provides a secure channel that extends beyond a hospitals' intranet to allow users in remote sites to work together?
   a. WAN
   b. VPN
   c. LAN
   d. d. Firewall

5. The OSI recommended protocol for using the Internet is:
   a. CDR
   b. TCP/IP
   c. ICD-10
   d. HTML

⊙ Evaluate Systems

To ensure that electronic systems meet end user needs and function as expected, the data relationships and the interfaces must be well defined during the initial planning cycle, and they must be built and tested in the system testing portion of the system development life cycle (Sandefer 2016, 380). Testing a system with realistic data helps the developers to find and correct design or implementation errors before the system is turned over to the user for system sign-off.

Systems Testing

During implementation, the hardware, software, and networks needed to use the new clinical systems are installed and tested. Databases are loaded with data, data relationships are created, and webpages are built. Documentation is created, errors and versions of software are tracked for project management reporting, and training is conducted. The system vendor may provide help for this testing, the end user may send a representative to take part, and definitely the system developers will participate. Because system testing is an iterative cycle, it is essential to track software versions, hardware names and type, network and database configurations, and errors found during testing. When major errors are found during testing, it is not unusual to have to roll back a change to an earlier state in order to fix the error so that testing can resume.

When the system is adequately tested by the project management team, pilot testing can be utilized by having small groups of end users test the system on live data. Initial pilot testing can be done by having these users process data in the new and existing systems. This parallel testing approach is time consuming and resource intensive, but it allows the system to be tested on real data without causing any problems for the users. However, it is usually the case that the new system is so different that parallel testing cannot be used effectively. In that case, pilot testing is accomplished by having a small group of users use the new system exclusively. Thus, a new coding system could be pilot tested in the Emergency Room on one of the slower days by a small well-trained group to minimize disruption. During this testing, support must be available in the form of developers and managers onsite to assist with questions and any bugs found.

Informatics personnel managing systems testing need to closely monitor timelines as it is easy to exceed the allotted time, budget, and resources for testing. Managers who have supported the project may be expecting frequent reports on progress because they know the system will go out to the user soon. The use of project management software like Gantt charts, which are a graphic tool used to plot tasks and timelines for project management (AHIMA 2014, 63) or Microsoft Project software can simplify project management and provide a mechanism for generating graphs and reports.

Interface Management

Computers communicate to each other and to humans using interfaces. These interfaces could be software programs, hardware, data definitions, or protocols. A common interface used for human-to-computer communication is the graphical user interfaces on computer systems, which allows the user to interact with the computer in a user-friendly way without having to learn system commands and type them in on a command line. An interface for software-to-software communication is the application program interface built into the operating system that allows information technology programmers' software to talk to the operating systems. Thus, a programmer can put the documented name of the operating system's API print function into a program and effortlessly send a report to the printer from within their code. Without APIs the same programmer would need extensive training and knowledge of the underlying operating systems. EHRs interface with lab, x-ray, pharmacy, registration, and transcription systems. For example, an application interface built into an Oracle database system allows the beginning clinical health data analyst to drag and drop table names, join tables, and create a data export for further statistical analysis.

With the abundance of interfaces available it is easy to see that interfaces used in healthcare development projects must be cataloged, documented, and managed. Many vendors now provide interface engine software to help with the management. Changes to interface code or hardware has caused many systems to fail, and it is very hard to track down these types of errors due to their complexity. Interface management starts during project management when the system is selected. Close scrutiny must be given to the interfaces available and how they will work with the existing systems. Failing to evaluate the interfaces provided by a vendor in this context can result in having to pay expensive contractor fees to get their developers to design additional interfaces. Even when the facility has an IT team in place with API development expertise, it is usually not feasible to write these types of APIs because the underlying code is proprietary. Correspondingly, the facility will need to assist the vendors by generating code that allows the vendors APIs to interact with existing clinical and administrative applications.

The mapping of interfaces would be part of the system design. Later, when they are built and tested changes to interfaces are recorded in the change management system. And after the system is in production change requests for interfaces should be examined by a special team of advanced informaticists. Diligence is needed in all phases because healthcare systems depend on the interoperability of data flowing through multiple interfaces, and even a small interface code change can bring down several ancillary systems in addition to the one in which the change was initiated.

Electronic Structure and Relationship of Health Data

Data for electronic health records are captured with interfaces and stored in databases. These databases must be designed to provide high-quality data that meets the end user's needs. As mentioned, the representatives of the end user should be involved in the initial design of the data flows and interfaces in order to accurately record what they expect the new system to provide. These requirements become part of the project management documentation and are used by the database designers and programmers to develop the system. They are also used to write the test scripts that will be run by the end user when they test and accept delivery of the final system.

To develop the system, a data dictionary is used to provide data consistency. The data dictionary is generated to record the name, data type, length, allowed values, where the data comes from, intended usage, and whether or not the data is required (Campbell 2004). Edit checks can be added to the database to enforce requirements for the data like "dosage must be less than 10 mg" (AHIMA 2014). The data dictionary is the blue print used by the database managers to create the database tables. After development, it is consulted by informatics personnel, e-HIM program managers, and database reporting specialists who write queries and generate reports. The data dictionary is an ongoing effort that is part of the maintenance cycle for managing electronic systems.

Concurrently with database creation, the existence of data relationships between data elements must be identified so that they can be modeled in the database. If one patient has many lab tests run in a day, then the relationship between patient and lab tests is one to many. When many specialists examine one patient that is a many to one relationship. Similarly, one bed is assigned to one and only one patient, which is called a one to one relationship. When these and other relationships are created in the database, the database management system will enforce constraints that prevent code accessing the database from assigning one bed to more than one patient, or disallowing a patient from being seen by multiple specialists. One initial problem with EHR systems was that multiple physicians' e-signatures were not allowed for one patient. In that case, two surgeons performing one operation on the same patient at the same time could not both sign off on the operative report.

Check Your Understanding 4.4

Answer the following questions.

1. Which activity would not happen during systems implementation?
   a. Install a new database server
   b. Test new database software
   c. Set up a new network system
   d. Design the new system

2. Which activity would not occur during the systems testing for a new database server?
   a. Install security system on database server
   b. Import data into the new database tables
   c. Create relationships between primary and foreign keys in the database
   d. Document end user needs

3. The main reason to track all hardware, software, and network configurations during system testing is that
   a. It is required by the Joint Commission
   b. Past configuration information is essential to finding testing errors
   c. The information may be forgotten
   d. It keeps the project manager busy

4. A pilot test of a new medication administration system would be conducted using
   a. All end users on all floors in the hospital with live data
   b. All end users on all floors in the hospital with the new and old systems running at the same time
   c. A small group of end users with live data
   d. a and c

Indicate whether each of the following is true or false.

5. Testing a system with realistic data helps developers to find errors in implementation.

6. It is not important to catalog the interfaces used in a software system.

⊙ Distributed Systems

Computer system networks can be classified as either **centralized** or **decentralized**. A **network** is a type of information technology that connects different computers and computer systems so they can share information (AHIMA 2014, 102). A centralized system is one in which the systems processing functions occur on a single computer. Conversely, in a decentralized system the processing functions are split or distributed among one or more machines in the network system. In most cases, all of the machines in the system are doing a portion of the overall work independently. In every case these distributed machines work together toward a common goal.

In a centralized system there is one component, such as a software program, shared by all users, all resources are accessible, and the system is homogeneous. That is, all machines in the system are built with the same technology, and software runs as a single process with a single point of control and failure. A centralized system is therefore working or it is not. If the system is a relational database, then the users can all share the data at the same time. There is no need for an interface because there is only one system.

In a **distributed system** there are multiple autonomous components that are not shared by all users and the software runs concurrently on different processors with multiple points of control and failure. A distributed system is a decentralized system. It is defined as a collection of independent computers connected through a network and managed by system software that enables the computers to coordinate their activities and to share system resources such that the users perceive the system as a single, integrated system (Steen 2007). Other machines may use the machines in this system so there is a need for interfaces between them and for request management.

Sophisticated software checks the load of machines on the network and assigns the workload to machines in the system to better balance out the load. These machines can be geographically close and connected by a LAN. Or they could be geographically distant and communicating over a WAN, which could in fact be several LANs connected by a phone system or satellite. For example, the Internet is a WAN. In any case, regardless of the connections, the goal of a distributed system is to make the system appear to the users as one computer.

Figure 4.4.   Distributed system

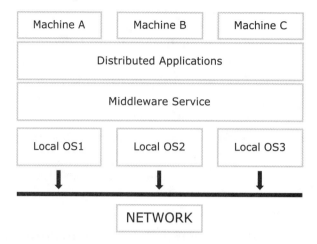

Figure 4.4 illustrates the typical architecture in a distributed system configuration. Notice that there are three machines in this configuration. Each machine has its own operating system (OS) and all the machines are connected via a network. The distributed applications run across all machines and access the **middleware**, that is software and hardware services that form a bridge between applications (Abdelhak et al. 2012, 272), in order to provide seamless application access to the users on Machine A (with Local OS1), Machine B (with Local OS2), and Machine C (with Local OS3). Thus the user on, say, Machine B may actually be running an application in Local OS3, but this is transparent to the end user.

Notice this definition implies that in a distributed system the data, computation, and users are all dispersed. Users communicate via a web-interfaced application to multiple computers containing separate data stores in order to perform healthcare data processing. Examples of distributed systems include the World Wide Web (WWW), an automatic teller machine (ATM), a LAN, a database management system, and an EHR system.

The goals of a distributed system are

- Resource sharing
- Openness
- Concurrency
- Scalability
- Fault tolerance
- Transparency

Resource sharing means being able to use the hardware, software, or data anywhere in the system (Emmerich 1997). This is often implemented with a client-server architecture that allows the client PC and the server to interact. In this scenario, described in detail later, the server acts as the resource manager allowing the client to access hardware (that is, a file server) or data anywhere in the system.

Openness means flexibility to extend and improve the existing system with minimal impact. System openness is achieved by interfaces and interoperability between systems, which can be difficult in a heterogeneous environment. It could mean adding new interfaces or modifying existing servers or interfaces. Additionally, the data representations in the multiple vendors' interfaces must be managed transparently for openness to occur. An open system supports interoperability between the systems in the distributed network.

Concurrent processes run simultaneously and access shared resources such as databases. Concurrent processes in transactions require special handling so that changes made by one process are not lost. For example, suppose two processes are working concurrently to update a bank account balance level. It should be the case that the addition of money is applied simultaneously with the withdrawal of funds so that the account is not overdrawn. Similarly, in a concurrent database all the changes should be processed and applied accurately so that reporting from that system preserves data consistency.

In the case of a distributed database, the data is stored on two or more machines and the **database management system (DBMS),** installed locally on each machine, is designed to keep track of data locations and coordinate data modifications. For example, a healthcare organization might consist of an acute-care hospital, an outpatient surgery center, and multiple remote clinics. Each facility has its own local applications and databases. All of the facilities are connected through a network that allows data sharing.

Scalability means the ability to support growth while maintaining the same level of service. The growth may occur for many reasons such as additional users, machines, and databases or expansion to another state or continent. In any case, users should not see a reduction of performance or reduced processing speed when the expansion occurs. Furthermore, scaling up should only require adding more processors, not redesigning the system. Note that while scalability should encompass adding more users and processes, even servers have an upper limit to the number of users that they can support, so this only works to a point.

Fault tolerant systems are highly available and remain in operation even when hardware, software, or network failures occur. This is usually achieved by having redundant systems and a good recovery plan. A redundant system could be a copy of the production server that is kept offline but updated frequently in case it needs to be switched out with the production server. Additionally, in a distributed system there is no single point of failure because resources, like data, are located across different servers, instead of centrally. Thus, if one server fails, the others should be able to continue without the users being aware of any disruption.

Transparency means the end user sees the distributed system as a single machine. This is often achieved with the addition of middleware. An example of this would be using the Internet to do online shopping. The user does not need to know how the order gets into the remote system or gets processed. Transparency makes the resources available, distributes them transparently, and provides openness and scalability while hiding network failures. Distribution transparency means the user does not have to know how the data are represented, where data are stored, or if the data have been replicated, moved, or updated to be more consistent. This can be difficult to achieve if the users are on different continents and there are some network failures that cannot be made transparent. Finally, it is difficult to be sure that system data was preserved in the event of a server failure. Transparency could include using web-based software to query a database in another state. The details of processing the request for data need not be known to the user nor does the location of the database matter.

Distributed systems depend on middleware to facilitate communication between multiple heterogeneous machines. A distributed system has the goal of appearing as a single system multiprocessor system to the users. In an ideal world, a distributed OS could be implemented by a cluster of machines connected by high-performance networks. In reality, this architecture is rarely seen. Instead, the machines in a distributed system are from various vendors, with different OSs and software installations. Middleware is the glue that allows messages to pass between the machines in the system.

Evolution of Distributed Systems

Distributed systems were not the model for systems processing in the past. In fact, in the 1960s, when computer use began to be popular in healthcare, computer processing was largely centralized. Programmers sat at machines, called terminals, which were physically connected to large mainframe host systems. The terminals were used for data entry but had almost no processing power, so all the work was done on the host machine. The need for faster and better processing to support data processing brought about the modification of terminals to have added processing capabilities. This allowed some of the system workload to be shifted to the terminals and was the beginning of the client-server architecture model. Several architectures that describe the configurations, relationships, and structures of the components in a computer system will be examined next.

Two-Tiered Systems

The client-server architecture model is a **two-tiered model** composed of several client computers that are used to capture and process the data. The servers in this configuration are powerful machines that have application software installed on them and in turn store the data captured by client machines. The clients could be notebooks, desktops, tablets, smart phones, or other computers in the network. There may be multiple servers in the network; and each of them works to process requests from the less powerful clients (Abdelhak et al. 2012, 272).

When a client machine sends a request to the server for a service, the host handles the client's requests, processes the data or performs the requested service, and then returns the results of that processing to the client. For example, the client can be a laptop computer that sends a request to the mainframe for data and the mainframe would package the requested data and send a network message back to the client containing that information. The diagram in figure 4.5 depicts the basic client-server two-tier architecture with a database server and the clients, the computer laptops, sending their data requests across a LAN.

Figure 4.5.   Two-tiered system

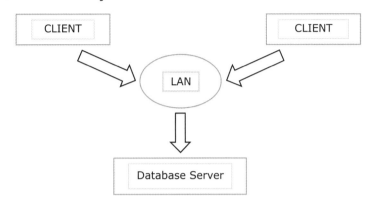

The users on a LAN can share printers, scheduling software, scanners, and files and can communicate by using network communication protocols. A single LAN has a limit as to how many PCs can be on the LAN. For example, a billing system at a physician's office might be on a LAN with 10 computers connected to a server. All the PCs on the network can share resources like printers and data files. And each of them can also execute software programs residing on their machines (such as Microsoft Word). The Ethernet is the most widely used LAN network, and it is a standard defined by the Institute of Electrical and Electronics Engineers (IEEE) as IEEE 802.3. The messages on an Ethernet are handled by all computers until they reach their final destination. The advantage of Ethernet communication is the high speed of data transmission, up to 100 megabits per second (Mbps). However, if one part of the network fails, the entire network has problems because some of the computers are not available to handle the messages.

Three-Tiered Architecture

The **three-tiered architecture** expands on the two-tier system with the addition of an application server that contains the software applications and the business rules. Another difference is that clients in this architecture are called "thin clients" because most of the processing is done on the server, and the client computer has very little software installed on it. The business rules on the application server are logical rules that are used for processing the data and as such they are determined by the business. For example, a business rule might be "Display lab values only if not in normal range" (Abdelhak et al. 2012, 272).

There are several advantages to a three-tiered architecture. First, the business rules can be easily modified with minimal impact on the system because they are located on a separate server. Second, the system is scalable; that is, clients and applications can easily be added. And finally, the technology of the machines in the system is flexible, which means that servers can easily be replaced with a different vendor's system with minimal impact on the system.

In the diagram of the three-tiered system in figure 4.6 below, the flow of data starts with the client application sending a request across the LAN to the application server.

Figure 4.6.   Three-tiered system

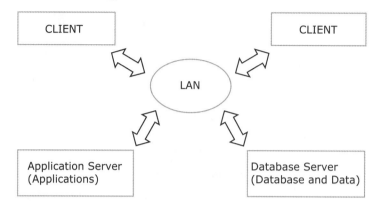

The application server processes the request and sends its own request for data across the network to the database server. When the database server returns the requested data to the application server it is sent back to the client. Thus the application server is acting as middleware by functioning as a bridge for data communication and data management between the client applications and the database server.

Web Services Architecture

A final computer structure called web services architecture (WSA) is needed for distributed computing in order to better integrate web-based healthcare applications with Internet protocols. It provides an environment that facilitates sharing of data behind a firewall across multiple systems using heterogeneous machines with different OSs (Sandefer 2016, 379). This would be used for all web-enabled client PCs in a facility to communicate with the EHRs and then again by the EHRs when they send and receive data from the various source systems.

To understand WSA one must first consider the nature of a web service. A web service is a software system that supports machine-to-machine communication. It is part of an XML-based message architecture system available over the Internet or an intranet, independent of OSs or programming languages. In this system a client browser sends a request, in the form of a message, to a web server. The message is then transported from the web browser client to the web server using http. The web server receives the message and passes it to a business objects component, which in turn contacts the database containing the requested data (W3C Working Group 2004).

Because the WSA is not tied to any particular OS or language, it can be implemented utilizing several open protocols or standards (TCP/IP, http, Java, and XML) with a variety of software applications in various languages running on disparate platforms to exchange data over the Internet. For example, many standard web services currently use these components: Simple Object Access Protocol (SOAP), Universal Description, Discovery and Integration (UDDI), and Web Services Description Language (WSDL).

The layers for WSA architecture implementation are Discovery, Description, Messaging, and Networking (W3C Working Group 2004). The Discovery layer is

Figure 4.7. Web services architecture layers

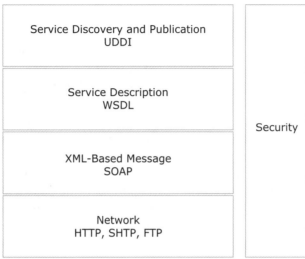

where the requestor PC sends a message to the web service requesting a description of the service provider's interfaces. The reply from the web service provider would contain a set of documents, called a service description, which includes interface descriptions, information about what messages the requestor client can expect to receive, descriptions of the types of the responses that the client might send back to the server, and a description of the service's semantics. For example, WSDL is a commonly used standard language.

Next, the Messaging layer describes the XML-based message format that will be transported from the web service. Specifically, it will outline what is in a request for service and what will be sent in the message. Generally, SOAP is the protocol used for the XML message. The Networking layer is where the basic functions of networking are handled. These could include error processing, sending and receiving messages, contacting hosts, and routing messages. Figure 4.7 summarizes this model which consists of the following layers: service discovery and publication, service description, XML-based message, network, and security.

Collaborative Computing

Collaboration means working together to achieve a common goal. Common goals can be achieved by collaborative computing, which allows users to harness the power of Internet-based collaborative software to work simultaneously on documents and presentations, attend web meetings, make plans using project management software, or create content in other media like wikis.

Examples of collaborative software include Google Docs, Dropbox, Microsoft NetMeeting, GoToMeeting, Webex, online calendars, project management software, videoconferencing (such as Adobe Connect), and instant messaging, among others. On the social front, collaborative software could be used for gaming, online dating, or social community sites like Facebook, LinkedIn, and Twitter. It could even include wikis when used for blogging, chatting, and surveys or creating social websites. Basically, collaborative computing occurs anywhere that individuals come together to work toward a common goal.

Medical work in general, in hospitals in particular, is highly collaborative due to the specialized nature of the medical treatment (Bardram and Christensen 2007). Collaborative computing is likely to be one of the solutions to the challenges in healthcare. For instance, a physician is trying to find a diagnosis of a patient. Traditionally, the physician can dictate the notes to a nurse to prepare the health record. During the radiology conference, the physician studies x-ray images with a radiologist. At the morning conference, the physician discusses proper medication with colleagues while browsing medicine catalogs. Later, the lab releases a blood sample result, and the physician must study it with a colleague while referencing recent publications. With collaborative computing it might be possible for many of these interactions to take place with minimal interference in the workflow. The physician might insert his or her own notes into the record, while using instant messaging to communicate with the nurse prior to rounds. The search for a medication and the implications of a laboratory result might take place within the EHR knowledge base, with different practitioners communicating using internal instant messaging or e-mail.

Cloud Computing

One area of interest in distributed information systems is the technology called cloud computing. See figure 4.8 for an illustration of cloud computing. Several advantages make cloud computing very attractive including the ability to access and use resources as they are needed without having to pay for them if they are idle and distributed computing in a distant or even several locations, which provides some redundancy for business continuity purposes (Sarna 2010, 2).

The concept of cloud computing is popular. Most businesses are in the process of determining whether or not they wish to move some, or all, of their information

Figure 4.8.   Cloud computing

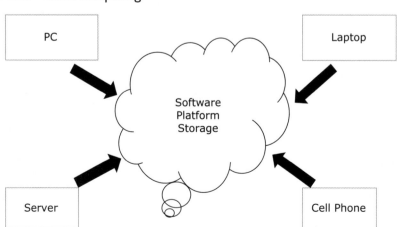

infrastructure to the cloud. In an effort to standardize what qualifies as cloud computing and what does not, NIST established five essential characteristics that define a cloud (Mell and Grance 2014). They are as follows:

1. **On-demand self-service**—Anyone with the appropriate permissions can make use of the resources without additional intervention.

2. **Broad network access**—Any capabilities available over the network can be accessed by a wide variety of interface devices (laptops, smart phones, and so on) using standard mechanisms.

3. **Resource pooling**—The cloud computing provider resources serve multiple consumers, usually independent of location, though these can be specified by the consumer.

4. **Rapid elasticity**—Service is provided on demand, meaning that more can quickly be provided when needed and reduced just as fast, so the consumer only pays for what they need and use.

5. **Measured service**—Use of resources in the cloud can be monitored, controlled, and reported, allowing for better management (Mell and Grance 2014).

NIST goes on to define three major cloud computing service models:

1. **Software as a service (SaaS)**—The highest level of cloud computing service models, SaaS enables access to the cloud computing provider's applications via a variety of devices, usually through an interface such as a web browser. The only part of the SaaS that might not be standardized is any consumer-specific application configuration settings.

2. **Platform as a service (PaaS)**—At this intermediate level of capability consumers create or acquire applications using programming languages and tools supported by the cloud computing service provider. Although the consumer does not control the underlying infrastructure, they do exercise more control over the applications.

3. **Infrastructure as a service (IaaS)**—This is the most minimal level of cloud computing where the infrastructure is provided, but the consumer controls the OS, storage, and applications. The consumer may also have control over networking components such as the firewall (Mell and Grance 2014).

Depending upon the particular application an organization may choose to use cloud computing services at all three levels, having responsibility and direct control for only the applications deemed most important or critical. Regardless of the service model, the deployment of the cloud may be distributed to organizations using one of these four models:

1. **Private cloud**—The cloud is accessible to only one customer and can be operated by the organization, a third party, or a combination of the two, at the customer's location or offsite. Healthcare organizations, especially larger ones, may choose this option due to the need for patient information security or if sensitive research is being conducted.

2. **Community cloud**—This cloud is supported for use by a "community" of users who share some trait, such as security needs, in common. One or more of the community may own and operate the cloud, or it may be operated by a third party or a combination of the two. A healthcare example of a community cloud might be the data infrastructure needed for an accountable care organization or that required by an HI exchange.

3. **Public cloud**—This cloud is open to the general public and owned by an academic institution, the government, or some other organization for the benefit of the public. As previously, the owner or a third party or some combination thereof can operate it, at any location.

4. **Hybrid cloud**—This consists of two totally separate cloud infrastructures (private, community, or public) that are unique but share standardized or proprietary technology facilitating data and application portability (Mell and Grance 2014).

Everything discussed to this point lays the foundation of cloud computing so potential consumers can understand their options, as well as what cloud service vendors are offering. In essence, this is the beginning of standards related to cloud computing. The following are benefits of cloud computing:

- ⊙ Scalability—the ability to use multiple servers and increase or decrease usage very quickly
- ⊙ Preconfigured OS images—including both Linux- and Windows-based servers
- ⊙ Virtual servers or physical servers—can be sized according to need with between one and four cores and one and four processors in a fault-tolerant RAID (redundant array of independent disks) configuration
- ⊙ Dedicated IP addresses—for cloud servers
- ⊙ Communication—extremely fast and without charge between services in the same cloud
- ⊙ Replication and distribution—for continuity or access over different geographic regions
- ⊙ Persistence—optional if a virtual server is used and it is shut down (Sarna 2010, 19)

One use of the cloud in healthcare is in the form of web-based EHRs. Providers access their cloud-based EHR applications via the Internet. This means that the hospitals and other facilities do not have to buy servers and storage. The provider may either purchase access to an EHR application or be able to access the application for free. One researcher conducted a case study on a cloud-based EHR that can be used for free with the standard advertising found in many free information services, or for a fee, without the advertising. This EHR also sells deidentified data as a part of the revenue stream, while maintaining their offerings in their own private cloud in order to comply with the privacy and security regulations in the Health Insurance Portability and Accountability Act (HIPAA) (Sarna 2010, 275–280). It is important to note several caveats not called out in this case study. Healthcare providers using this "free" EHR would need to understand how the vendor may or may not be in compliance with separate privacy and security laws in the provider's location. For example, some states have stricter security requirements or restrict the sale of even deidentified data. It is the responsibility of the provider to comply with laws that apply to them. Additionally, the provider would need to ensure that they will have access to the data should it be needed for legal purposes. In the case of pediatric records this can be a very long time, up to 20 or 21 years in the case of newborn records depending on the statute of limitations for the state (McWay 2016, 168).

Thus, when exploring cloud computing for a healthcare organization, several considerations must be investigated:

1. **Cost of ownership**—Using cloud computing can be more cost effective than maintaining a server onsite. Additional savings may be realized by reducing the number of employees and contractors needed for server maintenance, legacy system conversions, and upgrades.

2. **Dependability**—Cloud computing providers are dependable. They are up and running 24 hours a day, 7 days a week, every day of the year, which ensures access to much-needed items such as business applications, financial data, and help desk personnel. These providers also provide backup solutions, which relieve the facility of this chore and ensure business continuity in the case of a natural disaster such as a tornado, fire, or flood. Conversely, because the cloud is Internet-based, any disturbance that causes loss of Internet access will impact the system by disrupting connectivity. To keep the business running, redundant wireless hot points, leased lines, and fiber optics are recommended. Loss of Internet can come from malicious attacks by hackers or other sources. The cloud providers assist in this area by providing firewalls, which are protective boundaries between an intranet and the Internet that prevent unauthorized access from outside by filtering all incoming messages.

3. **Scalability**—Cloud systems can grow with the demands of the facility, which provides scalability for the business. This can be very important to companies that rely on web-based billing or sales for revenue. For example, if the size of the healthcare billing processing grows by 10 percent, due to the addition of additional outpatient services, then the cloud architecture would seamlessly provide additional computing power, storage, networking, and so on. Compare this to the amount of time, money, and meetings that would be required to plan a similar addition to resources if the healthcare facility had to add the resources themselves (that is, additional servers and PCs, extra networking, more software, and personnel to maintain the additional resources).

4. **Mobility**—Data streaming from the cloud allows for greater mobility because the Internet is accessible from multiple mobile devices, such as smart phones and tablets, PDAs, virtual desktops, or traditional laptops or PCs. For example, the CIO could work on his MS Excel report from home on his iPad by accessing data from the hospital's EHR system. When completed the report could be put into MS PowerPoint slides and presented through the cloud by using Internet meeting software.

5. **Future-proofing**—Computer hardware, software, and networking solutions begin their move toward obsolescence almost as soon as they are implemented, which can be costly. Cloud computing moves the cost of updating certain parts of the technology from the customer to the cloud provider, a substantial benefit given the rapid pace of the growth of Internet and other technologies.

6. **Security**—The security of the cloud application is paramount for healthcare providers to be able to ensure the privacy of individually identifiable healthcare data. Cloud computing service companies working with providers and others would be subject to all aspects of the HIPAA Privacy and Security Rules (Bellamy 2011).

A related issue is that the prevalence of cloud computing has created complex security management scenarios resulting from the challenges of maintaining interoperability between the various security, hardware, and software architectures present in the company's internal business systems, their distributed systems, their cloud system, or their cloud vendors' systems (Harvey and Harvey 2014). Cloud systems have complex architectures, which makes them challenging to maintain and secure. Information governance is problematic due to the diversity of the systems composing the cloud architecture and the fact that many of these systems are under the cloud vendor's control, and thus not subject to the same security and incident response policies as the healthcare facility who contracts their services (HIMSS 2015). Although the cloud provider is being paid by the healthcare entity, the entity must formally request that the cloud provider make changes in their security policies, procedures, interfaces, architectures, or protocols. Special consideration should be given to the details of this request for change process when the facility enters into the contract with their cloud vendor.

Many cloud services are accessed via the Internet. This exposes the cloud vendor's application interfaces and the users' cloud access software interfaces to hackers. In particular, risk exposure is created when syncing with the cloud provider to send the healthcare user's authentication information across the Internet for login. Automated electronic data transmission should be utilized when possible to provide standardized data transmissions packets. Because mobile devices are often used to access cloud servers, to mitigate the security risk the NIST suggests that a healthcare entities' mobile device security policy be the same as the organization's security policy with respect to system security, administration, and access restrictions. Mobile devices should have a customized security threat model in place due to the high level of risk presented by these devices. Indeed, the overall goal is to have one security architecture that can be used in all the healthcare facilities' systems because this facilitates the maintenance of security between these diverse systems.

Given that cloud computing, especially in the healthcare industry, is still very new, there are aspects that remain untested or still in development. These include issues very important to healthcare such as easy access to encrypted data (required for HIPAA compliance), as well as discoverability for legal purposes (Anthes 2010). For example, there is little legal precedent if the cloud provider is located within the United States, but the data center is in a different country or if the data is subpoenaed from the cloud provider instead of the healthcare provider (Anthes

2010). The bottom line for cloud computing in healthcare is the same as for all new technologies used in healthcare—users need to thoroughly investigate the pros and cons, seeking to protect patients and the organization, while maximizing productivity and efficiency.

Case Study: Bring Your Own Device

The IT company CDW provides healthcare and business IT solutions across North America. In the past, CDW employees primarily used Blackberrys, which simplified mobile device management. Increasingly employees were using a variety of mobile devices such as Android and Apple iOS smart phones. Some employee devices used were provided by the company and some were the employee's own devices that they brought in to use for work as part of the Bring Your Own Device (BYOD) program. In both cases, employees were required to have their device inspected and tested by the CDW security team. Many employees found that their devices were not supported so they were being denied network access, while those with approved devices were frustrated with the lengthy testing and approval process required.

CDW needed to provide employees with a more flexible BYOD program while still controlling all mobile devices in use at the company. After researching the choices, the company tested and adopted IBM's cloud-based enterprise mobile management software called MaaS360. This software's portal facilitated enrolling all the devices used at the company and increased the employees' BYOD device choices. Another benefit was that the employee could quickly self-check and self-enroll their mobile devices in two hours. Once enrolled, a mobile device's compliance with password and encryption policies could be monitored, device information could be remotely deleted to prevent theft, and the device location could be tracked. The company saved valuable IT time and the employees had a much smoother system for mobile device enrollment and security compliance monitoring.

(Case study adapted from Fiberlink, IBM 2016)

Chapter 4 Review Exercises

Answer the following questions.

1. The software and hardware services that form a bridge between applications are called
   a. Middleware
   b. Decentralized
   c. Fault tolerant
   d. Scalable

2. A type of systems architecture that has business rules on an application server is
   a. Two-tiered
   b. Client-server
   c. Three-tiered
   d. VPN

3. A distributed system that is seen by the end user as a single machine is said to be
   a. Shared
   b. Centralized
   c. Transparent
   d. Single processor

4. Which of the following describes the cloud service models where users interact with the service provider's applications from a web browser or client application without the customer having to buy the server or software license?
   a. Software as a service
   b. Platform as a service
   c. Infrastructure as a service
   d. Measured service

5. Which is not a reason that mobile devices are hard to secure?
   a. They have complex architectures
   b. Different security protocols are used in these systems
   c. They are accessed via the Internet
   d. They all use standard software

Discussion.

6. Give an example of four types of distributed systems and discuss the goals of a distributed system.

7. What are the differences between two- and three-tiered network architectures?

8. Give one example of middleware in healthcare and discuss the purpose of middleware.

9. Compare design models of distributed systems with respect to functionality.

10. Describe the development process of a distributed system.

11. Compare and contrast three major cloud computing systems.

REFERENCES

AHIMA. 2014. Health Data Analysis Toolkit. http://bok.ahima.org/PdfView?oid =107504.

AHIMA. 2014. *Pocket Glossary of Health Information Management and Technology.* 4th ed. Chicago, Illinois: AHIMA Press.

AHIMA. 2012. *Pocket Glossary of Health Information Management and Technology.* 3rd ed. Chicago, Illinois. AHIMA Press.

AHIMA e-HIM Workgroup: Best Practices for Electronic Signature and Attestation. (2009). Electronic signature, attestation, and authorship (Updated). *Journal of AHIMA, 80*(11) (November–December 2009: expanded online edition). http://library.ahima.org/xpedio /groups/public/documents/ahima/bok1_045551.hcsp?dDocName=bok1_045551.

Alkoshman, M.M. 2015. Unified modeling language and enhanced entity relationship: An empirical study. *International Journal of Database Theory and Application* 8(3):215–227.

Amatayakul, M. 2013. *Electronic Health Records: A Practical Guide for Professionals and Organizations.* 4th ed. Chicago, IL: American Health Information Management Association.

Andersen, P., A.M. Lindgaard, M. Prgomet, N. Creswick, and J.I. Westbrook. 2009. Mobile and fixed computer use by doctors and nurses on hospital wards: Multi-method study on the relationships between clinician role, clinical task, and device choice. *Journal of Medical Internet Research* 11(3):e32. doi: 10.2196/jmir.1221.

Campbell, R.J. 2004. Database design: What HIM professionals need to know. *Perspectives in Health Information Management* 1(6). http://library.ahima.org/xpedio /groups/public/documents/ahima/bok1_024637.hcsp?dDocName=bok1_024637.

Centers for Disease Control and Prevention. 2015. Healthcare-associated infections (HAIs). http://www.cdc.gov/hai/prevent/prevention.html.

Department of Health and Human Service, U. S. Food and Drug Administration. 2016. http://www.fda.gov/.

Department of Health and Human Services. 2015. Breaches affecting 500 or more individuals. https://ocrportal.hhs.gov/ocr/breach/breach_report.jsf.

Department of Health and Human Services. 2014. Annual report to Congress on breaches of unsecured protected health information for calendar years 2011 and 2012. https://www.hhs.gov/sites/default/files/ocr/privacy/hipaa/administrative /breachnotificationrule/breachreport2011-2012.pdf.

Department of Health and Human Services. 2006. HIPAA security guidance. http://www .hhs.gov/hipaa/for-professionals/security/guidance/.

Elliman, T., T. Hatzakis, and A. Serrano. 2008. Business Process Simulation: An Alternative Modeling Technique for the Information System Development Process. In *Innovations in Information Systems Modeling: Methods and Best Practices (Advances in Database Research).* Edited by Halpin, T., J. Krogstie, and E. Proper, 240–253. Information Science Reference. Hershey: PA: IGI Global.

Fiberlink, IBM. 2016. CDW Expands BYOD Program and Trims IT Support Time with MaaS360. https://static.ibmserviceengage.com/cs_maas360_mdm_CDW.pdf

Florida Center for Instructional Technology. 2013. *An Educator's Guide to School Networks.* University of South Florida. http://fcit.usf.edu/network/.

Halpin, T., J. Krogstie, and E. Proper, eds. 2008. *Innovations in Information Systems Modeling: Methods and Best Practices (Advances in Database Research).* Hershey: Information Science Reference.

Harvey, M.J., and Harvey, M.G. 2014. Privacy and security issues for mobile health platforms. *Journal of the Association for Information Science and Technology* 65(7):1305–1318. http://doi.org/10.1002/asi.23066.

HIMSS. 2011. Security of mobile computing devices in the healthcare environment. http://www.himss.org/ResourceLibrary/ResourceDetail.aspx?ItemNumber=10737.

International Standards Organization. 2016. ISO 9000—Quality Management. http://www.iso.org/iso/home/standards/management-standards/iso_9000.htm.

Kart, F., G. Miao, L.E. Moser, and P.M. Melliar-Smith. 2007. A Distributed e-Health System Based on the Service Oriented Architecture. Salt Lake City: IEEE International Conference on Services Computing.

Kim, Y., and M. Glassman. 2013. Beyond search and communication: Development and validation of the Internet self-efficacy scale (ISS). *Computers in Human Behavior* 29(4):1421–1429. http://doi.org/10.1016/j.chb.2013.01.018.

Kuan-Li, P., and H. Chin-Yu. 2014. Reliability evaluation of service-oriented architecture systems considering fault-tolerance designs. *Journal of Applied Mathematics* 1–11.

Lamport, L. 2001. Paxos made simple. *ACM SIGACT News* 32(2):18–25.

LeBlanc, M. 2016. Human Resources Management. Chapter 23 in *Health Information Management Concepts Principles, and Practices.* 5th ed. Edited by P. Oachs and A. Watters. Chicago, IL: AHIMA Press.

Mao, Y., F. Junqueira, and K. Marzullo. 2008. Mencius: Building Efficient Replicated State Machines for WANs. OSDI '08 Proceedings of the 8th USENIX conference on Operating Systems design and implementation, 369–384. Berkeley, CA.

McWay, D.C. 2016. *Legal and Ethical Aspects of Health Information Management.* 4th ed. Clifton Park, NY: Cengage Learning.

Mell, P., and T. Grance. 2011. *The NIST Definition of Cloud Computing.* National Institute of Standards. http://www.nist.gov/itl/csd/cloud-102511.cfm.

Microsoft Corp. 2016. What is a firewall? https://www.microsoft.com/en-us/safety/pc-security/firewalls-whatis.aspx.

Microsoft Corp. 2015a. *Chapter 2—Architectural Overview of the TCP/IP Protocol Suite.* https://technet.microsoft.com/en-us/library/bb726983.aspx.

Microsoft Corp. 2015b. *File Transfer Protocol (FTP): Frequently asked questions.* http://windows.microsoft.com/en-us/windows-vista/file-transfer-protocol-ftp-frequently-asked-questions.

Microsoft Corp. 2005. The TCP/IP model: TCP/IP. https://technet.microsoft.com/en-us/library/cc786900(v=ws.10).aspx.

Object Modeling Group Inc. 2005. Introduction to OMG UML. http://www.omg.org/gettingstarted/what_is_uml.htm.

Office of Disease Prevention and Promotion. 2015. National action plan to prevent health care-associated infections: Road map to elimination. http://health.gov/hcq/prevent-hai.asp.

Oscar, R. 2013. Using mobile technology to improve health-plan utilization and cut costs. *Employment Relations Today* 40(2):21–27.

PC Connection. 2016. Mobile Point of Care. http://www.govconnection.com/IPA/PM /Solutions/Healthcare/MPOC/ComputeronWheels.htm.

PC Magazine. 2015. Encyclopedia: Communication Protocols. http://www.pcmag.com /encyclopedia/term/40079/communications-protocol.

Pironti, J. 2006. May. Key elements of a threat and vulnerability management program. *Information Systems Audit and Control Association Member Journal.* http://www .iparchitects.com/wp-content/uploads/Key-Elements-of-a-Threat-and-Vulnerability -Management-Program-ISACA-Member-Journal-May-2006.pdf.

Reynolds, R.B. and M. Sharp. 2016. Health Record Content and Documentation. Chapter 4 in *Health Information Management Concepts Principles, and Practices.* 5th ed. Edited by P. Oachs and A. Watters. Chicago, IL: AHIMA Press.

Rodríguez, G., Á. Soria, and M. Campo. 2016. Artificial intelligence in service-oriented software design. *Engineering Applications of Artificial Intelligence* 53:86–104. doi: 10.1016/j.engappai.2016.03.009.

Saint, S., M.T. Greene, L. Damschroder, and S.L. Krein. 2013. Is the use of antimicrobial devices to prevent infection correlated across different healthcare-associated infections? Results from a national survey. *Infection Control and Hospital Epidemiology* 34(8):847–849. doi: 10.1086/671269.

Sandefer, R. 2016. Health Information Technologies. Chapter 12 in *Health Information Management Concepts Principles, and Practices.* 5th ed. Edited by P. Oachs and A. Watters. Chicago, IL: AHIMA Press.

Sarna, D.E.Y. 2010. *Implementing and Developing Cloud Computing Applications.* New York: Auerbach Publications.

Sayles, N.B., and Trawick, K.C. 2014. *Introduction to Computer Systems for Health Information Technology.* Chicago, IL: AHIMA Press.

Scarfone, K., M. Souppaya, and M. Sexton. 2007. Guide to storage encryption technologies for end user devices. *NIST Special Publication, 800.* http://nvlpubs.nist .gov/nistpubs/Legacy/SP/nistspecialpublication800-111.pdf.

Tanenbaum, A. S. and M. Van Steen. 2007. *Distributed Systems: Principles and Paradigms,* 2nd Ed. Amsterdam: Pearson.

Stirna, J. and A. Persson. 2008. EKD: An Enterprise Modeling Approach to Support Creativity and Quality in Information Systems and Business Development. In *Innovations in Information Systems Modeling: Methods and Best Practices (Advances in Database Research).* Edited by Halpin, T., J. Krogstie, and E. Proper, 68–88. Hershey: Information Science Reference. Hershey: IGI Global.

Thomas, G. 2007. Secure mobile device use in healthcare guidance from HIPAA and ISO17799. *Information Systems Management* 24(4):333–342. http://doi.org/10.1080 /10580530701586060.

US Food and Drug Administration. 2007. Draft Guidance for Industry and FDA Staff— Premarket Notification [510(k)] Submissions for Medical Devices that Include Antimicrobial Agents. http://www.fda.gov/MedicalDevices/DeviceRegulation andGuidance/GuidanceDocuments/ucm071380.ht.

Ventola, C.L. 2014, May. Mobile devices and apps for health care professionals: Uses and benefits. *P.T.* 30 (5):356–364.

Wager, K.A., F.W. Lee, and J.P. Glaser. 2009. *Healthcare Information Systems: A Practical Approach for Health Management*. 2nd ed. San Francisco: Jossey-Bass.

Zhao, J., P.O. de Pablos, and Z. Qi. 2012. Enterprise knowledge management model based on China's practice and case study. *Computers in Human Behavior* 28(2):324–330. doi: 10.1016/j.chb.2011.10.001.

ADDITIONAL RESOURCES

45 CFR 164.526 (**e**): Amendment of protected health information (2014).

Abdelhak, M., S. Grostick, and M.A. Hanken. 2012. *Health Information Management of a Strategic Resource*, 4th ed. St. Louis: Saunders.

Anderson, H. 2011. EHRs and Cloud Computing. InfoRiskToday. http://www .inforisktoday.com/interviews/ehrs-cloud-computing-i-1016.

Anthes, G. 2010. Security in the cloud. *Communications of the ACM* 53(11):16–18. http:// cacm.acm.org/magazines/2010/11/100630-security-in-the-cloud/abstract.

Bardram, J., and H. Christensen. 2007. Pervasive computing support for hospitals: An overview of the activity-based computing project. *Pervasive Computing, IEEE* 6(1): 44–51.

Bellamy, S. 2011. Is cloud computing for you? Five points to consider. *Computer World*. http://www.computerworld.com/s/article/9222249/Is_Cloud_Computing_for_You _Five_Points_to_Consider?taxonomyId=158andpageNumber=1.

Centers for Disease Control and Prevention. 2014. National and State Healthcare Associated Infections Progress Report. http://www.cdc.gov/HAI/pdfs/progress -report/hai-progress-report.pdf.

Davis, Z. 2011. Network operating system. *PCmag.com*.

Dean, T. 2009. Network operating systems. *Network+ Guide to Networks*. 421(483).

Emmerich, W. 1997. Distributed Systems Principles. http://www.cs.ucl.ac.uk/staff /ucacwxe/lectures/ds98-99/dsee3.pdf.

Glandon, L., D. Smaltz, and D. Slovensky. 2010. *Information Systems for Healthcare Management*. Chicago: Health Administration Press.

Gruman, G. 2008. What cloud computing really means. *InfoWorld*. http://www.infoworld .com/d/cloud-computing/what-cloud-computing-really-means-031.

Halpin, T. 2009. Object-Role Modeling. In *Encyclopedia of Database Systems*, Edited by Liu, L. and M. Tamer Ozsu. New York: Springer.

HIMSS. (2015). Cloud Computing Toolkit: Cloud Computing Privacy and Security 101. http://www.himss.org/cloud-computing-privacy-and-security-101?Item Number=10540.

Hugos, M., and D. Hulitzky. 2011. *Business in the Cloud*. Hoboken: Wiley.

Institute of Electrical and Electronics Engineers Inc. (IEEE). *IEEE 802.11TM Wireless Local Area Networks: The Working Group for WLAN*. http://www.ieee802.org/11/.

Keidar, I. 2008. Distributed computing column 34—Distributed computing in the clouds. *ACM SIGACT News* 39(4):53–54. doi:10.1145/1466390.1466402.

Schmidt, D. 2008. Software technologies for developing distributed systems: Objects and beyond. *Computer Society of India Communications*, 30–37. Special Issue on OO Technologies. Edited by Jana, D.

Simon, P. 2010. *The Next Wave of Technologies.* Hoboken: Wiley.

Thalheim, B. 2011. The Enhanced Entity-Relationship Model. In *Handbook of Conceptual Modeling*, Edited by Embley, D.W. and B. Thalheim, 165–206. Berlin Heidelberg: Springer.

Watfa, M. 2012. *E-healthcare Systems and Wireless Communications: Current and Future Challenges.* Hershey: IGI Global.

W3C Working Group. 2004, February. Group Note 11: Web Services Architecture. www.w3.org/TR/2004/NOTE-ws-arch-20040211/.

Data and Information

Learning Objectives

- Describe the types of data, as well as the relationship between data and information
- Practice using health information standards
- Create a data map for a given scenario
- Compare and contrast the methods of data collection
- Demonstrate the use of data quality practices
- Design appropriate data presentations
- Support and evaluate EHRs, HIEs, and RECs

KEY TERMS

Ad hoc standards
American National Standards Institute (ANSI)
Binary
Categorical data
Certification
Certification Commission for Health Information Technology (CCHIT)
Characteristics of data quality
Classification system
Code set
Concept

Concept identification
Consensus standards
Continuous data
Crosstabs
Data
Data cleaning
Data governance
Data mapping
Data Quality Management Model
Data set standard
Data standards
Data-interchange standard

De facto standards
Descriptive statistics
Discrete data
Equivalence
Expressivity
Forward map
Frequency
Government mandate
Health Information Technology for
   Economic and Clinical Health
   (HITECH) Act
Health Insurance Portability and
   Accountability Act (HIPAA) of 1996
Health IT Policy Committee
Health IT Standards Committee
Imputation
International Organization for
   Standardization (ISO)
Interval data
Narrative-text string
National Institute of Standards and
   Technology (NIST)

Natural language processing (NLP)
Negation
Nominal data
ONC-Authorized Testing and
   Certification Bodies
Ordinal data
Post-hoc text processing
Ratio data
Raw data
Reverse map
Semantic interoperability
Source
Standards development organizations
   (SDOs)
Structured data
Target
Temporal
Terminology
Transaction set
Transaction standard
Unstructured data entry
Vital statistics

Data and information are the resources that fuel the healthcare industry. Getting the right data or information to the right person at the right time is essential for the delivery of high-quality care as well as the financial well-being of healthcare provider organizations. Data can be entered into electronic health records (EHRs) to be used for clinical care, disease management, or disease prevention. They are also found in large data sets or data warehouses where clinicians, researchers, payers, and others access the data for a variety of purposes.

It is imperative that health informaticists understand the basics of data, the relevant data standards, issues involved with data collection, how to ensure the quality of the data, as well as concerns related to the analysis and presentation of data.

⊙ The Basics of Data

Data are the "dates, numbers, images, symbols, letters, and words that represent basic facts and observations about people, processes, measurements, and conditions" (AHIMA 2014b, 42). The term datum can be used as a singular noun to refer to specific bits of information. The term data is used as the plural noun in reference to many bits of information. Examples of singular datum include the patient's address, a single laboratory result, one blood pressure reading, the charge for one day in the hospital, and so on. Examples of plural data can include the entire set of entries for a single patient in the EHR or data sets such as the National Center for Health

Figure 5.1. Examples of singular and plural data

<u>**Singular data examples**</u>
Patient address: 123 Any Street, City, ST 10000
Hemoglobin level: 12.6 grams per deciliter
Blood pressure: 120/80 mm Hg
Room charge: $650 per day

<u>**Plural data examples**</u>
National Center for Health Statistics' National Hospital
Discharge Data Set, http://www.cdc.gov/nchs/nhds.htm
Centers for Medicare and Medicaid Services Medicare Provider Analysis and Review
File (MEDPAR), https://www.cms.gov/Research-Statistics-Data-and-Systems/
Statistics-Trends-and-Reports/MedicareFeeforSvcPartsAB/MEDPAR.html

Statistics' (NCHS) National Hospital Discharge Data Set (NHDDS), or all of the claims data in the Centers for Medicare and Medicaid Services (CMS) (see figure 5.1).

Data Related to Information

Although data are important, it is often difficult to utilize them effectively even for a single patient unless they are processed into information. So, how does the health informaticist get from individual data elements to information that can be used effectively and efficiently? Foremost is an understanding of the original purpose for which the data are used or collected. For example, data that are collected for clinical purposes may be, and often are, very different from data that are collected for reimbursement or research purposes. Clinical data are often very detailed, for instance, vital signs can be collected every 15 minutes in the intensive care unit (ICU), while the reimbursement data for the same patient will only include the more general diagnostic code. It is important to consider whether there are mandated or generally accepted **data standards** for the data. Data standards may be related to the data set, such as the data elements specified for the Uniform Hospital Discharge Data Set, or the allowable data values, such as a selection list being provided for the address data element of State. Standards such as the allowable data elements within a data set, the definitions of the different data elements, or the allowable data values, which constrain the data that can be entered into a field, ensure that the data is as accurate as possible. Another data standard is the NLM Value Set Authority Center (VSAC) from the US National Library of Medicine, in collaboration with the Office of the National Coordinator for Health Information Technology and the Centers for Medicare and Medicaid Services. The VSAC provides data on the 2014 Clinical Quality Measures (NLM 2016).

An additional consideration is the data collection method that was utilized. There are many different methods of data collection, such as keyboard, voice recognition, and automated methods, where data are transferred directly from digital thermometers, scales, blood pressure cuffs, and so on. The quality of the data must be assessed. It is difficult to produce good quality information when

Figure 5.2. Examples of data presentation

PATIENT X Cholesterol (normal is less than 200)

Date	Cholesterol level
January 2017	153
February 2017	168
March 2017	160
April 2017	174
May 2017	168
June 2017	181

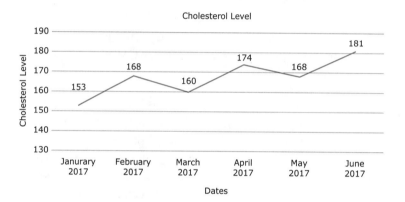

the data itself are of poor quality. It is also vital to understand the analysis that the data are intended to undergo or the analysis that was used to develop or produce the information. Finally, it is important to present the data so that it can be easily understood. Figure 5.2 presents total cholesterol levels for a patient in two different forms, tabular and graphical. It is generally easier to detect the rise of this patient's cholesterol levels using the graphical representation. Figure 5.3 presents these issues in the form of questions health informaticists can pose while they are working with data.

These and other concerns are important to address in order to ensure the data and information used in healthcare can be relied upon for all of the varied purposes. This chapter will examine these different aspects of data that are important to the production of information.

Data Format

Data collected for an electronic health record starts the data format life cycle as raw data. **Raw data** is an unformatted combination of text, symbols, and words. Data on patient names, diagnoses, admission, and healthcare payer typed into an Excel workbook would be considered raw data. Data that the user entered into a

Figure 5.3. Understanding data and information

Questions to Ask about the Data or Information

1. For which purpose or use was the data originally collected?
2. Are there any data standards related to the data?
3. How was the data collected?
4. What is the quality of the data?
5. How will the data be analyzed to produce information?
6. How can the data or information be presented so that it is meaningful to users?

webpage for electronic transmission to the electronic health records database is another example of raw data.

One example of raw data would be a comma delimited text string representing a patient's first name, last name, middle initial, and date of admission that was entered into a web-based form. For example, comma delimited text for these fields would be: "Green, Sue, A., Blue Cross, 02/12/15" This data would be transmitted by the webpage to a remote database where the data would be parsed by built-in database functions and user-generated database program code (such as Oracle SQL code). The data would then be imported into the correct database tables and become a formatted database field. Specifically, the text string "Green, Sue, A." would be broken apart and the portions delimited by the commas would be sent to three database table fields, which are last name (Green), first name (Sue), and middle initial (A.). Figure 5.4 presents the raw data transmission from text to webpage display and then to storage in the database table fields.

In general, a database field is one column in a database table that contains one type of information and is constrained by the field definitions. Field definitions

Figure 5.4. Raw data transmission

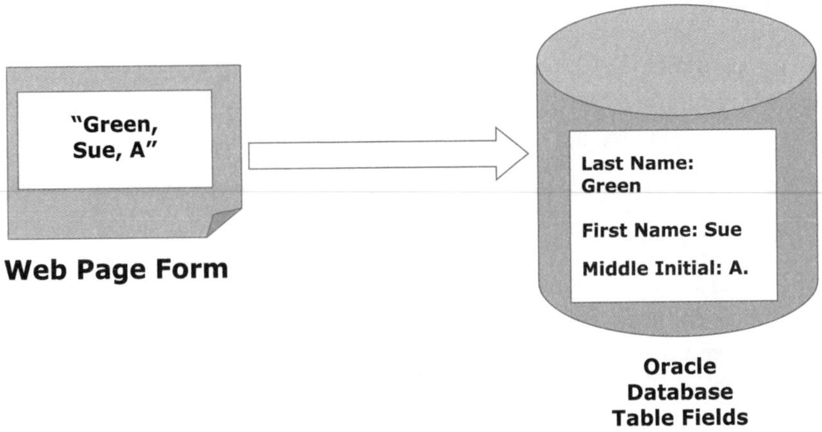

"Green, Sue, A"

Web Page Form

Last Name: Green

First Name: Sue

Middle Initial: A.

Oracle Database Table Fields

vary by database manufacture but most include constraints for what can be stored in the field that include allowable data formats, size of field, presence of index on the field, and whether or not the field is required. Users can also request that edit checks be added such as "must be < 10 mm." When the data are programmatically inserted into the database table field the database will automatically check to see if these constraints are violated. As an example, if a very long last name was inserted into a LAST_NAME field with field size of 25 then a warning would be issued. If the import program fails to check for the database's warning, results will vary but it many cases the last name would be truncated resulting in potential patient identification errors. Similarly, failing to insert data into a required field would generate a database error.

Next, the payer would be stored in a text field. To finish, the date of 02/12/15 would be placed in the data of admission field and reformatted to use the default date format set for that table such as MM/DD/YYYY. Allowable data types vary by database vendor and are discussed in the database vendors' documentation. Typical data types are character (variable, fixed length), number (float, integer, binary, and such), date, time, Boolean (which is a 1 or a 0), currency, XML, and **binary,** which is used to store graphs, text, video, and sound (Oracle 2015). A typical import error arises when the import codes erroneously attempt to insert data that are not a date into a field formatted as a date field. This data would not be inserted and the import program would receive an error code that can be explored by looking up the code in the database vendors' documentation.

Once all the data have been inserted into the database, it is common to run various reports to assess the number of admissions, diagnoses, payers, length of stay, and charges. The outputs of these reports provide useful information to healthcare managers, planners, coders, and researchers. Data that are present on these reports have been processed for meaningful use and are now in the form of information available for decision making.

⊙ Data Standards

Standards permeate our lives to the point where they are ubiquitous. Automobile travel would not be possible if there were no standards for the width of cars and trucks or highways. Data standards are necessary to support interoperable healthcare systems (González-Ferrer and Peleg 2015). This section will explore the healthcare data standards development process, as well as discuss the different types of standards needed to support health information for the healthcare industry.

Standards Development

One of the challenges encountered when working with healthcare data standards is understanding the process by which the standards are developed. However, it is not uncommon for informaticists to be asked to assist in the development of standards or policies and practices related to standards implementation and use. The four basic methods of standards development are ad hoc, de facto, government mandate,

Table 5.1.   Standards development methods

Standard Development Method	Definition	Example
Ad hoc	Agreed upon by a group of stakeholders with no formal adoption process.	The Logical Observation Identifiers, Names, and Codes (LOINC) and Digital Imaging and Communications in Medicine (DICOM) standards were developed using the ad hoc method by groups of interested experts.
De facto	A standard that evolves over time due to widespread, nonmandated adoption.	The Microsoft Windows operating system is a de facto standard due to its widespread adoption.
Government mandate	The government either develops the standards or specifies a certain standard be used for a purpose.	The code sets mandated by the government under the Health Insurance Portability and Accountability Act provisions are an example of governmentally mandated standards.
Consensus	Standards developed when stakeholders come together to reach formal agreement on the specifications.	Health Level 7 standards, developed by the HL7 organization and its members, are an example of consensus standards.

Source: Adapted from Hammond and Cimino 2001, 215–216.

and consensus. These four methods of standards development are not mutually exclusive. For example, there are many standards that were developed using the consensus method, which are now either de facto or governmentally mandated standards. Table 5.1 outlines the different methods and provides an example of each type of standard.

Whichever of these development methods is used, there are steps required for standards development. There are many different **standards development organizations (SDOs)** involved in creating and maintaining healthcare standards. The internationally recognized standards development body is the **International Organization for Standardization (ISO).** The United States representative to the ISO is the **American National Standards Institute (ANSI).** In order to promulgate a recognized standard, SDOs must be accredited by ANSI and, if applicable, the ISO. The ISO outlines a six-step standards development process:

1. Proposal—This is the stage in the process where there is a recognized need for a new standard. The stakeholders involved often vote or otherwise agree to the need for a new standard.

2. Preparatory—In this stage, a group of experts develops a draft of the proposed standard.

3. Committee—The original draft is reviewed and revised by the full committee of stakeholders until consensus is reached regarding the new standard.

4. Enquiry—The proposed standard is circulated throughout the entire organization for review and approval as a final draft standard.

5. Approval—The final draft standard is voted on again. At this stage, no substantive changes are allowed.

6. Publication—The standard is published with only minor editorial changes made if needed (ISO 2013).

Each standards development organization has its own process. For example, the Health Level Seven (HL7) organization outlines its standards development processes in its Governance and Operations Manual. The manual is very detailed, including guidance for the development of workgroups, as well as information gathering, balloting procedures for standards, and much more information (HL7 2013). Standards that are developed within a single organization may often undergo a much less formal process.

US Health Information Technology Standards

The Health Information Technology for Economic and Clinical Health (HITECH) Act enacted as part of the American Recovery and Reinvestment Act (ARRA) of 2009 established the **Health IT Standards Committee**, an official federal advisory committee (US Government 2009). The Health IT Standards Committee is "charged with making recommendations to the National Coordinator for Health IT on standards, implementation specifications, and certification criteria for the electronic exchange and use of health information" (HHS 2013).

Representatives on the Health IT Standards Committee come from across the healthcare industry and bring a variety of stakeholder viewpoints to the standards designation process. The Health IT Standards Committee has divided their work into different categories including Clinical Operations, Clinical Quality, Privacy and Security, and Implementation, among others (HHS 2010). The HIT Standards Committee assesses the policy recommendations of the **Health IT Policy Committee,** another federal advisory committee established under HITECH, and determines whether standards, implementation guidance or other assistance is needed for the healthcare industry (HHS 2012). Past, present, and future recommendations of the Health IT Standards Committee include standards for EHR certification for CMS's EHR meaningful use incentive program, as well as recommendations related to privacy and security, digital certificates, and so on (HHS 2012).

Prior to the HITECH Act, the majority of governmentally mandated health information technology standards were specified as a part of the **Health Insurance**

Portability and Accountability Act (HIPAA) of 1996. These standards included the Privacy Rule, the Security Rule, Transaction and Code Sets, as well as a provision for a National Provider Identifier (HIPAA 1996). Aside from the focus on privacy and security, the HIPAA standards were largely administrative in nature, supporting the efficient processing of claims to insurance companies and government payers for reimbursement. The increasing use of governmentally mandated standards serves to bring added complexity to healthcare data, while at the same time ensuring it is interchangeable and comparable.

Data Set Standards

One of the oldest types of data standards found in healthcare is the **data set standard.** An early example of the use of data set standards can be found in the London Bills of Mortality, which is an analysis of London's weekly mortality lists to generate mortality rates and life expectancy predictions (Graunt 1665). Data set standards have historically been established to assist in the tracking and understanding of important events such as births, deaths, hospital discharges, and so on. The United States considers events such as birth and death to be important enough that the data are designated as **vital statistics,** which are "data related to births, deaths, marriages and fetal deaths" (AHIMA 2014, 151).

Prior to computers, healthcare data set standards were established, usually by the government, to collect various types of data. These data set standards established the data elements or data variables to be collected and defined each data element. Medical or other records were carefully examined by clerical personnel. The data was abstracted and entered onto forms and mailed to the controlling governmental agency or entered into computer terminals and transmitted via dedicated lines. It is difficult to overstate the importance of these data sets as they often served as the foundation for public health management and other healthcare research.

Data set standards have evolved along with the information systems supporting them. Due to increased computerization, the time and money involved in establishing a new data set standard can be reduced. An example of a data set standard established because of increased availability of information systems is the ImmTrac immunization tracking registry in Texas (Texas Department of State Health Services 2010). This data set standard specifies required demographic and immunization fields, as well as preferred demographic, immunization, and provider fields (Texas Department of State Health Services 2010). Although the United States survived for many years without an immunization registry, the availability of this tool enables better management of health, healthcare, and even national defense in the face of emerging pathogens such as H1N1 or biological weapons such as anthrax.

Data set standards are foundational to healthcare information standards. They continue to evolve, now being used for quality management as with the Healthcare Effectiveness Data and Information Set (HEDIS) (Hazelwood and Venable 2016, 216) and for the continuity of patient care as with the Continuity of Care Document (CCD) (ASTM 2012). The need to collect and use explicitly defined data elements will not abate in the near future. Health informaticists should explore the different data sets standards that can meet a variety of healthcare information needs.

Classification, Code Set, and Terminology Standards

It is necessary, but not always sufficient, to have data set standards that specify and define the data elements that are collected regarding certain events. The existence of these standards supports researchers in their efforts to utilize the data and information effectively. Some data elements have such a large number of potential values that those values demand a standard themselves.

Among John Graunt's many accomplishments was that he analyzed the causes recorded for the deaths in the London Bills of Mortality (WHO 2011). This set the stage for what is now the widespread use of code sets, classification systems, and clinical terminologies. Code set is the term used by the Department of Health and Human Services (HHS) in HIPAA. HIPAA defines **code set** as "any set of codes used to encode data elements, such as tables of terms, medical concepts, medical diagnostic codes, or medical procedure codes. A code set includes the codes and the descriptors of the codes" (HIPAA 1996, 720). A **classification system** is defined as "a system that arranges or organizes like or related entities for easy retrieval" (AHIMA 2014b, 27). A **terminology** is defined as "a set of terms representing the system of concepts of a particular subject field" (AHIMA 2014b, 144). A terminology is often much more detailed than a classification system. This is because a terminology is intended to represent the details, while a classification system or code set is usually utilized to divide concepts into categories.

It is vital to have either mandated or de facto standards, whether it be a terminology or a classification system, for representing different concepts in healthcare. Both the human users and the computer processors need standards for enhanced understanding. What is a concept? At its most simple, a **concept** is an idea or "unique unit of knowledge or thought created by a unique combination of characteristics" (AHIMA 2014, 33). Concepts are not the same as words or terms. Consider, for example, the word "cold." This simple four-letter word can have many different meanings. The patient can report having a "cold." The patient can state that they feel "cold." It can be "cold" outside. If a code set, classification system, or terminology only focused on the term, the usage of any identifiers related to "cold" would soon become very confusing.

As the health information industry develops and researchers learn more about representing the complex world that is healthcare, it has become clear that it would be beneficial to have guidelines for classification and terminology standards. The most important guideline is to clearly articulate and focus the purpose of a classification or terminology (Hammond and Cimino 2001). This is not always as easy as it might seem. For example, the stated purpose for the International Classification of Diseases (ICD) was originally used for public health reporting and tracking. In the United States, ICD-10 is currently used for medical billing and coding (Pilato 2013; AHIMA 2012). For billing procedures, these codes are important to the hospitals' revenue with the ICD-10 charge codes linked to revenue codes stored in a database called a charge master, which contains both the ICD-10 codes and the procedures that map to each code (Pilato 2013).

Data Mapping

Data mapping is defined by ISO as "the process of associating concepts or terms from one coding system to concepts or terms in another coding system and defining their equivalence in accordance with a documented rationale and a given purpose" (AHIMA 2011). For the purposes of mapping, the term "coding system" is used very broadly to include classification, terminology, and other data representation systems. Mapping is necessary as the healthcare information systems and their use evolves in order to link disparate systems and data sets. This section will introduce basic mapping concepts for health informaticists.

As with coding, classification, and terminology systems, the creation of a map must begin with a clearly defined purpose for the map. Maps can be created for reimbursement, clinical care, or other purposes. It is important to note that the map created for reimbursement will be different from the clinical map, even if using the same coding or data sets. Any data map will include a source and a target. The **source** is the code or data set from which the map originates. The **target** is the code or data set in which one is attempting to find a code or data representation with an equivalent meaning. **Forward maps** are those that map from an older source code or data set to a newer target code or data set. A **reverse map** goes from a newer source code or data set to an older target code or data set. Maps must be specified as to their source, target, and direction for an understanding of the map.

The relationships in maps are often determined and defined by the purpose of the map. An example of types of map relationships could include:

- One-to-one—The one source entry has exactly one matching target entry.
- One-to-many—The one source entry has many potential target entry matches.
- No match—The source entry has no matches in the target system.

The level of equivalence can indicate the relationship between two code or data sets. **Equivalence** in a map is determined by the distribution of map relationships for a given map. For example, a map containing 50 percent one-to-one maps would have a higher level of equivalence than one containing 20 percent one-to-one maps (AHIMA 2011).

Transaction Standards

Health information **transaction standards,** also often called **data-interchange standards,** are standards for the transmission of health information data between two parties (AHIMA 2014, 146). These standards establish the means by which a sender transmits or communicates data or information to a receiver. The data required to complete a specified communication is termed a **transaction set,** which is the set of data transmitted during a transaction (Hammond and Cimino 2001, 220). These standards set out the technical format for the communication so the sender knows which data needs to be included in which format and the receiver knows which data to expect and in which format.

There are many different types of transaction standards, including X12 5010, National Council for Prescription Drug Programs (NCPDP), and the HL7 messaging standards, among others. The Accredited Standards Committee (ASC) X12 5010 standard is used by providers and insurance companies for claims processing. The NCPDP is used for e-prescribing. HL7 has a variety of standards, including their messaging standards, supporting the interchange of data between software applications and, ultimately, providers. Users should note that, though the transaction standards ensure both communicating parties understand the message type and the format, these standards do not interpret the content, nor do they constrain the use of the data on the receiving end. They are a transport mechanism only.

EHR Standards and Certification

All of the standards previously discussed are not sufficient to ensure adequate, standard, and usable EHRs. HL7 has an EHR functional model, in addition to the messaging standards already discussed. The EHR functional model has been adopted as the foundation of EHR standards. However, with no motivation or incentive to adopt standards, vendors or developers may ignore them or only adopt them in part.

In 2004, the **Certification Commission for Health Information Technology (CCHIT)** was established. CCHIT was an industry-wide initiative engaging a diverse group of stakeholders in a voluntary, consensus-based process that began certifying EHRs in 2006 (CCHIT 2015). **Certification** is "an evaluation performed to establish the extent to which a particular computer system, network design, or application implementation meets a specified set of requirements" (AHIMA 2014, 23). This proved to be a very valuable point of information for EHR purchasers, who could now determine which EHRs met the specified standards, which are always publicly available. In 2009, the certification of EHRs was codified in legislation and made a requirement for hospitals and physicians receiving payment by the CMS (US Congress 2009). The regulations implementing this section of the **Health Information Technology for Economic and Clinical Health (HITECH) Act** were extensive and incorporated many of the previously discussed standards while incorporating additional technical standards from the **National Institute of Standards and Technology (NIST)** (HHS 2010).

It is important to note that the standards and certification of the Office of the National Coordinator for Health Information Technology (ONC) are not all-encompassing and focus on the ability of a software product to enable a provider to demonstrate meaningful use of the product and qualify for payment incentives. In addition to the standards for EHR software, the legislation required the ONC to create an accreditation program to establish **ONC-Authorized Testing and Certification Bodies (ATCBs)** (HHS 2011). ATCBs are empowered to perform complete EHR or EHR module testing and certification. They utilize conformance testing requirements, test cases, and test tools developed by the NIST to determine whether the software complies with the EHR Incentive Program requirements for establishing meaningful use of an EHR. At the time this section was written, the number of EHR certification organizations had grown from one to six (HHS

2011). The ultimate goal of EHR certification to specified standards is **semantic interoperability,** that is, the ability to exchange data and information with its original meaning intact and understood by all receivers. CCHIT ceased operations in November 2014 citing fluctuating federal health IT programs rollouts as the primary reason for closure (Monegain 2014).

Check Your Understanding 5.1

Match the terms with the appropriate descriptions.

Standards Development

    a. Ad hoc
    b. Consensus
    c. Government mandate
    d. De facto

1. _____ Standards that are established by a group of stakeholders without a formal adoption process.

2. _____ Standards that have evolved over time to become universally used without a government or other mandate.

3. _____ Standards that are specified or established by the government for certain purposes.

4. _____ Standards that are developed through a formal process of comment and feedback by interested stakeholders.

Types of Standards

    a. Data set standards
    b. Classification standards
    c. Transaction standards
    d. EHR standards

5. _____ These are developed with the intent of ensuring adequate, standard, usable application software.

6. _____ Systems that arrange or organize like or related entities.

7. _____ These establish the means by which a sender transmits or communicates data or information to a receiver.

8. _____ These establish the data elements or data variables to be collected and define each data element.

Answer the following questions.

9. Which of the following standards includes the Privacy Rule, the Security Rule, Transaction and Code Sets, and provisions for a National Provider Identifier?

    a. LOINC
    b. DICOM
    c. HIPAA
    d. Health Level 7

10. Which of the following is a standard developed by consensus?
    a. LOINC
    b. DICOM
    c. HIPAA code sets
    d. Health Level 7

11. Which federal advisory board recommends standards to the National Coordinator for Health IT?
    a. HIPAA
    b. World Health Organization
    c. Health IT Standards Committee
    d. American National Standards Institute

⊙ Data Collection

The collection of healthcare data oftentimes must conform to the standards already described. Data can be entered by users via keyboard, handwriting, speech recognition, or direct feed from machines. However, data collection must also be carefully planned, keeping in mind the expected uses of the data and the needs and workflow of the users. Generally, data entry can be classified as either structured or unstructured. Figure 5.5 outlines questions that should be answered by organizations planning their EHR data collection efforts. Ultimately, the choices are usually between structured data entry, unstructured data entry, or a carefully considered combination of the two methods.

Structured Data Entry

The structured entry of healthcare data involves the use of templates and on-screen forms with the possible entry fields and the potential entries in those fields

Figure 5.5. Data collection considerations

- Why is the organization entering these data? Is it for patient care? To secure payment? To comply with a regulation?
- What data need to be entered? Is there a standard for the data?
- Who will enter the data? Will it be clinicians, nurses, ancillary staff, clerks, or a combination?
- What will be the most efficient method of data entry for each type of user?
- Under what circumstances will users enter data? Will they be rushed, or will they have adequate time? What will be the setting (admissions, emergency room, intensive care, or the patient's home)?
- What use does the organization expect to make of the data? Will they be used for patient care, reimbursement, quality improvement, or research?

Source: Fenton 2006

controlled, defined, and limited. **Structured data** can have many benefits including completeness, quality (Johnson et al. 2008), and accessibility of the data for a variety of purposes (van Mulligen et al. 1998). Structured data are often entirely appropriate and highly recommended for data entry when the options are limited or are required to conform to a specific standard. For example, the collection of race and ethnicity data is specified by the US government (US Census Bureau 2007). Although this could be a free-text field, the need to report data in conformance with the government standard has led most informaticists to limit the entries in the race and ethnicity fields. Structured data are often also highly desired for uses such as clinical decision support or quality measure reporting where false positives or false negatives could place either patients or organizations at risk (van Mulligen et al. 1998).

Structured data are not without its negative aspects. Some studies have suggested that structured data entry can slow down users, decreasing their productivity (Rosenbloom et al. 2011; Ash et al. 2007). In addition, structured data entry tools can be incomplete for user needs as well as inflexible when new or unexpected demands arise (Rosenbloom et al. 2011). Finally, structured data entry templates can be developed that insert a more complete narrative with a particular selection; however, the majority of structured data entry systems appear to be found in niche settings and specific clinical domains (Rosenbloom et al. 2011).

Unstructured Data Entry

Unstructured data entry is the use of free text or narrative data in the health record. In the paper record, a large amount of the data, especially the day-to-day progress notes, were unstructured. The clinician determines the level of detail entered and often the formatting used for the data entered in unstructured data entry. This enables the clinician to include the nuances and details that might otherwise be missed with the use of structured data entry. This is called **expressivity,** which is defined as "how well a note conveys the patient's and provider's impressions, reasoning, and thought process; level of concern; and uncertainty to those subsequently reviewing the note" (Rosenbloom et al. 2011).

The main drawback to unstructured data entry centers on the general inability to determine the completeness of the data (Fenton 2006) during the data entry process. Until methods can be developed that can assess the requirements for unstructured data relative to the document it is being used for (the type of patient, the setting of care, and such) this will remain a serious challenge when handling unstructured data.

Another challenge with unstructured data usage is the ongoing and increasing need to use the data in ways that require it to be structured. Health informaticists and linguists have been researching different methods of **post-hoc text processing,** which is using algorithms after data are entered. Some of the different methods that have been studied include searching for narrative-text strings or string patterns; concept identification or indexing; and combining concept indexing with negation or temporal algorithms to approach quite complex and sophisticated **natural language processing (NLP)** (Rosenbloom et al. 2011). NLP is "a technology that converts human language (structured or unstructured) into data that can be translated then manipulated by computer systems" (AHIMA 2014, 101). **Narrative-text string** or string pattern searches are similar to the "find" functionality used every day in software such as Microsoft Word or Adobe Reader. **Concept identification** methods map the text to standardized concepts using clinical terminologies with high levels of recall and precision (Rosenbloom et al. 2011). **Negation** and **temporal** issues are two that have proven to be obstacles for widespread use of NLP in the real-time clinical domain. Negation involves the ability of the processor to detect the differences between "no chest pain," meaning it is absent, and "chest pain," meaning it is present. Temporal means the computer can detect any time frames included when the concept is identified. For example, "past history of cancer" is very different from simply "cancer." NLP approaches vary by developer and software. Advances in the past four to five years, especially in the area of computer-based documentation systems, have been significant with expanded use, though anecdotal reports from clinical users are that NLP software can still pose challenges (Rosenbloom et al. 2011).

Whether an organization chooses structured or unstructured data entry depends upon the purpose of the data entry and the eventual uses of the data. Data entry acceptable for administrative purposes may not be adequate for clinical processes. Organizations must carefully investigate data entry when considering an EHR. Ultimately, each organization will need to make its own carefully considered decision when selecting data entry methods for its EHR (Fenton 2006).

Check Your Understanding 5.2

Answer the following questions.

1. In web-based healthcare forms structured data is often entered with a(n)
   a. Template
   b. On-screen form
   c. Text box for comments
   d. a and b

2. Which is a technology that converts human language into data that can be manipulated by computer systems?
   a. Concept identification
   b. Natural language processing
   c. Negation
   d. Expressivity

3. What is the main problem with using unstructured data for decision making?
   a. Cannot be stored in a database
   b. Lack of text-based processors
   c. Difficult to determine data completeness
   d. Takes more time to process the data

Indicate which type of data entry (s = structured; u = unstructured) applies to the pros and cons.

Pros

4. _____ The data will have detail and nuance.

5. _____ The data are easily used for analysis and reporting.

6. _____ It is easy to determine if these data are complete.

7. _____ These data usually reflect more of the clinician's thought processes.

Cons

8. _____ It usually takes more time to enter data using this method.

9. _____ It is more difficult to use this data for reporting or clinical decision support algorithms.

10. _____ This type of data entry tends to be very inflexible.

11. _____ It is difficult to determine the completeness of this data.

⊙ Data Measurement

The selection of the correct measurement scale to measure quantitative data is very important because it determines the type of statistical tests that can be conducted (Gravetter and Wallnau 2005, 16). The four scales of measurement in common use are nominal, ordinal, interval, and ratio. These four measurement scales represent two types of data, categorical and continuous. **Categorical data** (discrete), which includes nominal and ordinal scale data, represent mutually exclusive categories or labels. **Discrete data** is represented by whole numbers, such as the number of patients in the hospital or the number of discharged but not final billed charts. **Continuous data** such as interval or ratio scale data has equal intervals between the data points. Measurements of continuous data may contain fractions and decimals in the data.

Nominal data

Nominal data is a type of categorical data where the categories are simply names. Demographic data that is collected on a survey using check boxes is often nominal data. For example, gender represented by mutually exclusive male or female labels on check boxes, or marital status with choices like married, single, divorced, and such. Other nominal data frequently collected are age group, race/ethnicity, type of insurance payer and job category. Data collected for two patients on a nominal scale can be determined to be different, but the data analyst cannot add or subtract the data to compute the amount of difference because nominal data is not numerical. For that reason, nominal data is reported using percentages or frequency counts.

Ordinal data

In contrast, **ordinal data,** also called ranked data, are data where the names or labels have an order to them with meaning attached. The Likert rating scale where respondents select Strongly Agree (1) or Strongly Disagree (5) is an example of ordinal data (Gravetter and Wallnau 2005, 19). Likert scales are used for staging cancer, which is often represented as Stage I, Stage II, Stage III, or Stage IV. These are mutually exclusive categories; however, there is an order to the labels, with Stage IV cancer being more advanced than Stage I cancer. Data represented in an ordinal scale can be identified as different and a direction can be associated with that difference (higher or lower on the scale) but a numerical difference cannot be computed.

Interval data

Interval data is continuous numerical data that has equal intervals of ordered categories. This data is called continuous because there is an infinite number of possible data measurement values. Because the intervals between the data measurements are equal, these measurements can be compared to determine meaningful differences. Temperature in degrees Fahrenheit is interval data. Note the interval data has an arbitrary zero value, which does not indicate an absence of that value. This type of data can be compared to quantify the differences in two interval measurements.

Ratio data

Ratio data is a type of continuous numerical data. In addition to the equal intervals between data points that are found in interval data, ratio data have a true zero (0) point. An example of ratio data in healthcare would be weight. No human can weigh less than 0 pounds or ounces so this data element would be ratio. Data on age, length of stay, and charges are measured on a ratio data measurement scale.

Check Your Understanding 5.3

Match the terms with the appropriate descriptions.

    a. Nominal
    b. Ordinal
    c. Ratio
    d. Interval

1. _____ These data do not have a true zero and the distance between the data points is consistent.

2. _____ These data separate records into mutually exclusive categories in a meaningful order.

3. _____ These data have a true zero and the distance between the data points is consistent.

4. _____ These data separate records into mutually exclusive, named, categories with no order.

Answer the following questions.

5. Which are data represented by whole numbers such as number of beds in the facility?

    a. Interval
    b. Ratio
    c. Continuous
    d. Categorical

6. Which data would be found in a Likert scale on a survey?
   a. Ordinal
   b. Interval
   c. Nominal
   d. Ratio

7. Temperature in degrees Fahrenheit is an example of this data type.
   a. Nominal
   b. Ordinal
   c. Interval
   d. Ratio

8. This type of data typically has many measurements.
   a. Ordinal
   b. Continuous
   c. Discrete
   d. Nominal

9. This is the most important consideration regarding data collection.
   a. Standards
   b. Quality
   c. Purpose
   d. Method

⊙ Data Management

Data are an asset to an organization similar to the personnel, buildings, or other resources. As such, data require attention and maintenance to ensure the data are capable of supporting organizational needs and goals. The management of data is as important to a healthcare organization as the management of its buildings, capital equipment, and information technology infrastructure.

Data Governance

Data governance is an emerging practice in the healthcare industry. Definitions for data governance are that it is "the exercise of decision-making and authority for data-related matters" (Data Governance Institute 2013), or that it "is about establishing a culture where quality data is achieved, maintained, valued and used to drive the business" (Fisher 2009). Regardless of which definition one subscribes to, it is clear that any industry as reliant upon data as healthcare needs a plan for managing this asset.

Data Governance Process

As with most important healthcare processes, data governance is not a one-time effort, nor should it be "fast-tracked." It is important to take a considered approach, as the decisions made for data governance will have a long-term impact upon the organization. A suggested process follows:

1. Discover—Identify the databases or data sets or applications that store data; the relationships between the different data sets; the meaning of the data to

the organization; and who has responsibility for the data. This step requires the business users to be involved.

2. Design—Consolidation and coordination of organizational data and the environment focusing on consistency of any governing rules; consistency of the organizational data model; and consistency of the business processes. This step requires the involvement of the business users.

3. Enable—This step takes a considerable amount of time and effort, as this is when the new data governance standards are applied to each data source, business process, and application. It is recommended that the standards be deployed to the entire network, rather than embedded in each source, process, or application. Although this includes business users much of the responsibility falls on IT staff.

4. Maintain—A robust monitoring and reporting system is required to ensure that the data remains fit-for-purpose for the organization. The monitoring requires involvement from both business users and IT. The monitoring should be as automated as possible, with reporting to the responsible parties who then have the authority to make changes resulting in optimal standards and processes. Any changes must be documented so the data can be thoroughly understood when they are used.

5. Archive or Retire—It is important to ensure that the data that are no longer needed are retired in a methodical, considered fashion. This may involve complying with the legal requirements for maintaining the data, as well as understanding the different uses of the data within the organization (Fisher 2009, 146–161).

Data governance and stewardship are relatively new aspects of data management in healthcare organizations. Although the processes can be difficult and time consuming, they are essential to any organization wishing to maximize the use of their valuable data assets.

Data Quality

Assessing and understanding the quality of healthcare data is an extremely important and often overlooked aspect of managing data and information in healthcare provider settings. Ensuring that the data and information are correct has implications for the quality of patient care, reimbursement, and research. In short, it is important for all of the reasons providers document in patient records to begin with. For example, something as simple as the wrong patient weight could result in an incorrect drug dosage calculation and medication administration error. Rather than get bogged down in the details of studies regarding data quality, this section will discuss various aspects of data quality and draw from more general computer information systems theory to suggest methods for assuring high-quality data and information for healthcare.

Characteristics of Data Quality

Data quality can seem an overwhelming topic. There are many ways for data to be of poor quality and, in fact, the quality of the data can sometimes resemble the

Figure 5.6.   Data quality management model

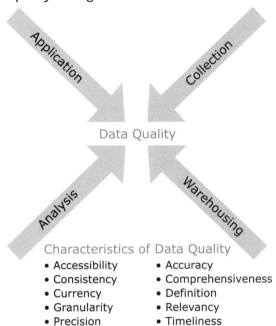

Source: AHIMA 2012

quality of patient care—it can vary according to the consumer. "Data are of high quality if they are fit for their intended uses in operations, decision making, and planning. Data are fit for use if they are free of defects and possess desired features" (Redman 2001, 73). This emphasizes that the data consumer and the use of the data are essential to any determination of data quality. In 1998, the American Health Information Management Association (AHIMA) Data Quality Management Task Force developed a **Data Quality Management Model,** most recently updated in 2015 (Davoudi 2015). The current model is seen in figure 5.6 and covers the different processes of data handling during which data quality should be addressed. The data handling processes are

⊙ Application—The purpose for which the data are collected

⊙ Collection—The processes by which data elements are accumulated

⊙ Warehousing—Processes and systems used to archive data and data journals

⊙ Analysis—The process of translating data into information utilized for an application (Davoudi et al. 2015)

In addition, 10 **characteristics of data quality** were identified and defined. The definitions and examples are provided in table 5.2. The 1998 model was updated in 2012. Though the fundamentals remain the same, understanding of how they can most effectively be implemented in healthcare continue to evolve.

It is important to understand that these processes and characteristics do not exist in a vacuum. Just as everyone who has a driver's license has to meet certain criteria, but not all drivers are equally accomplished, all data that meet these criteria may still not be appropriate or adequate. This is why the process of assessing data quality is so significant. Failure to address the quality of the data may mean that the massive increase in data collected and available due to the increased use of computers in healthcare has only resulted in an increase in poor quality data and, hence, decision making.

Table 5.2. AHIMA data quality characteristics, definitions, and examples

DATA QUALITY CHARACTERISTIC AND DEFINITION	HEALTHCARE EXAMPLE
Accuracy—The extent to which the data are free of identifiable errors.	The data element gender is completed for all patients and a random check of 500 records performed annually revealed only one demographic data element in conflict with the documentation.
Accessibility—Data items are easily obtainable and legal to access with strong protections and controls built into the process.	All persons with access to the EHR have the ability to search the master patient index and the search function is designed such that the wrong patient is rarely accessed.
Comprehensiveness—All required data items are included; ensures that the entire scope of the data is collected with intentional limitations documented.	Providers may decide that recording external cause data is not useful. If so, their data dictionary for the diagnoses data elements would need to include this as an intentional limitation.
Consistency—The extent to which the healthcare data are reliable and the same across applications.	Within the EHR, data such as allergies must be consistently displayed within different applications or screens to prevent confusion.
Currency—The extent to which data are up to date; a datum value is up to date if it is current for a specific point in time, and it is outdated if it was current at a preceding time but incorrect at a later time.	Patient age is generally current when the care is delivered. If age is not reentered the software needs to be have functionality to automatically update the age when appropriate.
Definition—The specific meaning of a healthcare-related data element.	Address as a data element label can mean the street address or it can mean the entire address to include city, state, and zip code.
Granularity—The level of detail at which the attributes and values of healthcare data are defined.	Adult weights are usually only recorded in pounds, possibly tenths of a pound. Newborn weights must be recorded in terms of ounces for accuracy.

DATA QUALITY CHARACTERISTIC AND DEFINITION	HEALTHCARE EXAMPLE
Precision—Data values should be strictly stated to support the purpose.	Diagnosis related group (DRG) values are carried out to four digits behind the decimal. It would be inaccurate to have the system only use two digits behind the decimal.
Relevance—The extent to which healthcare-related data are useful for the purposes for which they were collected.	Recording a primary diagnosis for hospital inpatients would be irrelevant because coding guidelines mandate collection of the principal diagnosis, which can be entirely different.
Timeliness—Concept of data quality that involves whether the data is up-to-date and available within a useful time frame; timeliness is determined by the manner and context in which the data are being used.	It would be inappropriate for blood pressure readings from ICU monitors to only be updated each hour.

Source: Davoudi et al. 2015

The Data Quality Assessment and Management Process

The process of data quality assessment is similar to and, in some instances, uses the same methods as healthcare quality assessment and management. This section will outline generally accepted steps to quality assessment through the lens of quality management. It has been explicated using examples from the healthcare industry.

Who Are the Data Consumers?

Any health informaticist tasked with assessing or managing data quality must first understand who the data consumers are. This involves making a list of all of the internal and external data consumers. Likely internal data consumers for healthcare data managers include patients, clinicians, administrators, and researchers. External data consumers might include payers, public health agencies, and law enforcement agencies. Once a complete list has been compiled the consumer list must be prioritized. This is an essential step. It will be impossible for the data manager to meet all of the needs of all of the data consumers. However, by enumerating all of the data consumers, data managers will begin documenting the full depth and breadth of data use in their organization.

What Are the Needs of the Data Consumers?

This step in the process is usually very challenging. Most data consumers do not understand their needs well enough to articulate them effectively. So, what is the data manager to do? Rather than asking what the data consumer needs, the data manager should ask the consumer to describe how they use the data, the

Table 5.3.   Data consumer needs assessment tool

Consumer:																									
Consumer needs						Product feature requirements										Gap analysis									
Primary Needs	Secondary Needs	Tertiary Needs	Translated Needs	Source	Unit of Measure	Accuracy	Accessibility	Comprehensiveness	Consistency	Currency	Definition	Granularity	Precision	Relevancy	Timeliness	Accuracy	Accessibility	Comprehensiveness	Consistency	Currency	Definition	Granularity	Precision	Relevancy	Timeliness

Source: Adapted from Redman 2001

decisions that are made, the potential consequences of a wrong decision, and so on. As an example, consider the data use of clinical decision support. Even within this seemingly single data use task there are nuances. Allergic drug reactions as well as preventive service reminders are each considered clinical decision support. However, allergic drug reactions are much more important because incorrect data could result in immediate, serious patient injury, even death. Although preventive service reminders are certainly important, they rarely, if ever, rise to the level of immediate injury or death. The person working with the consumers to determine their needs must explore each data use thoroughly.

The data manager must take a controlled and careful approach to collecting data that the data consumer needs. The initial steps of implementing a data quality process will not be quick. However, the data manager should better understand the needs of the various consumers upon completion of the template or similar tool. In addition, the data manager will now have a complete list of data consumer needs to carry forward for consideration by senior management if necessary. It would be usual and expected for senior management to become involved in data consumer needs prioritization efforts. Table 5.3 is an example of a needs and requirements collection template that might be used.

What Are the Required Features and Quality Characteristics?

After documenting the consumer needs, the functionality requirement associated with each quality characteristic needs to be identified. Building on the drug allergy reaction alert data use, each data quality characteristic will be examined in light of the functionality required. The following might be a partial list of the requirements:

⊙ Accuracy—The lists of drugs will need to utilize the current EHR data standard for pharmaceuticals. Allergies will need to be recorded as structured data or processed using an NLP algorithm after entry to be usable for drug allergy reaction processing.

⊙ Accessibility—The data entry methods for the allergies and drugs will be dependent upon the workflow of the organization and the abilities of the persons entering the data. This requires further study.

⊙ Comprehensiveness—Allergies are a required data element for the EHR. If the patient has no allergies the field should reflect "No allergies reported." If the clinician is not able to determine whether the patient has allergies the field should reflect "Unknown."

⊙ Consistency—Once recorded, an allergy should become a permanent entry in the patient EHR, which is always incorporated into the information presented to the clinician.

Once the functionality requirements are identified across all of the characteristics, the data consumer should review them to ensure they meet consumer needs. Seeing the requirements specified in this fashion may result in the consumer identifying additional, important uses that will also need to be specified using these methods.

The end result of the requirements and quality characteristics specification involves a dual examination of both the stringency of the requirements and a prioritization of all requirements. The most stringent requirement may not be at the top of the prioritization list, but it is the highest level of functionality required.

How Well Do Our Current Information Products Meet the Needs and Requirements?

After identification of the most important needs and requirements, it is now time to determine how well any current information products perform. There are several steps for this process:

1. Ask the data consumers.
2. Measure the data where possible and appropriate.
   a. Select a business process or operation that uses the suspect data.
   b. Determine a desired sample size and selection method.
   c. Decide on the assessment criteria. In healthcare we would like to strive for 100 percent accuracy or correctness; however, there may be instances in nonclinical data where data are "seriously flawed" or "flawed but acceptable."
   d. Establish the estimated impact by asking the people who work with the end data. Does flawed data impact patient care? Does it impact the ability to seek reimbursement? What are the impacts upon time, expenses, customer satisfaction, or other issues?
   e. Measure associated activities such as productivity and consumer satisfaction.
3. Include the results of the data measurement on the needs and requirements spreadsheet.

It is important to give in-depth consideration to documenting the data consumers' needs and concerns. Failing to do this can result in a product that does not meet the consumers' needs. Additionally, the consumers' representative has to sign off on the delivery of the final system, which must meet their functional specifications. Therefore, it is important to work closely with the data consumers to help them fully document the specifications of the new system. Another important consideration is how that functionality will be assessed. Consumers and information technologists are often challenged when designing tests of functionality. Additionally, consumers may be unfamiliar with the new technology that calls for integration into existing systems, which presents an additional layer of complexity for end user acceptance testing.

Where Are the Gaps and How Important Are They?

The data manager should now create a list of all of the gaps between the consumer needs and requirements and the current information products and performance identified in the previous steps. Once the gaps have been enumerated, the data manager can move forward with creating a priority list of areas or functionality needing attention. As always, this should not be done in a vacuum. The development of the list should be iterative, undergoing review by affected data consumers as well as senior management.

Check Your Understanding 5.4

Match the terms with the appropriate descriptions.

a. Accuracy
b. Accessibility
c. Comprehensiveness
d. Consistency
e. Currency
f. Definition
g. Granularity
h. Precision
i. Relevance
j. Timeliness

1. _____ The data are at the appropriate level of detail for the uses of the data.

2. _____ Each data element must be defined with a clear meaning and allowable values.

3. _____ All data required for the specified purpose are included. Any intentional limitations are documented.

4. _____ The data must be meaningful for the purpose.

5. _____ Data values are appropriate for a given time frame and then become obsolete.

6. _____ The exactness of the data is related to purpose of the data.

7. _____ The data must be able to be accessed or used within a given time frame as determined by the purpose of the data.

8. _____ Data items should be easily obtainable, legal to collect, and protected as necessary.

9. _____ Data values are reliable across applications, time, or other parameters as needed.

10. _____ Data that are valid, that is, within the allowable values, and are the correct values, not in error.

Indicate whether the following statements are true or false.

11. Data governance or stewardship is an optional function for data-rich healthcare organizations.

12. Business users of data can allow IT to be totally responsible for data governance activities.

13. Ongoing maintenance of the data governance processes is required to maximize use of the data asset.

14. Data are an important organizational asset similar to the equipment or the buildings.

15. Business users should be involved in data governance design.

16. The needs of the data consumers are important considerations for data governance.

⊙ Data Analysis

The increasing computerization of the healthcare industry has left many organizations awash in data. Effective data analysis plans, techniques, and processes are needed in order to turn the data into usable information.

Understanding the Data

The first, most essential step to analyzing any data is acquiring a thorough understanding of the data to be analyzed. This is best done by studying the data dictionary. The data dictionary is vital to understanding the data set. The data dictionary and minimum requirements are discussed in greater detail in Chapter 4.

The data dictionary may include information related to the originating source system, data owner, data entry date, and data termination date (AHIMA 2014a). In addition, the data dictionary should include any information regarding special processing utilized in the production of the data set. It is common for some data records to have missing values.

One part of understanding the data that can easily be overlooked is obtaining an understanding of the data collection methods. Laboratory data that are loaded directly into a laboratory information system and then transferred to an EHR automatically are likely to be of better quality than data that were entered manually. This holds for all data. Each time the data are handled or touched by a human the opportunity or likelihood of error increases. However, this understanding of the data collection can also be subtler. Consider the many claims databases that are used for research, quality measure development, and so on. Although these are often the most easily accessed, they may not always be the best. In ICD-10, the external cause codes (E-codes) were replaced by V, W, X, and Y codes that can be used for the entire treatment (Endicott 2014). Other hospitals code only the Principal Diagnosis and the Secondary Diagnoses, which will impact the reimbursement. Often these different methods of data collection are made for very pragmatic reasons such as coder workforce shortages. However, a failure to understand these differences when using large data sets from multiple organizations could result in false conclusions being drawn regarding the causes of injuries or the presence or absence of certain health factors.

Cleaning the Data

The largest part of any data analysis project should begin with cleaning the data. **Data cleaning,** sometimes termed data scrubbing, involves examining the data thoroughly to detect wrong or inconsistent data. This is a necessary task even if the data are drawn from a data set that is managed with a data quality program. When data are subset or transferred between data applications, the opportunity exists for the introduction of data errors.

The first step in data cleaning is to load or label the data. This process may be largely automated or users may have to perform it themselves. Either way, the data analyst needs to validate the data elements in the data set against the data dictionary.

Once the data are loaded and labeled, each data element needs to be examined. **Descriptive statistics,** also known as summary statistics, such as frequencies, mean, mode, range, and standard deviation, should be run for all continuous data elements. Table 5.4 is an example of descriptive statistical output for the continuous data element of age. Upon initial examination, the output seems fine, with a reasonable mean and median. However, continued examination of the output reveals a range of 268. Without looking at the minimum and maximum, the data analyst can tell that errors exist for this data element because 268 is not a valid entry for age. Either a negative age was entered for a patient or an incorrect, large entry was made for age. In this instance the minimum is 23.3, entirely reasonable, but the maximum is 291.3, not reasonable.

Correcting the continuous data element error first necessitates identifying the record(s) with the error. If available, it is always preferable to return to the source data to determine the correct value. If the source data are not available, the correct value may be imputed, or the incorrect record may have to be eliminated from the analysis.

Categorical data require a different method of examination for data cleaning purposes. Frequencies should be run on all categorical data elements. Table 5.5 is an example of a **frequency** for a categorical data element. A frequency is the number of times that a particular observation or value occurs in a data set. This type of output should prompt the data analyst to examine the data dictionary for the allowable values for this data element. Either the label for a valid entry was not captured correctly or there are a significant number of records with an invalid entry.

Table 5.4. Descriptive statistics for a continuous variable

Age	
Mean	60.834375
Standard Error	3.851114233
Median	66.4
Mode	N/A
Standard Deviation	21.78519191
Sample Variance	474.5945867
Kurtosis	−1.25981969
Skewness	−0.38286422
Range	268
Minimum	23.3
Maximum	291.3
Sum	2146.7
Count	32

Table 5.5. Frequency exploration of categorical data

Discharge Disposition	Count	Percent	Cumulative Percent
Home	100	33.33%	
Nursing Home	50	16.67%	50.00%
Rehabilitation	50	16.67%	66.67%
Died	50	16.67%	83.34%
99	50	16.67%	100.00%
			(rounding)
TOTAL	300	100%	

The relationships between the data elements may also prompt categorical data cleaning using **crosstabs**. Crosstabs serve to highlight any errors where there is an expected or explicit relationship between two data elements. Table 5.6 is

Table 5.6 Crosstab of categorical data

Procedures by gender	Male	Female	Total
Laparoscopy	200	350	550
Cardiac Catheterization	40	25	65
Arthroscopy	350	300	650
Hysterectomy	5	25	30
TOTAL	595	700	1295

an example of a crosstab analysis for two categorical data elements. The use of crosstabs for data cleaning is more ambiguous than the use of descriptive statistics or frequencies for single data elements. Often the data cleaning using crosstabs may not be done until the type of data analysis being attempted is known.

Correction of categorical data errors can be handled in a manner similar to continuous data errors. First the record with the error must be identified. However, unlike continuous errors where the only options are imputation or reviewing the source data, the correct categorical data can sometimes be deduced from other data element entries. For example, the records with the hysterectomy errors in table 5.6 could be examined to attempt to determine whether the procedure was incorrect or gender was incorrect. Other data that might provide a clue include preventive services such as a prostate exam or mammogram. The other options of imputation and reviewing the source data are also available.

The most sophisticated analysis is useless if the data that went into it are not cleaned because the statistical calculations will be impacted.

Imputation

When data are initially collected for a research study, the data set should be examined to determine if there are any missing data. Missing data values cause the data set to be incomplete. It must be addressed before statistical testing can be completed. Data may be missing due to errors such as data collectors not recording all the data in the data collection tool. Study participants may choose to not answer all the questions in a survey, which results in missing survey response data for those questions. Another scenario that generates missing data is that the data are collected, but later misplaced or destroyed due to physical destruction or to a system failure that affects the storage medium (for example, a computer crash). Healthcare studies using instruments to collect data may experience instrument failure. Natural disasters may cause data loss from physical destruction of equipment or damage to a lab. Participants in a study may decide to leave the study or may have changed circumstances and be unable to complete the study due to moving, having scheduling conflicts, or other personal situations. For a long survey, respondents may get survey fatigue and start skipping questions or they may not understand the questions.

The first step in addressing missing data is to determine what values are missing. For a small data set, the data can be examined by inspection (that is, looking at the data) to determine what is not present. In a larger Microsoft Excel spreadsheet, missing data would show up as blank cells, which can be located using the built-in Find and Select feature. For a very large data set, statistical software tools, like Statistical Package for the Social Sciences (SPSS), should be utilized to locate any missing data as they have a rich set of tools for this purpose. Graphing the data can assist in visualizing the data so that the location of missing data can be identified, and frequency tables will give the number of missing data items.

There are three common approaches to dealing with missing data. First, if question responses are missing for one participant researchers may decide not to use any of that participant's data in the data analysis (Green and Salkind 2013). This creates a problem if there are a lot of missing data because there will be a loss of data for the study. Thus, data analysts may decide to include the participant's other responses in the study, which should be noted in the study that the case was retained but excluded from some of the study calculations due to missing data for that response item (such as a survey question was skipped). This approach must be used judiciously because it could be the case that many participants skipped the same question due to a study design such as poor wording in the question or unclear directions. In this case the missing data are not randomly distributed and excluding it may skew the data (Cokluk and Kayri 2011).

Second, the missing data may be coded with an identifier like -9999 in order to be more easily located and dealt with during the data analysis. For example, statistical software can be programmed to exclude this user-defined value from calculation.

Third, depending upon the type of analysis, the missing values may be provided using a process called **imputation** in which missing data values are replaced (Cokluk and Kayri 2011). Imputation methods must be described fully and imputed values clearly labeled. For numerical data, the mean of all other values for that data item can be substituted for all the missing values. Other commonly used replacement values are simple calculated values such as the mean or median of points near the missing value, and complex predictive values calculated with regression. It should be noted that replacing too much data may also input bias into the study. All procedures used to replace missing data must be documented.

Check Your Understanding 5.5

Answer the following questions.

1. A data dictionary consists of
   a. The names, definitions, and attributes of data elements
   b. Synonyms for specific data variables
   c. All possible data elements in the healthcare industry
   d. Hints for using data elements

2. Once any records with data errors are identified, the data analyst should
   a. Delete the records with the errors
   b. Perform imputation to determine the correct values
   c. Determine whether the source records are available in order to validate the data
   d. Attempt to correct the data from the other data in the record

Indicate whether the following statements are true or false.

3. The first, most essential step to analyzing any data is acquiring a thorough understanding of the data to be analyzed.

4. Data cleaning is one of the smallest parts of a data analysis project.

5. Descriptive statistics include the frequencies, mean, and standard deviation.

6. A frequency is the number of times that a particular observation or value occurs in a data set.

◉ Data Presentation

Presenting the results of a data analysis effectively can be a challenge. The data output from an analysis may or may not be clear and easy to understand. When numbers are displayed incorrectly, they can encourage false assumptions about the data. Similarly, data sets with missing values can leave the analyst with questions that they cannot answer with statistical analysis (AHIMA 2014a). Whether presented with words, in tabular form, or in a graph or picture, it is imperative the presentation be clear.

Tables

A table is an organized arrangement of data, usually in columns and rows. Many different types of quantitative data can be displayed in tables. For examples of tables see tables 5.1 through 5.6. Tables should be used with care because the inclusion of too much data in a table can increase rather than decrease confusion.

If the decision is made to use a table, it is helpful to keep the following guidelines in mind:

- ◉ The table should be a logical unit that is self-explanatory and stands on its own.
- ◉ The source of the data in the table should be specified.
- ◉ Headings for rows and columns should be understandable.
- ◉ Blank cells should contain a zero or a dash.
- ◉ Formatting for headings and cell contents should be consistent so that the eye is not confused (Marc 2016, 540).

In some instances, a table can be the basis for a chart or graph to display the data.

Charts and Graphs

One of the benefits of a highly computerized world is that it is now relatively easy to generate charts and graphs for data analysis results. Charts and graphs can be very useful for emphasizing important points and conveying information about a topic. Guiding principles for the creation of charts and graphs include

- Distortion—The representation of numbers or percentages should be proportional to the quantities represented.
- Proportion and scale—Graphs should emphasize the horizontal and be greater in length than height. A general rule is that the y-axis (height) be three-quarters the x-axis (length) of the graph.
- Abbreviations—Any abbreviations used should be spelled out for clarity.
- Color—Color should be used as appropriate to the use of the graph. If the chart is going to be printed will it be printed in black and white or color?
- Text—The font and use of capitalization needs to be considered carefully. The use of all capital letters can sometimes be difficult to read (Marc 2016, 542).

Ideally, spatial representations with graphs will

- Support the interpretation of the data
- Allow data trends to be seen at a glance
- Present individual data points clearly
- Present differences in data between groups or over time
- Avoid presenting too much data in too small a space (Marc 2016, 542)

It is important to determine the best type of graph or chart for data display. For example, a pie chart would not be good for displaying data from two or more groups because a pie chart shows percentages for one variable only such as percentages of physician by specialty for the hospital. Data type is important when selecting a chart. For example, bar charts are used for nominal data, and line charts are best for displaying large amounts of data over time.

Data Visualization

Healthcare activities generate large amounts of data from electronic health records, computer physician order entry systems, digital radiology storage software, pharmacy, lab, and registration systems as well as numerous other healthcare applications. Healthcare professionals struggle with finding ways to analyze this mountain of data into meaningful, actionable information. Data visualization using graphs helps the data analyst to see the general shape of the data, which facilitates identifying skewed data, finding data outliers, exploring trends, and zeroing in on possible missing data points. For example, a Pareto bar chart displaying customer complaint categories from highest to lowest is an efficient visualization of the upper 20 percent of the customers' complaints, which if resolved will theoretically

Figure 5.7.   Pareto bar chart of complaint categories for a clinic

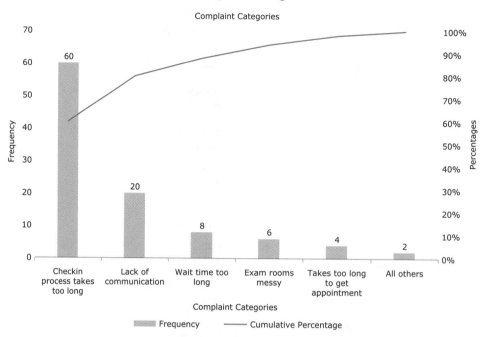

reduce the number of complaints by 80 percent (Shaw and Carter 2015). Figure 5.7 displays a Pareto chart of complaint categories for a hypothetical clinic.

Data visualization can be applied to many fields and purposes. Personal, public, and community health areas have been modeled using computers. In one study, academic analytical and text mining software was used by researchers to model document metadata as part of a medical and healthcare curriculum mapping study (Komenda et al. 2015). In a related study, the spatial component of epidemiological data was explored for disease patterns using HealthTracks web-based geographic information system software to graph demographic and healthcare data, such as community immunizations and notifiable diseases, for the purpose of identifying risk factors based on geolocation (Jardine et al. 2014).

In the personal injury area, Allscripts' software has been used to provide timelines for body mass and body maps showing sites of previous injury, while NodeXL software analyzed Twitter user data by searching for keywords like polio (Shneiderman et al. 2013). This type of data mining of large amounts of data can help guide medical researchers by uncovering new relationships in the data.

Another use of data visualization is to create data mapping. In a study on managing surgical outcomes, hierarchical mappings, called treemaps, of retrospective surgery data were evaluated as one way to help busy surgeons assess 30-day risk-adjusted surgical outcomes, surgical errors, and time to complete the surgery (Hugine et al. 2014). Results indicated that treemap visualizations were useful, but further research was needed into the optimal data displays for the data. Finally, even the federal government is embracing visualization tools; researchers wishing to explore population data should review the tools for mapping census data available at the US Census Bureau's website (US Census Bureau 2016).

Chapter 5 Review Exercises

Match the data display tool with its description.
- **a.** A horizontal or vertical arrangement of rectangular shapes that represents data from one or more groups or categories
- **b.** An orderly arrangement of values that displays data in rows and columns
- **c.** An arrangement of pieces in a circular shape that represents the component parts of a single group or variable
- **d.** One or more series of points connected by a line or lines to represent trends over time

1. _____ Table
2. _____ Bar chart
3. _____ Pie chart
4. _____ Line graph

Indicate whether the following statements are true or false.

5. The use of colors in graphs is an important consideration for graphs that will be printed.
6. Pareto charts can assist in identifying the top 20 percent of the recorded problems.
7. Data visualization methods can be applied to medical, healthcare, and geographic information systems and census and personal health data.
8. Age data collected by having the user type in their age in years (for example, 20.5 years) would be considered categorical.
9. Salaries collected in ranges of 0–25,000, 26,000–30,000, and such, are continuous data.
10. Imputation procedures for a research project do not need to be documented in the resulting paper.
11. Replacing too much data by imputation can bias your study.
12. Data standards are needed to facilitate interoperability of diverse systems.
13. Database data formatting for a table field includes the data type, size, and allowable content of the data field.
14. Structured data can come from webpage dropdowns and check boxes.

Discussion.

15. Describe the types of data, as well as the relationship between data and information.

16. Create a data map for exporting data from an electronic health record to the billing system. Discuss the data flow and the data standards used in your mapping.

17. Compare and contrast the methods of collecting structured and unstructured data. List one disadvantage of each type of data.

18. Design appropriate data presentation for displaying the professional certifications held by the HIM department staff. Justify the choice of your graph, list the possible certifications, discuss how the data would be graphed and presented.

REFERENCES

AHIMA. 2014a. Health Data Analysis Toolkit. http://bok.ahima.org/PdfView?oid=107504.

AHIMA. 2014b. *Pocket Glossary of Health Information Management and Technology.* 4th ed. Chicago, IL: AHIMA Press.

AHIMA. 2012. ICD-10 Toolkit: New toolkit provides resources to assist with the ICD-10 transition. *Journal of AHIMA* 83(3): 36–37.

AHIMA. 2011. Data mapping best practices. *Journal of AHIMA* 82(4):46–52.

Ash, J.S., D.F. Sittig, E.M. Campbell, K.P. Guappone, and Richard H. Dykstra. 2007. Some unintended consequences of clinical decision support systems. *AMIA Annual Symposium Proceedings* 2007:26–30.

ASTM. 2012. ASTM E2369—12 Standard Specification for Continuity of Care Record (CCR). *ASTM International.* http://www.astm.org/Standards/E2369.htm.

CCHIT. 2015. About certification commission for health information technology. http://www.cchit.org/about.

Cokluk, O. and M. Kayri. 2011. The effects of methods of imputation for missing values on the validity and reliability of scales. *Educational Sciences: Theory and Practice* 11(1):303–309.

Data Governance Institute. 2013. The DGI Data Governance Framework. http://www.datagovernance.com/the-dgi-framework/.

Davoudi, Sion, Julie A. Dooling, Barbara Glondys, Theresa D. Jones, Lesley Kadlec, Shauna M. Overgaard, Kerry Ruben, and Annemarie Wendicke. 2015. Data quality management model (2015 Update). *Journal of AHIMA* 86(10): expanded web version.

Department of Health and Human Services. 2011. HealthIT.hhs.gov: ONC-Authorized Testing and Certification Bodies. ONC-Authorized Testing and Certification Bodies. https://www.healthit.gov/policy-researchers-implementers/authorized-testing-and-certifications-bodies.

Department of Health and Human Services. 2010. Health Information Technology: Initial Set of Standards, Implementation Specification and Certification Criteria for Electronic Health Record Technology. Code of Federal Regulations. Vol. 75. No. 144, July 28, 2010. http://edocket.access.gpo.gov/2010/pdf/2010-17210.pdf.

Endicott, M. August 2014. Transitioning From E Codes in ICD-9-CM to V, W, X, Y Codes in ICD-10-CM. *Journal of AHIMA.* http://journal.ahima.org/2014/08/13/monthly-code-cracker-transitioning-from-e-codes-in-icd-9-cm-to-v-w-x-y-codes-in-icd-10-cm/.

Fenton, Susan H. 2006. Structured or unstructured? Options for clinician data entry in the EHR. *American Health Information Management Association,* March. http://bok.ahima.org/doc?oid=63115.

Fisher, T. 2009. *The Data Asset.* Hoboken: Wiley.

González-Ferrer, Arturo, and Mor Peleg. 2015. Understanding requirements of clinical data standards for developing interoperable knowledge-based DSS: A case study. *Computer Standards & Interfaces* 42 (November): 125–136. doi:10.1016/j.csi.2015.06.002.

Graunt, J. 1665. *Reflections on the Weekly [sic] Bills of Mortality for the Cities of London and Westminster, and the Places Adjacent but More Especially, Sofar as They Relate to the Plague and Other Mortal Diseases That We English-Men Are Most Subject Unto: With an Exact Account of the Greatest Plagues That Have Happened Since the Creation.* London: Printed for Samuel Speed.

Gravetter, Frederick J., and Larry B. Wallnau. 2005. *Essentials of Statistics for the Behavioral Sciences / Frederick J. Gravetter, Larry B. Wallnau.* Belmont, CA: Thomson/Wadsworth, c2005.

Green, S.B., and N.J. Salkind. 2013. *Using SPSS for Windows and Macintosh.* 6th ed. Upper Saddle River, NJ: Pearson.

Hammond, W., and J. Cimino. 2001. *Medical Informatics Computer Applications in Health Care and Biomedicine.* New York: Springer-Verlag.

Hazelwood, A.C. and C.A. Venable. 2016. Reimbursement Methodologies. Chapter 7 in *Health Information Management Concepts Principles, and Practices.* 5th ed. Edited by Oachs, P., and A. Watters. Chicago: AHIMA.

Health Level Seven International. 2013. HL7 Governance and Operations Manual. HL7, January 7. http://www.hl7.org/documentcenter/public_temp_F525E34A-1C23-BA17-0C7C0AA8A8F7ABCD/membership/HL7_Governance_and_Operations_Manual.pdf.

HIPAA. 1996. Health Insurance Portability and Accountability Act of 1996. Public Law 104-191. http://edocket.access.gpo.gov/cfr_2007/octqtr/pdf/45cfr162.103.pdf.

Hugine, A.L., S.A. Guerlain, and F.E. Turrentine. 2014. Visualizing Surgical Quality Data with Treemaps. *Journal of Surgical Research* 191(1):74–83. doi:10.1016/j.jss.2014.03.046.

International Organization for Standardization (ISO). 2013. ISO—Standards development processes—Stages of development of International Standards.

http://www.iso.org/iso/home/standards_development/resources-for-technical-work/support-for-developing-standards.htm.

Jardine, A., N. Mullan, O. Gudes, J. Cosford, S. Moncrieff, G. West, Jianguo X., G. Yun, and P. Somerford. 2014. Web-based geo-visualisation of spatial information to support evidence-based health policy: A case study of the development process of HealthTracks. *Health Information Management Journal* 43(2):7–16. doi:10.12826/18333575.2014.0004.Jardine.

Johnson, S.B., S. Bakken, D. Dine, S. Hyun, E. Mendonça, F. Morrison, T. Bright, T. Van Vleck, J. Wrenn, and P. Stetson. 2008. An electronic health record based on structured narrative. *Journal of the American Medical Informatics Association* 15(1):54–64. doi:10.1197/jamia.M2131.

Komenda, M., M. Víta, C. Vaitsis, D. Schwarz, A. Pokorná, N. Zary, and L. Dušek. 2015. Curriculum mapping with academic analytics in medical and healthcare education. *PLoS ONE* 10(12):1–18. doi:10.1371/journal.pone.0143748.

Marc, D. 2016. Data Visualization. Chapter 18 in *Health Information Management Concepts Principles, and Practices.* 5th ed. Edited by Oachs, P., and A. Watters. Chicago: AHIMA.

Monegain, B. 2014. CCHIT to shutter after 10 years. *Healthcare IT News.* November 3. http://www.healthcareitnews.com/news/cchit-ends-10-years-ehr-certification.

Oracle. 2015. Database Concepts: Oracle Data Types. https://docs.oracle.com/cd /B28359_01/server.111/b28318/datatype.htm.

Pilato, J. 2013. Charging vs. coding: Untangling the relationship for ICD-10. *Journal of AHIMA* 84(2):58–60.

Redman, B. 2001. *The Practice of Patient Education.* 9th ed. St. Louis: Mosby.

Rosenbloom, S.T., H. Denny, N. Xu, N. Lorenzi, W.W. Stead, and K.B. Johnson. 2011. Data from clinical notes: A perspective on the tension between structure and flexible documentation. *Journal of the American Medical Informatics Association* 18(2):181–186. doi:10.1136/jamia.2010.007237.

Shaw, P.L., and D. Carter. 2015. *Quality and Performance Improvement in Healthcare: Theory, Practice, and Management.* 6th ed. Amer Health Info Management Asn.

Shneiderman, B., C. Plaisant, and B.W. Hesse. 2013. Improving Healthcare with Interactive Visualization. *Computer* 46(5):58–66. doi:10.1109/MC.2013.38.

Texas Department of State Health Services. 2010. ImmTrac Electronic Data Reporting. http://www.dshs.texas.gov/immunize/immtrac.

US Census Bureau. 2016. *Visualizations.* http://www.census.gov/data/visualizations.html.

US Census Bureau. 2007. *Revisions to the Standards for the Classification of Federal Data on Race and Ethnicity.* https://nces.ed.gov/programs/handbook/data/pdf/Appendix_A .pdf.

U.S. National Library of Medicine (NLM). 2016. Value Set Authority Center. https:// vsac.nlm.nih.gov/.

US Congress. 2009. Health Information Technology for Economic and Clinical Health (HITECH) Act. Code of Federal Regulations. http://edocket.access.gpo.gov/2010 /pdf/2010-17210.pdf.

US Government. 2009. American Recovery and Reinvestment Act of 2009. http:// frwebgate.access.gpo.gov/cgi-bin/getdoc.cgi?dbname=111_cong _bills&docid=f:h1enr.pdf.

US National Library of Medicine. 2016. Value Set Authority Center. https://vsac.nlm.nih
.gov/.

van Mulligen, E.M., H. Stam, and A.M. van Ginneken. 1998. Clinical data entry.
Proceedings / AMIA Annual Symposium. AMIA Symposium, 81–85.

World Health Organization. 2011. History of the Development of the ICD. WHO. http://
www.who.int/classifications/icd/en/HistoryOfICD.pdf.

ADDITIONAL RESOURCES

Cimino, James J. 1998. Desiderata for Controlled Medical Vocabularies in the Twenty-
First Century. *Methods of Information in Medicine* 37(4–5):394–403.

Department of Health and Human Services. 2015. Health IT Standards Committee.
https://www.healthit.gov/FACAS/health-it-standards-committee.

Tang, P.C., M.P. LaRosa, and S.M. Gorden. 1999. Use of computer-based records,
completeness of documentation, and appropriateness of documented clinical decisions.
Journal of the American Medical Informatics Association 6(3):245–251.

Wager, K.A., F.W. Lee, and J.P. Glaser. 2009. *Health Care Information Systems*. 2nd ed. San
Francisco: Wiley.

Weir, C.R., J.F. Hurdle, M.A. Felgar, J.M. Hoffman, B. Roth, and J.R. Nebeker. 2003. Direct
text entry in electronic progress notes. An evaluation of input errors. *Methods of
Information in Medicine* 42(1):61–67. doi:10.1267/METH03010061.

Chapter

6

Understanding Databases

*By Susan White, PhD,
RHIA, CHDA*

Learning Objectives

- Identify the difference in flat data files versus relational databases
- Apply basic SQL commands to select data for reporting and analysis
- Utilize a data dictionary to understand data attributes
- Discover the role of data modeling in database maintenance and design

KEY TERMS

Cardinality
Clinical data warehouse
Column-delimited data
Comma-separated values (CSV)
Data dictionary
Data flow diagram
Data mart
Data model
Data table
Data warehouse
Database
Database management system
(DBMS)
Decision support databases
Diagram 0

Entity relationship diagram (ERD)
Extract, transform, and load (ETL)
Field
Flat file
Foreign key
Join
Method
Normalization
Object-oriented databases
Ontology
Primary key
Record
Relational databases
Select query
Structured Query Language (SQL)

Healthcare is a data-rich business. On the business side of healthcare, claims are generated and submitted for payment. Payment transactions are then sent back to the provider. On the clinical side of healthcare, countless diagnostic tests are performed and the results of those tests are provided back to practitioners and providers. Both operational and clinical data are used for healthcare services research and process improvement projects. The introduction of the electronic health record (EHR) and sophisticated electronic medical record systems increased the amount of data available in the healthcare setting exponentially. The Centers for Medicare and Medicaid Services' (CMS) meaningful use criteria, value-based purchasing programs, and the formation of Accountable Care Organizations (ACOs) and other payment reform policies are driving the need for providers to use the data produced during the delivery of care to help improve the efficiency and effectiveness of the healthcare system. If these goals are to be met, then the data must be organized in a way that allows analysis and reports to be produced accurately and in real time. Databases give structure to the raw data and facilitate the manipulation of data to achieve these goals.

⊙ Database Terminology

Prior to studying the various types of databases and database management systems (DBMSs), it is important to have a common set of terminology to describe the various components of a database. Databases may be envisioned as a collection of data tables. The most common form of a data table found in practice is a tab or worksheet within a spreadsheet.

Data tables include **records** or rows and **fields** or columns. For example, table 6.1 represents a table of patients and their associated appointments. The fields in this table represent data elements describing attributes of the appointment (provider, date, and time). A collection of fields that are related are placed in the same record. The records in this table represent the data describing the patient's appointment. Records in a data table may represent patient demographic information, attributes of a service provided to a patient, or even a diagnostic or procedural code (such as ICD-10) and its definition.

Sets of records include a common set of fields and those related to the same business purpose or focus are collected together into a data table. Common data tables found in healthcare include

- ⊙ Patient demographics
- ⊙ Physician specialty and licensure
- ⊙ Charge description master
- ⊙ Patient services

A collection of data tables is called a **database**. Databases can have a variety of structures and may be created and maintained using a **database management system (DBMS)**. A DBMS provides a method for adding or deleting data and also supports methods for extracting data for reporting.

Table 6.1. Patients and their appointments

PatientID	ProviderID	AppointmentDate	AppointmentTime
ABD239	SMI123	1/23/2016	9:00 a.m.
DIR235	SMI123	1/23/2016	9:30 a.m.
JKF764	SMI123	1/23/2016	10:00 a.m.

⊙ Types of Databases

To decide on the type of database that is most appropriate for storing data, the user must answer some key questions:

- ⊙ How many records will the database contain (currently and in the foreseeable future)?
- ⊙ How do the variables relate to each other?
- ⊙ What database tools are available for use?
- ⊙ How will the data be pulled or queried from the database?

The answers to these questions will drive the database type. There is typically not a right or wrong answer in database design. If the database is robust enough to hold all of the information required and extracting information is straightforward, then it should be considered a good quality design. The two most common types of data storage used in practice are flat files or data tables and databases. Databases may be further segmented into those that are relational or those that are not relational. Relational databases include tables that are related by common fields called keys. Nonrelational databases, including object-oriented databases, hierarchical databases, and Not Only SQL (NoSQL) databases, are used in healthcare because they allow flexibility in the storage and retrieval of nonstructured data such as images and free-text note fields commonly found in EHRs.

Flat Files

If the data structure is relatively simple, then a **flat file** or spreadsheet may be the right type of database. A flat file is a text file, usually delimited by a comma or tab, with one record found on each row. It has only one table of data. For instance, if a practice manager wished to track the number of records coded by each employee, then the flat file displayed in table 6.2 is sufficient.

This structure allows the manager to see who is the most or least productive and may be expanded by adding additional columns to track more days. A series of flat files or individual spreadsheets may be used to track other information about the employees such as credentials or continuing education (CEU) credits. If the number of additional attributes is small, then they may be added to the records displayed in table 6.2. If there is a large number of additional attributes, they may be stored in a second flat file.

Table 6.2.   Flat file

Employee	Monday	Tuesday	Wednesday	Thursday	Friday	Weekly Total
Anne	4	9	6	6	5	30
Nicholas	6	10	7	3	6	32
Zach	4	7	9	8	4	32

Table 6.3.   Comma-separated values

Employee, Monday, Tuesday, Wednesday, Thursday, Friday, Weekly Total
Anne,4,9,6,6,5,30
Nicholas,6,10,7,3,6,32
Zach,4,7,9,8,4,32

Flat file databases may be stored in a number of formats. Traditional spreadsheet tabs, such as those found in Microsoft Excel, are the most common format found in business applications. Flat files may also be stored in text files as columns of data or with the fields delimited by a character. Table 6.3 shows an example of the data depicted in table 6.2 stored as **column-delimited data** (a flat file database format where information is stored in text files as columns of data) or **comma-separated value (CSV)** file (a flat file database format where fields are delimited by a comma). Column-delimited data must be accompanied by documentation that lists the order and position of the variables so that the data may be interpreted properly.

CSV files may include the variable names in the first row. If not, then they too require documentation to identify the variables in each position.

Flat data tables have an intuitive two-dimensional format of rows and columns. The number of rows and columns is limited only by the software tool used to store and analyze the data. If a spreadsheet program is used to store the data, then formulas may be embedded into the table structure and are stored as part of the data table. A flat data table may be sorted or filtered to select particular values of the variables.

The two primary limitations of storing data in flat tables are first that the design does not allow relationships between variables in separate tables. This limits the ability to cross-check values for data integrity to those variables stored in the same table. For instance, if the charge description master (CDM) includes current procedural terminology (CPT) codes, the validation of the CPT code could only be accomplished by relating the CDM in one table to the CPT code table using the CPT code. The second limitation is that the same data element may need to be stored in multiple tables to allow for useful reporting. Data redundancy is not a good practice in database design and can cause serious data integrity issues when a variable is updated in one table, but not the others in which it is stored. If the tables used to store the various data elements need to be combined or must be validated against each other to ensure data integrity, then a relational database is a better choice.

Relational Databases

Relational databases were first conceptualized by Edgar F. Codd. He proposed that data should be stored in a way that allowed users to query and analyze data without having to restructure it (Codd 1970, 377). As an example, a data analyst wished to create a report of the number of patients served by zip code and clinical department. The data reside in two tables. One holds the patient demographic information. The second holds the information about the patient's visit, including the clinical department. If the database is stored in flat files, then the clinical department must be added to the first file or the zip code must be added to the second file. If the database is relational, then the two tables may be joined or linked using the patient identifier as a common data element.

In a relational database, data with a common purpose, concept, or source are arranged into tables. The relationship between the tables is displayed in an **entity relationship diagram (ERD)**. An ERD is defined as "a specific type of data modeling used in conceptual data modeling and the logical-level modeling of relational databases" (AHIMA 2014, 55). Figure 6.1 displays a simple ERD relating a patient information table to a table containing the dates of service for each visit for all patients. This ERD shows that the patient information and visit tables are related by the PatientID variable.

Relational databases are structured in a way that helps ensure data integrity. Notice that in figure 6.1, one variable in each table has an icon of a key next to it. These are the primary key in each of the tables. The **primary key** uniquely identifies the row in the database. PatientID uniquely identifies a row in the patient information table and AccountNumber uniquely identifies the row in the visits table. Properly defining the primary key field in a table prevents the adding of duplicate values of that field in the tables. A **foreign key** is a variable in one table that is a primary key in another table. In this example, PatientID is a foreign key in the visits table.

Figure 6.1. Entity relationship diagram

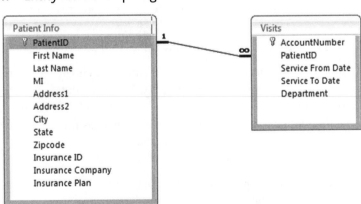

Table 6.4.   Cardinality

Cardinality	Table A	Table B	Explanation
One-to-one (1:1)	Patient ID Discharge status code	Discharge status code Definition	Each patient has only one discharge status code; each discharge status code has only one definition.
One-to-many (1:N or 1:∞)	Account number Patient name	Account number Diagnosis code sequence ICD-10-CM diagnosis code	Each account may have many associated diagnosis codes.
Many-to-many (N:N or ∞:∞)	Account number Bill type Bill date	Account number Bill type Bill date Payment amount	Each account may have multiple bill types and bill dates. Each bill type and bill date may have multiple payments.

The line extending in figure 6.1 from the PatientID variable in the patient information table to the PatientID variable in the visits table indicates that these two tables are related through the PatientID. Notice that the line has a 1 at the PatientInfo end and the infinity sign (∞) at the visits table end. These symbols represent the **cardinality** of the relationship between the two tables. Cardinality for each table refers to the number of elements in each table. Table 6.4 presents three types of relationship cardinality in relational databases:

1. One-to-one: Each row in one table relates to one and only one row in the other.
2. One-to-many: Each row in one table may relate to many rows in a second table; each row in the second table relates to only one row in the first table.
3. Many-to-many: Each row in one table may relate to many rows in a second table; each row in the second table may relate to many rows in the first table.

Carefully defining the variables in each table and the primary key fields for each table is the first step in ensuring data integrity. Data redundancy or duplication should be avoided in a relational database. The practice of **normalization** of a database prevents duplication of data elements and ensures the data all conform to a standard. There are three forms of normalization:

1. First Normal Form
   a. Eliminate repeating groups in individual tables
   b. Create a separate table for each set of related data
   c. Identify each set of related data with a primary key

2. Second Normal Form
   a. Create separate tables for sets of values that apply to multiple records
   b. Relate these tables with a foreign key

3. Third Normal Form
   a. Eliminate fields that do not depend on the key (Microsoft 2007).

Case Study: Normalizing Data Tables

In this case study, the flat data table included in table 6.5 will be converted to a relational database with a normalized form. When data are normalized, the data in one flat file may result in a number of tables.

The first normal form requires that the repeating groups be eliminated, separate tables be created for each set of related data, and each resulting table have a primary key. In table 6.5, the variables may be segmented into patient information (table 6.6) and service information (table 6.7).

The services table may be further broken down into a revenue code definition table, services by account number, and a CDM table. These are displayed in tables 6.7a, 6.7b, and 6.7c.

The final step in first-order normalization is to identify the primary key fields in each table. The primary key for the visits table is account number. The primary key in table 6.7a is a combination of the account number and the CDM item. The primary key in table 6.7b is the CDM item, and, finally, the primary key in table 6.7c is the revenue code.

By eliminating repeating rows, the tables now actually conform to the second normalized form. Recall that the second normalized form requires that separate tables be created for sets of values that apply to multiple records and that the tables be related with a foreign key.

The ERD displayed in figure 6.2 shows the relationships between the normalized tables. Notice that the field names were converted to single words by inserting an underscore between the words in the original variable names. It is best practice to use single-word variable or field names and table names to simplify the syntax for writing queries and reports.

The final step in normalization is to check the third normalized form. To conform to the third normalized form, all fields that do not depend on a key (primary or foreign) must be eliminated. The tables in figure 6.2 do not include any fields that do not depend on the key fields and therefore the tables are completely normalized.

Table 6.5.   Normalized data

MRN	Account number	Date of service	CDM item	Revenue code	Revenue code definition	HCPCS code	Units	Charge
123ABC	1	011011	L01	0300	LABORATORY OR LAB	36415	1	$ 55.75
123ABC	1	011011	L02	0300	LABORATORY OR LAB	84066	1	$ 51.50
123ABC	1	011011	L03	0301	LAB/CHEMISTRY	84153	1	$ 92.25
123ABC	1	011011	C01	0331	CHEMOTHER/INJ	96402	1	$ 168.50
123ABC	1	011011	D01	0636	DRUGS/DETAIL CODE	J9217	1	$ 507.77
987ZYX	2	010411	D02	0250	PHARMACY		6	$ 306.04
987ZYX	2	010411	S01	0270	MED-SUR SUPPLIES		1	$ 11.25
987ZYX	2	010411	S02	0270	MED-SUR SUPPLIES	A6257	1	$ 0.42
987ZYX	2	010411	L04	0305	LAB/HEMATOLOGY	85025	1	$ 107.00
987ZYX	2	010411	C02	0335	CHEMOTHERP-IV	96413	1	$ 495.00
987ZYX	2	010411	E13	0510	CLINIC	99213	1	$ 136.50
987ZYX	2	010411	D03	0636	DRUGS/DETAIL CODE	J2405	8	$ 50.65
987ZYX	2	010411	D04	0636	DRUGS/DETAIL CODE	J9305	100	$ 10,714.56
987ZYX	3	020611	S03	0270	MED-SUR SUPPLIES		1	$ 11.25
987ZYX	3	020611	S02	0270	MED-SUR SUPPLIES	A6257	1	$ 0.42
987ZYX	3	020611	E13	0510	CLINIC	99213	1	$ 136.50

Table 6.6.   Patient information

Patient_ID	Account_Number	Service_Date
123ABC	1	01/10/2011
987ZYX	2	01/04/2011
987ZYX	3	02/06/2011

Table 6.7.   Service information

			Services			
Account number	CDM item	Revenue code	Revenue code definition	HCPCS code	Units	Charge
1	L01	0300	LABORATORY OR LAB	36415	1	$ 55.75
1	L02	0300	LABORATORY OR LAB	84066	1	$ 51.50
1	L03	0301	LAB/CHEMISTRY	84153	1	$ 92.25
1	C01	0331	CHEMOTHER/INJ	96402	1	$ 168.50
1	D01	0636	DRUGS/DETAIL CODE	J9217	1	$ 507.77
2	D02	0250	PHARMACY		6	$ 306.04
2	S01	0270	MED-SUR SUPPLIES		1	$ 11.25
2	S02	0270	MED-SUR SUPPLIES	A6257	1	$ 0.42
2	L04	0305	LAB/HEMATO LOGY	85025	1	$ 107.00
2	C02	0335	CHEMOTHERP-IV	96413	1	$ 495.00
2	E13	0510	CLINIC	99213	1	$ 136.50
2	D03	0636	DRUGS/DETAIL CODE	J2405	8	$ 50.65
2	D04	0636	DRUGS/DETAIL CODE	J9305	100	$ 10,714.56
3	S03	0270	MED-SUR SUPPLIES		1	$ 11.25
3	S02	0270	MED-SUR SUPPLIES	A6257	1	$ 0.42
3	E13	0510	CLINIC	99213	1	$ 136.50

Table 6.7a.   Services

Services		
Account number	CDM item	Units
1	L01	1
1	L02	1
1	L03	1
1	C01	1
1	D01	1
2	D02	6
2	S01	1
2	S02	1
2	L04	1
2	C02	1
2	E13	1
2	D03	8
2	D04	100
3	S03	1
3	S02	1
3	E13	1

Table 6.7b.   Charge description master

Charge description master			
CDM item	Revenue code	HCPCS code	Unit charge
C01	0331	96402	$ 168.50
C02	0335	96413	$ 495.00
D01	0636	J9217	$ 507.77

Charge description master			
CDM item	Revenue code	HCPCS code	Unit charge
D02	0250		$ 51.01
D03	0636	J 2405	$ 6.33
D04	0636	J 9305	$ 107.15
E13	0510	99213	$ 136.50
L01	0300	36415	$ 55.75
L02	0300	84066	$ 51.50
L03	0301	84153	$ 92.25
L04	0305	85025	$ 107.00
S01	0270		$ 11.25
S02	0270	A6257	$ 0.42
S03	0270		$ 11.25

Table 6.7c.   Revenue codes

Revenue code	Revenue code definition
0250	PHARMACY
0270	MED-SUR SUPPLIES
0300	LABORATORY OR LAB
0301	LAB/CHEMISTRY
0305	LAB/HEMATOLOGY
0331	CHEMOTHER/INJ
0335	CHEMOTHERP-IV
0510	CLINIC
0636	DRUGS/DETAIL CODE

Figure 6.2.   Relationships between normalized tables

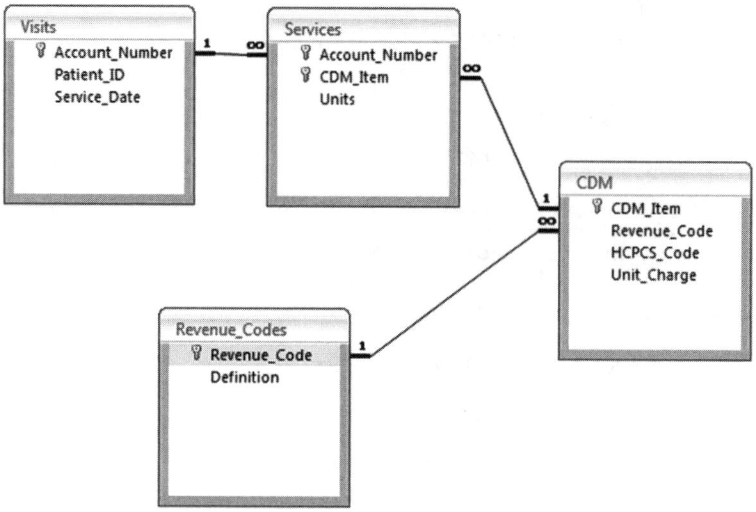

Source: Used with permission from Microsoft (2007).

Object-Oriented Databases

Object-oriented databases are designed to handle data types beyond text and numbers. Flat file and relational databases were developed to store data that fits into rows and columns. Object-oriented databases may be used to store images or videos. In healthcare, object-oriented databases may be used to store images from an MRI or an x-ray, or even an audio file capturing the heartbeat heard during a prenatal ultrasound. The building blocks of an object-oriented database are the objects, as opposed to the tables in a relational database system.

An object-oriented database stores two types of information about the object. The first element is the data itself (audio clip, image, video file, and such). The second element stored describes how to use the data and is called the **method**. Object-oriented databases are currently not used widely in practice, but the expansion of EHRs will require the storage of many objects beyond the simple rows and columns of numbers and text that may be stored in relational databases.

Database Management Software

To access and manipulate a database, it must reside in a software tool. The choice of database software depends on the type of database, the size of the database, and the complexity of the relationships between the database elements. Relational databases are found most often in practice. The most common relational database software applications include Microsoft Access, Oracle, and Microsoft SQL Server.

Microsoft Access is typically run from a workstation and is appropriate for smaller department-specific applications. It is also useful for prototyping larger enterprise-wide database systems. Once the number of users expands and Access can no longer efficiently accommodate the database, the database may require a more sophisticated software application. Microsoft offers a wizard that allows users to convert an Access database to a SQL Server database (Microsoft 2011).

Check Your Understanding 6.1

Answer the following questions.

1. Which database type stores both the data element and the method for its use?
   a. Relational database
   b. Object-oriented database
   c. Hierarchical database
   d. Flat file database

2. A primary key
   a. Uniquely identifies a record
   b. Contains only numerical values
   c. May be repeated across rows
   d. Represents the relationship between two fields

3. Microsoft Access in an example of:
   a. Relational database management software
   b. A spreadsheet program
   c. A program to manage flat data files
   d. A querying language

Indicate whether each of the following is true or false.

4. The fields in a data base represent the rows of the database.

5. The records in a database are the rows of data in the database.

⊙ Data Dictionary

A **data dictionary** is a tool that provides metadata or data about data. For example, the data element of First Name might include metadata such as the field length, that it is an alphanumeric field, and that the field is required. A key focus of a data dictionary is "to support and adopt more consistent use of data elements and terminology to improve the use of data in reporting. A data dictionary promotes clearer understanding; helps users find information; promotes more efficient use and reuse of information; and promotes better data management" (Dooling et al. 2014, 7).

A data dictionary should document the following attributes (or metadata) for the fields in a data table at a minimum:

⊙ Field name

⊙ Table name

⊙ Description of the field

⊙ Data type (numerical or text, field length)

⊙ Data frequency (required field or not)

⊙ Primary or foreign key

⊙ Valid values

⊙ Data source

⊙ Field creation date

- ⊙ Field termination date
- ⊙ Update frequency

The data dictionary in table 6.8 documents the contents of the CDM table found in the normalization example. The details included in this table allow a user with little or no knowledge of the contents of the table to understand the fields present and their various roles.

⊙ Structured Query Language (SQL)

Structured Query Language (SQL) is the programming language that is used to manipulate data in a relational database. SQL is sometimes pronounced "sequel." SQL fulfills many roles in a DBMS:

- ⊙ SQL is an interactive query language. Users type SQL commands into an interactive SQL program to retrieve data and display it on the screen, providing a convenient, easy-to-use tool for ad hoc database queries.
- ⊙ SQL is a database programming language. Programmers embed SQL commands into their application programs to access the data in a database. Both user-written programs and database utility programs (such as report writers and data entry tools) use this technique for database access.
- ⊙ SQL is a database administration language. The database administrator responsible for managing a minicomputer or mainframe database uses SQL to define the database structure and control access to the stored data.
- ⊙ SQL is a client/server language. Personal computer programs use SQL to communicate over a network with database servers that store shared data. This client/server architecture has become very popular for enterprise-class applications.
- ⊙ SQL is an Internet data access language. Internet web servers that interact with corporate data and Internet application servers all use SQL as a standard language for accessing corporate databases.
- ⊙ SQL is a distributed database language. Distributed DBMSs use SQL to help distribute data across many connected computer systems. The DBMS software on each system uses SQL to communicate with the other systems, sending requests for data access.
- ⊙ SQL is a database gateway language. In a computer network with a mix of different DBMS products, SQL is often used in a gateway that allows one brand of DBMS to communicate with another brand (Groff et al. 2010, 6).

The role of SQL as an interactive query language is described in more detail in the following section. The other roles of SQL are beyond the scope of this text, but health information management (HIM) professionals should be aware that SQL is far more than just a tool used to extract data from a relational database.

SQL commands that may be used to retrieve data follow a basic structure that allows nonprogrammers to understand and write queries. For example, a SQL command to collect all of the visits for a particular patient from a visits table is

SELECT * FROM visits WHERE patient_id = '987ZYX'

Table 6.8.   Data dictionary

Field Name	Table	Description	Data Type	Field Length	Data Frequency	Key?	Valid Values	Data Source	Field Creation Date	Field Termination Date	Update Frequency
CDM item	CDM	CDM item code	Text	20	Required	Primary	Alpha-numeric	Finance	01/01/1900		N/A
Revenue code	CDM	UB-04 revenue code	Text	4	Required	Foreign	Valid revenue code	HIM	01/01/1900		Annual
HCPCS code	CDM	CPT/HCPCS Level II	Text	5		Foreign	Valid HCPCS	HIM	01/01/1900		Annual
Unit charge	CDM	Charge per unit	Currency	10	Required		>= $0.00	Finance	01/01/1900		Annual

The results of the query are the two records displayed in table 6.9.

This is called a **select query**. The purpose of a select query is to pull records that meet a certain criterion from a particular table or combination of tables. The words SELECT, FROM, and WHERE are capitalized in the query because they represent keywords or instructions in the SQL command.

In this case, the two visit records for patient 987ZYX were selected from the three records found in the visits table. The query may be modified to present the records in a particular order. For instance, the records in the previous example may be sorted by descending service date by revising the query to include an ORDER BY statement:

> SELECT Visits.Account_Number, Visits.Patient_ID, Visits.Service_Date
>
> FROM Visits
>
> WHERE Visits.Patient_ID="987ZYX"
>
> ORDER BY Visits.Service_Date DESC;

The ORDER BY clause states that the results of the query should be sorted by descending service date. The results of this query are presented in table 6.10.

A select query may be used to combine data from two or more tables by defining a **join**. For example, a SQL query to select all of the patients that received the medical supply with the CDM item code S02 would require the services table be joined to the visits table. The relationship between these tables is found in the ERD displayed in figure 6.2. The tables must be combined or joined based on the Account_Number field. When more than one table is included in a query, the fields are referenced by both the table and the field name concatenated together and delimited by a period. For example, when referring to the field Account_Number in the visits table, the user would reference the field as Visits.Account_Number. The following select query will find the patients who received CDM item S02:

> SELECT Visits.Account_Number, Visits.Patient_ID, Visits.Service_Date, Services.CDM_Item, Services.Units
>
> FROM Visits INNER JOIN Services ON Visits.Account_Number = Services.Account_Number
>
> WHERE Services.CDM_Item="S02";

In this query, the SELECT statement includes the fields that are desired; the FROM statement includes the two tables (Visits and Services) as well as how those two tables should be related (Account_Number). Finally, the WHERE statement indicates that only rows where the CDM_Item is equal to S02 in the services table. The results of this query are presented in table 6.11.

A SQL command may also be used to summarize data. In the above example, a count of the number of visits for each patient may be generated with the following query:

SELECT Visits.Patient_ID, Count(Visits.Service_Date) AS CountOfService
_Date
FROM Visits
GROUP BY Visits.Patient_ID;

Table 6.9. Select query

Account_Number	Patient_ID	Service_Date
2	987ZYX	01/04/2011
3	987ZYX	02/06/2011

Table 6.10. Select query example results

Account_Number	Patient_ID	Service_Date
3	987ZYX	02/06/2011
2	987ZYX	01/04/2011

Table 6.11. Join query example results

Account_Number	Patient_ID	Service_Date	CDM_Item	Units
2	987ZYX	1/4/2011	S02	1
3	987ZYX	2/6/2011	S02	1

Table 6.12. Count of service dates

Patient_ID	CountOfService_Date
123ABC	1
987ZYX	2

This query includes the familiar SELECT and FROM keywords, but notice that there is now a GROUP BY statement. When a query is used to summarize data the summary statistic and the field that designates the group to be summarized must be designated. In the example, the SELECT statement includes a command that creates a count of the number of service dates, Count(Visits,Service_Date), and stores that result in a new field called CountOfService_Date. The GROUP BY portion of the query states that the counts should be presented by Patient_ID. The result of this query is presented in table 6.12.

Check Your Understanding 6.2

Answer the following questions.

1. SQL is an acronym for
   a. Sequential Query Language
   b. Structured Query Language
   c. Selective Question Language
   d. Sequential Question Language

2. SQL is used to manipulate
   a. Data in a relational database
   b. Data in a flat file database
   c. A data warehouse
   d. Unstructured data

3. What keyword is missing from this SQL statement:
   SELECT name, birthdate WHERE month(birthdate) = 12
   a. BY
   b. FROM
   c. LIST
   d. GROUP

4. Which of the following SQL keywords results in an aggregation of data?
   a. FROM
   b. SELECT
   c. GROUP BY
   d. WHERE

5. A field reference of visits.patient_id refers to:
   a. A field called visits in the patient_id table
   b. A table called patient_id in the visits database
   c. A field called patient_id in the visits table
   d. A row with a value of 'patient_id' in a field called visits

---

⊙ Data Modeling

A **data model** is a representation of the data to be stored in a database and the relationships between the tables and data fields. Prior to the design of the database, the business process to be supported by the database must be modeled. This may be accomplished through the use of process and data flow diagrams. The components of a database, discussed previously in this chapter, are designed and assembled in a way that supports the business process requirements. Data modeling may be carried out using either an object-oriented or an entity relationship approach. The entity relationship approach will be outlined here.

There are two important outputs to the data modeling process. The first output is the ERD, a graphical representation of the tables in the database and their relationships.

The second output is the data dictionary. The data model serves as the basis for the database structure and design as documented by the ERD and data dictionary.

The process of data modeling includes three steps: the conceptual model, the logical model, and the physical data model. The conceptual model includes a mapping of the business requirements for the database using nontechnical terms that end users can understand. A database that does not meet the need of the end users is of no value, so they must be involved in the design process at the earliest stage. The conceptual data model is independent of the type of database that will ultimately be used to store the data. The conceptual data model may be mapped using a context-level **data flow diagram**, which maps out the database's boundary and scope. Figure 6.3 shows a context-level data flow diagram for the claims database example used earlier in this chapter. Notice that the diagram does not include any field or table information. It simply displays the general categories of data and their roles in the business process. The details regarding the actual database structure are fleshed out in the logical modeling step.

The logical model is the next step in database modeling. During this phase the tables start to take shape. The fields are not defined, but the basic contents of the tables and how they relate are defined. In the claims data example, the tables are

- Patient information
- Visit for each patient
- Services provided to patient
- Charge for services

The relationships between the tables may be mapped out in a **Diagram 0** data flow diagram. A Diagram 0 data flow diagram expands on the context diagram and adds details regarding the tables and their relationships. Figure 6.4 displays a Diagram 0 for the claims database example.

The final step in the database modeling process is to determine the physical model. This includes mapping out the tables, keys, and relationships using an ERD as well as determining the DBMS and hardware to house the database. The ERD for this example is displayed in figure 6.2. At this point in the modeling process a database type may be selected. Because this database requires multiple tables that

Figure 6.3. Context-level data flow diagram

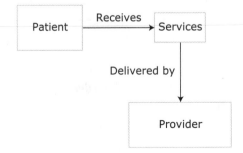

Figure 6.4. Diagram 0

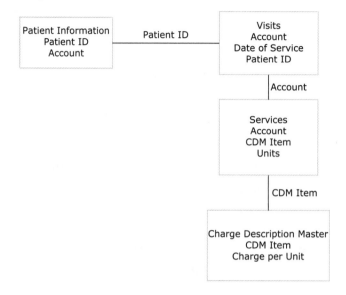

may need to be linked together for reporting purposes, a relational database is the best choice for this business process. There are a number of DBMSs that support relational database structures. Some examples include

- ⊙ Microsoft Access
- ⊙ Microsoft SQL Server
- ⊙ Informix
- ⊙ Oracle
- ⊙ MySQL

The choice of specific DBMS software should be based on the size and scope of the database as well as the budget for the project.

The physical model also includes a specification of the computer hardware that will be used to house the database. The amount of storage or disk space required for the database should be determined prior to selecting any hardware platform. Estimating the space required for the database currently and for the foreseeable future will help determine the appropriate hardware and software to select for implementation of the database.

Check Your Understanding 6.3

Answer the following questions.

1. Which phase of data modeling includes a description of the business process?
   a. Physical model
   b. Logical model
   c. Conceptual model
   d. Final model

2. Which phase of data modeling describes the relationship between the data tables?
   a. Physical model
   b. Logical model
   c. Conceptual model
   d. Final model

3. What is one of the two outputs from a data modeling process?
   a. ERD
   b. SQL
   c. NDC
   a. DBMS

4. Which portion of the data modeling process maps out the relationships between the tables?
   a. Context-level data flow diagram
   b. Conceptual model
   c. Diagram 0
   d. Diagram 2

5. The choice of which DBMS to use depends on:
   a. Physical data model
   b. Conceptual data model
   c. Size and scope of the database
   d. Availability of physical space

⊙ Data Warehouses and Data Marts

Arraying data into databases for storage and retrieval is the first step in using data for decision making. The case study in this chapter was a very simple database designed to hold information about the services provided to a patient. Clinical and operational databases may be found in various departments throughout a healthcare facility, including

- ⊙ Patient accounting
- ⊙ Clinical departments
- ⊙ Pharmacy
- ⊙ Clinical trials
- ⊙ Marketing
- ⊙ Quality measurement
- ⊙ Finance
- ⊙ Patient experience

Combining these data sources into a **data warehouse** is an effective method of making the data accessible to a wider audience of users. A data warehouse must be designed in a way that maintains sufficient detail so that the data is useful for research and analytic purposes and related in a way that supports real-time access to the data by users. Data warehouses are snapshots of a variety of databases found throughout a company that are combined for the purpose of reporting and analysis. The data warehouse does not include the "live" or transaction data that are used for business operations, but instead are populated by periodic downloads from the live database. A **clinical data warehouse** is a database that facilitates accessing data from many databases in one query for reporting (AHIMA 2014, 26). The frequency of refreshing the clinical data warehouse depends on the volatility of the underlying data (how often it changes) and the need for timely reporting.

The key requirements for a data warehouse and business intelligence system (DW/BI) include:

1. The DW/BI system must make information easily accessible.
2. The DW/BI system must present information consistently.
3. The DW/BI system must adapt to change.
4. The DW/BI system must present information in a timely way.
5. The DW/BI system must be a secure bastion that protects information assets.
6. The DW/BI system must serve as the authoritative and trustworthy foundation for improved decision making.
7. The business community must accept the DW/BI system to deem it successful (Kimball and Ross 2013, 3).

Although these requirements were not specifically written about clinical or healthcare data warehouses, all of the requirements still apply. The last requirement, acceptance by the business community, is key. If the data warehouse is not accepted as the source of truth for data used to drive operations, then there is no reason for it to exist. Data warehouses can often become unwieldy and difficult to navigate for end users. To avoid this issue, departments often construct **data marts**, which are well-organized, user-centered searchable databases containing information drawn from a data warehouse to meet the users' specific needs (such as specific data in the database) (AHIMA 2014, 43).

Data marts offer a convenient method of accessing the most relevant data elements for a particular use case or department, but they represent a challenge in terms of data and information governance. As such, they are not generally accepted in large organizations as a good solution for long-term data needs.

Data warehouses and data marts are both methods used to bring complex data from multiple sources to a common database for end user analysis. The data is moved from the source to the data warehouse via a process that is called **extract, transform, and load (ETL)**. Extracting data is the process of copying the data into the ETL system for manipulation (Kimball and Ross 2013, 19). Once the data are extracted, it is essentially part of the data warehouse. Because data may come from multiple systems, the transform step ensures the data are compatible. Any data mapping, correction, or translation occurs during this step. The final step in moving data from the source to the data warehouse is the load step. This is the step when the data are physically loaded into tables that make up the data warehouse. Once the ETL process is mapped out and built, it is often scheduled to occur at regular times such as nightly or weekly. The data in the data warehouse are then essentially a snapshot in time of the data in the source systems at the time of the ETL process.

Decision support databases are a common example of a data warehouse. These databases are found in many healthcare entities and may include claims data, financial data, and quality data combined in one database to support both internal and external reporting. One of the unique challenges in combining clinical data is that any release of that data may be subject to HIPAA regulations if it includes any of the protected health information fields such as dates or Social Security numbers (45 CFR Parts 160, 162, and 164). Any efforts to combine data into a clinical data warehouse should include the involvement of a compliance officer or other professional with knowledge of the rules and regulations surrounding deidentification of data and the release of identifiable data.

Much of the time and effort invested in compiling a clinical data warehouse is used to clean and combine the data. Although clinical data is singularly focused on healthcare and patient information, the coding systems may or may not be consistent. For instance, pharmacy databases may include the National Drug Code (NDC) or may only include an inventory or CDM code that only has meaning inside a particular facility or system of facilities. The mapping between code sets and standardization of coding systems is an age-old issue in healthcare data. The concept of common **ontology** or system of categories as a method of combining data that may be categorized by clinical classification systems such as ICD and CPT codes as well as those categorized by clinical nomenclatures such as Systematized Nomenclature of Medicine Clinical Terms (SNOMED CT) has emerged. An effective ontology is "a theory of those higher-level categories which structure the biomedical domain, the representation of which needs to be both unified and coherent if it is to serve as the basis for terminologies and coding systems that have the requisite degree and type of interoperability" (Smith and Ceusters 2007). A properly designed ontology may allow the automated combining of data from many sources. Such a system would speed the design and delivery of new clinical data warehouses.

Case Study: Stanford Translational Research Integrated Database Environment (STRIDE)

The Stanford School of Medicine has an extensive clinical data warehouse called STRIDE (Stanford Translational Research Integrated Database Environment) that stores data that supports clinical and translational research (Stanford Center for Clinical Informatics 2013). STRIDE includes data from both hospitals affiliated with Stanford. The hospitals use different billing systems and yet the

(Continued)

warehouse is designed to combine the data sets across the facilities. In January 2013, the STRIDE warehouse included

- 1.85 million pediatric and adult patients with clinical and demographic data (1994 to present)
- 21.5 million Clinical Encounters (1994 to present)
- 40 million ICD-9 coded inpatient and outpatient diagnoses (1994 to present)
- 25 million ICD-9 and CPT-coded inpatient and outpatient clinical procedures (1994 to present)
- 3.1 million radiology reports (2005 to present)
- 1.3 million surgical pathology reports (1995 to present)
- 21 million transcribed clinical documents (2005 to present)
- 145 million laboratory test numerical results (2000 to present)
- 14 million inpatient pharmacy orders (2006 to present)
- 99,000 dates of death drawn from hospital and Social Security Administration records

Clinical data warehouses like Stanford's STRIDE are becoming widespread as the technology to support the storage and access of huge volumes of data.

One project that shows tremendous promise in facilitating the combining and sharing of clinical data is an NIH-funded study called Informatics for Integrating Biology and the Bedside (i2b2) (Murphy et al. 2010). The mission of the project is to provide researchers with a framework to combine medical record and clinical research data. The data are stored in a deidentified format so that researchers can analyze the data to develop hypotheses and perform initial analyses to investigate the likelihood for the availability of patient cohorts for clinical trials. I2b2 facilitates the sharing of large amounts of standardized clinical data and yet protects the identification of individual patients and may be implemented using either an Oracle or a Microsoft SQL Server database.

Chapter 6 Review Exercises

Answer the following questions.

1. DBMS is an acronym for
   a. Database manipulation standards
   b. Database management standards
   c. Database management system
   d. Database manipulation system

2. A flat file database is a
   a. Database that only has simple data tables
   b. Database with only one table
   c. Database that contains records with a large number of fields
   d. Database manipulation system

3. An entity relationship diagram is used to display
   a. The update schedule for data
   b. The flow of data to reports
   c. The relationships between tables in a database
   d. The number of records in each table

4. A one-to-one (1:1) relationship describes which aspect of the relationship between two tables?
   a. The number of matching fields
   b. The cardinality
   c. The number of key fields
   d. The number of rows in each table

5. Patient and social security number is an example of what kind of relationship?
   a. 1:1
   b. 1:N
   c. N:1
   d. N:N

6. Which normal form eliminates repeating groups of values?
   a. First
   b. Second
   c. Third
   d. Fourth

7. Which of the following attributes are not included in a data dictionary?
   a. Valid values
   b. Data type
   c. Update frequency
   d. Size of table

8. Which of the following SQL statements will select all columns and rows from the table visits?
   a. SELECT patient_id FROM visits
   b. SELECT * FROM visits WHERE service_date = #1/1/2010#
   c. SELECT * FROM visits
   d. SELECT account, count(patient_id) FROM visits

9. The field reference cpt.code in a SQL query refers to
   a. The database named cpt.code
   b. The field code in the table named cpt
   c. The field cpt in the table named code
   d. The table named code found in the database named cpt

10. Which phase of data modeling includes the selection of the database type?
    a. Physical model
    b. Logical model
    c. Conceptual model
    d. Final model

REFERENCES

45 CFR Parts 160, 162, and 164. HIPAA Transactions and Code Sets, Security Rule, Privacy Rule, Breach Notification for Unsecured Protected Health Information. Department of Health and Human Services.

AHIMA. 2014. *Pocket Glossary of Health Information Management and Technology.* 4th ed. ed. Chicago, Illinois: AHIMA Press.

Codd, E.F. 1970. A Relational Model of Data for Large Shared Data Banks. Edited by P. Baxendate. *Communications of the ACM* 13(6):377–387.

Dooling, J., P. Goyal, L. Hyde, L. Kadlec, S. White. 2014 Health Data Analysis Toolkit. Chicago: AHIMA.

Groff, J., P. Weinberg, and A. Oppel. 2010. *SQL: The Complete Reference.* 3rd ed. New York: McGraw-Hill/Osborne.

Kimball, R., and M. Ross. 2013. The Data Warehouse Toolkit: The Definitive Guide to Dimensional Modeling. 3rd ed. Indianapolis: Wiley.

Microsoft. 2011. How to Convert an Access Database to SQL Server. Microsoft Support. http://support.microsoft.com/kb/237980.

Microsoft. 2007. Description of the Database Normalization Basics. Microsoft Support. http://support.microsoft.com/kb/283878.

Murphy, S., G. Weber, M. Mendis, V. Gainer, H. Chueh, S. Churchill, I. Kohane. 2010, March. Serving the enterprise and beyond with informatics for integrating biology and the bedside (i2b2). *Journal of the American Medical Informatics Association* 17(2):124–130.

Smith, B., and W. Ceusters. 2007. Ontology as the Core Discipline of Biomedical Informatics: Legacies of the Past and Recommendations for the Future Direction of Research. In *Computing, Philosophy, and Cognitive Science—The Nexus and the Liminal.* Edited by G.D. Crnkovic and S. Stuart, 104–122. Cambridge: Cambridge Scholars Press.

Stanford Center for Clinical Informatics. 2013. Clinical Data Warehouse Projects— SCCI Stanford Medicine. Stanford Center for Clinical Informatics. https://clinicalinformatics.stanford.edu/projects/cdw.html.

ADDITIONAL RESOURCES

Inmon, B. 1992. *Building the Data Warehouse.* Wiley and Sons.

Chapter 7

Introduction to Research

Learning Objectives

- Develop a personal vocabulary of research related terms
- Apply the steps in the research process
- Articulate the role of the EHR in healthcare research
- Relate the principles of research design
- Examine statistical analysis tools
- Select the means of appropriate data analysis
- Choose the appropriate means for data visualization

KEY TERMS

Alternate hypothesis
ANOVA
Applied research
Basic research
Cause and effect
Clinical outcomes assessment
Control Group
Correlational research
Dashboard
Data analysis
Data mining
Data retrieval

Data visualization
Dependent variable
Descriptive research
Descriptive statistics
Double-blind study
Experimental research
Export
External validity
Field studies
Forecasting
Historical research
Hypotheses

Import	Quantitative research
Independent variable	Quasi-experimental
Inferential statistics	Random sampling
Institutional Review Board (IRB)	Reliability
Internal validity	Research
Metadata	Research question
Mixed methods research	Retrospective research
Natural experiments	Sample
Nonexperimental research	Scatterplots
Null hypotheses	Structured Query Language (SQL)
Placebo	t-test
Population	Validity
Predictive analysis	Variable
Qualitative research	Vulnerable subjects

Research is

> an inquiry process aimed at discovering new information about a subject or revising old information. Investigation or experimentation aimed at the discovery and interpretation of facts, revision of accepted theories or laws in the light of new facts, or practical application of such new or revised theories or laws; the collecting of information about a particular subject (AHIMA 2014, 129).

As a result of a HITECH act modification, research is considered to be "a systemic investigation, including research development, testing and evaluation, designed to develop or contribute to generalized knowledge" (Congress 2009). Using the patient record for research purposes is considered to be a secondary use of the information.

Using patient information for research purposes is quite appealing due to the capabilities of the EHR to capture or manipulate data in ways that were not previously available or that were time consuming and difficult to obtain. For example, tracking just one patient's blood pressure over several episodes of care, using paper charts, would require abstracting the readings from each of the records for the individual encounters. By contrast, with an EHR and electronic data exchange, the underlying databases could be queried across episodes of care and even different healthcare organizations for a specific period of time for one patient. Utilizing the EHR, the possibilities for accessing this same information for groups of patients such as different age groups, presence of other specific diagnoses, medications and treatment provided, and so on, are almost limitless.

There are regulations specifically for using patient identifiable information for research purposes. The HIPAA privacy rule requires prior patient authorization for internal use or for the disclosure of patient information for research use unless one of several exceptions are met or if approved by a privacy board or the organization's

Institutional Review Board (IRB) (45 CFR 160.514(d)). Situations that do not require patient authorization include

- ⊙ Reviewing the information to plan for research to include developing the research question or hypothesis but maintaining the patient information within the covered entity;
- ⊙ Studying those who are no longer living; and
- ⊙ Using only a limited data set where data has been deidentified (removing any information that could be used to identify the individual; AHIMA 2014) also referred to as anonymized data.

The HIPAA Privacy Rule's minimum necessary standard requires covered entities to use the minimum PHI necessary for the research project (45 CFR 164.502(b); 45 CFR 164.514(d)). The minimum necessary standard must be followed even when the use of the patient information is authorized or a waiver has been granted. HIPAA is the primary federal regulation that addresses the use of this information, but the Federal Policy for Protection of Human Subjects, also called the Common Rule, must be considered when support for the research has been provided by the federal government and includes entities such HHS and Veterans Affairs (45 CFR 46.111(a)(7)). The Common Rule is a set of regulations regarding human research and testing governed by the IRB (AHIMA 2014, 31). Researchers must also be compliant with state laws that cover the access and use of patient data, which are, in some instances, more stringent or cover particular types of data such as for HIV or genetics.

⊙ Principles of Research Design

Consistent with the definition of research to find new information, research can be divided into two major types: basic research and applied research. **Basic research,** which may also be referred to as pure or theoretical, is done with a "focus on the development and refinement of theories" (AHIMA 2014, 15) but not necessarily to identify a solution to the problem. **Applied research**, also referred to as practical or clinical research, "focuses on the use of scientific theories to improve actual practice" (AHIMA 2014, 10). Moreover, it is common for the initial research on a new topic to involve exploratory studies designed to evaluate current practices for the emerging topic (Dolezel and Moczygemba 2015).

For either basic or applied research, addressing the research design before a study begins provides "structure of the study ensuring that the evidence collected will be relevant and that the evidence will unambiguously and convincingly answer the research question; the design includes a detailed plan that, in a quantitative study includes controlling variance" (AHIMA 2014, 129). One component of the overall research design is the research approach. There are three types of research approaches used for conducting research inquiries: quantitative, qualitative, and mixed methods. Researchers must consider the purpose of the study when selecting the research approach (Layman and Watzlaf 2009, 194). To test a hypothesis where numerical data can be collected for statistical analysis, a quantitative research approach is indicated. Conversely, qualitative studies to gather information would be appropriate to explore the perceptions of individuals or groups in a new area or regarding a shared experience.

Quantitative Research

Quantitative research aims to test a theory by defining specific, measurable study variables, collecting and analyzing data on those variables, and conducting statistical tests to examine the relationships among the variables (Creswell 2011). Quantitative research is used extensively in healthcare studies. To begin, quantitative researchers first conduct extensive literature reviews to establish the importance of the research topic, to understand what previous research has been conducted, and to define the study variables and methods based on the evidence-based work of previous researchers. Data collected for the study are generally numerical. Quantitative researchers seek to collect large amounts of data from many participants on the explicitly defined study variables. An example of a quantitative study would be Safian's study on the factors influencing students to enroll in HIM programs in which a survey was used to collect data from closed ended questions (Safian 2012). This study determined that career opportunities were the biggest factor in the decision to enroll in a medical billing and coding undergraduate program.

Qualitative Research

Qualitative research involves investigating nonnumerical observations such as words and perceptions (Forrestal 2016, 565). Often the qualitative study does not start with defining a hypothesis to be proved or disproved in the study, or by defining specific variables to be examined (Creswell 2011, 16). Instead, the research questions are broad, open-ended questions such as, "What motivated you to study health information management?" Qualitative studies aim to analyze the data for emerging themes that can be used to derive meaning (Creswell 2011, 16). The nonnumerical data analyzed in these studies can be words, gestures, actions, pictures, recordings, activities, or perceptions of the study participants gathered from open-ended questions asking their opinions (Layman and Watzlaf 2009).

Usually, data are collected on a small group of participants (Creswell 2011, 16). A common way to analyze the data is to look for themes in the respondents' answers to the research questions. In one qualitative study, the researchers collected data on the opinions on health information exchanges, e-prescribing, and personal health records of individuals who were invited to participate in focus groups (Cochran et al. 2015). Qualitative analysis was conducted using transcribed audio data. For example, NVivo qualitative statistical software was used to identify common themes, which were compiled for each of the discussion categories: HIE, e-Rx, and PHR. Results indicated respondents were concerned about privacy and security, cost of implementation, and quality of care (Cochran et al. 2015, 1).

Mixed Methods Research

Mixed methods research studies utilize data collection and data analysis methods from both quantitative and qualitative research in one study. The major part of the mixed methods study may be either quantitative or qualitative. These studies are more complicated to undertake than a quantitative or qualitative study, but the combination of the two approaches provides a more in-depth picture of the phenomenon under study (Creswell 2013, 534). A common form of mixed method studies begins with a largely quantitative component followed by a smaller qualitative component such as a study to record customer satisfaction with 25 closed questions asking the user to rate their satisfaction on various factors followed by four or five written response questions.

For example, a mixed methods study on the benefits of telemedicine in rural communities explored hospital staff perceptions on the benefits of telemedicine (Potter et al. 2016). Data were collected with surveys, phone interviews, and site visits. Descriptive and thematic data analysis was conducted. Survey respondents reported tele-emergency was beneficial to rural communities, while interviewees indicated that telemedicine improved the hospitals image in the community (Potter et al. 2016, 1).

Experimental Research

Random sampling is a sampling method utilized to select an unbiased group of study participants (AHIMA 2014, 125). **Experimental research** is conducted using random sampling to assign participants to either an experimental or a control group (Forrestal 2016, 585). A **double-blind study** is one in which neither the participants nor the researchers know who is in the control group and who is in the study group. During the study, one group is subjected to the study treatment, and the other group, called the **control group**, is not given the study treatment. It should be noted that administering treatment, or an intervention, can mean providing a new type of physical therapy, having participants listen to educational videos on coding practices, or giving them a medication. By contrast, the control group in these studies would use the existing type of physical therapy, would not listen to the video on new coding practices, and would be given a **placebo** that does not contain the new medication. Results from both groups are then compared to determine the effectiveness of the treatment. Experimental research can be used to give strong evidence of **cause and effect,** which means that researchers can state with some confidence that the variable under study caused, or did not cause, the effect under study (Layman and Watzlaf 2009, 115).

There are many **nonexperimental research** studies conducted where there is no random selection of participants nor is there any random assignment of participants to study groups. Quasi-experimental, historical, descriptive, correlational, and qualitative are all nonexperimental studies. **Historical research** studies inspect past events like the events leading up to AHIMA's adding the Clinical Health Data Analyst credential. Researchers conducting **descriptive research** collect and analyze data to describe the population characteristics (Huck 2012). Data results typically include summary statistics (that is, mean, median, mode, range, and standard deviation) and frequency calculations for data characteristics (for example, percentage of males and females). Qualitative studies were described above.

Correlational Research

The results of a **correlational research** study indicate the existence, direction, and strength of relationships between two numerical variables (Huck 2012). Results of these studies can show that two variables are strongly or weakly related, or that they both increase (positive relationship) or decrease (negative relationship) together. A **variable** is something that may have different values (Huck 2012). Correlational studies cannot be used to establish causation, only experimental studies can give strong evidence of cause and effect (Layman and Watzlaf 2009, 115). With correlational studies, it may be that some variable outside the study caused the event. For example, researchers in a 2010 correlational study investigated the relationship between the patient's comprehension of their reasons for being admitted to the hospital from the Emergency Room (ER) and their overall satisfaction with the care received (Downey and Zun 2010). Results indicated that ER wait times were not a major determinant of their satisfaction with their care, and that most would return to the ER if necessary.

Quasi-Experimental

Quasi-experimental studies are appropriate when the study variables cannot or should not be manipulated (Forrestal 2016, 586). This could occur because study variables cannot be changed (that is, age, race, gender) or should not be changed as they are integral to the study (that is, patients with certain diseases, facilities that are using a HIE). **Retrospective research**, also called case control research, is quasi-experimental because the phenomenon under study occurred in the past. These types of studies are common in healthcare. Some examples of retrospective studies are researchers' examining postoperative infection rates at a facility, calculating the rate of coding errors for each medical coder, or evaluating the usage levels of electronic health records from usage data collected over the last five years. Other types of quasi-experimental studies are field studies and natural experiments. A **field study** is done outside the laboratory or place of work. For example, researchers could have observed nurses' handwashing techniques in the field at a one-day surgery center. During a **natural experiment,** researchers have no control over the phenomenon under study. They do have the study planned but are waiting for the event to occur naturally, such as a study to evaluate the effects of an increase in physicians' copayments on primary care physician visits (Jakobsson and Svensson 2016). The natural experiment research plan includes gathering existing data on the primary care physician visits then gathering data on the visits during the time frame of the study (when the higher copays are in effect) and comparing them. It is easy to discern that studies conducted to quantify the consequence of changing policies and procedures are also natural experiments, as are studies that measure the facility's process for restoring computers systems after a hardware system failure.

Clinical Outcomes Assessment

Healthcare outcomes are results or what follows medical interventions by the providers of care. **Clinical outcomes assessment** is "research that seeks to improve the delivery of patient care by studying the end result of healthcare services" also referred to as outcomes analysis (Forrestal 2016, 577). Many healthcare studies are conducted to assess clinical outcomes. The information gained by these studies is very important to improving quality of care along with controlling costs. The EHR affords new opportunities for tracking and assessing patient data. The Health Resources and Services Administration (HRSA), a resource for providers to aid in the development of their EHR, indicates that there are four steps for measuring clinical processes and outcomes. The steps are to:

- Identify the intervention or processes for improvement,
- Select the appropriate measures to evaluate the focus of the assessment,
- Establish a baseline of current practices using the selected measures, and
- Monitor and reassess the outcomes once the changes have been made to determine the effect on the outcomes (HRSA 2016).

The primary purpose of clinical outcomes assessment is improved patient care, which is accomplished by providing information for clinical decision making and evaluating and improving the performance of clinicians. Clinical outcomes assessment data can also be utilized as justifications for pay for performance and to assist potential patients in the selection of a clinician.

IRB Processes and Procedures

Prior to conducting any type of research involving human subjects, researchers must obtain **Institutional Review Board (IRB)** approval from the IRB office where the study is being conducted (HHS 2016). The IRB approval process provides review, oversight, and guidance to the researchers and is mandatory for federally funded programs (AHIMA 2014, 80). The Office for Human Research Protections (OHRP) of the Department of Health and Human Services monitors compliance of IRB offices with the federal regulations governing research with human subjects. Most institutes have their own IRB compliance office and researchers may need to submit two IRB applications if they are not conducting the study at their place of employment. For example, an educator wishing to conduct research at a university hospital needs to apply to their university's IRB office and the hospitals' IRB office. Upon applying for IRB approval, the researcher selects the type of IRB application that is exempted, expedited, or requires a full board review. Exempted applications would include utilizing deidentified data such as past patient data but with all identifiers removed (that is, deidentified computer report). Expedited submissions are used when the study potentially poses some risk to human subjects, and full board review and approval submissions deal with studies not in the first two categories or dealing with vulnerable subjects (21 CFR Parts 50 and 56: US Food and Drug Administration). **Vulnerable subjects** in the context of research studies are children, pregnant women, human fetuses, neonates, mentally disabled individuals, educationally or economically disadvantaged, prisoners or persons with incurable or fatal diseases (21 CFR Parts 50 and 56: US Food and Drug Administration). The study participants in these categories require additional consideration or protection. Whether the research is exempted or not, researchers must obtain informed consent from the subjects signifying that they understand the nature of the study, study risks, and that the study data will be deidentified. Participants should be informed that they may opt out of the study at any time.

Check Your Understanding 7.1

Match the terms with the appropriate descriptions.
- **a.** Research
- **b.** Applied research
- **c.** Quantitative research
- **d.** Qualitative research
- **e.** Experimental research

1. _____ Process aimed at discovering new information about a subject
2. _____ Tests a theory by defining measurable variables and collecting and analyzing data on those variables
3. _____ Practical or clinical research
4. _____ Research aimed at investigating nonnumerical observations such as images
5. _____ Research conducted by randomly assigning participants to an experimental or a control group

Answer the following questions.

6. Which is the type of research that gives the strongest evidence of cause and effect?
   - **a.** Experimental
   - **b.** Nonexperimental
   - **c.** Correlational
   - **d.** Descriptive
   - **e.** Predictive

7. Which is research that examines the existence, strength, and direction of the relationship between two numerical variables?
   - **a.** Historical
   - **b.** Evaluation
   - **c.** Correlational
   - **d.** Descriptive

Steps in the Research Process

There are fundamental steps that should be followed when embarking on research. For clarification, these steps will be illustrated for a hypothetical quantitative correlational study. Before examining the research process, basic terminology related to the process steps must be reviewed. As mentioned previously, a variable is an attribute that may have different values. Quantitative studies have independent and dependent variables. As an illustration, consider the research question "Does providing additional training on a new EHR system increase the physicians' utilization of the system at this facility?" The **independent variable** is the variable that researchers believe will cause change in the **dependent variable,** which is the variable being measured. In the case of the EHR training, receiving the additional training (independent variable) is expected to cause a change in the level of utilization of the new EHR system (dependent variable), which is being measured. If the study results were graphed, the values on the x-axis would be the independent variables and the y-axis values would be the dependent variable, usually frequency values, because the value of y (level of utilization) is determined by the value of x (did or did not receive the training).

The research process steps will be illustrated for a hypothetical quantitative correlational study. Initially, the quantitative researcher will generate a quantitative purpose statement, which is a sentence that describes what the study is examining, and identifies the independent and dependent study variables, the participants, and the study site. Research textbooks should be consulted when defining the purpose statement as many provide templates as guidelines (Creswell 2011, 123–124). For example, the following is a template for a purpose statement:

> The purpose of this study is to test (the theory) by relating (the independent variable) to (the dependent variable) for (participants) at the (research site) (Creswell 2011, 123).

For the correlational study, using the template, the purpose is to relate age (independent variable) with number of ER visits (dependent variable) for patients (participants) at Valley General Hospital (research study site) (Creswell 2011).

Determine Research Question

Next, a quantitative **research question** will be generated. All quantitative studies have one or more research questions. The research questions restate the research problem and name the independent and dependent variables, participants, and research site, but with a narrowed focus. This study will use a relationship research question. The research question for this study will be "How does the age relate to the number of ER visits for patients at Valley General Hospital during the study period?"

Some researchers may also advance **hypotheses** that are their predictions of the results that are often based on findings from their extensive literature review. The **null hypothesis** indicates there is no association between the independent and dependent variable (AHIMA 2014, 104). The **alternate hypothesis** indicates there is an association between the independent and dependent variable (AHIMA 2014, 7). For this study, the research hypothesis will be "The greater the age of the patient, the more ER visits they will have at Valley General during the study period." Formally, the null hypothesis is tested as "There is no difference between age and number of ER visits at Valley General in the study period." The alternate hypothesis is tested as "There is a difference between age and number of ER visits at Valley General in the study period."

Define Study Variables and Their Data Types

Structured data collected for a study can have four levels of measurement: nominal, ordinal, interval, or ratio (AHIMA 2014, 21). Nominal and ordinal data are expressed in categories, while ratio and interval data are continuous data (White 2016, 512). The selection of data measurement levels for data representation is an important part of a study because it determines what type of statistical tests can be conducted.

For this study, the independent study variable is age and the dependent variable is number of ER visits. To further define age, the researcher must decide on how to represent the data for age. The researcher could use categorical ordinal age groups like 20–25 years, 26–30 years, and so on. Or he could record age as a continuous number such as 20.5 years or 48 years. To simplify data collection, age will be a continuous variable and number of ER visits will be a discrete counting number. Studies also typically collect demographic data about their participants, so the researcher will add two demographic variables to collect race and gender, and they will be nominal variables.

Identify Sample and Population

The **population** is the universe of phenomena, objects, people, or data under investigation from which a sample is taken (AHIMA 2014, 116). A **sample** is a group of patients selected to represent the population and that sample is tested using **inferential statistics** techniques that allow the researchers to make statements about the populations characteristics based on the sample's characteristics (AHIMA 2014, 78). For this study, suppose the ER manager says that her staff is very busy but she will try to provide the sample data for the study by having the staff collect data on 30 patients a day, with each shift surveying 10 patients. Because it is always possible that the study sample is not representative of the population, at this point data should be obtained on the age groups, gender, and race of all the ER patients seen during the study period.

Data Collection Methods

Types of data collection methods include census, sample, questionnaires (survey), observation, and interviews. These are defined as:

- Census—a survey that collects data from all members of a population
- Sample—a subset of the population selected for study
- Survey—self-reported research where the individual is the data source
- Observation—method of collecting data by watching research participants
- Interview—member of the population being studied responds to oral questions (AHIMA 2014, 22, 82, 106, 133, 141)

In the example, the study period is determined to be one year. Survey data may be collected by e-mailing the survey, calling the participant on the phone, interviewing the participant, or sending them a link for a web-based survey. For this study, a paper survey is used to collect data in the ER, and retrospective record reviews are used to determine how many visits the patients in the sample have during the study year. Researchers also need to decide how to handle return visits by people who have already been surveyed. Researchers should decide if they want to collect a new form for previously surveyed participants returning to the ER. For accuracy, data could be collected each time a participant comes back. However, unless this is communicated to the data collection staff in the ER, valuable data may be lost.

Data Collection Instruments

The data collection instruments provide the means for consistency in obtaining the data in a required format (AHIMA 2014, 80). For example, an instrument could be a web-based online survey, or a paper form for the respondents to fill out. This is important as data collection issues, such as failing to define the study variables can result in unusable survey responses. For this study, a query will be run to export the data for age, ethnicity, gender, date, and time of the ER visit from the electronic ER registration system. The data will be collected by the ER staff for at least 10 patients on each shift. Researchers will enter the deidentified data into an Excel spreadsheet. In this way, the online survey can facilitate obtaining structured survey data for analysis.

Check Your Understanding 7.2

Mark the answer as true or false.

1. The independent variable is the variable being measured.
2. The dependent variable is the one the researcher believes will cause a change.
3. Hypotheses are predictions of the study outcome by the researcher.
4. The sample is a subset of the population of interest in the study.
5. Survey data may be collected by e-mailing the survey, calling the participant on the phone, interviewing the participant, or sending them a link for a web-based survey.

Answer the following questions.

6. Which is the data collection method for self-reported research where the individual is the data source?
    a. Survey
    b. Observation
    c. Interviews
    d. Census

7. What is not a characteristic of the alternate hypothesis?
    a. It is a statement of the researcher's working hypothesis
    b. It is a prediction of the study outcome
    c. It indicates no association exists between the independent and dependent variables
    d. It indicates an association exists between the independent and dependent variables

⊙ Data Analysis

Data analysis is defined as "the methods that help to describe the facts, detect patterns, develop explanations and test hypotheses" (AHIMA 2014, 42). In order to conduct data analysis, the reliability and validity of the data must be evaluated. The statistical analysis software must be selected or purchased, and the statistics tests must be selected. After these preliminaries, descriptive and inferential statistics can be generated using the statistical software and the correct statistical tests.

Reliability and Validity

Research should be valid and reliable. **Reliability** of instruments is when they give similar results on repeated administration of the test. **Validity** is the extent to which an instrument measures what it is supposed to measure (AHIMA 2014, 151). **Internal validity** is a characteristic of the study design (Forrestal 2016, 588). Threats to internal validity come from factors inside the study that interfere with proving that the study outcome is the result of the independent variable (Forrestal 2016, 588). Common threats to internal validity are due to

- History—a current event occurring during research affects the outcome
- Maturation—subjects mature during study
- Testing—taking repeated tests affects scores
- Instrumentation—lack of consistency in data collection or changing instruments
- Statistical regression—subjects selected due to extreme scores tend to have scores that regress toward the mean with repeated observations
- Differential selection—individuals selected with certain characteristics for control and experimental groups
- Attrition of subjects—subjects leave during the study
- Diffusion of treatment—participants learn who is in the control group and who is in the treatment group (Forrestal 2016, 588).

External validity threats come from outside the study such as the selection bias where the characteristics of the participants are so narrow that results cannot be generalized, or the setting characteristics of participants prevent generalization. For example, a study of the challenges of underprivileged teenagers growing up on a Caribbean island would have selection bias due to the specific selection characteristics and the unique setting that would prevent generalization to teenagers in the United States.

If the study instrument is the Excel data collection worksheet then validity could be established by having the instrument reviewed by an experienced researcher, and by conducting a pilot study using the instrument. To establish internal validity, the researcher must control for confounding variables that could influence the study outcome, which could be done by controlling for the common threats to internal validity, for example, making sure the data collection procedures are consistent and not selecting subjects with extreme scores. With respect to external validity, the sample will be compared to the population of ER visitors to determine if it is representative. However, it is still a small sample from one ER for only one year, thus this will be listed as a study limitation.

Select Statistical Analysis Software

Commonly used statistical software includes Microsoft's Excel, Statistical Package for Social Sciences (SPSS), SAS, and R software. The choice of software used by the researcher may be limited by the research budget and the lack of availability of the more expensive software. Specifically, R software is free but has a steep learning curve, Excel is moderately priced, and the remaining statistical analysis software requires expensive licensing that requires renewal each year. Nevertheless, for large data sets the licensed software provides many advantages in terms of usability, ease of running the tests, and results output in a more usable format.

Microsoft Excel

Microsoft (MS) Excel is a spreadsheet product that comes with the installations of Microsoft Office for Windows or Macintosh computers (Microsoft 2013). There is a free Excel add-in that can be enabled to easily conduct statistical tests. Many web-based survey tools, like SurveyMonkey, offer the users the ability to export their data to MS Excel. MS Excel is a good choice for analyzing smaller data sets. See figure 7.1 for an example of a MS Excel datasheet.

SPSS

The Statistical Package for the Social Sciences (SPSS) is an IBM product consisting of a family of products for data analysis, reporting, import, and export. SPSS is widely used in research and it supports imports and exports from a large variety of systems in many different formats (SPSS 2016). There are three editions of SPSS: Standard, Professional, and Premium. The Standard edition provides the basic analytics that would be used for most projects. The Premium version is designed for enterprise-wide data analysis needs. SPSS usage requires purchasing a license each year. SPSS can be used to perform sophisticated statistical tests

Figure 7.1.   Excel datasheet

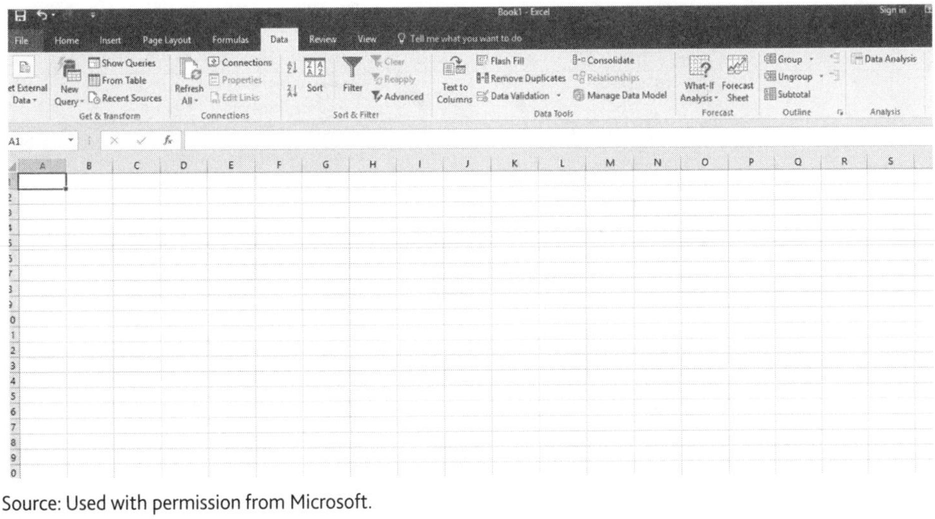

Source: Used with permission from Microsoft.

such as factor analysis, binomial, multinomial, and logistic regression as well as predictive analytics. SPSS has customers in medical, academic, insurance, banking, government, manufacturing, and survey and marketing fields.

SAS

SAS®, Statistical Analysis Software, has a large set of integrated enterprise solutions for performing advanced analytics, business and customer intelligence, data, decision, performance and risk management. SAS has a large programming language set that can be used to load and analyze a large variety of data (SAS Institute Inc. 2011). It is used globally and has a large user group. Uses in healthcare include studies on readmission, health outcomes, and patient safety.

R software

R statistical software is a free open source software program, based on the R programming language developed at Bell Labs, which can import and export data to a large variety of statistical software (R Core Team 2016). Currently, there are many free resources for learning R (CRAN 2016). Initially the software is downloaded and installed on the user's PC with versions available for Windows, Mac OS, and Linux operating systems. R has a significant learning curve because many of the commands are entered at a command prompt, which may be unfamiliar to some users. However, there are many tools to assist the user such as a free development environment called RStudio that can be downloaded (RStudio 2016). There is also an active R user community (Jackson 2014). In healthcare, R has been used to explore duplicate record sets (Haenke Just et al. 2016), and to compare EHR Incentive Program attestations from rural and urban facilities (Sandefer et al. 2015). Figure 7.2 shows RStudio.

Figure 7.2. RStudio

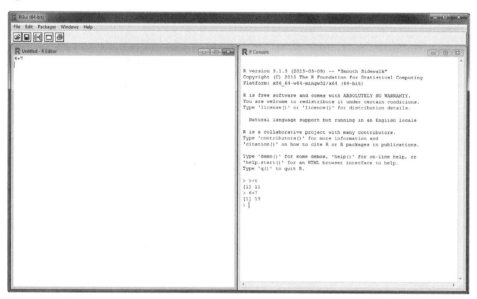

Source: Used with permission from RStudio.

Stata

Stata data analysis and statistical software was developed by StataCorp, who also publishes a peer-reviewed quarterly statistical journal focused on Stata use (StataCorp 2016). Stata provides basic and advanced statistical analysis and has a rich set of data graphing tools. There are Stata products available to handle small, moderate, and large data sets on Windows, MAC, and Unix platforms. Uses of Stata in healthcare include predicting 30- to 120-day readmissions for Medicare patients (Ostrovsky et al. 2016) and facilitating the development of innovative predictive models developed for cardiac prevention studies (Barkhordari et al. 2016).

Determine Statistical Formulas to Use or Statistical Tests to Conduct

To select the correct statistical test for inferential statistics, the independent and dependent variables' data types and numbers must be considered, as well the purpose of the study. A statistical textbook should be consulted as failing to select the correct test can affect study validity (White 2016, 513). For example, in the current example of age and number of ER visits there are two variables (bivariate) both of which are numbers and the aim is to determine the existence and strength of a relationship between the two variables, therefore Pearson's correlation is an appropriate test. Pearson's correlation generates a value between −1 and +1 that indicates the strength and direction of the correlational relationship. For example, a value of 0 indicates no relationship, while values of −1 and +1 indicate strong negative and positive relationships, respectively.

Compute Descriptive Statistics

Descriptive statistics are used to analyze study variables like age and number of ER visits because they can describe the features of the data; but they are not used for hypothesis testing. In many studies the descriptive (summary) statistics generated are frequency distributions, and the mean, median, mode, standard deviation, and variance.

Measures of Central Tendency

Specifically, continuous variables may be analyzed using measures of central tendency, which are the mean and median (White 2016, 520). The mean is the arithmetic average, which is computed by adding up the values in the data set and dividing by the number of values in the data set. The median is the middle value, which is computed by first arranging the values from smallest to largest, then either picking out the middle value (if the number of values is odd) or averaging the middle values (if the number of values is even).

Outliers are values that have very high or very low values in comparison to the rest of the values in the data set. Outliers can influence the mean to "move" toward the outliers. If an outlier is very high, the mean will be artificially high. In this case the researcher may wish to report the median instead of the mean because the median is not influenced by outliers (White 2016, 520).

The mode is reported for categorical data. It is the most frequently occurring value. A data set may have no mode, one mode, or many modal values. For example, the data set {1, 2, 3, 4, 5, 6, 7, 7, 7} has one mode, which is the value 7, because it occurs the most frequently (three times).

Measures of Spread

For continuous variables, the variance, standard deviation, and range are utilized to calculate the spread of the data, which is the distance from the mean of the data set. Variance is computed as the average of the square of the distance from the mean. The standard deviation is calculated by taking the square root of the variance. The range is the difference between the largest and the smallest value in the data set. For example, the range for the data set {1, 2, 3, 4, 5, 6, 7} is 7−1 or 6.

Compute Inferential Statistics

Inferential statistics can be computed using rates and proportions or simple linear regression or by computing a value for the strength of a relationship between two variables or with other advanced statistical tests (White 2016, 526–530). For the example under consideration in this chapter, a bivariate correlational test can be conducted in Excel or SPSS to determine the strength and relationship between age and number of visits to the ER per year.

Explicitly, the statistical test would be a Pearson's correlation test, which in Excel is calculated with the CORRELL function. This function generates an r correlation coefficient, which can be 0 (no correlation), 1 (strong positive relationship), −1 (strong negative correlation), or somewhere in between. In determining the strength of the relationships, the absolute value of r is utilized and the closer to zero the weaker the relationships. The conditions for the test are met because both age and number of ER visits are numbers, and data have been collected for both variables. For example, a Pearson's correlation r value of −0.98 indicates a strong negative correlation, a value of 0.85 indicates a strong positive correlation, and a value close to 0 indicates no correlation.

Similarly, in SPSS the data must be prepared, which means that initially variables loaded into SPSS need to be coded and labeled. Once the coding is done, SPSS has many built in functions and features that automatically generate output and graphs (Green and Salkind 2013, 69). After loading the data, the user runs a bivariate correlation on age and number of ER visits. The SPSS output window will display a correlations table containing the Pearson's r correlation value, which is .672 and the significance will be given by Sig. (2-tailed) as .098. A significance value greater than .05 indicates there is no statistically significant correlation between the variables. A significance value less than or equal to .05 indicates there is a statistically significant correlation between the variables, and variables that are related will increase or decrease together. For this test, the significance is .098, which is much greater than .05 so the variables Age and Number of ER Visits are not significantly correlated. The conclusion is that Age is not related to the number of ER Visits.

Check Your Understanding 7.3

Match the terms with the appropriate descriptions.

    a. Reliability
    b. Internal validity
    c. External validity
    d. Validity

1. _____ Threats to the study like poor data collection instruments

2. _____ Test instrument gives consistent results on repeated administration

3. _____ Threats to the study such as selection bias

4. _____ Extent to which an instrument measures what it is supposed to measure

Indicate whether each of the following is true or false.

5. SAS is a Microsoft product that can be used for data analysis and statistics.

6. SPSS is an IBM product widely used in research.

7. R is a free open source statistical software program where users type commands at a command prompt

8. The type of statistical test is dependent on the data types of the independent and dependent variables, the number of independent and dependent variables, and the purpose of the study.

⊙ Advanced Data Analysis

Advanced data analysis is growing in popularity due to the amount of Big Data now being analyzed in healthcare. Advanced data analysis includes trend, forecast, and predictive analysis, as well as data mining and epidemiological applications of data analysis. Big Data are data sets so large that new tools for analysis are necessary to explore them (Patena 2016, 750).

Trend Analysis

Trend analysis can be conducted with scatterplots (Green and Salkind 2013, 236), t-tests (Green and Salkind 2013, 145), or One-Way Analysis of Variance (ANOVA) testing (Green and Salkind 2013, 163). **Scatterplots** are graphs that show correlation between variables; the x-axis displays the independent variable and the y-axis shows the dependent variable. Scatterplots are generated by most correlation tests, and the values of 0, −1, and +1 indicate no relationship, perfect negative relationship, and perfect positive relationship, respectively. Scatterplots are excellent visualization tools and are present in many research studies. Figure 7.3 shows a scatterplot for hypothetical data on age and length of stay in the hospital.

Figure 7.3. Scatterplot for age and length of stay

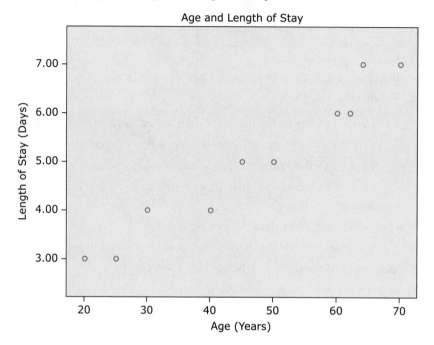

Visual examination of this scatterplot shows an upward trend indicating that as age in years increases so does length of stay in the hospital.

A **t-test** compares a mean to a test statistic to determine how they are related. It can be used to compare current data to a company benchmark. For example, is the current average ER wait time more or less than the facilities desired value of 40 minutes ER wait time? Trends can also be determined using an Analysis of Variance (**ANOVA**) test to compare two or more means to see if they are equal, or if at least one of them is different. There are several types of ANOVA tests. A commonly used ANOVA test is the one-way between-subjects ANOVA, this test should be used when there is one independent variable and one numerical dependent variable (Huck 2012, 217). It is called one-way because only the levels of one factor, the independent variable, are used when putting the participants into the three groups. For example, if a participant takes a high, low, or no dose of Vitamin C then the three levels of this factor are used to create the three groups according to level of Vitamin C usage. The ANOVA test could then be conducted to determine if there was any difference between the groups with respect to number of days to develop cold symptoms (the dependent variable) (Green and Salkind 2013, 163).

While the ANOVA test can indicate that two or more of the Vitamin C groups differ significantly, it does not indicate which of the two groups are different (Green and Salkind 2013, 167). To determine which groups are different, an additional post hoc test must be conducted. For example, Dunnett's C test is a post hoc comparison for the one-way ANOVA test that is available in SPSS (Green and Salkind 2013, 168).

Predictive Analysis

Predictive modeling is "a process used to identify patterns that can be used to predict the odds of a particular outcome based on observed data" (AHIMA 2014, 112). This input data is usually historical as well as current data. **Predictive analysis** predicts future outcomes and is often used for simulating future scenarios that help managers optimize their outcomes. Researchers in a study designed to evaluate predictive and descriptive analysis for use in optimizing nursing staffing patterns at a small rural hospital determined that their predictive tools helped managers to maintain optimal nursing staffing levels (Ramsey 2014). The use of predictive analytics is increasing because it can offer managers a way to model what-if scenarios in order to select the best paths (Minsker 2015).

Forecasting

Forecasting is calculating or predicting some future event or condition through study and analysis (AHIMA 2014). Forecasting in healthcare predicts health disease episodes or health events like number of admissions, life expectancies, or disease outcomes for one individual (Soyiri and Reidpath 2013). Forecasting is a commonly conducted test. For example, SPSS has a Forecasting selection on the dropdown menu. Forecasting can be done using several mathematical models such as time series analysis where data collected over time are analyzed to find trends, cycles, and seasonal changes in the data.

One study described how forecasting was utilized to determine peak asthma times (Soyiri et al. 2013). First, two years of retrospective data were collected from the National Health Service in England on hospital admissions where the primary diagnosis was asthma and the admissions occurred between January 1, 2005, and December 31, 2006 (Soyiri et al. 2013, 2). The binary dependent variable was days of peak demand for admissions for asthma, that is days where there were 40 or more asthma admissions (Soyiri et al. 2013, 2). Data were analyzed with multiple regression in order to develop a multivariate model to predict the days of peak demand for asthma visits to the ER.

Data Mining

Data mining is "the process of extracting and analyzing large volumes of data from a database in order to find patterns in the data" (AHIMA 2014, 43). Tools for data mining include IBM SPSS data modeler, Oracle data mining, SAS Enterprise Miner, HP Vertica Analytics Platform, and Microsoft Analysis Services. For smaller data sets, the R statistical tool has data mining packages. Data mining has been used to explore family history (Hoyt et al. 2016), to explore factors associate with decubitus ulcers (Dheeraj et al. 2015), and to identify fall-related injuries (Luther et al. 2015).

Artificial neural networks (ANNs) are "predictive computer models that use interactive learning to process multiple inputs in order to detect patterns" (AHIMA 2014, 102). Thus, their behavior is similar to the human nervous system neurons. ANNs have been used in radiology, cardiology, and neurology (Hoyt et al. 2016, 2). Regarding data mining, researchers used ANNs to analyze digital medical family history data on approximately 2,400 participants (Hoyt et al. 2016, 2). Results from data analysis with ANNs were compared to previous cross-tabulations results for the same data, and they were determined to be sufficiently correlated indicating that ANNs are useful tools for detecting patterns in data.

Researchers aiming to develop an improved model for predicting decubitus pressure ulcers utilized R statistical software to compare the results from four data mining models on four years of data (Dheeraj et al. 2015). The data mining models examined were logistic regression, decision trees, random forests, and multivariate regression splines. Results indicated that the random forest model, a special type of decision tree, was the most predictive of pressure ulcers for this data set (Dheeraj et al. 2015).

Statistical text mining (STM) was utilized to identify fall-related injuries in EHRs (Luther et al. 2015). Data were collected for visits related to falls (n=1653) at the Veterans Health Administration ambulatory care clinics. Data from the VHA EHRs were extracted for two days after the ambulatory clinic fall visit, and this data was annotated by three clinicans to mark text related to the falls. A statistical software package called RapidMiner was used to develop a statistical model that correctly predicted 87 percent of the visits for falls (Luther et al. 2015). This result is important because using data mining, persons at risk for falls can be more easily identified and offered fall-prevention information (Luther et al. 2015).

Epidemiological Applications

Epidemiological studies are concerned with finding the cause and effect of diseases (AHIMA 2014, 54). Public health informatics involves studying epidemiological data for large numbers of people around the world. Finding a data mining tool that works in remote locations can be challenging due to lack of reliable Internet connectivity. R has an EpiTools package that provides basic programming for epidemiological problems. Also, EPI-Info is freeware available from the US Centers for Disease Control and Prevention (CDC) that facilitates data collection, analysis, visualization, and reporting (CDC 2016). Using this software, advanced statistical analysis and geographic information system mapping can be quickly and easily accomplished. Additionally, it works well in remote locations with sporadic Internet connectivity (CDC 2016).

Check Your Understanding 7.4

Match the terms with the appropriate descriptions.

   a. Scatterplots
   b. Predictive analysis
   c. t-test
   d. ANOVA

1. _____ Graphs that show correlation
2. _____ Compare two means of two data sets to determine the relationship
3. _____ Compare means of four data sets to determine the relationship
4. _____ Calculating the odds of an outcome

Answer the following questions.

5. Data mining is
   a. The process of extracting large volumes of data to look for patterns
   b. A test for bivariate relationships in quantitative variables
   c. An epidemiological application for analysis
   d. a and b

6. Health forecasting can not predict
   a. The number of admissions in the future
   b. Life expectancies
   c. Disease outcomes
   d. The number of admissions last year

7. Which of the following is not a data mining tool?
   a. SPSS Data Modeler
   b. SAS Enterprise Miner
   c. Microsoft Analysis Services
   d. Microsoft Excel

⊙ Data Visualization

Data visualization refers to the representation of data pictorially with graphs and other visual displays. Representing the data with graphs helps the researcher to get an overview of the features of the data. Viewing graphs, it is easier to detect outliers, spot trends, and see the skew of the data. When selecting the type of graph, recall that the data type determines what graphs can be created. If categorical data was used, the bar chart, pie charts, and frequency tables are appropriate.

Microsoft Excel

Under the insert tab, MS Excel provides a large array of graphs. After selecting the data, the user can decide to use the Recommended Charts, or select from pie, bar, line or PivotCharts. Pie charts can be created to show the percentage of the whole, such as the percentages of medical specialties in the hospital (for example, OB/GYN, MED/SURG, Cardiology). A line chart is a good choice for displaying large amounts of data over time. PivotCharts can be utilized to summarize large amounts of data according to several factors. For example, charges can be summarized by age and Length of Stay (LOS). Figure 7.4 shows a PivotChart for total charges by payer class and age group.

SPSS

In addition to the aforementioned basic graphing suite, SPSS offers geospatial analytics, bulk imports for large data sets, and reports that can be posted to the

Figure 7.4.   PivotChart of total charges

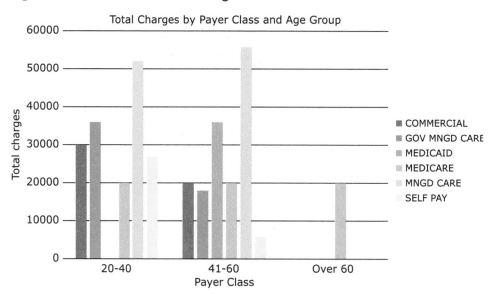

web. SPSS offers visualization custom chart examples with details on how to do the customization at their website (IBM Corp. 2016). The IBM SPSS Modeler has added functionality that allows the user to use their data to create geospatial maps. The visualization can be modified by changing the coordinate system, displaying the data in layers or generating predictions of what will happen at a given location in the future such as disease outbreaks.

R software

Using R, the user can create graphs often with one line of code. In R, the command plot() can be used to create a scatterplot. There is also a more advanced graphics package called ggplot2 that can be installed in order to generate univariate and multivariate graphs for numbers and categorical data in addition to the basic graphs available with the built-in package.

Dashboards

Dashboards are portals that allow the user to display statistics and data from multiple sources on one screen, which allows the data relationship to be more easily visualized. Dashboards can be programmed to code areas that are failing (with different colors) so that the user can quickly identify problem areas. They are becoming more popular in healthcare and are present on many government websites as well. Figure 7.5 presents CMS Medicare chronic conditions data with a dashboard from their website.

Figure 7.5.   CMS Medicare chronic conditions dashboard

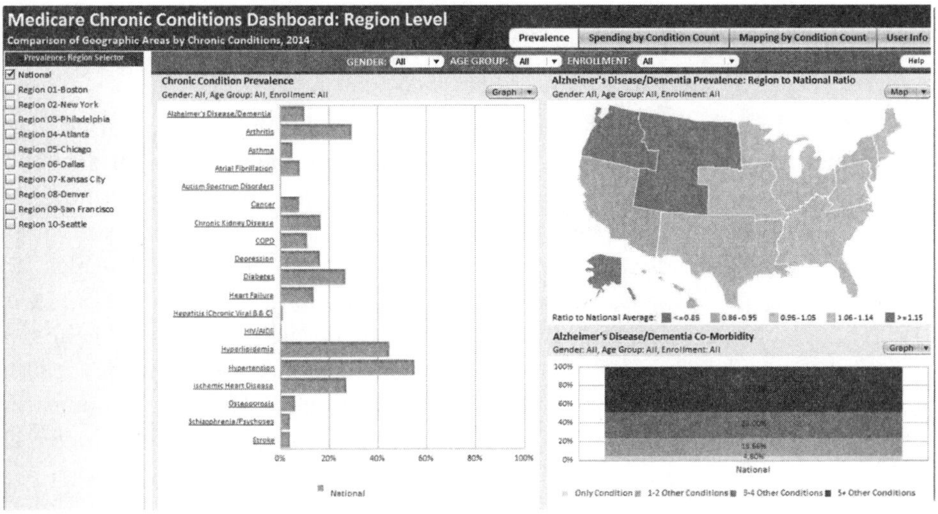

Source: CMS 2016

Check Your Understanding 7.5

Match the terms with the appropriate descriptions.
- **a.** Excel
- **b.** SPSS
- **c.** R software

1. _____ Microsoft spreadsheet tool that produces PivotCharts
2. _____ Tool with Data Modeler for creating geospatial graphs
3. _____ Free software that can create graphs from one line of code

Indicate whether each of the following is true or false.

4. Dashboards are portals that allow the user to display statistics and data from multiple sources on one screen.
5. Excel integrates easily with R software.
6. A line chart is a good choice for displaying percentages of the whole.

⊙ Data Retrieval

Data retrieval is the process of obtaining data from a healthcare database (AHIMA 2014, 44). Initially, researchers collect data that is then analyzed and stored in a data repository. This repository could be a part of one of the statistical software packages mentioned thus far, or it could be in a database system like Microsoft Access, Oracle, DB2, or SQL Server. After the data are stored, users want to get the data out of the system and use it for reporting, or export it to another system. The process of getting the data out of the system is called data retrieval. To accomplish data retrieval, data languages and tools must be used.

Languages and Tools

Data can be imported and exported from statistical software and other data repositories by using built-in tools. Data are loaded into the system with the built-in **import** function. This can be done in one step by selecting the import function then picking the correct data type from the one listed on the statistical software's dropdown. Common data types for import are text or comma delimited files. To get the data out of one system, the **export** functionality is used. For example, in SPSS, the data can be exported in a variety of formats such as an Excel file or to a Microsoft Access database. Other databases could be connected as well or the user can save the data file and import it manually to the other system. For example, the SPSS Save Data pop-up lists a variety of file types that can be imported such as SPSS, tab or comma delimited, Excel, dBase, Stata, and SAS.

SQL: Microsoft Access, Oracle, IBM DB2, SQL Server

The most common language used for data retrieval is **Structured Query Language (SQL),** which is used to query relational databases to retrieve the data for display. The basic principles for using SQL commands with databases were developed by IBM (Dolezel 2015a). The syntax for the data retrieval commands are available in the database documentation, and there are numerous resources that can assist the beginning database reporter. Of course, the syntax of these statements used for retrieval will differ across the systems, but MS Access, Oracle, DB2, and SQL Server all use a query language, which is a language used for retrieving data from a database, and the retrieval statements are similar. One SQL data retrieval query can be used to gather data from one or more tables located in one or more databases, and these databases may be in another building, town, or country. They can be small or large, or even, with some bridging tools installed, from a different database vendor.

For relational databases, the SELECT statement is used for data retrieval. The following syntax for the SQL Select command is:

> Select [columname1, columname2, etc.]
> From [tablename1, tablename2, etc.]
> Where [condition]
> [other optional conditions]; (Dolezel 2015a)

Therefore, if you have created a table named "mytable" then typing "Select * from mytable" into a command window would direct the database to retrieve data from an IBM DB2 database table called "mytable," and the same statement would work for an Access or Oracle table. In fact, this query would select all data from the table, which may not be optimal for a large table. For this reason, data retrieval statements have a WHERE clause specifying conditions that must be met in order to retrieve the data.

For example, "SELECT * from mytable WHERE charges > 50000" would select all the database table rows where the charges field had a value greater than

50,000. Additionally, the SELECT statements typically have many other filters added to group and order the data, and the Boolean operators () can be added to create complex functions (Dolezel 2015a). Data retrieved from running these queries can be displayed to the screen, stored in a table or sent to a file for later viewing. These queries can be stored inside the database in database packages, which reside permanently on the database server, and the packages can be invoked later from other software to generate a report or data export based on the code in the package. These newer tools simplify database reporting such that the beginning health informatics user can quickly create basic data analytics reports.

SPSS Data Explore Function

SPSS has a useful procedure called the Explore function. This procedure generates summary statistics and boxplot, stem and leaf plots, normality and spread plots for quantitative variables. The advantage is that a variety of statistics is available using one procedure. This is useful for experienced users as they can quickly check for data skewness, examine normality tests, and glance at plots to see the shape of the data. Because SPSS sends all output to the output window, the results of running the Explore procedure can easily be saved for later review. However, the beginning SPSS user may find the multipage output to be overwhelming, thus more value may be derived from doing these tests individually.

Check Your Understanding 7.6

Match the terms with the appropriate descriptions.
- a. Data retrieval
- b. Import
- c. Export
- d. Structured Query Language

1. _____ Obtaining data from a database
2. _____ Used to query a database for reporting
3. _____ Putting data into a database
4. _____ Getting data out of a database

Indicate whether each of the following is true or false.

5. The SQL statement for data retrieval is the Update statement.
6. SPSS has an EXPLORE function that will generate summary statistics and several useful graphs.

⊙ Data Reporting

Healthcare data analysis typically generates multiple reports that can be evaluated for performance monitoring, trend analysis, and other related quality improvement and management activities. MS Excel is often used for graphing and to create Pivot tables. Users with large data sets or databases in several geographic locations may wish to purchase a commercial reporting system.

Tables, Charts, and Figures from Statistical Software Results

Table, charts, and figures from statistical software results can be exported to PDF, Microsoft Word documents, or MS Excel. The exported data can be used for reporting or as input for further analysis in another system. For example, MS Excel data on length of stay by Diagnosis Related Group (DRG) can be imported into SPSS and analyzed to determine if any trends exist. Users wishing to select just one graph for use as a document or MS PowerPoint will find this ability present in almost all of the statistical software. In the SPSS output window, chart images are selectable and they can be copied as images and pasted into a MS Word document. MS Excel graphs, tables, and MS PivotCharts are easily copied to a document as well.

Reporting Software

Many database management systems have their own built-in reporting software. However, most of these systems are designed to be used by the database administrators for monitoring and maintenance. For that reason, an important first step before writing any code or using any reporting tools is to understand what data and databases a facility has available. This can be found in the metadata catalogs for the database system. **Metadata** is information about the data in the database, typically this is maintained at the system level and the user level (Dolezel 2015b). It is essential the user contact the database administrator (DBA) who is assigned to their project prior to designing a report and work with them to explore the metadata. Metadata information includes the names of all tables, objects, fields, indexes, primary and foreign keys, usernames, and privileges for the database. To create a report, it is best to work with the DBA to identify the table names and fields needed to query for your report. The DBA can also help informatics specialists to optimize queries and in particular the queries where data comes from two or more tables, called table joins, giving attention to not causing the database to become bogged down.

Users with large databases and heavy reporting needs often decide to purchase a separate reporting system from a vendor such as Crystal Reports by SAP, Microsoft SQL Server Reporting Services, and IBM's Hyperion system. Database reporting can also be conducted using Microsoft Access reporting wizards and SQL command line. The PC user can import Excel data for a reporting and print or save the report output.

Presentation Software

Presentation software is used to disseminate ideas at conferences and during lectures. The use of graphs and text allows the speaker to convey the main points of their study to their audience. In particular, the tables and graphs from a data report, together with statistical software results can be used in reports or in presentation slides. Adding a data visualization element to a presentation is a way to engage the audience. Copying and pasting data results to the presentation are a quick, easy way to summarize a large amount of information in an understandable format. PivotCharts are especially useful for summarizing large amounts of complex data. Attendees at a presentation can get PDF copies of the presentations for later review.

Recommending Organizational Action

An inventory of all the knowledge repositories to record the name, location, user base, administrator, and content of the repository can provide a useful index to the current data stores. For example, PubMed may be used as a knowledge repository. The content should be specified down to the level of the data dictionary details of each data element in each repository. Data from the knowledge repository inventory should be placed in an enterprise wide knowledge management metadata database so that it can be tracked and updated on a regular basis. This step is essential to understanding the data stored in each system.

Second, the report names, report content, when they are run, who requested the report, and how the results are disseminated should add to the metadata utilized by the healthcare facility. Recording the information about the facilities reports is important as this can help top management identify issues with data integrity as well as issues with reports. Specifically, it is common for the queries that underlie these reports to summarize the detail data in such a way that the summation misrepresents the actual data. This could be from misusing a database function, errors in the query code or data type conversion issues (for example, number stored as character incorrectly converted). Decisions based on misrepresented data are most likely incorrect.

Another frequent issue in complex reporting involving the same data element being stored in multiple locations is that the data are not updated in the same way in all locations. In the simplest case, this could occur when two departmental systems update the same field and the data then flows into the EHR. A second way that data integrity can be compromised occurs when data marts are used. To understand this, it is important to know that running large queries for reporting slows down a database. Moreover, an error in the coding of the SQL reporting query can even cause the database processing to effectively be hung up with nothing being run. To facilitate reporting while not impacting database performance, a data mart is created for reporting. For example, the accounting department may want to see specific data from multiple tables in several databases, but they do not want to run 20 queries to do this. The DBAs will create a data mart (that is, set of tables) for use by the accounting department for reporting. The benefit here is that accounting can efficiently run their reports with little or no access to the main database tables, but they cannot make any changes to the data. Of course, the downside is that the DBAs have to put data into these tables frequently or the data becomes old, and this creates the problem originally mentioned of updates running against several data marts not updating the data the same way or at the same time. In fact, if the lag in updating is great enough, one department may make uninformed decisions that flow into another department's data mart and wipe out the original data.

Chapter 7 Review Exercises

Match the research type with its description.

- **a.** Quantitative
- **b.** Qualitative research
- **c.** Mixed methods
- **d.** Retrospective

1. _____ Tests a theory by defining measurable variables and collecting and analyzing data on those variables

2. _____ Case control study examining past events

3. _____ Study with both open and closed questions

4. _____ Nonnumerical data is analyzed to investigate group interactions

Indicate whether the following statements are true or false.

5. When conducting research, the HIPAA Privacy Rule's minimum necessary standard must also be followed even when the use of the patient information is authorized or a waiver has been granted.

6. Research must be compliant with state laws and must be IRB approved.

7. The alternate hypothesis states that there is no difference between the independent and dependent variable.

8. The researcher should always check to see if the sample is similar to the population.

9. Changing data instruments or researchers could affect the study validity.

Discussion.

10. A study on the correlation between age and hours of social media use per week is being conducted among physicians at your hospitals. Apply the steps in the research process to this study:

⊙ Determine the research question

⊙ State research hypotheses

⊙ Define study variables and their data types

⊙ Identify sample and population, data collection

⊙ Conduct data analysis

For each step, state in one or two sentences what you would do at that step.

11. Discuss the role of the EHR in healthcare research and give at least two examples.

12. Select two statistical data analysis tools mentioned in the chapter that would be suitable for data mining on large amounts of quantitative data. Describe why you selected those tools with respect to their data collection, data analysis, and data graphing functionalities.

13. Select four data visualization tools mentioned in the chapter. Create a table listing their advantages and disadvantages.

REFERENCES

21 CFR Parts 50 and 56: U.S. Food and Drug Administration. FDA Policy for Protection of Human Subjects. 1991.

45 CFR 46.111(a)(7): Research—Protection of human subjects, including protecting confidential information. 2006.

45 CFR 164.502(b): Minimum necessary requirement. 2016.

45 CFR 164.514(d): Other requirements relating to uses and disclosures of protected health information. 2016.

AHIMA. 2014. *Pocket Glossary of Health Information Management and Technology.* 4th ed. Chicago, IL: AHIMA Press.

Barkhordari, M., M. Padyab, F. Hadaegh, F. Azizi, and M. Bozorgmanesh. 2016. Stata modules for calculating novel predictive performance indices for logistic models. *International Journal of Endocrinology and Metabolism* 14(1):1–5. doi: 10.5812/ijem .26707.

Centers for Disease Control and Prevention. 2016. Epi info. https://www.cdc.gov /epiinfo/index.html.

CMS. 2016. *Medicare Chronic Conditions Dashboard: Regional Level.* https://www.cms.gov /Research-Statistics-Data-and-Systems/Statistics-Trends-and-Reports/Dashboard /Chronic-Conditions-Region/CC_Region_Dashboard.html.

Cochran, G.L., L. Lander, M. Morien, D.E. Lomelin, C. Reker, and D.G. Klepser. 2015. Consumer opinions of health information exchange, e-prescribing, and personal health records. *Perspectives in Health Information Management* (Fall):1–12.

Comprehensive R Archive Network. 2016. www.cran.rstudio.com.

Creswell, J.W. 2011. *Educational Research: Planning, Conducting, and Evaluating Quantitative and Qualitative Research.* 4th ed. Upper Saddle River, NJ: Pearson.

Department of Health and Human Services (HHS). 2016. Institutional Review Boards (IRBs). http://www.hhs.gov/ohrp/.

Dheeraj, R., S. Xiaogang, P.A. Patrician, L.A. Loan, and M.S. McCarthy. 2015. Exploring factors associated with pressure ulcers: A data mining approach. *International Journal of Nursing Studies* 52(1):102–111. doi: 10.1016/j.ijnurstu.2014.08.002.

Dolezel, D. 2015a. How to use relational databases: Data retrieval with Structured Query Language. *Journal of AHIMA* 86(11):22–27.

Dolezel, D. 2015b. Metadata offers roadmap to structured data. *Journal of AHIMA* 86(2):44–46.

Dolezel, D., and J. Moczygemba. 2015. Implementing EHRs: An exploratory study to examine current practices in migrating physician practice. *Perspectives in Health Information Management* Winter:1–15.

Downey, L.V., and L.S. Zun. 2010. The correlation between patient comprehension of their reason for hospital admission and overall patient satisfaction in the Emergency Department. *Journal of the National Medical Association* 102:637–643.

Forrestal, E. 2016. Research Methods. Chapter 19 in *Health Information Management Concepts Principles, and Practices.* 5th ed. Edited by P. Oachs and A. Watters. Chicago, IL: AHIMA Press.

Green, S.B., and N.J. Salkind. 2013. *Using SPSS for Windows and Macintosh.* 6th ed. Upper Saddle River, NJ: Pearson.

Haenke Just, B., D. Marc, M. Munns, and R. Sandefer. 2016. Why patient matching is a challenge: Research on Master Patient Index (MPI) data discrepancies in key identifying fields. *Perspectives in Health Information Management* (Spring):1–20.

Health Resources and Services Administration. 2016. *How do we measure and improve clinical processes and outcomes?* http://www.hrsa.gov/healthit/toolbox/ruralhealthittoolbox/patientquality/measureprocesses.html.

Hoyt, R., S. Linnville, S. Thaler, and J. Moore. 2016. Digital family history data mining with neural networks: A pilot study. *Perspectives in Health Information Management* (Winter):1–14.

Huck, S.W. 2012. *Reading Statistics and Research.* Boston, MA: Pearson Education.

IBM Corp. 2016. IBM SPSS Statistics for Windows (Version 24) [Computer Software]. Armonk, NY: IBM Corp.

Jackson, J. 2014. R programming language gaining ground on traditional statistics packages. *PC World* (Aug 20).

Jakobsson, N., and M. Svensson. 2016. The effect of copayments on primary care utilization: Results from a quasi-experiment. *Applied Economics* 48(39): 3752-3762. doi: 10.1080/00036846.2016.1145346.

Layman, E.J., and V.J. Watzlaf. 2009. *Health Informatics Research Methods: Principles and Practice.* Chicago, IL: AHIMA.

Luther, S.L., J.A. McCart, D.J. Berndt, B. Hahm, D. Finch, J. Jarman, P.R. Foulis, W.A. Lapcevic, R.R. Campbell, R.I. Shorr, K.M. Valencia, and G. Powell-Cope. 2015. Improving identification of fall-related injuries in ambulatory care using statistical text mining. *American Journal of Public Health* 105(6):1168–1173. doi: 10.2105/AJPH.2014.302440.

Microsoft (2013). Excel [Computer Software]. Redmond, WA: Microsoft.

Minsker, M. 2015. Peek into the Future. *CRM Magazine* 19(4):22–26.

Ostrovsky, A., L. O'Connor, O. Marshall, A. Angelo, K. Barrett, E. Majeski, M. Handrus, and J. Levy. 2016. Predicting 30- to 120-day readmission risk among medicare fee-for-service patients using nonmedical workers and mobile technology. *Perspectives in Health Information Management* (Winter):1–20.

Patena, K. 2016. Employee Training and Development. Chapter 24 in *Health Information Management Concepts Principles, and Practices.* 5th ed. Edited by P. Oachs and A. Watters. Chicago, IL: AHIMA Press.

Potter, A.J., M.M. Ward, Nabil Natafgi, F. Ullrich, A.C. McKinney, A.L. Bell, K.J. Mueller. 2016. Perceptions of the Benefits of Telemedicine in Rural Communities. *Perspectives in Health Information Management* (Summer):1–13.

R Development Core Team. 2011. *R: A Language and Environment for Statistical Computing.* Vienna, Austria: the R Foundation for Statistical Computing. http://www.gbif.org /resource/81287.

Ramsey, K.S. "Using Predictive and Descriptive Models to Improve Nurse Staff Planning and Scheduling" (masters thesis, University of Tennessee, 2014). trace.tennessee .edu/cgi/viewcontent.cgi?article=4033&context=utk_gradthes.

RStudio. 2016. *Welcome to R Studio.* https://www.rstudio.com/.

Sandefer, R.H., D.T. Marc, and P. Kleeberg. 2015. Meaningful use attestations among US hospitals: The growing rural–urban divide. *Perspectives in Health Information Management* (Spring):1–10.

Safian, S. C. 2012. Factors influencing students to enroll in health information management programs. *Perspectives in Health Information Management* (Summer):1–18.

SAS Institute Inc. 2011. Statistical Analysis Software (Version 9.4). Cary, NC: SAS Institute Inc. http://www.sas.com/en_us/industry/health-care-providers.html.

Soyiri, I.N., and D.D. Reidpath. 2013. An overview of health forecasting. *Environmental Health and Preventive Medicine* 18(1):1–9. doi: 10.1007/s12199-012-0294-6.

Soyiri, I.N., D.D. Reidpath, and C. Sarran. 2013. Forecasting peak asthma admissions in London: An application of quantile regression models. *International Journal of Biometeorology* 57(4):569–578. doi: 10.1007/s00484-012-0584-0.

SPSS. 2016. IBM Analytics. http://www.ibm.com/analytics/us/en/technology/spss/.

StataCorp. 2016. *Resources for learning Stata.* http://www.stata.com/links/resources-for -learning-stata/.

US Congress. 2009. Health Information Technology for Economic and Clinical Health (HITECH) Act. *Code of Federal Regulations.*

White, S. 2016. Healthcare Data Analytics. Chapter 17 in *Health Information Management Concepts Principles, and Practices.* 5th ed. Edited by P. Oachs and A. Watters. Chicago, IL: AHIMA Press.

ADDITIONAL RESOURCES

45 CFR 160.502: Uses and disclosures of protected health information: General rules. 2016.

Absten, J. 2016. Tools and technologies. *Industrial Engineer.* 48 (2):56–57.

ComputerWorld. 2016. Learning R for beginners with our PDF. http://www .computerworld.com/article/2884322/learn-r-programming-basics-with-our-pdf .html.

ITBusinessEdge. 2015. SQLCourse—Lesson 3: Selecting Data. www.sqlcourse.com /select.html.

Lau, F.Y. 2004. Toward a conceptual knowledge management framework in health. *Perspectives in Health Information Management* 1(8).

National Library of Medicine. 2010. Comparative effectiveness research (CER). https://www.nlm.nih.gov/hsrinfo/cer.html.

Sheridan, P.T., V. Watzlaf, and L.A. Fox. 2016. Health information management leaders and the practice of leadership through the lens of Bowen theory. *Perspectives in Health Information Management* (Spring):1–36.

Chapter 8

Implementing Healthcare Information Systems

KEY TERMS

Accountable Care Organization (ACO)
American Recovery and Reinvestment Act (ARRA)
Application service provider (ASP)
Chief information officer
Computers-on-wheels (COWs)
Functionality
Hybrid
International Organization for Standards (ISO)
Legacy data

Meaningful use
ONC-Authorized Testing and Certification Bodies (ATCBs)
Physician champion
Practicality
Reputation
Request for information (RFI)
Request for proposals (RFP)
Stakeholders
Usability
Use case

The successful implementation of healthcare information systems (HISs) is becoming integral to the success of healthcare organizations of all types and sizes. HISs are extremely complex, support all aspects of healthcare delivery and are very susceptible to error when implemented poorly or utilized by untrained users. This chapter discusses the many aspects of HIS implementation, focusing on the important human elements. Ultimately, it is vital to remember the purpose of the HIS or electronic health record (EHR) is "to handle the medical information necessary for patient care and improve the efficiency and accessibility of that information" (Corrao et al. 2010).

⊙ Leadership, Roles, and Strategic Planning

Key to successful implementation of an EHR is strong leadership from a variety of roles at different levels in the organization, as well as ensuring the HIS is aligned with the strategic goals of the organization. Lack of leadership from the top of the organization or from key roles in the organization could result in inadequate resources for or other fatal flaws in the implementation. Alignment with the organizational strategic plan is required to ensure system **stakeholders** (persons, roles, or organizational units with a vested interest) can use the EHR to accomplish their goals.

Leadership

Top leadership in healthcare organizations can vary from a single, primary owner in a solo practice to a large board of trustees in a nonprofit healthcare organization to a board of directors in for-profit corporations to state and federal officials of government-run healthcare organizations. Top leadership implements the strategic direction of the healthcare organization through five primary activities:

- ⊙ Select and work with the chief executive officer (CEO)
- ⊙ Establish the organization's mission, vision, and values
- ⊙ Approve strategies and budget to implement the mission
- ⊙ Maintain quality of care
- ⊙ Monitor results for compliance with the goals, laws, and regulations (Griffith and White 2010)

The extent of these activities or the ways in which they are manifested differs by organizational setting and size; however, the overall role of top leadership related to EHR implementation is to establish the strategic goals for the organization, identify initiatives that will be enabled by or benefit from an EHR, and provide resources to achieve those goals.

The governing body delegates responsibility for the daily operations of the healthcare organization to the senior management team through the CEO. Senior management support from the chief financial officer (CFO), **chief information officer** (CIO), who is responsible for managing all the information resources for the company (AHIMA 2014, 25), chief nursing officer (CNO), chief medical officer (CMO), and chief medical information officer (CMIO) (collectively known as the C suite) is also essential to the success of EHR initiatives. In this setting, physicians and office managers can provide leadership by employing project management skills to set up timelines, budgets, and tasks using a planning tool. Administrative and clinical staff can be directed to assist in discussions of current and future workflow and how to handle record location during the transition to the new system. Due to the lack of standard guidelines on data migration to EHRs, the clinic leadership should decide how much data to move and document how to locate all parts of the chart (that is, paper and electronic) during and after the paper data has been moved to the new system.

A study of EHR implementation in clinics identified several themes among the physicians migrating existing data to the new EHRs: the need for advanced planning of the data migration, the need to involve clinical staff in planning, and the difficulty determining how much data to move to new systems or other issues (Dolezel and Moczygemba 2015). Migrating data to a new system is a costly, time-consuming process that disrupts the workflow of the clinical practice. The current workflow should be documented, and the future workflow should be diagrammed (Dolezel and Moczygemba 2015). Policies and procedures are needed to standardize the migration processes, and staff training must be planned and conducted. A steering committee should be established to provide guidance for the data migration to the new system (Dolezel and Moczygemba 2015).

In organizational strategic planning, the top leadership sets the organization's direction, defines key relationships with all stakeholders and positions the organization through its missions, values, services, and partnerships. To develop the strategic plan, top leadership engages senior management and key stakeholders to identify, prioritize, and implement strategic opportunities to achieve the long-term vision of the organization. Many strategic opportunities in healthcare are likely to require the implementation or enhancement of an EHR to achieve the organization's goals.

In high-performing healthcare organizations, there is high employee satisfaction, strong earnings, and high quality of care (Griffith and White 2010). The EHR facilitates excellent care, but it is not essential, and high-performing healthcare organizations have built a culture and operational infrastructure of excellence first, and moved later to automate the supporting patient record (Griffith and White 2010). This serves to support the contention that successful implementation of an EHR is more dependent upon the people and other factors than the latest and greatest technology.

Implementation of an EHR is a journey toward goals that are aided by technology. The organization must establish its goals and determine whether the path toward those goals can be assisted with the implementation of an EHR. Most healthcare organizations have some EHR components already in place. It is important to maintain the perspective that an EHR is one of many organizational assets that can be used to enable the healthcare organization's mission and services. Other factors such as knowledge of the regulatory environment and healthcare financing initiatives may also facilitate identification and achievement of strategic goals.

For example, one organizational goal may be to participate in the Medicare **Accountable Care Organization (ACO)** program. An ACO is "an organization of healthcare providers accountable for the quality, cost, and overall care of Medicare beneficiaries who are assigned and enrolled in the traditional fee-for-service program" (AHIMA 2014, 2). The goal is to achieve higher quality at lower costs with Medicare paying incentives to ACOs that meet quality measures and achieve cost savings. ACOs will require accurate, timely, and well-coordinated health records and effective information flow in order to achieve the quality and cost-savings goals. It is possible to achieve the requisite information flow with paper records, but coordinating information across multiple providers and healthcare organizations will be greatly facilitated with an EHR. Consider the example of ordering a laboratory test for a patient in the ACO. To check with all other providers and organizations in the ACO to be sure that the test has not recently been completed would be very labor intensive without an EHR; multiple sites would have to be contacted by telephone, fax, or e-mail, and there could be delays as the information was retrieved from the paper records. With an EHR, immediate access to lab results would be available to the provider at the time they determined that they needed the information in order to diagnose or treat the patient in a timely manner. In this example, it is not likely that the provider would delay ordering the test while all other providers in the ACO were contacted, and the lack of timely access to an EHR would result in duplicate testing.

Another goal for a healthcare organization may be to become the community leader in quality measures. Collecting and reporting quality measures is facilitated by timely access to accurate and complete patient information so they can be reported to the Centers for Medicare and Medicaid Services (CMS), the Joint Commission, and other quality monitoring organizations. It is possible to report quality measures without an EHR, but electronic capture, analysis, and reporting will facilitate the timeliness and accuracy of the data.

Historically, the business case for the acquisition of an EHR has not been as straightforward as compared to business planning for other types of technology. Benefits of a full-fledged EHR often accrue to the payers, rather than the entities that invest in the technology. For example, the physician office must pay for the EHR and associated technology. However, if the patient requires fewer visits then the physician will ultimately lose money; however, the payer will enjoy higher profits. Additionally, some of the benefits of health IT such as provider convenience, patient satisfaction, and improved communication are not easily captured on the bottom line (Garrido et al. 2004). Strategic planning for health IT must consider both financial and nonfinancial benefits.

Federal initiatives are changing the business case. The Office of the National Coordinator for Health Information Technology (ONC) Federal Health Information Technology Strategic Plan for 2011 through 2015 noted that the lack of capital for small- and medium-sized providers has slowed acceptance of EHRs and widespread health information exchange (HIE). The ONC also noted that there was a lack of skilled health IT professionals to support providers as they transition from paper records to EHRs (Office of the National Coordinator, DHHS 2011). These barriers are being addressed through the Merit-Based Incentive Payment Systems, which is a part of the Medicare Access and CHIP (Children's Health Insurance Program) Reauthorization Act of 2015 (CMS 2015a).

The purpose of the American Recovery and Reinvestment Act of 2009 (ARRA) was to create jobs to promote economic recovery, to help individuals affected by the recession, to provide investments for economic recovery, transportation and environmental improvements and to help stabilize local government budgets (AHIMA 2014, 9). The ARRA provided a federally funded EHR incentive program that provides additional weight to the business cases for implementing a fully functioning EHR. In 2011, healthcare organizations and providers became eligible for incentive funding for implementing and using EHRs meaningfully and will begin to incur penalties for not doing so by 2016 (US Congress 2009). In general, the 2011 incentive funds did not fully cover the cost of implementing the EHR, but the additional funding opportunity needed to be considered in the EHR planning business case (Dimick 2011). In 2015, the MACRA Quality Payment Program changed Medicare payments by rewarding healthcare practitioners for providing higher quality care using either Merit-based Incentive Payments (MIPS) or Alternative Payment Models (APMs) (CMS 2015a). The MIPS program focused on quality care, resource utilization, improving clinical practice, and meaningful use of EHR technology. Moreover, the Alternative Payment Model program, which starts in 2019, will provide financial incentives for providers with Medicare patients.

Several studies have provided data regarding EHR implementation. A statewide survey of over 2,300 physicians in Rhode Island determined that 81 percent of those surveyed were using EHRs, which is a significant increase from 54 percent reported usage of EHRs in 2011 (Wylie et al. 2014). Providers perceptions were that the EHRs improved quality and facilitated billing. Results varied with older physicians indicating less usage of EHRs. Conversely, younger doctors with larger practices, hospital or primary care practice, or more Medicaid patients reported higher usage of EHRs (Wylie et al. 2014). A related study exploring the usage of electronic health records among US physicians determined that adoption by other healthcare organizations and perceived success by competitors were strongly associated with increased EHR usage (Sherer et al. 2016). These researchers also uncovered associations between age, with older doctors being less likely to adopt EHRs, and practice characteristics, with organizations being more likely to adopt EHRs than physician practice groups (Sherer et al. 2016). Organizational leaders should be aware of these studies as they work to help prepare the organization for this shift from paper to electronic health records.

Strategic Planning Roles

The requirements for strategic planning will vary by the size and type of the healthcare organization, or their systems, and their settings. The scope of strategic planning is broader now and includes planning for social media, consumer informatics, value-based purchasing, as well as ongoing EHR maintenance. Planning for the small physician practice may be accomplished in a less formal manner than the methods required for a large healthcare facility or system. In any setting, it is imperative for top leadership to support the implementation of the EHR and for all key stakeholders to be involved in the planning process. Table 8.1

Table 8.1. Strategic planning roles

Role	Inpatient environment	Physician practice
Leadership	Governing body (Board) Senior administrative leadership Senior clinical leadership	Physician
Internal stakeholders	Medical staff Nursing Laboratory Radiology Pharmacy Respiratory Case management Other clinical departments Finance information systems Health information management Patient access Patient financial services	Physicians Physician extenders Nursing Medical assistants Other caregivers Administrative support staff Scheduling Insurance verification Coding Billing
External stakeholders	Patients Payers Licensing and accrediting organizations Health information exchanges	Patients Payers Licensing and accrediting organizations Health information exchanges

identifies leadership and stakeholder roles in the inpatient environment and in the small physician practice. This table may be used as a starting point to identify the leadership and stakeholders across the full spectrum of sizes and types of healthcare organizations.

Internal Stakeholders

The support of internal stakeholders, which includes clinicians—physicians, nurses, pharmacists, therapists—and others who use clinical information to care for patients is critical to successfully implementing the EHR. They must be involved in the entire process in order to ensure the needs of the users are fully addressed, the most appropriate system is selected, and the implementation is successful.

Three levels of communication within and among internal stakeholders have been noted to be important to successful EHR implementation: between executive leadership and internal stakeholders, stakeholder to stakeholder, and among the executive leadership, stakeholders, and vendors (Yoon-Flannery et al. 2008). The importance of this communication and active listening between all parties cannot be overstated. There have been a number of barriers to the adoption of the computerized provider order entry (CPOE) system, which is an electronic prescribing system (AHIMA 2014, 32), reported to offer opportunities for improved communication. For example, physicians may be reluctant to adopt CPOEs because of resistance to change and concerns about consumer engagement, despite the fact the patients may not report any significant decrease in satisfaction after CPOE implementation (Charles et al. 2014). Executive leaders should consider working with physicians to select a physician champion that can be involved in CPOE planning, vendor meetings, system testing, and system implementation as one way to address these physician's perceptions of decreased consumer engagement.

Although it is important to involve physicians due to their responsible role in patient care, it is also important to remember that all internal stakeholders perform vital functions and all types of stakeholders need to be involved in any EHR implementation.

External Stakeholders

External healthcare organization stakeholders include actual and potential patients, payers, HIEs, as well as licensing and regulatory organizations. Involving patients is especially important if the healthcare organization is considering a patient portal to facilitate patient access to their personal health information within the healthcare organization's EHR. However, other external stakeholders should also be considered. For example, payers may begin requiring quality measures or other data from providers, while regulatory organizations can require specific technological standards. For example, specific standards must be used for effective HIE or for submitting Joint Commission core measures. Healthcare organizations must also ensure that systems selected will be able to effectively exchange information with all necessary external stakeholders such as other treatment providers or pharmacies.

Development of Leadership Management Plans

When creating a leadership management plan, it is important to ensure that the plan is in alignment with the mission and vision statements for the organization. First, top management support of the plan is essential to the success of the change activity (Garrido et al. 2004). Second, it is critical that the leadership management plan support the organization's goals or it will result in an unusable final work product (Denić et al. 2014). Moreover, employees must be prepared for change well in advance of the actual implementation, which requires multiple scheduled activities designed to make them comfortable with the transition process and the new system or processes.

Planning for change is complex. At the highest level change is a multifaceted interrelated set of processes that consist of establishing the necessity for change, implementing the change, and returning the company to a new status quo (Hord and Hall 2015). Various models have been proposed for managing change, such as Lewin's Change Model, Kotter's Change Model, and Systems Thinking. Change has been abstracted as being conducted by change agents who send directions to change recipients (Armenakis et al. 2007). Factors related to managing change have been examined by several researchers. Change fatigue, change stress, and the effect of internal and external factors on organizational change has been examined (Torppa and Smith 2011).

However it is viewed, like any major leadership activity, the cycle of change must be governed in order to avoid disarray and to facilitate arriving at the intended change goals with minimum disturbance to existing personnel and existing workflows (Stevens 2013). Foremost, when creating plans for HI systems, it should be noted that acquiring and implementing the HI system is a lengthy and expensive process that spans several years. For example, it is typical for the procurement of the system alone to take a year or more, and the planning and design to consume the second and third year (Amatayakul 2012). Thus, any leadership management plan for HI management is effectively a change management plan.

The HIT Technology Project

It is advisable to use formal project management methodologies together with project management software (for example, Microsoft Project), document management, and change management for managing the phases of an HI technology project. At a casual glance, it may seem that a leadership management plan for HI would focus on acquiring and implementing the HI system itself. However, due to the pervasive nature of these systems, adopting the HI technology requires reengineering the facility's hardware, software, and networking systems, acquiring new human resources, and training existing personnel (Campbell and Gilman 2010). Thus, to manage HI technology both the organizational and the technical needs must be considered by the top leadership. This is accomplished during several project phases, which are planning, designing, selecting, implementing, testing, evaluating, and supporting.

The initial involvement of leaders at the organizational level may be considered to occur in a preplanning phase after the project is approved. In the preplanning phase, strategic decisions are made to determine the project scope, establish a project team, set project deadlines, and establish a project budget. Consideration is given to the scope of the project and the need for consultants. It may be necessary to hire additional human resources or to provide space for the team to work and meet. Forming a testing team for quality management is indispensable.

During the planning and design, leaders would facilitate as-is and to-be business process modeling. For as-is modeling, documentation on the current processes affected by the change would be created or updated, and current information and workflow would be mapped. Information flow is especially important because information in an organization flows up and down the chain of command, within and between functional units, and in and out of the facility. Failing to map information flow may result in delivering a system that is not interoperable. With to-be modeling the new system would be designed, then a map from the old to the new systems would be created.

During system selection senior leadership would be present for functional specification design and vendors' system demonstrations and would provide the final authorization for purchasing the systems. They may also participate in the final handoff testing, and their approval would be needed to set up ongoing maintenance contracts.

Disaster and Recovery Planning

When a system is in operation, it becomes necessary to consider contingency planning to handle unexpected occurrences. In fact, the HIPAA Security Rule mandates the creation of a business contingency and a disaster plan (HIPAA 1996). **Disaster planning** is defined as a plan for protecting electronic personal health information (ePHI) in the event of a disaster that limits or eliminates access to facilities and ePHI (AHIMA 2014, 48). HIPAA requires a disaster recovery plan that addresses activation, assessment, containment, and an emergency mode operation (HIPAA 1996). Specifically, what would the steps be to handle the disruption to business processes if a natural disaster such as a flood, hurricane, or tornado damaged the HI system? In this digital age, one solution to preserving company data from loss is cloud-based data storage offered by offsite storage vendors. Although many savvy managers are aware of the need to ensure their business entities are HIPAA compliant when handling ePHI, it is doubtful that these managers know the level of the vendors' obligations for disaster recovery. The vendors' contracts often contain clauses that release them from obligation in the event of a natural disaster. These issues raise concerns with top managers about their lack of control over their cloud data.

Recovery planning is a plan for recovering data and restoring business operations to normal levels after a disaster or disruption occurs. HIPAA requirements include having a data backup plan for routinely saving and restoring data (HIPAA 1996). It might address something as simple as bringing systems back up after a power outage, or restoring data on one server. Or, recovery planning could mean moving IT operations to a redundant recovery site complete with duplicate servers, networking, PCs, and other systems. Clinical systems will need specific recovery plans. For example, Joint Commission requires laboratories to have a disaster plan outlining their response for the four days after the event (Scungio 2014). Similar to the facility recovery plan, the lab's recovery plan must be tested annually. Having policies and procedures in place for handling disasters and facilitating recovery is necessary to prevent disruptions to the business, to mitigate loss of data, and to ensure that the facility can recover without significant loss of data.

Check Your Understanding 8.1

Indicate whether the following statements are true or false.

1. The purpose of the EHR is to handle the medical information necessary for patient care and improve the efficiency and accessibility of the information.
2. Successful implementation of an EHR is not significantly dependent upon the human factors but rather on the most recent and advanced technology.
3. Input from internal stakeholders is essential for a successful EHR implementation.
4. Top leadership for a healthcare organization implementing an EHR always includes a board of directors.

5. Leadership management plans should be aligned with the facilities' mission statements.

6. Failing to map information flow between existing systems can result in a final system that is not interoperable.

7. HIPAA does not require the creation of business contingency or disaster plans.

8. Employees do not need any preparation for big changes, most are eager for change.

9. During the planning and design leaders would facilitate as-is and to-be business process modeling.

10. Laboratories do not require that a disaster recovery plan be in place.

⊙ Systems Development Life Cycle

It can be very helpful to have a framework for considering the processes and stakeholders in the development and implementation of health IT. The **systems development life cycle** (SDLC) includes four primary phases: planning and analysis, design, implementation, and maintenance and evaluation (Amatayakul 2016, 388). The framework is depicted in figure 8.1. It can be used as the framework for a wide range of initiatives, from small health IT projects to the transition to a complete EHR. Within a full-blown EHR implementation, many different SDLC processes may be occurring at the same time at various levels of the implementation. The entire SDLC process begins with the identification of a need and ends when the benefits of the system no longer outweigh costs, at which point the life cycle would begin again.

Planning and Analysis

Implementing an EHR represents a significant investment in time and money for healthcare providers and organizations of all sizes and types. Selecting the right product requires an investment in advanced planning to guide the selection process. Once a strategic decision is made to explore the use of technology to solve a business need, the planning and analysis phase of the SDLC is initiated. It is in this phase of life cycle development that the organization first defines the goals and scope of the project, taking into account the unique needs and characteristics of the organization including the size, complexity, and scope of services provided. The focus in this phase is on defining the organization's business problem and the resources that may be needed to develop the project. The resources to be defined in this phase include people, time, and funds. The specific technology is not included here. It will be addressed in a later phase.

An in-depth assessment of the needs of the user and their functional requirements must be accomplished in this planning and analysis phase. The assessment should include widespread participation from all end-users of the technology to ensure

Figure 8.1. Systems development life cycle

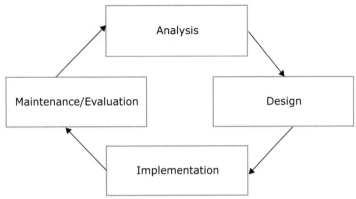

that the key stakeholder's needs and gaps in present technology and processes are clearly defined. The current system(s) and the user's response to the system should be analyzed to identify opportunities for improvement.

Areas to be addressed in the assessment include

- Identification of the technology currently being used and how it is used
- Analysis of current work and data flow processes
- Efficiency assessment of current technology and workflow
- User proficiency in using the current technology
- Timeliness and availability of data and information
- User satisfaction with the current system and processes
- Patient satisfaction, if applicable
- How the use of technology is expected to
  - Increase efficiency
  - Enhance quality
  - Meet other goals of the users

It is possible that the planning and analysis phase may reveal that the business problem is actually caused by issues with the workflow, processes, procedures, or training and that new technology may not be required or that the technology being used is obsolete. If a business need for a technology solution is identified, the planning and analysis phase is also the time to carefully consider whether it is technologically, financially, and operationally feasible to undertake the implementation of new technology to solve the business need.

The planning and analysis phase creates the blueprint for the project. This phase must take into account the unique characteristics of the organization to ensure that there is a strong foundation upon which to build the system and that the system is aligned with the healthcare organization's strategic goals.

Design

Once a determination is made that new systems or technologies are required, the design phase begins. In this phase, a project manager should be designated and a project steering committee of key stakeholders established to oversee and manage the project. The role of the steering committee is to plan, organize, coordinate, and manage the design and acquisition of the new technology. The role of the project manager is to lead the steering committee and keep the project on track.

The steering committee should be comprised of key stakeholders, including physicians, nurses, and other clinical disciplines and administrative personnel who will use the system. It is important that all groups who have an interest in the system be represented on the steering committee, including individuals who have expertise in information technology. Organizations that lack internal expertise in information management may choose to contract with an IT consultant to join the steering committee and assist throughout the life cycle of the project.

Define the System Goals

The goal of a systems implementation is very important to the ultimate design. Each organization will have goals aligned with its vision and mission. At the same time, goals can originate from external sources, too. For example, ONC is authorized to test and certify EHRs, and EHR modules (Office of the National Coordinator, DHHS 2015). To support this effort, ONC offers a list of certified Health IT products that have been thoroughly tested and given a certification identification number (Office of the National Coordinator, DHHS 2016).

Examples of system goal statements include

- Facilitate the exchange of information throughout the integrated delivery system by establishing a single EHR for the enterprise.
- Enable the physicians in a large multispecialty clinic to create and exchange information electronically from multiple locations, including the hospital, clinic offices, and at home using a wide variety of devices including smart phones and tablets.

These goal statements should align with the strategic goals of the organization and should serve as measures of performance throughout the SDLC.

Define Project Objectives and Scope

The project objectives and scope should be clearly defined. Projects may range from a limited scope, such as managing an upgrade to an existing application, to the much larger project of leading a complete assessment of the organization's information management needs and implementation of an enterprise-wide EHR.

Determine and Prioritize the System Requirements

Once the goals have been developed and evaluated against the organization's strategic goals, the specific requirements should be identified and prioritized. As an example, the goal to enable the physicians to create and exchange information electronically from multiple locations will require specifically defining the information they need as well as the methods they will use to create and exchange information.

The foundation of requirements needs to begin with any defined regulatory requirements. Any additional requirements can be determined by interviewing individual users and by establishing focus groups. In many cases, the users are unable to clearly identify their specific requirements, so vendor demonstrations or exploratory site visits to similar organizations may be necessary to develop their system requirements. Defining and prioritizing the functional and technical requirements requires the clear identification of the current state workflow analysis and development of the future state workflow. The Agency for Healthcare Research and Quality (AHRQ) has a *Health Information Technology Evaluation Toolkit* that includes educational presentations, research compilations, tools, and examples of how to use the tools available via the Internet (AHRQ 2012). Utilizing a framework such as the AHRQ tool can be very helpful for many organizations. This part of the process is of vital importance. Failure to assess workflow and requirements adequately can result in the purchase of software that will not meet user needs.

Screen the Marketplace for Potential Vendors

Once the project objectives and scope are defined, research should be conducted to identify potential vendors. The definitive resource for identifying an EHR solution or multiple solutions is the ONC Certified Health IT product list (ONC HSS 2016). The ONC issues EHR certification criteria to ensure compliance with the CMS EHR Incentive Program, also known as **meaningful use** (MU) which provides financial incentives to eligible professionals and hospitals who treat Medicare and Medicaid patients for adopting certified EHRs (AHIMA 2014, 91).

To ensure EHR software is certified appropriately, the ONC has designated **ONC-Authorized Testing and Certification Bodies (ATCBs)**. ATCBs are empowered to perform complete EHR or EHR module testing and certification. ATCBs utilize conformance testing requirements, test cases, and test tools developed by the National Institute for Standards and Technology (NIST) to determine whether the software complies with the EHR Incentive Program requirements for establishing MU of an EHR (ONC, HHS 2015).

Other sources of information may include trade shows and conferences operated by groups such as the American Health Information Management Association (AHIMA), Health Information Management Systems Society (HIMSS), and the American Medical Informatics Association (AMIA). There is also an abundance of EHR vendor information available on the Internet; however, consumers should take care to use official sources such as CMS, ONC, and AHRQ websites. Vendor information may also be obtained by contacting similar healthcare facilities to determine the technology they utilize.

There are usually two types of EHR software to consider: best of fit and best of breed. Best of fit refers to a single EHR product that provides a comprehensive integrated solution. For example, a physician practice may wish to select the best fit from among EHR vendors that offer a practice management system and clinical documentation as one system. Best of breed refers to products selected from a variety of vendors. Best of breed allows the user to find products that most closely meet their needs and preferences. However, best-of-breed products may not be interoperable with other software. Best of breed results in acquisition of separate software solutions for various operational and administrative functions.

Develop and Distribute the RFI or RFP

Once the requirements have been defined and documented, the organization should determine if they wish to initiate a **request for information (RFI)** or a **request for proposals (RFP)**. The RFI is used to ask vendors for information about their products and services. It is often used to obtain information from a large number of vendors to narrow the field of vendors to whom a RFP will be issued. The RFP is a more formal request to vendors to provide specific information about how they can meet the organization's specific requirements. In the RFP, the organization should describe the goals and priorities for the IT acquisition including technical and functional requirements.

A proposal committee of key stakeholders may be established at this point to assist in the RFP process. Similar to the project steering committee, the proposal committee should have broad representation of internal stakeholders, including all departments that will use or be affected by the EHR system. Representatives may include a **physician champion**, clinical departments (nursing, laboratory, radiology, and such), pharmacy, health information management, information technology, compliance, privacy and security, legal, finance, and purchasing. The physician champion is a physician tasked with the responsibility of representing the views of the physician users. AHIMA has published an RFI/RFP template, which provides guidance for organizations. The entire RFI/RFP Practice Brief and Template are found in appendixes C and D of the online resources for this book.

A vendor's response to an RFP will generally include a summary of all costs related to the project: hardware and software acquisition, technical support, consulting, staff training, and implementation services. The detail in the RFP allows for comparison across vendors on the proposed solutions. The RFP may also serve as the basis for the final contract, which is the legal agreement between the vendor and the organization.

Evaluate Vendor Options

Once the responses to the RFP are received, a side-by-side comparison of the proposals should be conducted. A matrix to compare the various vendor's proposals may be useful in facilitating the evaluation of the options. Appendix E provides an example of how an evaluation matrix might be used to compare different vendors across the required functionality. In evaluating options, it should be determined how the software will be delivered, whether in an **application service provider (ASP)** model whereby application services are accessed via the Internet or as an onsite application.

Hold Vendor Demonstrations

Based upon the results of the RFP comparison matrix, organizations will generally select three to five vendors to provide demonstrations of their technology. Demonstrations should be on a live system with internal stakeholders present to explore if and how the technology can meet the end users' needs. Users should have the opportunity to ask for demonstrations of specific tasks and processes that will be used after the software is implemented. A selected, diverse sample of stakeholders should have a hands-on experience with the product during the demonstration.

Make Site Visits and Check References

Many organizations will elect to send members of their project steering committee or proposal committee to visit one or more potential vendor sites where the technology is in operation so they can obtain detailed information from end users who have had the technology in place to support their business processes. Extensive reference checks with organizations that have used the vendor's products are recommended. Due to the evolving nature of the technology, it is recommended that both long-term and short-term users of the vendor's technology be contacted.

Vendors should also be asked to provide data regarding their customer satisfaction ratings and their customer service records. For example, KLAS reports provide a source of information about the potential vendors. KLAS is a company that evaluates vendor performance based upon input from providers about the technology and provides the results of their evaluations for a fee.

Evaluate Vendors

Given that EHRs are expensive, it is important for organizations to evaluate any potential vendor thoroughly. This is a part of good governance and is often referred to as "due diligence." Persons in an organizational position with decision-making power must exercise that power carefully. One model for selecting an ambulatory EHR vendor suggests evaluating the goals of the clinic or practice as it relates to following four aspects of the EHR:

- **Functionality** addresses the features of the EHR product, including patient encounter documentation, automating and facilitating office workflow, decision support during patient encounters, and reporting that supports care management and template customization.
- **Usability** addresses the speed and ease of use, including goals about tasks that must be done fast, computer literacy of the practice staff, and the methods by which data will be entered.
- **Practicality** addresses costs including goals about price, internal resources to maintain the EHR, whether the EHR is integrated or interfaced with the practice management systems, and interfaces with labs.
- The **reputation** of the vendor should also be evaluated, including determining how long they have been in business and what systems they have in operation, conducting site visits with the vendor's customers, and conducting other due diligence checks (Louisiana Health Care Quality Forum 2009).

Rank Vendors and Costs

Once the vendors have been evaluated, a ranking system should be used to assess the vendors on the functionality of the system and estimated cost. It is unlikely that one vendor will have all of the desired functionality at the lowest price. Organizations may have many requirements above and beyond the required criteria. The additional requirements should be prioritized so that a ranking system can be developed and utilized to assist in decision making. The top vendor should be selected and contract negotiations initiated based upon the overall ranking.

Conduct Contract Negotiations

The Centers for Medicare and Medicaid Services (CMS) developed the Doctor's Office Quality–Information Technology (DOQ-IT) program to assist physician practices with EHR implementation activities (CMS 2015a). The DOQ-IT materials suggest that organizations request language changes to make the contracts more "equal." DOQ-IT contracting guidelines advise that purchasers look at a number of specific issues, including hardware and software, support, interfaces, training, implementation, and disaster recovery and planning (Anon 2009). The language should be clear and understandable with specific terms defined. One important way an organization can protect itself is to include the vendor response to the RFP in the contract. This is where the vendor stipulated, usually with great specificity, what they could provide.

One of the challenges encountered in HIT and EHR contracting has been the insertion of "hold harmless" clauses in contracts. These clauses were designed to indemnify software vendors for malpractice or injury claims when the software may have been at fault or even to prevent healthcare providers from disclosing errors, bugs, design flaws, and other HIT-software-related hazards (Goodman et al. 2011). The 2011 American Medical Informatics Association Board Position Paper maintained that these clauses are unethical because they protect corporations at all times, sometimes to the detriment of patient safety and quality of care (Goodman et al. 2011). In 2014, new requirements were added to the EHR certification program. Only a few vendors have been able to meet the newly added requirements, and those few did so at the expense of not providing other requested usability and workflow modifications (Payne et al. 2015). Moreover, the vendors that did provide the necessary enhancements did so at the expense of not providing requested usability and workflow modifications (Payne et al. 2015). This has prompted the AMIA Task Force to recommend simplifying the certification process. This is becoming a widespread and recognized concern as evidenced by the 2012 Food and Drug Administration Safety and Innovation Act, which charges the Food and Drug Administration, the ONC, and the Federal Communications Commission with developing "a report that contains a proposed strategy and recommendations on an appropriate, risk-based regulatory framework pertaining to health information technology, including mobile medical applications, that promotes innovation, protects patient safety, and avoids regulatory duplication" (FDA 2012). As of 2016, EHRs are not under FDA regulation, but the FDA has begun regulating some mobile medical applications such as those intended to regulate an infusion pump, measure blood glucose or blood oxygen levels, or display digital x-ray images (FDA 2012).

Implementation

Implementing a new system or technology represents a significant change to any size or type of healthcare organization. Establishing a comprehensive project plan and schedule is required. This is often accomplished by an implementation team. This implementation team will generally include members of the project steering committee and the proposal committee, but will also include additional user representatives and individuals with the expertise to deploy the new system. The implementation team must forecast and senior management must dedicate the resources needed for the implementation.

It is also recommended that the implementation team include at least one champion, someone who is known and respected in the organization, who sees the new system as necessary to the achievement of the organization's goals, and who is passionate about implementing it. In many healthcare organizations, the EHR champion will be a highly regarded physician who assumes a leadership role with the medical staff and with other system users. The champion must also have strong verbal communication skills. The champion will often have to find ways to motivate many different people to utilize the new technology. Effective communication is critical to successful implementation.

Project Implementation Plan

It is important to have a project implementation plan for an EHR implementation project, just due to the size and scope. The project implementation plan should include the following elements:

1. Major tasks identified
2. Major milestones set
3. Estimated duration of each task
4. Dependencies among activities (for example, if one task must be completed before another can be started)
5. Resources and budget (including staff who will be devoted to the project)
6. Responsible individual or group for each task and milestone
7. Target dates for each milestone
8. Measures for evaluating completion and success (Wager et al. 2009)

A longer list might be utilized for an EHR or HIT implementation plan. It is important to remember that the plan often has to be modified as the project progresses. This should not be considered failure. It may be beneficial to think of the implementation as an opportunity to learn for the next implementation or upgrade.

Workflow and Process Analysis

The workflow process and analysis completed in the assessment phase of the system life cycle development documented the "as-is" of the healthcare practice. It is important to plan how technology either can or, of necessity, will evolve into the new workflows and processes. For example, in a hospital, doctors or nurses may be required to enter orders that were once entered by unit clerks. This is because the new system will generate alerts for possible contraindications or provide other knowledge the clinician may need to deliver appropriate care. If this new and additional work is not acknowledged and accounted for, the clinicians may become frustrated. Conversely, the new system may include tools that change the communication methods, that is, inboxes or alerts for abnormal lab results or other needed notifications that used to require phone calls. Everyone involved in the communication, unit clerk, diagnostic technician, and receiving clinician, including the physician, needs to be involved in the planning for these new flows.

Install System Components

Before a project can go-live the hardware and software must be installed. This will include ensuring that there is adequate network infrastructure to support the new system and that required interfaces are built. Depending upon the penetration and use of information technology that already exist in the organization, this can be a minor upgrade or it can be a major part of the project, such as installing computers-on-wheels (**COWs**), self-contained rolling carts containing a computer for access to the EHR on each unit. It is recommended that a test of the system's effectiveness be piloted in a small unit before the entire system is installed. This will allow for an evaluation of the system and the opportunity to address any issues or concerns.

Train Staff

Training is essential to the successful implementation of any new system. The vendor's role in training should have been defined in the contracting process. The implementation team must define who needs to be trained, who should do the training, how much training is required, and how the training will be accomplished.

The AHRQ Health Information Technology research portfolio recommends demonstration systems (Dixon and Zafar 2009). These are systems entirely separate from the planned production system. They allow clinicians and other users to practice prior to system implementation. In many cases, vendors will supply training as a part of the implementation. Whether the vendors provide the training, the organization builds a demonstration system, or other methods are used, training is important and cannot be ignored.

Convert Data and Test the System

One of the decisions that should already have been made is the extent to which the organization will convert or incorporate **legacy data**, as well as the methods for doing so. Legacy data are existing data, some of which are on paper and some of which may already be digital. Whatever the current format, they must be converted to a format that is compatible with the new product or system. It is recommended that the process or product be tested to ensure that it will allow the data to be converted using a limited amount of data at first. All data should be backed up and cleaned prior to the conversion. There are processes outside the scope of this chapter that describe data cleaning in detail.

The amount of data to be converted should have been defined in the planning process but it is recommended that only as much data as must be accessed in the new system be converted. Very often this decision must be made with both clinical and administrative staff having input. Data conversion can be time consuming, expensive, as well as impact system response time, thus the pros and cons of conversion should be considered carefully. At a minimum, conversion should be scheduled outside of peak periods. Following the conversion, steps must be taken to validate that the data were successfully converted. Chapter 5 of this book includes steps and processes for data quality checking.

Communicate Progress

Throughout the system implementation, stakeholders should be kept apprised of the project status. This is important to ensure the various users begin to understand the project and do not get the feeling that it is happening in a vacuum. Communication can be accomplished through formal and informal methods including reports to major committees, e-mail blasts, updates in a newsletter, or posts on the company's website. The methods of communication will vary with the size and complexity of the organization and the project, but as many channels of communication as possible should be used to ensure that all stakeholders have timely and accurate information about the project. It is impossible to overcommunicate with a project of this impact and scope.

Plan for Go-Live Date

The go-live date is the date that the organization transitions from the old system to the new or initiates the transition from a paper to an electronic system. The targeted go-live date was identified when the project implementation plan was initiated.

The go-live date should be selected for a time period when workload is lower. In the inpatient setting, the date should be one for which there is a historically low census. In academic medical centers, the go-live would need to occur when interns, residents, and fellows are not in the first month of their training. Organizations could also decide to defer elective admissions and surgeries during the go-live time frame to ensure optimal deployment of staff and minimal interruption to patient care. In the ambulatory setting, organizations may elect to reduce the patient workload for a period immediately prior to, during, and following the conversion to allow time for training, learning the new system, and becoming proficient in using the system. Reducing the census or ambulatory workload has an economic effect that should be planned for as part of the implementation process.

Support and Evaluation

Changes will have to be made as any new system is implemented. The implementation team must respond quickly to identified problems or concerns to ensure that users remain confident in the system and feel supported by the organization. A specific individual or group should be assigned to address issues and the end users should be advised to contact that person or group to report any problems or concerns.

Table 8.2.   Sample HIT evaluation measure

Measure	Quality Domain(s)	Data Source(s)	Notes	Potential Risks
Preventable adverse drug events (ADEs)	Patient safety Quality of care	Chart review Prescription review Direct observations May also consider patient phone interviews Instrumenting the study database EMR	Need to distinguish between ADEs and MEs can be divided by stage of medication process: • Ordering • Transcribing • Dispensing • Administering • Monitoring Can be assessed in both inpatient and outpatient settings. ADEs are: • Idiosyncratic reactions • Drug-diagnosis interactions	Preventable ADEs are relatively common, especially if there is no clinical decision support (CDS) at the time of drug ordering. Many drug–drug and drug–diagnosis interactions can be avoided if CDS tools are available at the time or ordering of medications. Keep track of alerts that fire in a system with CDS, understanding that in a system without CDS those alerts will not be available; we can get an upper bound for preventable ADEs. It is hard to define what is meant by a "preventable ADE." Some idiosyncratic reactions are not preventable and it is impossible to predict who will get what reaction.

Source: AHRQ 2009.

The implementation committee should establish a formal process to collect data regarding all reported problems to identify patterns and trends and opportunities to improve the system. AHRQ has published a *Health Information Technology Evaluation Toolkit* (AHRQ 2012). This toolkit is very helpful when developing monitors. It includes the consideration of feasibility of collecting the measure, as well as the science behind a measure. Table 8.2 is a sample measure found in the toolkit. In one study on CPOEs, a team of researchers focused on evaluating CPOE and recommend 18 measures, including percentage of system downtime, mean response time, percentage of orders entered by physicians, percentage of orders entered as miscellaneous, and others (Sittig et al. 2007). As can be seen from this limited CPOE example, there are many measures that can be monitored for an EHR implementation. The entire team should participate in setting the measures, the most current research from resources such as the ONC and AHRQ websites should be utilized, and, most important, the measures must be pertinent to the practice and the setting.

The implementation committee should be careful to establish a mechanism to identify any unintended adverse consequences. This is made easier with the publication of the *Unintended Consequences Guide (UCG)* published by RAND under contract with AHRQ (Jones et al. 2011). The guide is web-based and includes introductory information regarding the overall evaluation of health information technology. The main reason for this site, though, is to assist in the identification of unintended adverse consequences. It does this by educating users on why these consequences can and do occur, as well as providing a template to assist with the identification and tracking of unintended consequences. An example of the Issues Log workbook, found in the section Identify Unintended Consequences, can be found in appendix F of this book. It is important to monitor unintended consequences to protect patient safety and ensure user satisfaction.

Maintenance and Evaluation for EHRs, HIEs, and RECs

After EHRs, HIEs, or RECs are in operation, the ongoing maintenance and evaluation of these systems must be considered. Regional extension centers, provided by the ONC, are designed to help doctors implement EHRs (National Learning Consortium 2015). The ONC has been instrumental in the development of standards, policies, and innovations in the field of HIE evaluation and maintenance (Dullabh et al. 2013). A recent case study evaluation of five HIEs in different states emphasized the importance of governance, stakeholder engagement, provider engagement, and long-term planning to establish sustainability for the HIEs after the initial start-up funding has been spent. Provider engagement was deemed especially important for ACOs and patient-centered medical homes (Dullabh et al. 2013).

The ONC managed the federally funded initiative to implement Regional Extension Centers (RECs) in order to provide primary care physicians (PCPs) in rural areas with the ability to have electronic health records. Specifically, this program provided assistance with identifying needs and selecting, procuring, and connecting the system (Lynch et al. 2014). A descriptive study of 62 RECs from

2010 to 2013 indicated that over 130,000 PCPs were in the program, and almost half achieved meaningful use of these systems (Lynch et al. 2014).

Similarly, EHRs must have support contracts in place and they must undergo regular planned evaluation. Like any HI system in operation in a healthcare facility, regular updates must be applied to the system, antivirus and malware must be installed, backups must be maintained, and the system must be reevaluated regularly to ensure the privacy and security of ePHI is being maintained. This reevaluation would include making sure that the system is meeting the original goals as set forth in quality and technical measures by the project team working in conjunction with top management.

⊙ Transition to a Complete EHR Process

The implementation of an EHR does not mean that paper patient records will cease to exist or that the use of paper in healthcare organizations will be a thing of the past. The continued need or requirement to utilize paper in conjunction with an EHR has a name. Patient records that are maintained in both paper and electronic formats are known as **hybrid** records. These records are the most difficult to manage because what is in paper and what is electronic may be constantly changing, while the organization will have to comply with the regulations for both paper records and EHRs. A study of 14 sites from across the United States found that continued use of paper was due to one of the following reasons:

- ⊙ Old uses are still valued;
- ⊙ New uses of paper have been identified; or
- ⊙ Sometimes paper may be best (Dykstra et al. 2009).

Advantages of Hybrid Records

A hybrid health record contains a combination of paper and electronic records (AHIMA 2014). Additionally, hybrid records may also contain scanned images of paper records like emergency room reports, or lab and x-ray results. The old uses of paper that are still valued run from the psychological, including the familiarity of paper, which creates a level of comfort, to the social, where clinical activities are organized around paper documents such as intensive care unit flow sheets, and then to a natural resistance to or failure to change, meaning that paper is printed because that is the way it has always been done.

The new uses of paper include the ability of paper to "fill the gaps" left by incompletely developed or implemented EHR software or functions that have yet to be standardized. One example is the advance directives of patients. Very often the EHR will include an advance directive indicator of Yes, No, or Unknown, but the advance directives will often be maintained in hard copy or, at most, scanned and retained as a PDF document. It is also standard for the downtime system to be paper based (Dykstra et al. 2009).

A paper patient record can be better than an EHR as paper is very versatile. In addition to the forms approved for the record, sticky notes can facilitate much clinical communication. Paper checklists and reminder lists are standard tools for healthcare. Although most of the regulatory hurdles to paper have been addressed, some states may still require paper for specific purposes. States may require paper copies of documents for informed consent or resuscitation status (Dykstra et al. 2009).

Challenges When Handling Hybrid Records

The use of patient records that are part paper and part electronic is the most complicated because the requirements, regulations, and constraints of both types of records must be met. This especially becomes problematic when the patient record format may be constantly changing, as is the case with an organization involved in the active implementation of an EHR system.

There are several disadvantages to hybrid records. First, one disadvantage is the complexity of locating data in the health record when part is scanned in from paper and part is in an electronic system (Mitchell 2011). For example, a nurse looking for a lab report needs to call the results to the physician. First, she looks at the electronic system and sees that the lab values are not in that system. Next, she looks at the paper chart and sees some scanned lab reports but does not find the one she is looking for. She will still need to call the lab and get a paper copy of the lab report. Thus, the complexity of locating hybrid data in two systems and the possibility of errors with scanned data entry must be addressed by the facility. It is essential that a mapping of the location of all the hybrid records documents be created and circulated or the clinical and administrative staff will have problems finding the paper and electronic parts of the patient records.

Second, a significant challenge exists with the definition of the legal health record. This is the official record that healthcare organizations release when it is requested by a third party such as an attorney or insurance company via the Release of Information department. Maintaining this definition can mean the creation of a "cheat sheet" to indicate which format is used for the different data and information types. To be on the safe side, many organizations spend considerable time and money printing the records from both systems (Mitchell 2011). This results in increased cost and time to maintain and compile the complete record.

A further complicating issue is the fact that when paper records exist clinicians wishing to avoid using the electronic records may start creating their own copies of records that are subsequently used to make treatment decisions. For example, a physician may use a paper printout of the health record that he printed off when making treatment decisions. In addition, changes, updates, deletions, and corrections to hybrid systems are difficult to propagate. The nature of the hybrid systems is that the paper document must be updated first then that update must be scanned or entered manually into the electronic system. This creates an opportunity for errors to be introduced along the way and presents additional challenges in the management of updates or addendums because they must be maintained in two places (Dimick 2008).

Creating reports in hybrid systems is difficult. The person wishing to create a report from a hybrid health record must collect data from two different systems.

Depending on the tool available in the electronic systems, it may be possible to generate and export report data. However, the scanned data will have to be printed out and manually entered into a reporting tool, unless the source system (such as lab or x-ray) provides some query and export functionality to assist in the collection and aggregation of the data. In either case, the data in these two systems must be cross-referenced to assure that they correctly integrated into the electronic data set. This process adds yet another layer of complexity to quality measure reporting.

Check Your Understanding 8.2

Indicate whether the following statements are true or false.

1. The specific technology to be acquired is determined during the planning and analysis phase of the SDLC.

2. It is possible to communicate too much information to stakeholders about the progress or a project.

3. A request for information (RFI) is used to ask vendors for information about their products and services in order to narrow down the vendors to whom a request for proposals (RFP) will be issued.

4. Patient records that are maintained in both paper and electronic formats are known as hybrid records.

5. The ONC has been instrumental in the development of standards, policies, and innovations in field of HIE evaluation and maintenance.

6. Regional Extension Centers were funded in order to provide primary care physicians (PCPs) in rural areas with the ability to have electronic health records.

7. Creating reports in hybrid systems is difficult because the data is in two different systems.

Answer the following questions.

8. The role of a project manager is to
   a. Lead the steering committee
   b. Decide which technology should be acquired
   c. Keep the project on track
   d. a and c only

9. Which of the following does the FDA regulate?
   a. Electronic health record systems
   b. Mobile medical device systems such as blood glucose monitors
   c. Document management systems
   d. Computer physician order entry systems

⊙ Usability

The **International Organization for Standards (ISO)** is a worldwide nongovernmental organization that develops and publishes international standards. The ISO is a network of the national standards institutes of countries that enable consensus to create solutions to meet business requirements and the broader needs of society (ISO 2012).

In standard 9241-11, the ISO defines the usability of a product as "the extent to which a product can be used by specified users to achieve specified goals with effectiveness, efficiency and satisfaction in a specified context of use" (ISO 2012). This means that usability cannot be measured as a property of the product itself, but only in relation to the context of its use: the physical and social conditions in which the product is being used (Svanaes et al. 2008). The usability measures proposed by ISO are

1. effectiveness or the extent to which the goals, whatever they may be, of the users are achieved (often this is measured as task completion);

2. efficiency or the resources needed to achieve the goal (for information technology this is usually measured as completion time); and

3. the user's subjective assessment of the product (Svanaes et al. 2008).

For medical informatics users, candidate tasks range from patient scheduling to clinical care to data reporting necessary for quality management and beyond. When using an EHR, efficiency might mean reducing common tasks to the fewest clicks or screens possible so that time and effort are not wasted. A user's subjective assessment may be more difficult to accomplish with a full-blown EHR, but this input can be well worth the trouble to ensure a high-quality product. Usability in healthcare IT must be considered in context because of the great diversity of users, their tasks, and the work environments (Svanaes et al. 2008). The healthcare delivery system is highly specialized, with many different interpretations for usability. The software developers and EHR vendors are responsible for a large portion of the usability of the systems.

Researchers in a AHRQ-funded study interviewed various EHR vendors to determine their practices related to EHR usability (McDonnell et al. 2010). The EHR vendors expressed a commitment to developing usable EHR products for the market; however, formal usability testing, user-centered design processes, and development personnel with expertise in usability engineering are still rare (McDonnell et al. 2010).

Use Cases

A **use case** is a scenario based on how a user will utilize information in a given information system (AHIMA 2014). Use cases are utilized to create use case diagrams showing the to-be processes and how the user will interact with them. First, the abstracted logical use case diagram is translated into a systems model and that becomes the blueprint from which HI developers will design the new system for maximum usability. For example, the home care use for one system describes how doctors and nurses communicated effectively to generate a Medicare patient care plan for treatment and billing (Campbell 2016). CMS provides guidance for developing a comprehensive chronic care management plan for all patients, which would contain:

⊙ A problem list

⊙ Expected outcome and prognosis

⊙ Measurable treatment goals

⊙ Symptom management

⊙ Planned interventions

⊙ Medication management

⊙ Community/social services ordered

⊙ A description of how services of agencies and specialists outside the practice will be directed/coordinated

⊙ A schedule for periodic review and, when applicable, revision of the care plan (CMS 2015b).

In a related effort, mobile health use cases are being developed for emergency rooms and patients likely to experience adverse events (Campbell 2016). Many other use cases have been created by the HIMSS Interoperability Maturity Model (IMM) Task force. For example, readmission tracking is an important activity because facilities maintain statistics on patients who are readmitted within 30 days of the original discharge from the facility as this may reflect on the quality of care provided as well as impact reimbursement. The HIMSS IMM use case for readmissions tracking includes data on receiving and exchanging clinical data, reporting clinical results, and referring the patient (HIMSS 2011).

The flow of the readmission process is detailed starting with the patient's admission to the inpatient facility, transfer to a skilled nursing facility, and the subsequent readmission through ER back into the inpatient facility. Finally, this use case contains other use cases, which are patient referral use case, exchanging clinical data use case, and receiving clinical data use case. This nesting of related use cases is a common practice.

EHR Vendors and Usability

One challenge for EHR implementation is that there are no standards for EHR vendors to collect and report usability issues that might impact patient safety (McDonnell et al. 2010). Usability is considered to be a competitive differentiator so little collaboration occurs between vendors.

Usability experts were allowed to review the interview findings and made the following recommendations regarding EHR usability:

1. Standards in design and development
   a. Increase the diversity of users surveyed for predeployment feedback. It was noted that most vendors use volunteers, hardly an unbiased sample.

Most people who would volunteer enjoy testing technology and are not representative of the typical end user.

b. Support an independent body for vendor collaboration and standards development. As with much of healthcare, the health IT market does not meet the criteria for a full free market. All parties do not have equal access to information. Specifically, the buyer has a limited ability to determine whether the product meets their needs and, if they decide incorrectly, the cost of purchasing a different product is substantial.

c. Develop standards and best practices in use of customization during EHR deployment. Some customization is necessary to support the needs of different healthcare organizations and different users within those organizations. However, more information is needed to understand which and how much customization is of benefit and which is not.

2. Usability testing and evaluation

a. Encourage formal usability testing early in the design and development phase as a best practice.

b. Evaluate ease of learning, effectiveness, and satisfaction qualitatively and quantitatively. In essence, use the measures promulgated by the ISO. Be sure to include qualitative or contextual information.

3. Postdeployment monitoring and patient safety

a. Decrease dependence on postdeployment review supporting usability assessments. An EHR's usability is pervasive throughout the software. Although smaller issues can often be corrected after deployment, major usability issues, which may be more of a threat to patient safety, will be much more difficult to fix.

b. Increase research and development of best practices supporting designing for patient safety. Specifically, designing for patient safety needs to be incorporated from the beginning. Currently, vendors appear to monitor and design for patient safety in the late stages or during the release cycle.

4. Certification programs should be carefully designed and valid. Usability is complex and any certification would need to reflect that complexity. Assisting the EHR vendors to create usable products requires a process that identifies usable products, establishes and disseminates standards, and encourages innovation (McDonnell et al. 2010).

As with many other aspects of health information technology, the industry is learning that standards and collaboration are necessary in order to provide the support required to deliver safe, high-quality patient care.

EHR Usability Testing and Assessment

EHR usability and the evaluation of that usability is a part of implementing an effective, efficient EHR system. It is necessary to have a basis of understanding or a framework for examining the usability of systems.

ISO standard 25062 specifies the format for reporting usability testing. The format allows comparisons across technologies and includes the following elements:

- ⊙ "The description of the product
- ⊙ The goals of the test
- ⊙ The test participants
- ⊙ The tasks the users were asked to perform
- ⊙ The experimental design of the test
- ⊙ The method or process by which the test was conducted
- ⊙ The usability measures and data collection methods
- ⊙ The numerical results" (ISO 2012).

It would also be important to include a description of the use context of the test as described previously. This is because healthcare has multiple settings. Good usability for the ambulatory setting would be different than good usability for the acute care setting and so forth.

A framework for EHR usability, called TURF (Tasks, Users, Representations, and Functions) defines usability as how useful, usable, and satisfying a system is for the intended users to accomplish goals (Zhang and Walji 2011). TURF is based upon ISO 9241-11, but differs in some selected definitions ("effective" in the ISO and "useful" in TURF and "efficient" in ISO and "usable" in TURF). Under TURF, a system is usable if it is easy to learn, efficient to use, and error tolerant. Learnability is defined as the ease of learning and relearning, which can be measured by the amount of time and effort required to become skilled in performing the task (Zhang and Walji 2011). Other important components of the framework include efficiency, the amount of effort required to accomplish a task, and error tolerance, the ability of the system to prevent errors and recover from errors that do occur (Zhang and Walji 2011). The TURF framework may be used to objectively measure usability and for evaluating and redesigning existing technologies to reduce the number of task steps and the time required to complete tasks. It will be very valuable as a method for organizing and discussing EHR usability. For example, the researchers applied the TURF framework in the analysis of a task to maintain an active medication allergy list, and reduced the task from 187 steps to 82.

With EHR implementation reaching significant levels across the United States and the world, the usability of these systems can no longer be ignored. The threat to patient safety and the waste of resources, especially clinician time, make a focus on EHR usability an imperative.

Check Your Understanding 8.3

Indicate whether the following statements are true or false.

1. Usability cannot be measured as a property of a product itself, but only in relation to the context of its use.

2. The heterogeneous nature of the healthcare system requires that products be evaluated and tested for usability in the actual healthcare setting in which they will be deployed.

3. Learnability is not an important component of EHR usability.

4. Poor usability is generally not included as a threat to patient safety.

5. Use case diagrams are a blueprint for data flow in a HI system.

6. The International Standards Organization has well recognized standards for usability.

7. The users' perceptions of the systems' usefulness and ease of use are a big part of determining system usability.

Case Study: HIS Implementation

Implementing any HIS is challenging. One ongoing challenge is how to implement a system according to best practices that protect the privacy and security of PHI while allowing consumers access to their information. Increasingly patient portals have been used to engage consumers in their healthcare, which has been shown to provide positive outcomes. This case study examines best practices for maintaining pediatric health information in a patient portal that was implemented by Vanderbilt University Medical Center (VUMC) in Tennessee.

As a first step, the leadership of the organization that is implementing the system must familiarize themselves with state and federal laws and regulations for protecting the privacy of the pediatric consumers' data. Policies and procedures must be created that address the spectrum of today's blended and extended families. For example, same-sex parents, foster parents, and guardians. VUMC is a sprawling academic medical center with six hospital systems having facilities spread across the state. In December 2013, there were approximately 17,722 pediatric accounts in the patient portal guarded by the HIM department.

HIM professionals worked with VUMC's general counsel to establish best practices for compliance with privacy laws and regulations. Each minor between the age of 0–17 years needed to complete and sign a paper application, which was witnessed by the VUMC representative and a parent or legal guardian with proper identification. Rules were created for verifying the documentation of parents, legal guardians, stepparents, and such. Parents had to apply for their own portal account. After the application was processed and approved, the minor was linked to their parent or legal guardian. Additionally, state laws for minors vary by state. Tennessee grants minors attaining the age of 13 years some rights. Thus, there were separate applications for minors between 13 and 17 years that needed to be signed by the minor and a parent or guardian in order for both parties to see the teens account. However, teen parents may not access their minor child's account until the minor child is 18 years old.

(Continued)

Several other issues must be addressed by the organization's leadership, such as what information to put in the pediatric portals. At VUMC, each individual department decided what to export to the portal. For example, VUMC's portal did not have radiology results available. Each hospital in the six VUMC hospital system had a different policy regarding when access to the accounts must be renewed.

This case study is important because it underscores the role of leadership in a system implementation. Specifically, top leadership carefully approached providing consumer-centered healthcare that complies with laws for privacy of PHI. They informed themselves regarding state and federal privacy laws and regulations, and considered the complex nature of the evolving family structure in the context of providing access to the minors' portal data. They systematically proceeded to develop policies and procedures that provided best practices for implementing their pediatric portal. (Case study adapted from Sherek and Gray 2014.)

Chapter 8 Review Exercises

Match the term with its description.

a. Persons, roles, or organizational units with a vested interest can use the EHR to accomplish their goals

b. A plan for protecting electronic personal health information (ePHI) in the event of a disaster that limits or eliminates access to facilities and ePHI

c. An organization of healthcare providers accountable for the quality, cost, and overall care of Medicare beneficiaries

d. Formal request to vendors to provide specific information about how they can meet the organization's specific requirements

e. Application services are accessed via the Internet

f. Data in the old system that needs to be put into the new system

1. _____ Stakeholder

2. _____ Accountable care organization

3. _____ Request for proposal

4. _____ Disaster planning

5. _____ Application service provider

6. _____ Legacy data

Indicate whether the following statements are true or false.

7. During the planning and design leaders would facilitate as-is and to-be business process modeling.

8. The systems development life cycle includes four primary phases: planning and analysis, design, implementation, and maintenance and evaluation.

9. HIPAA requirements include having a data backup plan for routinely saving and restoring data.

10. Clinical labs do not have to have specific recovery plans.

Discussion.

11. What are roles of leadership related to healthcare information systems implementation. Why are they needed?

12. Create a strategic plan for implementing a new e-prescribing system. The plan should state two project goals and describe the project duration and how to determine if the project goals are met.

13. Describe the system development life cycle for an EHR implementation. Discuss two activities that occur in each step.

14. Describe and analyze four issues associated with the benefits of paper versus EHR.

15. Compare and contrast the advantages and disadvantages of hybrid records.

16. Discuss the impact of usability on EHR utility.

17. Define disaster planning, state why a facility needs a disaster plan, and analyze two issues related to disaster planning.

REFERENCES

AHIMA. 2014. *Pocket Glossary for Health Information Management and Technology.* 4th ed. Chicago: AHIMA.

AHRQ. 2012. Health Information Technology Evaluation Toolkit. https://healthit.ahrq.gov/health-it-tools-and-resources/health-it-evaluation-toolkit-and-evaluation-measures-quick-reference.

Amatayakul, M. 2012. *Electronic Health Records: A Practical Guide for Professionals and Organizations.* 5th ed. 2013 update. Chicago, IL: American Health Information Management Association.

Amatayakul, M. 2016. Health Information Systems Strategic Planning. Chapter 13 in *Health Information Management Concepts Principles, and Practices.* 5th ed. Edited by P. Oachs and A. Watters. Chicago, IL: AHIMA Press.

Armenakis, A.A., J.B. Bernerth, J.P. Pitts, and H.J. Walker. 2007. Organizational change recipients' beliefs scale: Development of an assessment instrument. *The Journal of Applied Behavioral Science* 43(4):481–505. doi:10.1177/0021886307303654.

Campbell, S. 2016. USE CASE: Of standards development. *Journal of AHIMA* 87(1):24–29.

Campbell, T. and C. Gilman. 2010, September. Workforce transformation in the world of an EHR. AHIMA. http://bok.ahima.org/doc?oid=106023.

Centers for Medicare and Medicaid. 2015a. Quality Payment Program: Delivery System Reform, Medicare Payment Reform, and MACRA. https://www.cms.gov/Medicare/Quality-Initiatives-Patient-Assessment-Instruments/Value-Based-Programs/MACRA-MIPS-and-APMs/MACRA-MIPS-and-APMs.html.

Centers for Medicare and Medicaid. 2015b. Chronic Care Management Services. https://www.cms.gov/Outreach-and-Education/Medicare-Learning-Network-MLN/MLNProducts/Downloads/ChronicCareManagementTextOnly.pdf.

Charles, K., M. Cannon, R. Hall, and A. Coustasse. 2014. Can utilizing a computerized provider order entry (CPOE) system prevent hospital medical errors and adverse drug events? *Perspectives in Health Information Management* (Fall): 1–16.

Corrao, N.J., A.G. Robinson, M.A. Swiernik, and A. Naeim. 2010. Importance of testing for usability when selecting and implementing an electronic health or medical record system. *Journal of Oncology Practice* 6(3):120–124. doi:10.1200/JOP.200017.

Denić, N., V. Moračanin, M. Milić, and Z. Nešić. 2014. Risk management in information system projects. *Upravljanja Rizicima Projekta Informacijskih Sustava* 21(6):1239–1242.

Dimick, C. 2011. Meaningful use: Notes from the journey. *Journal of AHIMA* 82(10):24–30.

Dixon, B.E., and A. Zafar. 2009. Inpatient computerized provider order entry (CPOE): Finding from the AHRQ Health IT Portfolio. Rockville, MD: AHRQ National Resource Center for Health IT under Contract No. 290-04-0016. https://healthit.ahrq.gov/ahrq-funded-projects/emerging-lessons/computerized-provider-order-entry-inpatient/inpatient-computerized-provider-order-entry-cpoe.

Dolezel, D., and J. Moczygemba. 2015. Implementing EHRs: An exploratory study to examine current practices in migrating physician practice. *Perspectives in Health Information Management* Winter:1–15.

Dullabh, P., L. Hovey, P. Ubri, R. S. Catterson, and A. Jha. 2013. Evaluation of the State Health Information Exchange Cooperative Agreement Program. https://www.healthit.gov/sites/default/files/casestudysynthesisdocument_2-8-13.pdf.

Dykstra, R.H., J.S. Ash, D.F. Campebell, K. Sitting, J. Guappone, J. Carpenter, A. Richardson, A. Wright, and C. McMullen. 2009. Persistent paper: The myth of going paperless, 158–162. AMIA Annual Symposium Proceedings/AMIA Symposium.

Garrido, T., B. Raymond, L. Jamieson, L. Liang, and A. Wiesenthal. 2004. Making the business case for hospital information systems—A Kaiser Permanente investment decision. *Journal of Health Care Finance* 31(2):16–25.

Goodman, K. W., E. S. Berner, M. A. Dente, B. Kaplan, R. Koppel, D. Rucker, D. Z. Sands and P. Winkelstein. 2011. Challenges in ethics, safety, best practices, and oversight regarding HIT vendors, their customers, and patients: a report of an AMIA special task force. *Journal of American Medical Informatics Association* 18:77-81. doi:10.1136/jamia.2010.008946.

Griffith, J.R., and K.R. White. 2010. *Reaching Excellence in Healthcare Management.* Chicago: Health Administration Press.

HIMSS. 2011. Security of Mobile Computing Devices in the Healthcare Environment. http://www.himss.org/ResourceLibrary/ResourceDetail.aspx?ItemNumber=10737.

HIPAA. 1996. Health Insurance Portability and Accountability Act of 1996. Public Law 104-191. http://edocket.access.gpo.gov/cfr_2007/octqtr/pdf/45cfr162.103.pdf.

Hord, G.E., and S.M. Hall. 2015. *Implementing Change: Patterns, Principles, and Potholes.* Boston, MA: Allyn and Bacon.

ISO. 2012. About ISO. http://www.iso.org/iso/home/about.htm.

Jones, S.S., R. Koppel, M.S. Ridgley, T.E. Palen, S. Wu, and M.I. Harrison. 2011. *Guide to Reducing Unintended Consequences of Electronic Health Records.* Prepared by RAND Corporation under Contract No. HHSA2902006000171, Task Order #5. Rockville, MD: Agency for Healthcare Research and Quality. https://www.healthit.gov /unintended-consequences/.

Louisiana Health Care Quality Forum. 2009. *Electronic Health Record Resource Toolkit Volume 1: The Adoption Process.* http://lhcqf.org/lapost-old/images/stories/White%20 Papers/EHR%20Resource%20Toolkit%20Vol.%201-Adoption%20Process.pdf.

Lynch, K., M. Kendall, K. Shanks, A. Haque, E. Jones, M.G. Wanis, M. Furukawa, and F. Mostashari. 2014. The Health IT regional extension center program: Evolution and lessons for health care transformation. *Health Services Research* 49(1pt2):421–437. doi:10.1111/1475-6773.12140.

McDonnell, C., K. Werner, and L. Wendel. 2010. *Electronic Health Record Usability.* Rockville, MD: Agency for Healthcare Research and Quality.

Mitchell, R.N. 2011. Hybrid medical records are here to stay. *For the Record (Great Valley Publishing Company, Inc.)* 23(2):20–23.

National Learning Consortium. 2015. *Regional Extension Centers: Advising Providers in All Phases of Electronic Health Record Implementation.* https://www.healthit.gov/providers -professionals/regional-extension-centers-recs.

Office of the National Coordinator, DHHS. 2016. Certified Health IT Product List. https://www.healthit.gov/policy-researchers-implementers/certified-health-it -product-list-chpl.

Office of the National Coordinator, DHHS. 2015. What Is ONC-Authorized Testing and Certification Body (ONC-ATCB)? https://www.healthit.gov/providers -professionals/faqs/what-onc-authorized-testing-and-certification-body-onc-atcb.

Office of the National Coordinator, DHHS. 2011. Federal Health IT Strategic Plan (2011–2015)—Overview. https://www.healthit.gov/sites/default/files/utility/final -federal-health-it-strategic-plan-0911.pdf.

Payne, T. H., S. Corley, T. A. Cullen, T. K. Gandhi, L. Harrington, Gilad J. Kuperman, J. E. Mattison, D. P. McCallie, C. J. McDonald, P. C. Tang, W. M. Tierney, C. Weaver, C. R. Weir, and M. H. Zaroukian. 2015, Report of the AMIA EHR 2020 task force on the status and future direction of EHRs. *Journal of American Medical Informatics Association.*doi: http://dx.doi.org/10.1093/jamia/ocv066.

Scungio, D. J. 2014. Disaster and the laboratory: Preparation, response and recovery. *Medical Laboratory Observer* 46(6):34–36.

Sherek, P.D., and E. Gray. 2014. Case study: Managing pediatric health information in a patient portal. *Journal of AHIMA* 85(4):46–47. http://bok.ahima.org /doc?oid=300411.

Sherer, S.A., Chad D. Meyerhoefer, and Lizhong Peng. 2016. Applying institutional theory to the adoption of electronic health records in the U.S. *Information and Management* 53(5):570–580. doi: doi:10.1016/j.im.2016.01.002.

Sittig, D. F., and H. Singh. 2013. A red-flag-based approach to risk management of EHR-related safety concerns. *Journal Of Healthcare Risk Management: The Journal Of The American Society For Healthcare Risk Management* 33 (2):21-26. doi: 10.1002/jhrm.21123.

Stevens, G. W. 2013. Toward a process-based approach of conceptualizing change readiness. *The Journal of Applied Behavioral Science.* http://jab.sagepub.com/content/early/2013/02/07/0021886313475479.abstract.

Svanaes, D., A. Das, and O.A. Alsos. 2008. The contextual nature of usability and its relevance to medical informatics. *Studies in Health Technology and Informatics* 136:541–546.

Torppa, C.B. and K.L. Smith. 2011. Organizational change management: A test of the effectiveness of a communication plan. *Communication Research Reports* 28(1):62–73. doi:10.1080/08824096.2011.541364.

US Congress. 2009. Health Information Technology for Economic and Clinical Health (HITECH) Act. United States Code. http://www.hhs.gov/hipaa/for-professionals/special-topics/HITECH-act-enforcement-interim-final-rule/index.html.

US Food and Drug Administration (FDA). 2012. Food and Drug Administration Safety and Innovation Act. US Code. http://www.fda.gov/RegulatoryInformation/Legislation/SignificantAmendmentstotheFDCAct/FDASIA/ucm20027187.htm.

Wager, K.A., F.W. Lee, and J.P. Glaser. 2009. *Health Care Information Systems: A Practical Approach for Health Care Management.* 2nd ed. San Francisco, CA: Jossey-Bass.

Wylie, M.C., R.R. Baier, and R.L. Gardner. 2014. Perceptions of electronic health record implementation: A statewide survey of physicians in Rhode Island. *American Journal of Medicine* 127(10):1010.e21-7. doi: 10.1016/j.amjmed.2014.06.011.

Yoon-Flannery, K., S. O. Zandieh, G. J. Kuperman, D. J. Langsam, D. Hyman, and R. Kaushal. 2008. A qualitative analysis of an electronic health record (EHR) implementation in an academic ambulatory setting. *Informatics in Primary Care* 16 (4):277-284.

Zhang, J., and M.F. Walji. 2011. TURF: Toward a unified framework of EHR usability. *Journal of Biomedical Informatics* 44(6):1056–1067. doi: 10.1016/j.jbi.2011.08.005.

ADDITIONAL RESOURCES

Bass, Alison. 2003. Health-Care IT: A big rollout bust. *CIO.* http://www.cio.com/article/2442013/infrastructure/health-care-it--a-big-rollout-bust.html.

Behravesh, B. "Understanding the end user perspective: A multiple-case study of successful health information technology implementation" (dissertation, Pepperdine University 2010). http://cdm15730.contentdm.oclc.org/cdm/ref/collection/p15093coll2/id/59.

Dimick, C. 2008. Record limbo: Hybrid systems add burden and risk to data reporting. *Journal of AHIMA* 79(11):28–32.

Han, Y.Y, J.A. Carcillo, S.T. Venkataraman, R.S.B. Clark, R.S. Watson, T.C. Nguyen, H. Bayir, and R.A. Orr. 2005. Unexpected increased mortality after implementation of a commercially sold computerized physician order entry system. *Pediatrics* 116(6):1506–1512. doi:10.1542/peds.2005-1287.

NCCD. 2013. The University of Texas Health Science Center School of Biomedical Informatics. https://sbmi.uth.edu/.

US Food and Drug Administration. 2016. Examples of MMAs the FDA regulates. http://www.fda.gov/MedicalDevices/DigitalHealth/MobileMedicalApplications/ucm368743.htm.

Healthcare Informatics and Decision Support

By Joanne D. Valerius, PHD, RHIA, MPH, Sue Biedermann, MSHP, RHIA, FAHIMA, and Diane Dolezel, EdD, RHIA, CHDA

Learning Objectives

- Interpret the use of decision support systems (DSSs) in healthcare settings
- Compare and contrast the potential and limitations of DSSs in research
- Use data visualization processes to facilitate decision making
- Analyze the trends that demonstrate quality, safety, and effectiveness of patient care using statistical analysis of healthcare data
- Evaluate administrative reports using department software tools

KEY TERMS

Clinical analytics
Clinical decision support system (CDSS)
Computer-assisted coding (CAC)
Computerized provider order entry (CPOE)
C-suite
Data analytics

Decision support system (DSS)
Electronic patient portals
HL7 FHIR®
Knowledge management (KM)
Natural language processing (NLP)
Unintended consequences

Decisions are a part of daily living. Through repetition, rules, and regulations for safety and well-being, along with ongoing input from our environment, humans automatically respond to situations and make instant decisions. For example, a fuel warning alert tells us to refuel. Ignoring warnings can result in being harmed. A red oil light might mean severe engine damage could occur if it is not addressed immediately. Traffic lights flash warnings of when to walk, when to stop walking, or when to go (green), slow down (yellow), and stop (red), which prevent pedestrians from being harmed. Additionally, laws and regulations must be followed to avoid penalties. In a complex, changing environment decisions must be adapted to environmental changes, and those environmental adaptations may affect future decisions.

Healthcare is a complex system that is constantly adapting to external and internal forces. Making decisions in healthcare may be instantaneous, such as the decision to perform cardiopulmonary resuscitation (CPR), which relies on automatic responses and trusted clinical protocols. Or, the decisions may involve long-term healthcare solutions with multiple factors that need human interaction as well as electronic interpretation of data.

This chapter will examine the many ways that administrative and clinical electronic **decision support systems (DSSs)** impact the healthcare environment and the organization. A DSS is

> a computer-based system that gathers data from a variety of sources and assists in providing structure to the data by using various analytical models and visual tools in order to facilitate and improve the ultimate outcome in decision-making tasks associated with nonroutine and nonrepetitive problems (AHIMA 2014, 45).

An administrative DSS supports organizational decisions using data sources that could include reimbursement, utilization of services, and aggregate patient sociological data. Similarly, **clinical decision support systems (CDSSs)** can include alerts in the electronic health record such as an allergy to medications and reminders for preventive healthcare services, as well as links for providers to find references or order sets. A CDSS is an interactive program that assists clinicians in making patient care decisions (Sandefer 2016, 373).

Knowledge management (KM) is a dynamic way to transform discrete electronic health data into easily distributed information to provide context for decision making (O'Dell 2016, 641). In the ever-changing healthcare system, the focus is on the ability of organizations to enhance quality of patient care. Use of KM systems to support decisions at many levels in the healthcare organization is essential. Understanding how to extract, or "mine," the patient data from databases, data stores, and discrete electronic health documentation is key to providing feedback to improve patient care. Additionally, data can be derived from evidence-based knowledge or data extracted from data.

The role of electronic resources in guiding the human decision-making process is evolving with the development of new applications that enable improvements in patient safety and in the provisioning of quality healthcare. As an example, the increased use of CDSSs has improved the quality of patient care.

The definition of CDSS is a system to measure the success of information in providing the

1. Right information
2. To the right person
3. In the right format
4. Through the right channel
5. At the right time (Osheroff et al. 2009).

The challenge to an organization is to analyze any computerized system to determine how these components can be provided. Each organization must be able to define the architectural components of their system and to determine the interoperability of their software programs in order to provide the "rights" for their CDSS. At the same time, interoperability requires a consensus on the standards that organizations will use to exchange electronic data with other CDSSs. The OpenCDS consortium is working with multiple facilities to develop standard CDSS tools and resources that support HL7 FHIR (OpenCDS 2016). Participating organizations includes Alabama Department of Public Health, HP Advanced Federal Healthcare Innovation Lab, University of Utah, and the Veterans Health Administration, to name a few (OpenCDS 2016). **HL7 FHIR** (Fast Healthcare Interoperability Resources) "is a next generation standard Framework created by HL7" that combines parts of previous versions of HL7 and CDA (clinical documentation architecture) product lines and uses current web standards with a particular focus on the implementation (HL7 2015). Clinical and administrative problems are solved with FHIR components in many contexts such as phone apps, the cloud, and EHR-based data sharing.

⊙ Knowledge Management

This section presents **KM** systems, which are systems used to capture and disseminate electronic information for use in decisions at multiple levels of an organization. Knowledge management subsystem functions include the evaluation of organizational needs (at high levels or discrete department, clinical levels), the processing of appropriate information gathered based on the needs of an individual or the organization, the mining of the data, and the dissemination of the data as processed information. For instance, individual patients can mine their information through patient portals that allow patients to graph their lab results over time. When visiting a primary care provider, that information can be discussed for better understanding of a persistent problem (such as repeated, unexplained urinary tract infections). A researcher may mine systems of data collected from questionnaires such as CMS Quality Assurance and Practice Improvement surveys of patients with end stage renal disease (ESRD) (CMS 2016). Financial administrators may wish to use this same data to analyze claims for those with ESRD.

Figure 9.1.   A conceptual knowledge management framework in healthcare

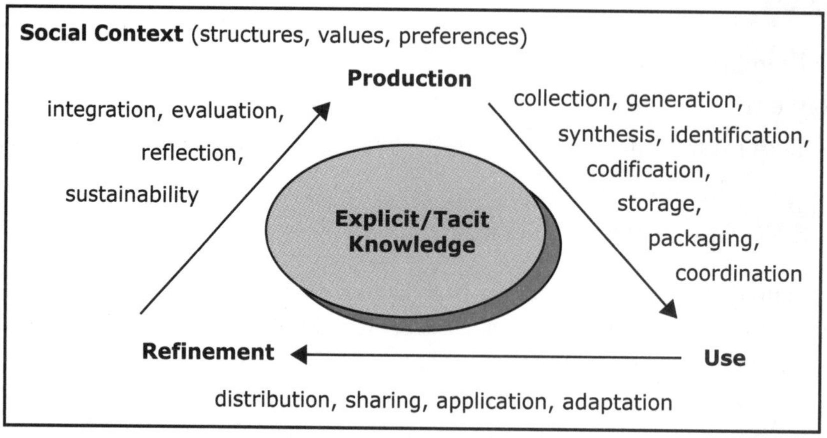

Source: Lau 2004, 3.

A model of KM was utilized to determined that

a. "a knowledge artifact, that is, codified knowledge is in a format that is insufficient for fully effective knowledge use by practices (e.g., digital medical records);

b. a number of interdependent processes are necessary to manage knowledge;

c. there are social and technical dimensions to these processes as a result of knowledge being tacit (e.g., that knowledge conveyed in apprenticeships relationships) and being explicit (e.g. objects such as procedure manuals);

d. action emanates from the tacit dimension of knowledge and KM processes engaged in pursuit of organization's mission" (Orzano et al. 2008).

Figure 9.1 is one conceptual model of KM illustrating the complexity inherent in KM. This includes the interdependencies of human relationships, which are essential to the success of any program. This model relies on the human resources to collaborate and build systems that meet the expectations of organizational performance. Applied to any healthcare environment, it demonstrates an effective means to improve the quality of healthcare by accessing every employee and system in the organization. It reflects the importance of relationships, trust, and practice (social context) while having expectations for accessible technology and systems to generate needed information for decision making.

Check Your Understanding 9.1

Indicate whether each of the following is true or false.

1. An electronic decision support system (DSS) can support a healthcare organization with both administrative and clinical decisions.

2. A CDSS is a subset of a DSS.

3. A CDSS's primary use is for financial decision makers in an organization.

4. Analyzing electronic databases and discrete information is also coined as data mining.

5. Computer software programs naturally talk to one another, therefore, organizations can assume data systems are integrated.

6. When using data mining, considerations regarding clinical as well as financial decisions can be applied.

⊙ Administrative Uses of Decision Support Systems

Not all decisions in healthcare immediately affect the patient's safety or the quality of care delivered, but they do affect the patient's encounter with the healthcare system. For example, the process of coding a diagnosis for reimbursement affects the patient. In the most advanced systems, a code could be generated from **natural language processing (NLP)** technology systems, which are sophisticated electronic systems reading the structured word-processed document. NLP is "a technology that converts human language (structured or unstructured) into data that can be translated then manipulated by computer systems" (AHIMA 2014, 101). This process, also known as **computer-assisted coding (CAC)**, has dramatically changed the medical coding processes. CAC is "the process of extracting and translating dictated and then transcribed free-text data (or dictated and then computer-generated discrete data) into ICD and CPT with menu driven prompts evaluation and management codes for billing and coding purposes" (AHIMA 2014, 33). However, the critical analysis of a coding specialist is needed to review the medical record to validate a final decision for medical claims. Reminders and alerts about correct coding procedures also provide clues for decision making for the coder. Reminders to choose more specific codes, alerts that certain codes cannot be utilized for the principal diagnosis, and other reminders have increased the reliability and accuracy of coded data.

Decision support tools like NLP, reminders, and alerts are a part of the many administrative DSSs that affect the workflow of information processing. These alerts inform the patient that their claim is processed and advise the healthcare organization that the claim will be paid. Informatics professionals rely on DSSs that can assist in daily operations. Through electronic portals, providers can be sent reminders that can help the organization with value-based healthcare decisions. The reminders are built from the laws, rules, regulations, internal policy and procedures, and accreditation standards that healthcare organizations must follow. These tools for completing quantitative and qualitative analysis on an electronic record assist the health information specialist in completing these processes.

The **C-suite** includes executive management, such as chief operating officer or chief information officer, as well as department managers and public health agencies. C-suite members rely on data collected and analyzed to make decisions about managing current programs, developing new programs, providing public information for the improvement of safety for patients, and increasing the quality of overall healthcare. DSSs provide financial as well as clinical information for administrative decision making. Reliance on DSS and other systems, like data warehouses and national repositories, have the potential to inform administrators of opportunities to improve efficiency and effectiveness in healthcare, which impacts the quality of healthcare for patients. Electronically generated reports and dashboards provide textual information as well as visual displays of specific data from the data warehouses. The more electronically readable, or structured, the data are, the greater the usability for decisions. Administrators will rely on the employees who can mine and statistically interpret the metadata, databases, and repositories that are rich informatics tools. This use of statistical analysis of data to make business decisions is called **data analytics** (White 2016, 510). Similarly,

Figure 9.2. Preventive care from Veterans Health Administration HealtheVet Blue Button example

VA Wellness Reminders			
Source:	VA		
Last Updated:	06 March 2016 @ 1134		
Wellness Reminder	**Due Date**	**Last Completed**	**Location**
Body Mass >25 Alert	DUE NOW	UNKNOWN	DAYT29
Colon Cancer Screening	13 Aug 2016	13 Aug 2012	DAYT29
Influenza Vaccination	13 Aug 2016	13 Aug 2011	DAYT29
Pneumonia Vaccination	DUE NOW	UNKNOWN	DAYT29
Control of Your Cholesterol	13 Aug 2016	13 Aug 2011	DAYT29
Eye Exam for Diabetes	13 Aug 2016	13 Aug 2011	DAYT29
Foot Exam for Diabetes	13 Aug 2016	13 Aug 2011	DAYT29
HbA1c for Diabetes	13 Aug 2016	13 Aug 2012	DAYT29
Elevated Blood Pressure Alert	DUE NOW	13 Aug 2009	DAYT29
Lipid Measurement (Cholesterol)	DUE NOW	13 Aug 2009	DAYT29
Comments	Learn more about these Wellness Reminders by visiting My HealtheVet. Please contact your healthcare team with any questions about your VA Wellness Reminders.		

Source: Adapted from Blue Button, Veterans Health Administration, 2016. http://www.va.gov/BLUEBUTTON/docs/VA_My_HealtheVet_Blue_Button_Sample_Version_12_10.pdf

clinical analytics is mining discrete patient healthcare data such as laboratory results, medication, genetics, or population health data to make clinical decisions or to aid in translating data for research or further healthcare treatment.

Information available to the public provides consumers with the material necessary to make intelligent decisions about where to seek healthcare organizations or individual clinicians who will meet their standards for care or will be covered by their healthcare insurers. Websites such as HealthGrades (http://www.healthgrades.com/), the Leapfrog Group (http://www.leapfroggroup.org/), and Hospital Compare (http://www.hospitalcompare.hhs.gov/) provide consumers with comparable information on hospitals and physicians. Social media websites, such as Facebook and Twitter, provide more direct person-to-person evaluations of healthcare experiences.

Electronic patient portals provide access to personal health information and may be available through the patient's healthcare organization. These portals provide patients with opportunities to view results of exams and treatment, and they provide alerts for preventive care. Figure 9.2 shows an example of these types of reminders from the Veterans Health Administration Blue Button portal. Patients will need training on how to access their portals in order to facilitate patient engagement, and to make patients aware of their responsibility in their own care. Determining if a patient has access to a computer, a mobile application, or other technology will be important to patient outcomes because these tools can provide alerts for the patients. Electronic communication systems must provide protections for patients' rights to privacy that are compliant with all federal Health Insurance Portability and Accountability Act (HIPAA), state rules and laws. Moreover, the importance of looking at organization-wide information systems as a way to provide meaningful information and enhance patient safety is imperative.

Case Study : Patient Engagement

Patient engagement has been shown to increase compliance with medication schedules and to reduce the number of missed office visits, which improves clinical outcomes. Patient portals, mobile applications, and other electronic and web-based tools are being studied for associations with increased patient engagement. This case study describes how a patient portal system facilitated patient engagement and medical compliance, while providing an easy, free way for the patient to refill medication, and obtain and update copies of their medical records.

Two retired US army veterans use VA Blue Button as a way to maintain up-to-date copies of their medical records and to communicate with their physician's office. They also use the system for online prescription refills and

(Continued)

secure messaging to providers. The veterans especially like the ability to view, download, and print their medical information so that they can have this documentation ready in case of a medical emergency. Another benefit of the system is that they are less likely to forget to refill their medications or go to appointments due to the system's reminders and the user-friendly interface. In their opinion, the best feature is the cost, which is free to veterans.

This case study illustrates a success story for a patient portal that serves a large audience of veterans that includes many retired and physically challenged individuals. It provides online access to up-to-date copies of the patients' records, which is essential in case of an emergency. Organizations wishing to create their own portal should use the VA Blue Button system as a model. System developers should study the usability and security features.

(Source: Adapted from Peterson 2014)

Check Your Understanding 9.2

Indicate whether the following statements are true or false.

1. Most electronic patient portals are currently designed to allow patients to review their entire medical record.

2. Systems that extract discrete and unstructured data from the EHR to assist in the coding process are known as natural literacy programs.

3. The use of CAC has eliminated the coding specialist positions.

4. Social media sites and more structured sites can provide persons with information about healthcare satisfaction.

5. The skill to mine data is needed in administrative and clinical analytics.

⊙ Clinical Decision Support Systems (CDSSs) to Improve Safety and Quality of Patient Healthcare

Electronic health record vendors and healthcare IT teams continue to build reminders and alerts that are intended to support the goals of patient safety and quality of healthcare. The health record is the primary communication tool for a healthcare team. Using CDSS tools to improve documentation in the health record is intended to improve patient safety and overall quality of healthcare. Alerting a clinician of a potential medication interaction or a nurse of a missed medication administration will contribute to the care of the patient. In addition, a CDSS can aid a healthcare provider in making decisions about treatment that can be used for an individual.

Regarding the quality of CDSSs, the ONCs Standards and Interoperability Framework, called Health eDecisions initiative, in collaboration with CMS is continuing their work of integrating CDSS standards with electronic quality measurement standards (ONC 2014). They have developed a use case for CDSS business rules and a use case for CDSS support guidance. These use cases are now part of the rule Voluntary 2015 Edition Electronic Health Record (EHR) Certification Criteria; Interoperability Updates and Regulatory Improvements (45 CFR 170 (a)(10)). Health eDecisions are developing a Clinical Quality Framework (ONC 2014). Up-to-date information on clinical protocols and disease management can be incorporated into EHRs, often reflected by alert systems. CDSSs are viewed as applications that have a direct impact upon patient care and patient safety.

Disparity in Access to Information for CDSSs

One goal of a CDSS is to eliminate provider bias for care. For instance, if a provider believes that a patient will not comply with medical management based on age, race, sexual preference, or other characteristics, information about options for treatment or medications may be withheld from them. A system-wide EHR could be used to objectively determine a patient's need for services. Alerts sent to patients and to providers simultaneously based on clinical protocols and using electronic data extraction could reduce bias. In developing these systems, however, patient literacy needs to be considered because low literacy levels may mean that the patient is not understanding their treatment plan as presented by the physician or the nurse.

Providing patients with information related to their healthcare diagnoses contributes to improved care (Lopez et al. 2011). Regulatory agencies are now recommending the use of HIT systems and chronic disease management to aid in addressing disparities. For example, as the LGBT communities have become more open, it is critical for the needs of patients from these communities to be understood by the healthcare systems serving them. The IOM is part of the leadership working to decrease this disparity affecting the LGBT communities (IOM 2011). One movement is to increase the number of choices for gender self-identification in demographic data. The University of California in Riverside now has gender choices of Male, Female, Trans Male/Trans Man, Trans Female/Trans Woman, Gender Queer/Gender Nonconforming, or Different Identity (CBS News 2015).

Finding the best way to communicate with a patient will be essential to the selection of CDSSs that meet everyone's needs for information. Not all patients will have computers, apps on their mobile devices, or other technology to respond to alerts. Healthcare organizations that seek ways to engage patients in their healthcare should develop strategies that reduce discrimination or disparities based on lack of electronic technology availability (Gold et al. 2015; Tieu et al. 2015). The body of research that examines ways to engage patients continues to grow. The Office of the National Coordinator for Health Information Technology provides ongoing easily accessible guidance to patients and healthcare organizations (ONC 2015b).

The Joint Commission (JC) encourages focused efforts in areas where significant health disparities occur (Haider and Pronovost 2011). Disparities in healthcare continue to plague healthcare delivery systems and negatively impact patient safety and quality of care. Although equity in healthcare delivery has been emphasized in national reports and guidelines from the Institute of Medicine, AHRQ, US Department of Health and Human Service Office of Minority Health, the Pew Institute, and the National Library of Medicine, it is evident that this ongoing divide needs to be lessened (NLM 2016; Rapporteur 2013; Plain Language Action and Information Network 2011; HHS 2015).

Many HIT factors can influence ongoing patient care. However, typical root causes emphasize the communication issues that interfere with patients accessing and complying with healthcare providers. In an area where consumers are encouraged to access their EHR, it is imperative that the tools for doing this will be available. If an alert system is in place, it is only as good as the access to the system. As decision support tool access for one community is improved, the potential for increased patient safety and quality of healthcare for others improves as well.

The CDSSs need strong leadership and executive management directives to develop strong, inclusive, patient-focused systems that also influence the efficiency and effectiveness of resources. Key to the advancement of a stellar CDSS is also the inclusion of clinician champions to lead the process. But clinicians are not the only practitioners who need to be included. Any department utilizing an electronic clinical system, such as pharmacy, radiology, nursing, and so on, needs to be a part of a dynamic team to lead the organization to a successful system. End users of the system that need to be involved include HIM administrators, quality assurance administrators (and individuals within the department who manage quality assurance), and patients.

Research about Decision Support Systems

Research on the use of DSS should be examined in order to understand how their implementation and uses can support or be a barrier to the effective use of DSS. Informaticists who are involved in DSS will want to explore the plethora of articles that explore this area. Below are a few examples of the use of decision support tools (DSS or CDSS).

Long-Term Care

CDSS systems can be used in acute or non–acute-care settings. One ongoing area of clinical concern in nursing homes is the issue of pressure ulcers. Pressure ulcers are often painful and hard to heal once developed, and they can be a costly problem. A CDSS tool, On-Time QI for Pressure Ulcer Prevention (On-Time PrU) sought to design a program "to leverage the knowledge of certified nursing assistant (CNA) staff and promote proactive care coordination and planning using IT" (Hudak and Sharkey 2011). The research shows that it took 12 to 18 months to implement this program at a nursing home (Hudak and Sharkey 2011). At-risk residents were reported on a Trigger Summary, which identified known risk criteria such as nutrition, incontinence, and others. The On-Time PrU focused on quality improvement processes. An important part of this CDSS tool was the integration of IT into the normal workflow of those caring for the patient (Hudak and Sharkey 2011). Further development of CDSS tools like the On-Time PrU benefit patient quality and safety and satisfaction of care, and reduce the cost of healthcare in this environment.

Genomics and Personalized Medicine

The need for CDSS in genomics and personalized medicine is burgeoning. As more is known about the human genome and treatment of diseases, the impact of CDSS will grow. The use of CDSS is complicated when protocols change for treatment, and the knowledge is not uniformly communicated. The need for national and international data repositories of knowledge content is inevitable. The use of standard language such as Health Level 7 (HL7), the Systemized Nomenclature for Medicine (SNOMED), Logical Observation Identifiers Names and Codes (LOINC), Unified Medical Language System (UMLS), and others continues to be of importance in this area. Additionally, how information is collected so that it can be retrieved uniformly is of concern. The Nationwide Health Information Network (NHIN), now called the eHealth Exchange, recognizes that CDSSs are important to the effective use of health information technology (ONC 2015a).

Current national and international informatics standards to support the national CDSSs may conflict. However, many organizations continue to work collaboratively to reduce the conflicts in order to further the exchange of healthcare information and to support a national infrastructure. The government agencies include the Office of the National Coordinator, the Agency for Healthcare Research and Quality (AHRQ), the Veterans Health Administration, and the US Department of Health and Human Services along with many other governmental and nongovernmental agencies seeking to improve the secure exchange of health information to improve patient safety and reduce the cost of healthcare. The need for standards continues to be a high priority for all stakeholder organizations.

It is useful to visualize the use of CDSS in various treatment areas. In one retrospective study, an enterprise-level CDSS was utilized to mine over 800 patient records for signs of sepsis (Amland and Hahn-Cover 2016). The goal was to reduce the time between diagnosis and treatment for sepsis because delayed treatment can cause fatalities. Results were positive, the CDSS correctly classified 92 percent of the sepsis cases (Amand and Hahn-Cover 2016). In personalized medicine, mining techniques are being refined to examine the association between patient traits and patient response to non-small-cell lung cancer, which can inform clinicians of the most promising treatment course (Kureshi et al. 2016). To increase HIV screening, a customized EPIC electronic record screen was used with a suite of CDSS tools to help Emergency Department physicians obtain consent for and process HIV tests for adults (McGuire and Moore 2016). In the second year of the HIV pilot program, 97 percent of the targeted patients were being tested. Personalized healthcare for type 2 diabetics over 60 years was effectively managed utilizing a CDSS that sent diet and exercise messages to cell phones and to a web site (Lim et al. 2016). After six months, these patients had good glycemic and lipid control (Lim et al. 2016). One agency that is driving CDSS use is the Agency for Healthcare Research and Quality (AHRQ 2016). They support the use of patient-centered outcomes and CDSSs by developing CDSS tools and funding research (AHRQ 2016).

Specific skill sets are important for working with researchers to translate personalized and genomic information into meaningful information. Figure 9.3 presents skills that are identified as important. Continuing to develop skills in research will impact the advancement of the HIM professional in projects that relate specifically to decision support.

Figure 9.3. Skills for HIM professionals in the post-genomic era

---

Current Skills to Apply

- Policy and procedure development for managing patient health information to ensure its accuracy, integrity, privacy, and security (including investigating and resolving problems that may arise in the development of phenotype and genotype databases that involve breaches of patient information)
- Knowledge of EHR database systems design and their maintenance
- Knowledge of forms design, computer input screens, and clinical documentation tools and guidelines
- Knowledge of implementing industry standards for data sharing and interoperability
- Developing standardized healthcare data sets
- Knowledge of coding and classification systems
- Experience with organizational compliance to laws, rules, and regulations for licensure and accrediting agencies
- Knowledge of maintaining a master patient index and master client index
- Developing policies and procedures for release of medical information

Skills to Develop

- Statistics for data analysis, including calculus-based probability and statistics; statistical programming languages (SAS, S-Plus, R)
- Information science
- Computer science
- Knowledge of genetics

Source: Mendoza 2010.

Computer-Assisted Coding (CAC) in All Healthcare Settings

A report from the American Health Information Management Association (AHIMA) discussed the implications of ongoing changes in CAC (including the changing role of the coding specialist to more of an editor, using critical thinking and decision-making skills; Bronnert et al. 2010–2011). NLP has created advances in extracting key information that can be used to identify possible codes. Code numbers are used as secondary data for the revenue management cycle but also for data mining for registries, research studies, and administrative planning purposes. Accurate coding not only influences the capture of reimbursable claims, but also impacts the entire use of informatics for those secondary purposes.

CAC DSSs need to be designed so that the designated record set to be utilized for coding diagnoses and procedures is clearly utilized. This calls for a system that can track when appropriate documentation is entered into the electronic system.

Additional tools such as this will assist in the coding process, lessening the need for physician queries. A CAC total package will include decision support tools of reminders and alerts that will contribute to meeting the government regulations related to the meaningful use of EHRs (Bronnert et al. 2010–2011). Overall, this report suggests that CAC can function to support the coding process in the following ways:

- ◉ Streamline the coding workflow
- ◉ Support clinical documentation improvement programs
- ◉ Facilitate data mining
- ◉ Create problem lists for physician review and validation
- ◉ Provide Recovery Audit Contractor (RAC) audit trails (Bronnert et al. 2010–2011)

An important focus of CAC is the reduction in compliance risk because of the KM tools that are embedded in the system. Built-in fraudulent billing alerts, for instance, assure managers that misrepresentation for financial purposes is reduced or eliminated. Encoding systems will provide a magnitude of resources and references that provide up-to-date coding changes and appropriate application of the current and future payment and reimbursement models.

Community Mental Health

In an attempt to increase patient involvement in their care, a community mental health clinic compared the use of an electronic DSS to set goals with patients during care planning to promote shared decision making and greater awareness. The researchers found that case managers who used the system were more satisfied than those who did not. Client satisfaction in the process, however, did not improve with the DSS (Woltmann et al. 2011). The result of this study illustrates that although a DSS can contribute to easing an operational function like goal setting in mental health settings, it does not necessarily have the same effect on patient satisfaction with their care. In this case, the management may need to determine if the DSS is appropriate for use or engage more patient input to improve the tool.

In another mental health study, EHR-based tools were used to screen for bipolar disorder for patients with depression (Gill et al. 2012, 289). A screening instrument from the World Health Organization (WHO) Composite International Diagnostic Interview (CIDI) was used as a clinical decision support tool embedded into the EHR to assist clinicians. When a patient with a diagnosis of depression was seen at an office visit, the screening tool automatically displayed for use. They found that "widespread use of the CDSS tool and a higher rate of diagnosis and medication prescription suggest that an EHR-based CDSS can be useful in improving the detection of bipolar disorder in patients with depression" (Gill et al. 2012, 289). Developing tools that are easily available to clinicians can improve the quality of care and patient safety.

Mobile technology may allow for greater patient engagement. As evidenced by one study, some success was noted with improved patient engagement with the use of mobile technology for remote monitoring of bilingual diabetic patients with depression from low-income areas.(Ramirez et al. 2016). CMS reimbursement changes for eligible providers to receive payment for services via telecommunication systems in lieu of an in-person encounter supports the use of this technology (Mera et al. 2014).

Unintended Consequences of Clinical Decision Support Systems

When change occurs, such as reengineering a workflow or introducing a new technology, one cannot anticipate all of the repercussions that might occur from it. Human–computer interaction for many clinicians, informaticists, end users, workflow managers, and others has been smooth after implementation of an EHR, while others have struggled with the change process. Additionally, research in this area is finding that there are unanticipated and undesirable issues or problems, often described as **unintended consequences** of implementation (Ash et al. 2007). Electronic systems, and the humans who interact with them, are not error free, and new systems may inadvertently introduce new documentation errors, communication issues, and a dependence on the system that is unrealistic. One area that may not be considered is the shift in power, control, and autonomy affecting the provider–patient relationship.

In a preliminary study of **computerized provider order entry (CPOE)**, unintended consequences affecting clinicians during early implementation of the EHR were reported (Ash et al. 2007). CPOE consists of electronic prescribing systems that allow physicians to write prescriptions and transmit them electronically. This qualitative research provided a better understanding of the impact of the change in workflow and frustrations that impeded successful CPOE implementations (Ash et al. 2007). The AHRQ, tasked with research to improve the quality of patient care, published a publicly available Unintended Consequences Guide (Jones et al. 2011). The Unintended Consequences Guide uses the framework in figure 9.4 to illustrate the variety of issues that must be considered related to unintended consequences, as well as the iterative nature of the process, which is never truly finished.

Figure 9.4.   ITSA framework

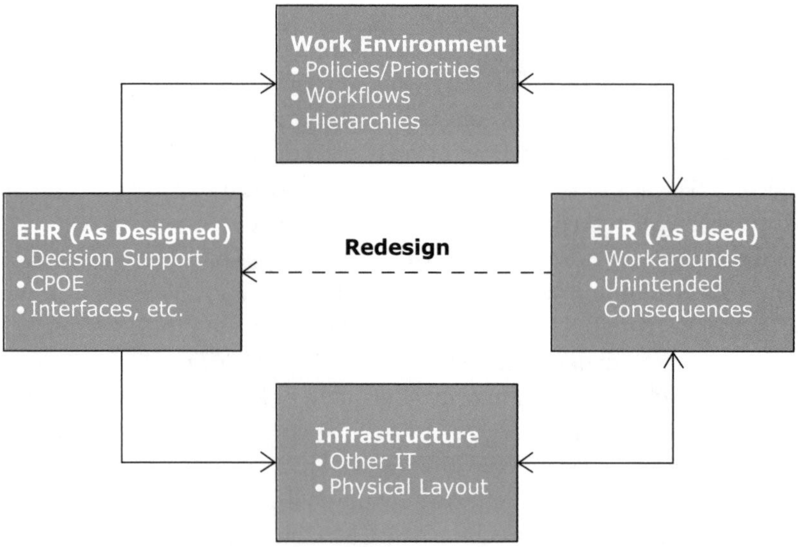

Source: Jones et al. 2011

As discussed previously, alert systems, patient bias, issues of patient engagement and connectivity to information, and basic human resistance to change will continue to perplex those analyzing data into usable information to make changes in the safety and quality of healthcare. The ever-changing dynamic nature of healthcare is consistent, and unintended consequences are to be expected.

Check Your Understanding 9.3

Indicate whether each of the following is true or false.

1. Disparity in healthcare cannot be improved with DSS.
2. ONC provides ongoing guidance and is easily accessible to patients and healthcare organizations.
3. Demographic data must include choices for transgender patients to ensure data granularity.
4. CMS will reimburse some connective technology expenses for patient care.
5. Health eDecisions is working on a clinical quality framework for CDSSs.

⊙ Quality

Unintended consequences of CPOE implementation have impacted quality of healthcare as found in some studies. Workflow and electronic system issues can seriously and negatively impact quality of care when implementing new electronic systems. The importance of analyzing workflow prior to, during, and after implementation cannot be emphasized enough. As project teams study the implementation of a system, it is essential to consider the precise timeliness of needed information. Reflecting on current practice (what works and what does not), human relationships (trust and effective communication), and the infrastructure of systems and human resources helps in completing a successful implementation that can impact patient safety and quality.

What continues to plague DSSs is the ability to have just-in-time information so decisions critical to patient care can be made in a timely manner. Determining who can turn alerts "off and on" and what happens when a clinician ignores an alert are other details that need to be determined. It is not only important to involve clinicians, information technology (IT), quality professionals, and others in the process of determining the policies and procedures for the facility. It is also imperative to involve legal counsel in this process. Some organizations have implemented CDSS committees in order to assist the setting up alerts, review their effectiveness, review issues, and ultimately ensure the most effective CDSS (Kuperman et al. 2005).

One of the areas that tends to be difficult to establish for some healthcare organizations is the definition of the legal health record and the implications of ignoring or working around alerts. If metadata is allowed in discovery, subpoenaed, and found admissible in a court of law, the decisions made to ignore alerts may find new legal ramifications. The court system will need to decide if and how the lack of alerts, content of DSS, and ignoring or working around alerts have affected the quality of care of a patient. As court decisions are made related to these issues, the power and autonomy concerns will be impacted. In a practice brief on defining the legal health record, AHIMA states,

> At a minimum the EHR should include documentation of the clinician's actions in response to decision support. This documentation is evidence of the clinician's decision to follow or disregard decision support. The organization should define the extent of exception documentation required (e.g., what no documentation means) (AHIMA 2011).

As health informatics and information management professionals, knowledge about the legal system, the legal health record, and the access to metadata is needed as DSSs and CDSSs are developed and utilized. Knowledge of laws, regulations, rules, and accreditation standards is essential to not only protect the safety of the patient, but also the healthcare organization.

⊙ The State of the Art

Although there has been great progress in the use of CDSS, several barriers to adoption remain. A government report on CDSS design noted barriers to achieving efficient CDSS usage that included issues with inconsistent terminology, missing codes for data, low adoption of built-in order sets, poor screen design, too many nonspecific alerts, and lagging system updates, which necessitated workarounds. They recommend establishing committees to validate data quality, appropriateness of order sets, rules for alerts, and screen layout (HHS 2011). Data in the CDSS must be complete and accurately coded or the alerts and reminders will not be triggered. A related report emphasized planning information workflow and the five CDSS Rights which are right information, people, format, channel, and workflow (Campbell 2013).

When designing and testing CDSS systems, informatics must address potential healthcare IT safety issues that can result from poorly designed and implemented systems (NQF 2016). For example, too many alerts will result in a clinician ignoring or disabling the alert systems (NQF 2016). CDSS content should be updated on a schedule and as needed when new information becomes available, such as drug–drug interactions. Quality measures must be developed and used to monitor the appropriateness of built-in orders. Built-in order sets usability must be examined and order sets should be updated or removed (NQF 2016). Guidance for safe CDSS use can be derived from the ONC's Safety Assurance Factors for EHR Resilience (SAFER) guidance, which advocates downtime policies, standard coding of data, clinician involvement, and regular reviews of system logic and rules (HHS 2014).

A remaining concern for informaticists, clinicians, IT professionals, and others is the intention of those using the DSS. For example, consider a hard stop alert intended to stop a clinician from ordering two medications that will interact; savvy clinicians may find ways to override the alert. This may be warranted by their intimate knowledge of the patient's current health situation. The art of medicine demands that the clinician have that independence to think critically about treatment. However, protecting the integrity of the legal health record by enforcing basic policies and procedures about tools such as alerts is essential. Clearly documenting who has the rights and responsibility to change alert tools further protects the facility. Conducting quality audits of alert overrides, for instance, can provide information that impacts patient safety.

In the future, the CDSSs may be affected by

- Social risks—well-trained informatics personnel need, multidisciplinary leadership require, CDSS policies and procedures evolving
- Technical risks—system interface interoperability, system upgrades and maintenance must be scheduled
- Coding changes—coded data in the system needs frequent updates, legacy data must also be preserved for reporting, allergies must be up to date across systems
- Patient identification—challenging with data from multiple systems needing to be reconciled in CDSS (ONC 2016)

DSSs, whether clinical or administrative, call for creative individuals to continue development and to manage the knowledge that is needed to keep current. This is time intensive and costly. Large academic hospitals, government facilities such as the Veterans Affairs Medical Centers, and large healthcare enterprises have traditionally taken the lead in development, research, and evaluation of systems. The benefits of the collective work provide smaller healthcare systems with hope for accessing DSSs that will also enhance their administrative and patient safety goals.

Chapter 9 Review Exercises

Indicate whether each of the following is true or false.

1. DSSs can serve both administrative and clinical decision making.
2. Disparity between healthcare and the data for making decisions may create conflict.
3. ONC strives to educate patients and healthcare organizations to understand ways to engage patients with their EHR information.
4. Unintended consequences of the EHR can be eliminated.
5. Providing the right information at the right time is a formula for improvement of decisions in patient care.
6. Social media, as well as established research sites, are ways patients evaluate healthcare.
7. Healthcare organizations need to consider the literacy of patients when trying to engage them in their healthcare.
8. NLP and CAC can assist medical coding specialists in workflow.

9. NLP and CAC will replace medical coding specialists.

10. CDSSs focus on the contractual decisions that are needed for administrative decisions.

Discussion.

11. Discuss the use of DSSs in healthcare settings.

12. Compare and contrast the potential and limitations of DSSs in research.

13. Identify data visualization processes to facilitate decision making.

14. A coding manager for a large hospital has been given an annual administrative report generated by a CDSS describing coding productivity for the year. How should the coding manager evaluate the report using department software and other tools?

REFERENCES

45 CFR 170(a)(10). 2015. Voluntary 2015 Edition Electronic Health Record (EHR) Certification Criteria; Interoperability Updates and Regulatory Improvements. https://www.law.cornell.edu/cfr/text/45/part-170/subpart-C.

AHIMA. 2014. *Pocket Glossary for Health Information Management and Technology*. 4th ed. Chicago: AHIMA Press.

AHIMA. 2016. Clinical Documentation Improvement Toolkit. Chicago. AHIMA. http://bok.ahima.org/PdfView?oid=301829.

Agency for Health Research and Quality. 2016. *Health Information Technology—Best Practices Transforming Quality, Safety and Efficiency*. https://healthit.ahrq.gov/ahrq -funded-projects/clinical-decision-support-cds.

Amland, R.C., and K.E. Hahn-Cover. 2016. Clinical decision support for early recognition of sepsis. *American Journal of Medical Quality* 31(2):103–110. doi: 10.1177/1062860614557636.

Ash, J., D. Sittig, E. Poon, K. Guappone, E. Campbell, and R. Dyskstra. 2007. The extent and importance of unintended consequences related to computerized provider order entry. *Journal of the American Medical Informatics Association* 14(4):415–423. doi:10.1197/jamia.M2373.

Bronnert, J., B. Cassidy, S. Eichenwald-Maki, H. Eminger, J. Flanagan, M. Morsch, K. Peterson, K. Phibbs, P. Resnick, R. Schichilone, and G. Smith. 2011. CAC 2010-11. Industry outlook and resources report. AHIMA.

CBS News. 2015, July 30. *California colleges will now ask students to pick from 6 genders*. https://ucrtoday.ucr.edu/30352.

Centers for Medicare and Medicaid. 2016. End State Renal Disease (ESRF) Center. https:// www.cms.gov/Center/Special-Topic/End-Stage-Renal-Disease-ESRD-Center.html.

Department of Health and Human Services, Office of the National Coordinator. 2014. Safety Assurance Factors for EHR Resilience (SAFER). https://www.healthit

.gov/sites/safer/files/guides/safer_organizationalresponsibilities_sg002_form_0.pdf.

Department of Health and Human Services, Office of the National Coordinator. 2011, May. Decision support evaluation tools clinical decision support design. https://www.healthit.gov/sites/default/files/cds/3_5_5_decision_support_evaluation_tools.pdf.

Gill, J., Y.X. Chen, A. Grimes, and M. Klinkman. 2012. Using health record–based tools to screen for bipolar disorder in primary care patients with depression. *Journal of American Board of Family Medicine* 25:283–290. doi:10.3122/jabfm.2012.03.110217.

Gold, M., M. Hossian, and A. Manqum. 2015. Consumer engagement in Health IT: Distinguishing rhetoric from reality e*GEMS* 3(1):1190. doi: http://dx.doi.org/10.13063%2F2327-9214.1190.

Haider, A., and P. Pronovost. 2011. Health information technology and the collection of race, ethnicity, and language data to reduce disparities in quality of care. *The Joint Commission Journal on Quality and Patient Safety* 37(10):435–436.

HL7. 2015. FHIR implementation standards. http://www.hl7.org/implement/standards/fhir/summary.html.

Hudak, S., and S. Sharkey. 2011. *California Healthcare Foundation. Trendspotting: How IT Triggers Better Care in Nursing Homes*. http://www.chcf.org/.

Jones, S.S., R. Koppel, M.S. Ridgely, T.E. Palen, S. Wu, and M.I. Harrison. 2011. *Guide to Reducing Unintended Consequences of Electronic Health Records. Prepared by RAND Corporation under Contract No. HHSA290200600171, Task Order #5*. Rockville, MD: Agency for Healthcare Research and Quality. https://healthit.ahrq.gov/sites/default/files/docs/publication/guide-to-reducing-unintended-consequences-of-electronic-health-records.pdf.

Kuperman, G.J., R. Diamente, V. Khatu, T. Chan-Kraushar, P. Stetson, A. Boyer, and M. Cooper. 2005. *AMIA Annual Symp Proc.* 415–419. PMCID: PMC1560425.

Kureshi, N., S.S. Abidi, and C. Blouin. 2016. A predictive model for personalized therapeutic interventions in non-small-cell lung cancer. *IEEE Journal of Biomedical Health Inform* 20(1):424–431. doi: 10.1109/JBHI.2014.2377517.

Lau, F. 2004. Toward a conceptual knowledge management framework in health. *Perspectives in Health Information Management* 1:8.

Lim, S., S.M. Kang, K.M. Kim, J.H. Moon, S.H. Choi, H. Hwang, H.S. Jung, K.S. Park, J.O. Ryu, and H.C. Jang. 2016. Multifactorial intervention in diabetes care using real-time monitoring and tailored feedback in type 2 diabetes. *Acta Diabetol* 53(2):189–198. doi: 10.1007/s00592-015-0754-8.

Lopez, L., A. Green, A. Tan-McGrory, R. King, and J. Betancourt. 2011. Bridging the digital divide in healthcare: The role of health information technology in addressing racial and ethnic disparities. *The Joint Commission Journal on Quality and Patient Safety* 37(10):437–445.

McGuire, R., and E. Moore. 2016. Using a configurable EMR and decision support tools to promote process integration for routine HIV screening in the emergency department. *Journal of the American Medical Informatics Association* 23(2):396–401. doi: 10.1093/jamia/ocv031.

Mendoza, M.C.B. 2010. HIM and the path to personalized medicine: Opportunities in the post-genomic era. *Journal of AHIMA* 81(11):38–42.

Mera, M., C. Gonzalez, and D.M. Lopez. 2014. *Towards an Intelligent Decision Support System for Public Health Surveillance—A Qualitative Analysis of Information Needs.* Amsterdam: IOS Press.

National Library of Medicine. 2016. Health literacy and cultural competence. https://www.nlm.nih.gov/hsrinfo/health_literacy.html.

National Quality Forum. 2016, February. Identification and prioritization of HIT patient safety measures. http://www.qualityforum.org/Publications/2016/02/Identification_and_Prioritization_of_HIT_Patient_Safety_Measures.aspx.

O'Dell, R.M. 2016. Clinical Quality Management. Chapter 21 in *Health Information Management Concepts Principles, and Practices.* 5th ed. Edited by P. Oachs and A. Watters. Chicago, IL: AHIMA Press.

Office of the National Coordinator for Health Information Technology. 2015a. *What Is eHealth Exchange?* https://www.healthit.gov/providers-professionals/faqs/what-ehealth-exchange.

Office of the National Coordinator for Health Information Technology. 2015b. *Patient Education and Engagement.*

Office of the National Coordinator for Health Information Technology. 2014. *Two Significant S&I Framework Milestones: The Health eDecision Initiative Close-Out and Clinical Quality Framework Launch.* https://www.healthit.gov/buzz-blog/electronic-health-and-medical-records/interoperability-electronic-health-and-medical-records/standards-interoperability-framework-milestones-health-edecision-initiative-closeout-clinical-quality-framework-launch/.

OpenCDS. 2016. http://www.opencds.org/.

Orzano, J.A., C.R. McInerney, D. Scharf, A.F. Tallia, and B.F. Crabtree. 2008. A knowledge management model: Implications for enhancing quality in healthcare. *Journal of the American Society for Information Science and Technology* 59(3):489–505.

Osheroff, J.A, J.M. Teich, D. Levick, L. Saldana, F.T. Velasco, D.F. Sittig, K.M. Rogers, and R.A. Jenders. 2009. *Improving Outcomes with Clinical Decision Support: An Implementer's Guide.* Chicago: HIMSS.

Peterson, H. 2014. US Department of Veterans Affairs. The Blue Button is literally a life saver. http://www.va.gov/health/newsfeatures/2014/september/the-blue-button-is-literally-a-life-saver.asp.

Plain Language Action and Information Network. 2011. Federal Plain Language Guidelines.

Ramirez, M., S. Wu, H. Jin, K. Ell, S. Gross-Schulman, L. Myerchin Sklaroff, and J. Guterman. (2016). Automated remote monitoring of depression: Acceptance among low-income patients in diabetes disease management. *JMIR Mental Health* 3(1):e6.

Rapporteur, L.M. 2013. *Health literacy: Improving health, health systems, and health policy around the world—Workshop summary.* Washington, DC: National Academies Press.

Sandefer, R. 2016. Health Information Technologies. Chapter 12 in *Health Information Management Concepts Principles, and Practices.* 5th ed. Edited by P. Oachs and A. Watters. Chicago, IL: AHIMA Press.

Tieu, L., U. Sarkar, D. Schillinger, J.D. Ralston, N. Ratanawongsa, R. Pasick, and C. Lyles 2015. Barriers and facilitators to online portal use among patients and caregivers in a safety net health care system: A qualitative study. *Journal of Medical Internet Research* 3(17). doi: 10.2196/jmir.4847.

Veterans Health Administration. *Blue Button.* http://www.va.gov/bluebutton/.

White, S. 2016. Healthcare Data Analytics. Chapter 17 in *Health Information Management Concepts Principles, and Practices.* 5th ed. Edited by P. Oachs and A. Watters. Chicago, IL: AHIMA Press.

Woltmann, E., S. Wilkniss, A. Teachout, G. McHugo, R. Drake. 2011. Trial of an electronic decision support system to facilitate shared decision making in community mental health. *Psychiatric Services* 62(1). http://ps.psychiatryonline.org/doi/abs/10.1176/ps.62.1.pss6201_0054.

ADDITIONAL RESOURCES

Agency for Healthcare Research and Quality. 2016. *National Healthcare Disparities Reports.* Publication No. 10-0004. March. Washington, DC. http://www.ahrq.gov/research/findings/nhqrdr/index.html.

AHIMA. 2011. Fundamentals of the legal health record and designated record set. *Journal of AHIMA* 82(2). http://library.ahima.org/xpedio/groups/public/documents/ahima/bok1_048604.hcsp?dDocName=bok1_048604.

Ahmadian, L., M. van Engen-Verheul, F. Bakhshi-Raiez, N. Peek, R. Cornet, and N.F. de Keizer. 2011. The role of standardized data and terminological systems in computerized clinical decision support systems: Literature review and survey. *International Journal of Medical Informatics* 80(2):81–93. doi:10.1016/j.ijmedinf.2010.11.006.

Beeler, P.E., E.J. Orav, D.L. Seger, P.C. Dykes, and D.W. Bates. 2016. Provider variation in responses to warnings: Do the same providers run stop signs repeatedly? *Journal of the American Medical Informatics Association* 23(e1):e93-98. doi: 10.1093/jamia/ocv117.

Berner, E. 2009. *Clinical Decision Support Systems: State of the Art. Agency for Healthcare Research and Quality.* Rockville, MD. Publication number: 09-0069-EF.

Berner, E.S. 2002. Ethical and legal issues in the use of clinical decision support systems. *Journal of Health Information Management* 16:4.

Campbell, E., D. Sittig, K. Guappone, R. Dykstra, and J. Ash. 2007. Overdependence on technology: An unintended consequence of computerized provider order entry. *AMIA Annual Symposium Proceedings* 9: 94–98.

Campbell, R. J. 2013. The five rights of clinical decision support: CDS tools helpful for meeting meaningful use. *Journal of AHIMA* 84(10): 42–47.

Fossum, M., G. Alexander, M. Ehnfors, and A. Ehrenberg. 2011. Effects of a computerized decision support system on pressure ulcers and malnutrition in nursing homes for the elderly. *International Journal of Medical Informatics* 80:607–617. doi:10: 1016/ j.ijmedinf.2011.06.009.

Han, Y.Y., J.A. Carcillo, S.T. Venkataraman, R.S.B. Clark, S. Watson, T.C. Nguyen, H. Bayir, and R.A. Orr. 2005. Unexpected increased mortality after implementation of a commercially sold computerized physician order entry system. *Pediatrics* 116(6):1506–1512.

Kaplan, B. 2001. Evaluating informatics applications: Clinical decision support systems literature review. *International Journal of Medical Informatics* 64(1):15–37.

Kawamoto, K., D. Lobach, H. Willard, and G. Ginsburg. 2009. A national clinical decision support infrastructure to enable the widespread and consistent practice of genomic and personalized medicine. *BMC Medical Informatics and Decision Making* 9:17. doi: 10:1186/1472-6947-9-17.

Kesselheim, A.S., K. Cresswell, S. Phansalkar, D.W. Bates, and A. Sheikh. 2011. ANALYSIS and COMMENTARY: Clinical decision support systems could be modified to reduce "alert fatigue" while still minimizing the risk of litigation. *Health Affairs* 30:122310–122317.

Kohn, L.T., J.M. Corrigan, and M.S. Donaldson. 2001. *Crossing the Quality Chasm: A New Health System for the 21st Century.* Washington, DC: Committee on Quality of Health Care in America, Institute of Medicine.

Learned Hand, J. *The T.J. Hooper*, 60 F.2d 737, 740 (2d Cir. 1932).

US Government. 2012. Food and Drug Administration Safety and Innovation Act. US Code. http://www.gpo.gov/fdsys/pkg/BILLS-112s3187enr/pdf/BILLS -112s3187enr.pdf.

Chapter 10

Health Information Interoperability

Learning Objectives

- Describe the history of health information exchange (HIE) in the United States
- List and define the different types of HIE organizational structures
- Explain the advantages and disadvantages of the different types of HIE consent models
- Analyze the issues and challenges encountered when securing provider and consumer acceptance of HIE
- Describe the difference between population and public health
- Discuss the use of HIE in relationship to Accountable Care Organizations

KEY TERMS

Accountable Care Organization (ACO)
Aggregated HIE
Cooperative HIEs
Data liquidity
Data segmentation
Federated HIE
Health information exchange (HIE)
Interoperability

No-consent
Opt-in
Opt-in with restrictions
Opt-out
Opt-out with exceptions
Population health
Public health

The increased adoption of electronic health records (EHRs) and other health information technology has resulted in ever-increasing amounts of health data and information. Although this data and information is expected to be extremely useful and beneficial in the settings where created, the usefulness and benefits should increase if the data and information can be made available when and where they are needed.

The ubiquitous sharing of healthcare data and information was termed **data liquidity** by a group focusing on the need to think beyond EHRs (Penfield et al. 2009). They recommended two actions to improve the flow of healthcare information. First, the market needs to focus on **interoperability**, the ability of different systems to work together seamlessly. In health information, interoperability is expected to include transmitting the meaning of the data. The second action focused on the need for payment reform, so that participating providers are not penalized, but are rewarded for freely sharing health information (Penfield et al. 2009).

This chapter will explore the evolution of health information exchange (HIE) in the United States, its structural and organizational issues, efforts supporting national implementation, as well as provider and consumer perceptions. It will conclude with a discussion of the population health and public health benefits resulting from health information exchange.

The key to any "interoperability" or "health information exchange" is the existence of complete, publicly available standards. This chapter will not try to examine the many different technical standards that are evolving at a rapid pace. Readers are encouraged to refer to the latest ONC and CMS regulations and guidance, which can be accessed at the www.healthit.gov website.

⊙ Health Information Exchange

Health information exchange (HIE) is defined as "exchange of health information electronically between providers and others with the same level of interoperability, such as labs and pharmacies" (AHIMA 2014, 68). For the remainder of this chapter the acronym HIE will be used to refer to the organization while the words "health information exchange" will be used to refer to the action of exchanging the information.

Health information exchange is becoming commonplace in the United States since it was included in the provisions of the Health Information Technology for Economic and Clinical Health (HITECH) sections of the American Recovery and Reinvestment Act (ARRA) (US Government 2009). The legislation is being implemented via the Centers for Medicare and Medicaid Services EHR Incentive Program, which pays providers for their meaningful use (MU) of EHR technology. The plan for MU included the articulation of three stages so that providers could adopt EHRs and increase the functionality and interoperability over time. Stage 1 of MU requires providers to have the ability to perform health information exchange (HHS 2010). Initially, Stage 2 of MU increased the requirements for health information exchange in multiple ways. Eligible providers (EPs) needed to participate in generating and transmitting prescriptions electronically; provide patients with the online ability to view, download, and transmit their health information; submit electronic data to immunization registries; and use secure electronic messaging to communicate with patients on relevant health information (CMS 2012).

In 2015, Stage 2 and 3 requirements were streamlined to address providers' comments (CMS 2015b). In the revised requirement, providers can select the measures for reporting that are a better fit for their professional needs, and starting in 2015 the reporting period maps to the calendar year and the reporting period is extended to 90 days (CMS 2015b). Patient action was added to Stage 2 patient engagement measures, and providers can utilize EHRs for care improvement (CMS 2015b). From 2105 to 2017 other changes include a reduction in objectives to 10 objectives for professionals, reduced from 18, and 9 objectives for hospital, lowered from 20 (CMS 2015a). For stage 3 in 2017 and later, application program interfaces with increased data access and public health reporting are required, and there are 8 objectives for professionals and hospitals, with 60 percent of these measures referencing interoperability (CMS 2015a). Additionally, health information professionals will need to perform CMS measures reporting. These stage 3 requirements are optional for 2017, but providers should began using them in 2018.

The Office of the National Coordinator for Health Information Technology (ONC) was providing assistance for establishing HIEs with the State Health Information Exchange Cooperative Agreement Program. When it was available, the ONC funding mechanism supported "states' efforts to rapidly build capacity for exchanging health information across the health care system both within and across states" (ONC, DHHS 2012). However, as the grant funding dwindles, HIEs struggle to be sustainable. This section will discuss health information exchange; the history, challenges, and clinical and financial benefits; provider and consumer perceptions, and sustainability; as well as anticipated future efforts.

History of HIE

Health information exchange was conceived prior to the HITECH legislation. Networks titled community health management information systems (CHMISs) were first established in 1990 through grants from the Hartford Foundation (Vest and Gamm 2010). CHMISs focused on the development of a centralized repository of clinical, demographic, and eligibility data. They experienced significant obstacles as they preceded the advent of widespread, reasonably priced, standards-based high-speed Internet access. Expensive hardware, software, and network connections were required for CHMISs, the lack of data standardization was an obstacle, and both patients and providers expressed privacy concerns (Vest and Gamm 2010).

A few years later saw the emergence of community health information networks (CHINs). These commercial initiatives focused on financial savings, with little emphasis on the public health benefits that might accrue. CHINs encountered problems when competitors limited the data sharing functionality to prevent any perceived loss of competitive advantage, the ability of vendors to charge fees, and differences in the fees charged different participants raised questions regarding any financial benefits (Vest and Gamm 2010). The main lesson from CHINs was that the benefits could not be assigned to one small group (in this instance, providers); they must be spread and shared across the healthcare industry.

The late 1990s and 2000s saw the rise of the regional health information organization (RHIO) in the healthcare industry. RHIOs are the immediate precursor to the HIE. An RHIO is "a neutral, third-party organization that facilitates information exchange between providers within a geographical area" (Vest and Gamm 2010). The obstacles to RHIO success were less about the technology. These organizations continued to experience problems identifying a sustainable business model, assuring privacy and security of the data, and overcoming the issue of competitor distrust. These same problems exist for HIEs today.

However, the HITECH legislation and MU regulations now mandate HIE functionality and its use. Researchers have proposed the following considerations for the continued development of US HIEs. They include

- Adopting an improved business model—perhaps with the increased use of quality incentives

- Acknowledging the public health benefits of health information exchange— this might include improved registries for chronic conditions and much better biosurveillance

- Monitoring health information exchange activities so both providers and consumers trust that private health information is private and secure

- Setting state borders as the standard geographic unit for HIEs (now operationalized by ONC) (Vest and Gamm 2010)

The CMS Health Information Exchange Objective for EHR incentive for 2015 to 2017 requires that a summary of care record be sent by all eligible providers when a patient is transferred to another care setting or to another provider (CMS 2015c). The care record must use certified EHR technology (CEHRT) and must be transmitted for more than 10 percent of patient care transfers or referrals (CMS 2015c). Summary of care documents must include the current problem, medication, and allergy list. Additional fields are name, provider, procedure, lab, demographic, and care plan items (CMS 2015b).

Structure and Adoption

Health information exchanges can have different technical and organizational structures. Given their history, no one superior structure has emerged. It is reasonable to presume that HIE operations will become standardized in the future; however, the industry is still evolving related to HIEs.

Structure

There are two main technological approaches to HIEs. The first is an **aggregated HIE**. The aggregated HIE combines all of the data into a centralized repository with a master patient index (MPI) or record locator service. The different HIE participants query, or send a request to, the repository to obtain demographic, clinical, or other information (Hess 2011). The aggregated HIE might be preferred by persons or local governments trying to maximize the public health benefits of HIEs; however, they present greater risks to the privacy and security of data. All of the data, some of it very detailed and potentially sensitive, must flow to the centralized repository.

The second type of HIE model is a **federated HIE**. Federated HIEs are designed as provider-to-provider networks using the Internet for connectivity, with no central repository of data (Hess 2011). A central entity maintains the MPI or record locator service, which is used to determine where patients have been treated previously and where their health information might exist. Providers send requests for data information directly to other providers. This type of arrangement may require an additional step; however, given the distributed maintenance of the data it is viewed as having stronger privacy and security protection.

The technical structure of the HIE is separate from the organizational structure of the HIE. HIEs tend to be one of three types: public, cooperative, or private. Public HIEs are entirely supported by state government agencies or are semi-independent, with governmental financial backing (Hess 2011). There is some consideration of HIEs as a public good, such as the road system (Vest and Gamm 2010). The case for the long-term governmental support of HIEs is, unfortunately, not an easy one to make. The occurrence of natural disasters supports the public health benefit claims. Examples include Hurricane Sandy in New Jersey where many were relocated for an extended period of time. Sandy also significantly impacted New York City with hurricane damage to many structures including healthcare facilities, evacuations of patients and others, and loss of power and public transportation for an extended period of time affecting millions of people.

Cooperative HIEs arise when relationships are formed for the purpose of exchanging information between what are otherwise competing healthcare providers (Hess 2011). Sometimes these HIEs struggle with financial viability and sometimes they are quite successful. Often the difference rests on the community or geographic region's concerns. For example, hospitals in Austin, Texas, came together to form the Integrated Care Collaborative (ICC). The original goal was to address mutual concerns related to "drug shopping" and the excessive use of area emergency rooms (ERs) (ICare 2016). Because all of the hospitals with ERs could easily see potential financial advantages, they agreed to contribute money to establish the HIE. The ICC has received governmental funding under the HITECH initiatives and is expanding its operations to other providers.

The third HIE model is the private HIE. This type involves a single, integrated delivery system (IDS) that connects all of its different providers with an "internal" HIE. One example is the Veterans Health Administration (VHA). For years VHA had aggregated their patient data; however, as the World War II veterans aged and began retiring or spending large parts of each year in different regions of the country, the need to transmit or exchange the data became a high priority (Tsai and Rosenheck 2012). Over a decade or more VHA established the data and other standards that allowed them to be a pioneer in health information exchange. They are now undertaking efforts to include non-VHA data from non-VHA providers in their health information exchange efforts (Tsai and Rosenheck 2012).

One additional, very important, aspect of structure and management for an HIE is the consent option chosen. Each HIE must determine how patients and consumers will consent or not consent to have their data and information transmitted by or included in HIE operations. A white paper prepared for the Texas Health Services Authority describes five generally accepted models for defining patient consent to participate in an HIE (Gray 2011). Each will be described here with the main points for each option described in table 10.1.

The **no-consent** model does not require any agreement on the part of the patient to participate in an HIE. HIEs that have adopted this model operate in states that explicitly allow this model via legislation such as Indiana and Delaware (Gray 2011). The major benefit of this option is that providers can be more certain that any data and information they are receiving is complete. This ensures they are not trying to make clinical decisions using incomplete data. However, this consent option does not mean patients have no rights. The HIEs using this option usually allow consumers to deny access to their data and information even if it is technically included in the HIE. This is the easiest consent option to administer as patients and consumers must take action to deny access. Providers must include the fact that they participate in an HIE in their Health Insurance Portability and Accountability Act (HIPAA) Notice of Privacy Practices that patients receive at their first visit (Gray 2011).

The **opt-out** model allows for a predetermined set of data to be automatically included in an HIE, but a patient may still deny access to information in the exchange. This model allows the consumer to prevent their data and information from inclusion in the HIE. Inclusion or exclusion is all or nothing for this option, that is, either all of the patient's information is included or it is all excluded. Issues to address in this model include the following:

- ⊙ Who will collect the necessary information for patients to opt out?
- ⊙ How will the opt-out information be communicated to the HIE and to other providers?
- ⊙ What processes can be implemented to handle cases where a patient changes his mind? (Gray 2011).

The **opt-out with exceptions** model makes the patient's information available in the exchange, but "enables the patient to selectively exclude data from an HIE, limit information to specific providers, or limit exchange of information to exchange for specific purposes" (Gray 2011). Although this option is understandably attractive to patients, it is not yet clear how to implement this model from a technical standpoint, that is, it is very resource intensive. As well as raising questions about the completeness of the data, this option presents many of the challenges the opt-out model does (Gray 2011).

The **opt-in** model requires patients to specifically affirm their desire to have their data made available for exchange within an HIE. This option provides up front control for patients because their data cannot be included unless they have agreed. Disadvantages of the opt-in model are primarily the administrative complexity of implementing such an approach. Issues the HIE must address include the following:

- ⊙ Who will obtain the consent?
- ⊙ Will one consent suffice for participation in the system as a whole or must each provider obtain consent for his or her own patients?
- ⊙ What process will be used to communicate the patient's consent?
- ⊙ What happens if a patient wants to withdraw his consent? Can his data be removed from the HIE or will the withdrawal of consent only be effective for data developed after the withdrawal of consent was given? (Gray 2011).

Table 10.1.   Health information exchange consent options

OPTION	PROS	CONS
No-consent model: does not require any agreement on the part of the patient Unknown: Notice requirements to patients; interface with an HIE requiring consent	Easier to administer; addresses provider concerns about incomplete information	Lack of patient control
Opt-out: a predetermined set of data are automatically included, unless the patient "opts-out" or denies access to the information.	Automatic inclusion of data for more complete data for providers, yet patients can restrict use	Procedures for documenting opt-out so providers know about it are unclear
Opt-out with exceptions: patient can choose level of participation. • Selective exclusion of personal health information (PHI) • Limited to certain providers • Limited to exchange for certain purposes	Much more patient control	Very, very difficult to implement
Opt-in: patients choose to include their data in an HIE. It is an all-in or all-out choice.	Patient has complete, up-front control; provides an opportunity to educate patients; may provide better record matching	Obtaining and communicating consent; questions as to how consent be revoked or withdrawn
Opt-in with restrictions: patient agrees up front, but can determine which data is shared, which providers can access it, or the purposes for which it can be accessed.	Patient control up front and very detailed	Very, very difficult to manage

The **opt-in with restrictions** model allows patients to restrict how much data and what data is available. They may enable access for certain doctors or only for certain data elements or purposes (Gray 2011).

As of this writing there is no single mandated consent option for HIE implementation. It is imperative that HIEs choose wisely as the ease of provider implementation, as well as consumer confidence in the HIE, may be impacted by the option chosen.

Adoption

The adoption of HIEs is a part of the national initiatives to help healthcare adopt 21st century information technology. Specifically, the HITECH legislation provided funding for the State Health Information Exchange Cooperative Agreement Program (ONC, DHHS 2013). This section will explore levels of adoption of HIEs, how HIEs are used, as well as costs, benefits, and evaluation, concluding with the expected interaction between the states and the federal health information exchange.

Research reveals moderate levels of HIE adoption at 30 percent of all US hospitals (McCann 2014). Medicaid's shift to managed and accountable care payment systems are predicted to create a need for the type of coordinate care that is facilitated by HIEs. Lack of standards, lack of interoperability and poorly designed interfaces continue to be barriers (McCann 2014). Rural hospitals are lagging in adoption of HIEs due to cost constraints and staffing shortfalls (Kim et al. 2016). These and other surveys of operational HIEs reveal a continued concern regarding sustainability and financial viability, with questions about clinical benefits remaining.

Overall, HIEs at the federal and state levels are focusing on a public–private collaborative structure. Although the National Health Information Network (NHIN) was established and supported by the Office of the National Coordinator, management of national health information exchange efforts was transferred to Healtheway, Inc. on October 10, 2012. Healtheway, Inc. states it is "is a community of public and private exchange partners who share information based upon a shared set of 'rules of the road' and a trust agreement, called the Data Use and Reciprocal Support Agreement (DURSA)" (Healtheway, Inc. 2012). State HIEs will become members of Healtheway, Inc., which will establish and support a portfolio of nationwide health information network standards, services, and policies (Healtheway, Inc. 2012).

The Health Level Seven organization has developed Fast Healthcare Interoperability Resources (FHIR), which use a set of resources that can be combined into systems for mobile phones, cloud-based systems and EHRs (HL7 2015). FHIR is based on a framework that allows the users to integrate existing resources. It is purported to be easy to implement and use (FHIR 2015). As of 2016, FHIR has not replaced HL7 or X12 standards. As technical standards, policies, and procedures are constantly changing, the reader is directed to the ONC website for the most up-to-date information (ONC 2016b).

The fact that HIEs and interoperability have been mandated as a significant part of MU and are supported by funding does not provide one with any information regarding usage of the HIE, or financial or clinical benefits. Usage refers to the manner in which providers utilize HIEs. It is important to understand how HIEs are used within clinician workflow to continue to improve functionality and value. The most common type of HIE use is "encounter-based" (Vest et al. 2012). Studies have shown HIEs are often queried for information when patients are seen in clinics and report a history of other clinical care such as a physician visit or hospital stay (Frisse et al. 2012; Vest et al. 2012). Both studies reported unanticipated impacts upon workflow. For example, the Frisse research team found clinicians reporting additional work when sorting through their clinical data, the data from the HIE, and any paper forms (Frisse et al. 2012). Organizational factors rather than the HIE technology may impact use. For example, if the emergency department is not fully staffed the personnel may not take the time to query the HIE. Yet another study found that usage varied by user and workplace setting. Physicians and others under significant time pressures used the system less than nurses, public health, and other workers (Vest and Jasperson 2012). As with other new technologies, effective incorporation of HIE data and the processes for health information exchange into the delivery of high-quality healthcare will need to develop over time.

Evaluation of the use and utility of HIEs is imperative as the country continues to implement them. One researcher who performed a meta-analysis summarized his findings with the statement, "The extent of clinical HIE benefits to date is dependent upon the context of the HIE" (Joshi 2011). For example, though a community such as Baltimore, Maryland, might reap significant benefits by tracking patient usage of ERs via an HIE, the physicians in the ER actually see an increase in their work or, at the least, experience a potential delay in the timing of care delivery. Likewise, the benefit of the surveillance of epidemic or outbreaks is related to the size of the exchange system (Joshi 2011). HIEs can be used to improve patient care or it can have little impact upon patient care. Implementation and context makes a difference.

The relationship between cost savings and utilization of health information exchange is complex because cost savings from HIE systems do not always come back to the payers. One study did quantify an annual savings of $1.07 million in an emergency department utilizing health information exchange (Frisse et al. 2012). This is particularly noteworthy because a related study also points out that the perverse incentives in the US healthcare industry payment models have providers paying for HIT implementation and health information exchange efforts, while patients and payers reap the efficiency (financial) and quality benefits (Pevnick et al. 2012). Development and evolution of HIEs is likely to continue for the foreseeable future. The final structures, technical and organizational, along with ultimate clinical and financial benefits, remain to be determined.

Stakeholder Perceptions

The ultimate success or failure of HIEs is dependent upon two important factors: (1) providers or users accessing the HIE and using the data and information; and (2) patients or consumers allowing their data and information to be transmitted across the HIE. This section will explore these factors.

Providers or Users

HIEs do not operate in a vacuum and must be supported by the healthcare organizations in a geographic region for success. Aside from the national mandate, health information exchange implementation will be more successful if the organizations believe it can bring value to themselves and their constituents. The value may be in the form of financial benefits, such as reduced duplicative laboratory testing, or enhancing the organizational reputation for technology use that contributes to the quality of patient care. Conversely, the organization may have concerns such as legal liability or loss of competitive advantage.

Of course, within each organization participating in an HIE are the users who must access the HIE in order for the benefits to be achieved. As described previously, the HIE is either a central data repository of existing patient data or an index linked to historical patient data. Thus, any provider wishing to access data must request it from the HIE. It is important to understand how users, the physicians and nurses who use the HIE in their day-to-day work, feel about HIEs.

Similar to organizational stakeholders, clinicians perceive significant positive value from an HIE. In particular, clinicians noted benefits with HIE participation including better decision making, improved treatment planning, enhanced medication tracking, and an enriched physician–patient relationship (Hincapie et al. 2011). Given that HIEs are still evolving, many do not transmit or share complete EHR data due primarily to interoperability or inability to use the data by the receiver of the information. A consistent clinician request was for additional information to be included in the HIE (Gadd et al. 2011; Hincapie et al. 2011). One study focused on analyzing usage to evaluate HIE utility. As might be expected with most systems, usage ranged from minimal to intensive, sometimes depending upon the setting, sometimes depending upon the type of user (Vest and Jasperson 2012). The main take-away is that HIEs are similar to other HIT and will require human factors analysis and studies of usability to maximize utility.

The perceptions of organizational and provider participants in HIEs are important and will play a vital role in their success or failure. The potential benefits in terms of patient health management are expected to accrue to society or geographic regions.

Consumer Perceptions

Consumers and patients must agree to participate and have their data included in HIEs in order for them to be successful. In some ways it seems odd that this might even be a concern. After all, many consumers use social media, such as Facebook, to share intimate personal information. Similarly, they use mobile banking and shop online as well as use other advanced technologies that put their data out on the Internet. However, health data and information is considered to be sensitive, especially if it is related to conditions such as substance abuse, addiction, or sexually transmitted diseases. That said, easing access to health information or moving it across cities, regions, and countries could be of significant benefit to patients. HHS OCR and ONC guidance says that the consumer may request the method the provider communicates with them using a variety of methods such unencrypted e-mail or texting.

Data segmentation can be used to tag patient information so that selected portions of the record can be shared (CMS 2015d). Sensitive data like substance abuse treatments can be held private while other data is shared. Providers can receive alerts if they try to access data tagged as having re-disclosure restrictions (CMS 2015d). Patients may be more likely to seek treatment for AIDs, mental health, or other socially sensitive health problems. HITECH notes that the Health Information Technology Policy Committee (HITPC) recommends data segmentation, and suggests furthers studies to assess this methodology (CMS 2015d). HL7 has international standards for segmentation of sensitive health information (CMS 2015e).

As stated previously, the Stage 2 MU standards have an increased emphasis on engaging consumers in their healthcare, with criteria calling for providers to offer patients ability to view, download, and transmit their health information online and to use secure electronic messaging to communicate with patients on relevant health information (CMS 2012). These requirements are consistent with findings that 51 percent of consumers trust their physicians' practice over a health plan, hospital, or the government to regulate the privacy and security of their electronic health information (Dhopeshwarkar et al. 2012). In a different study more than 75 percent indicated they might use personal health record (PHR) services to manage their electronic information with more than 80 percent supporting the electronic sharing of health information via an HIE (Patel et al. 2012). Between 78 and 80 percent of cancer patients, who often require sustained continuing care, perceived patient information access to their own records, as well as the sharing of information between providers, to be important functionality for EHRs (Beckjord et al. 2011). The consistent, most important concern for these various consumers was the privacy and security of their data and information (Dhopeshwarkar et al. 2012; Beckjord et al. 2011; Dimitropoulos et al. 2011; Patel et al. 2012). Chapter 15 covers consumer informatics thoroughly; however, these findings demonstrate that consumers understand the benefits and are willing to be involved if the tools are available.

Future Efforts

The ONC has focused on HIE efforts to increase systems interoperability and add public health measures. Additionally, HIEs are not able to provide complete, accurate point-of-care data. Consumer mediated exchange, where the consumer is empowered to manage their personal health information, may seem to be easy to achieve in the digital age. But, in reality, hybrid records and lack of interoperability pose significant challenges to consumers wishing to assume more control over their health data exchange.

There are several barriers to consumer engagement in HIEs. First, patients have historically been conditioned to see the physician as an authority figure and may be intimidated about asking to control their own data (ONC 2012). Many patients are not aware that physicians do not readily share information among themselves for patient care. Conversely, physicians are concerned that giving patients access to too much information may cause unnecessary concerns, increase office phone calls, result in misunderstandings about physicians' chart entries, and invite litigation. Moreover, consumers who attempt to collect their data from the HIE and place it in their PHR can face numerous technical challenges. Tethered PHRs connected to hospital portals will only provide data from that hospital's portal. Entering data into untethered PHRs may be a manual process, as these systems typically do not accurately parse and import clinical data. And neither of these PHRs will provide seamless data exchange with other healthcare systems such as your physician's office EHR. It follows that consumers who are not tech savvy may feel that the effort of managing their PHI outweighs the perceived benefits.

A government report indicated that 70 percent of all medical decisions are affected by clinical lab results (ONC 2013a). The report highlights three successful approaches that are used by these providers. The first approach is facilitating data exchange between the lab's Laboratory Information System (LIS) and the provider's electronic system. With this approach, lab results are electronically transmitted to the providers' system. For example, this approach is used for 98 percent of the Delaware Health Information Network's providers (ONC 2013). The second approach is storing lab results in a repository for later reporting. For example, during a typical 10-day period the Maryland Chesapeake Regional Information System for Our Patients receives lab results from 32 to 46 acute care hospitals, which are then stored for later reporting (ONC 2016a). The third approach comes from companies providing services to HIEs for translating local lab codes to the universal standard LOINC codes and providing outreach and training to providers. Other service providers conduct workshops and arrange outreach activities.

The HITECH Act of 2009 provided funding for HIEs, but the ultimate goal was that the HIEs would be sustainable (Khurshid et al. 2015). Results on the return on investment (ROI) of HIEs are mixed. One study reported that 66 percent of the respondents indicated their HIEs had positive ROIs, and 33 percent did not report positive ROIs (Khurshid et al. 2015). Unfortunately, only one-fourth of the respondents indicated that they used metrics to calculate their HIEs' investment return. ROI metrics used included savings in labor, reducing duplication of tests and procedures, and improving communication, coordination, and health outcomes (Khurshid et al. 2015).

A related article exploring the decline and the future of HIE efforts reported that there were a total of 106 HIEs across the nation in 2016, down 11 percent from 119 in 2012 (Adler-Milstein et al. 2016). Among these HIEs, approximately 50 percent indicated they were sustainable, an increase from 24 percent reported in 2012, and an additional 9 percent were covering most of their costs (Adler-Milstein et al. 2016). These concerns about sustainability raise the question of whether or not communities and states can take on the burden of supporting the HIE's multimillion dollar operational costs. HIEs seeking finances would be advised to develop a paying customer by expanding their service offering beyond data transmission, perhaps by charging for data analytics and decision support services (Adler-Milstein et al. 2016).

Check Your Understanding 10.1

Match the HIE consent terms with the appropriate descriptions.

- **a.** No consent
- **b.** Opt-in
- **c.** Opt-in with exceptions
- **d.** Opt-out
- **e.** Opt-out with exceptions

1. _____ Data are automatically included, though the patient can limit the data to specific types.

2. _____ Does not require any agreement on the part of the patient.

3. _____ Data are automatically included unless the patient chooses not to participate at all.

4. _____ Patient agrees up front but can limit the data included.

5. _____ Patients choose to include their data in an HIE. It is an all-in or all-out choice.

Indicate whether each of the following is true or false.

6. Stage 3 meaningful use characteristics include more focus on patient engagement.

7. Issues with HIE adoption are lack of consensus on standards and poorly designed interfaces.

8. HIE interoperability is mandated by meaningful use.

9. HIE data can be directly uploaded to a PHR.

⊙ Aggregating Health Information

As described in the previous section, moving health information between providers for healthcare benefits patients as they seek and receive care in a variety of settings. However, the need also exists to move the detailed information from EHRs into central locations, or aggregate it, for other purposes. This section will discuss the aggregation of patient health data or information for population health and for public health.

Population Health

Population health can be defined as the level and distribution of disease, functional status, and well-being of a defined group of people with specified characteristics (Friedman and Parrish 2010). The specified characteristics might be treatment by a given physician organization or admission to a given hospital with a defined time frame (Friedman and Parrish 2010). This differs from public health because public health usually refers to all of the inhabitants of a given neighborhood, city, region, state, country, or the world. Population health is not usually charged with responsibility for vital statistics but focuses on overall well-being of the specified group of people.

Population health initiatives are being pursued by healthcare organizations to meet the goals of the Medicare Accountable Care Organization regulations (HHS 2011). **Accountable Care Organization (ACO)** contracts issued under these regulations attempt to provide financial incentives for reductions in unnecessary treatment, such as procedures and hospitalizations, while ensuring quality outcomes improve (Gourevitch et al. 2012). An ACO is an organization of accountable care participants, the participants are "individuals or groups of ACO provider(s)/ suppliers that are identified by a" tax ID number (AHIMA 2014, 2). Research has revealed that many diseases result from a combination of individual behavioral factors (smoking, physical activity, and so on), the environment (pollution, access to health food, and so on), and social factors (housing, education, and so on) (Hardcastle et al. 2011). Thus, prevention strategies such as smoking cessation and the promotion of physical activity within a given population can measurably improve the health of a given population. The ACO regulations reward providers for helping their populations make healthy choices while reducing the use of healthcare services (Gourevitch et al. 2012).

Value-based care initiatives like reducing the number of ER visits, and reducing the number of readmissions are goals of population health management systems (Yeager 2016). Data from many sources, such as the physicians' quality reporting system, clinical EHRs, or insurance company databases, are aggregated and analyzed to determine the best way to individualize preventive interventions for reducing the number of hospital admissions and the number ER visits (Yeager 2016). Benchmarks from registries for diabetes or CHF provide guidance for population health goal setting (Yeager 2016). Interfaces must be in place to facilitate data flow between disparate systems. The patient should be surveyed to determine their healthy behaviors at home (for example, diet, exercise, medication compliance). Return on investment calculations and monitoring care outcomes against benchmarks are essential to demonstrating population health preventive program success (Yeager 2016).

In 2017, the Merit-Based Incentive System (MIPS) for Medicare Part B will be in use for providers (HcPro 2016). MIPS will consolidate three programs including the Physician Quality Program Reporting System (PQRS) and the Value Based Modifier for PQRS and Medicare into a single 0- to 100-point value-based performance scale with four categories (HcPro 2016). The intent is that MIPS will replace meaningful use for physicians with a merit-based system focused on patient care using interrelated technologies. It is projected that Medicare reimbursement adjustments will began under the MIPS system in 2019 (HcPro 2016).

Ambulatory care settings are challenged to the staff and manage the interdisciplinary care teams necessary to meet ACOs needs for providing collaborative care and reporting on care outcomes (Haas 2016). In this setting, staffing complexities arise because the documentation is encounter based, patients are seen for care a few hours a week in a clinic, and healthcare providers direct the patient and the patient's family in the provisioning of care (Haas 2016). When providing ambulatory care, the care givers may need to become involved in helping patients secure transportation to appointments or get in for a visit sooner in order to prevent them from going to the emergency room. Healthcare providers in ambulatory clinics may need to provide medication education then follow up with phone calls to encourage compliance with medication schedules. Poor health literacy, patient isolation, and physical limitations are also challenges to providing effective care for the ambulatory population (Haas 2016).

Community-based preventive interventions for cardiovascular disease and cancer prevention focused on health education, counseling, and web navigation help were determined to be a cost-effective method for promoting preventive healthcare in vulnerable populations like the poor, elderly, children, or minorities (Kyounghae et al. 2016). Success was measured as lower blood pressure, glucose, and weight, increased screening for cancers, and increased levels of exercise. Examples of specific interventions were medication safety for the elderly, bilingual workshops on the importance of cancer screening, and diabetes self-management weekly meetings (Kyounghae et al. 2016).

These developments are important for the health information management profession because HIM is likely to be the one charged with ensuring that ACOs and value-based systems are able to aggregate and use the organizational healthcare data as needed. This might mean activities such as establishing a centralized data warehouse or virtual data locator service; ensuring that all of the necessary data elements are standardized; protecting the privacy and security of the aggregated patient data; assuring the quality of the data; and, not least, manipulating and presenting the patient data to clinicians who provide the care and those who make the organizational decisions. In short, aggregated patient information is vital to population health and the success of the CMS ACOs.

Public Health

Public health exists at many different levels in healthcare. It is defined as the study of the health of populations in large areas like states or countries (AHIMA 2014, 122). At its broadest, the World Health Organization (WHO) promulgates the International Classification of Diseases (ICD) to track the causes of mortality and morbidity across the entire planet. This is not as academic as it might seem because new strains of influenza emerge each year, HIV originated in the 20th century, and traveling across the globe within hours makes it possible to spread disease in a very short time. For example, Ebola hemorrhagic fever is a deadly disease, found primarily in Africa, that has spread to the United States carried by people who were infected. Ebola is transmitted to humans from wild animals, it then spreads through direct contact with the body fluids (for example, blood, sweat) of the infected person (CDC 2015). The first case of Ebola in the United States occurred in New York City in 2014 when a medical aid worker, who had traveled to Guinea, was diagnosed (CDC 2015). Healthcare providers are at risk of getting Ebola especially when protective gloves and gowns are not worn, there is no approved vaccine and the recovery period can last several years (CDC 2015).

Each country, in turn, performs its own public health surveillance, usually required by law. States and usually counties and large cities also have public health systems, which may have separate requirements. Generally, the requirements include a predefined list of notifiable diseases or treatments such as immunizations that healthcare providers must report to healthcare authorities. A list of notifiable diseases, conditions, treatments, or laboratory results required to be reported to the US Centers for Disease Control and Prevention are included at appendix E. Examples of the information in this table include diseases that require immediate, extremely urgent notification such as anthrax and small pox. Then there are those that require immediate (Ebola), urgent (diphtheria and measles), and standard notification (botulism and hepatitis). For each condition further guidance is provided for which cases in these disease categories require notification by indicating the time frame of the condition with statements such as confirmed and probable cause, confirmed cause, all cases prior to classification, and so on. This reporting is essential to maintaining the public health whether through outbreaks of diseases such as H1N1 (avian) flu or fungal meningitis contracted by patients across the country after being treated with tainted medicine.

Historically, public health data reporting was done via entirely separate systems, such that hospitals reported with one format using one system, while physicians reported using entirely separate methods (Shapiro et al. 2011). Eleven potential use cases have been identified where health information exchange can be used to improve public health (Shapiro et al. 2011). Each type of use case is listed here, along with more explanation of the benefits of health information exchange.

1. Mandated Reporting of Laboratory Diagnoses: The cornerstone of public health surveillance, this reporting is resource-intensive when performed manually. Electronic reporting is difficult if local modifications require initial and ongoing custom interfaces. An HIE could assist with transmission and standardizing message formats.

2. Nonmandated Reporting of Laboratory Data: Not all diseases that might have public health significance are required to be reported, for example, influenza and gastrointestinal illnesses. HIEs could be set up to cooperate with the appropriate health authorities to support improved illness and prevention efficacy tracking.

3. Mandated Reporting of Physician-Based Diagnoses: As stated above, physician reporting is separate from laboratory and hospital reporting. Further, compliance ranges anywhere from 9 percent to 99 percent depending upon the disease, provider training, and provider perception of the benefits. Effective use of HIE could ease the reporting burden on physicians while greatly increasing its reliability and validity.

4. Nonmandatory Reporting of Clinical Data: HIE could assist with syndromic surveillance monitoring of nonreportable, nondiagnostic data such as the chief complaints from emergency departments or sales of over-the-counter medicines. Combined with reportable data and analyzed using the latest software, public health authorities could detect and address outbreaks earlier and more effectively.

5. Public Health Investigation: Public health authorities often become aware of cases that require investigation. With the availability of HIE these authorities could use their legislated authority to perform these investigations.

6. Clinical Care in Public Health Clinics: In some jurisdictions public health authorities are required to provide healthcare. Having access to an HIE would enable these providers to access patient data needed for clinical care purposes.

7. Population-Level Quality Monitoring: A regional HIE that included all of the providers of a region (not an ACO) could measure the quality of care delivered to members of the community, as well as the relevant outcomes.

8. Mass-Casualty Events: If the HIE were designed to receive ongoing admission-discharge-transfer messages from registration systems, local disaster authorities could be empowered to allow designated centers to query the HIE in response to requests from families and loved ones of persons who are missing.

9. Disaster Medical Response: The VHA was one of a handful of large healthcare providers with internal health information exchange that was utilized to make their patients' data available soon after Hurricane Katrina destroyed the New Orleans physical infrastructure. Obviously, exchanging the data and having it exist in multiple locations results in redundancies that can be very beneficial in an emergency.

10. Public Health Alerting: Patient Level: The use of health information exchange could make it easier for the public health authorities to track and ensure patients with designated conditions, such as tuberculosis or antibiotic-resistant organism infections, are tracked and treated appropriately when presenting for healthcare by new providers.

11. Public Health Alerting: Population Level: HIEs could assist with provider alerts related to outbreak trends or necessary preventive services. If patients were also allowed access to an HIE portal they could receive the same alerts and information for their given areas. This might help control the outbreak, spread, or prevention of selected diseases and conditions (Shapiro et al. 2011).

Several researchers have documented the real benefits associated with HIEs. One set of researchers determined that bidirectional health information exchange between public health and clinical practice could improve decision making and public health for infants with pertussis (Fine et al. 2010). Researchers in Louisiana sought to address the incidence of HIV/AIDS, using a bidirectional public health information exchange to facilitate the identification of patients with HIV/AIDS who had been lost to follow-up. When the patients reported to any ambulatory or inpatient facility, the clinicians were alerted to attempt to reengage the patients in clinical care. It was successful for 82 percent of the patients (Herwehe et al. 2012).

The studies just reviewed demonstrate that the theory of HIE use in public health can become the reality. With regulations and careful controls to prevent abuses of patient-level information, the use of health information exchange holds the promise of improved health and higher quality care for all citizens.

Case Study: Information Interoperability

This case study illustrates the need and importance of interoperability with respect to transferring healthcare data for treatment. Specifically, documentation of an allergy was not transferred between systems before surgery and reconciliation of information was not performed in time to prevent a serious event.

A 50-year-old man with a history of substance abuse suffered a gunshot wound resulting in paraplegia. He presented in the emergency department at Hospital B in the evening with pain and fever after having been previously seen at four hospitals, including Hospital A where he left against medical advice. Medical records obtained from Hospital A by the emergency department staff at Hospital B where he had gone for treatment indicated that he previously had antibiotic treatment for sepsis.

Subsequently, the ED staff diagnosed the patient with sepsis resulting from decubitus ulcers, he was started on an IV, given vancomycin and piperacillin and admitted to Hospital B. The next day he became unresponsive, underwent a code blue, and was transferred to ICU in a coma. The diagnosis was massive rupture of red blood cells due to a reaction to the antibiotics vancomycin and piperacillin. The result was brain injury and an unresponsive state necessitating discharge to a long-term care facility. The ICU eventually received records from the other hospitals that documented a previous cardiac arrest cause by an allergic reaction to the same antibiotics. Unfortunately, when the ED staff asked the patient about allergic reactions, he reported that he had a blood transfusion reaction and this was transcribed as a statement indicating the patient had no allergies.

With better systems interoperability between Hospitals A and B, data recorded at the first hospital would be available within minutes at the other hospital. Lacking built-in systems interoperability, the ED staff could have called the other hospitals to get a verbal report of allergies and treatments. The allergy could then have been entered into Hospital B's systems (adapted from Reider 2015).

Chapter 10 Review Exercises

Answer the following questions.

1. True or False: The public health benefits of HIE are the same as the population health benefits of HIE.

2. Which of the following is not a potential public health benefit of HIE?
   a. Financial payment reform
   b. Disaster medical response
   c. Public health alerting
   d. Nonmandated reporting of laboratory data

Match the population or public health use of data to the correct example.

    a. The Accountable Care Organization monitors whether smokers are receiving counseling.

    b. The system ensures patients receive critical medications after a tornado.

    c. Confirmed cases of HIV must be reported to the Department of Health.

    d. The schools are being notified that there is an influenza outbreak in the state.

  3. _____ Mandatory laboratory result reporting

  4. _____ Population health monitoring

  5. _____ Disaster medical response

  6. _____ Public health alerts

Discussion.

  7. Describe the history of health information exchange (HIE) in the United States.

  8. List and define the different types of health information exchange organizational structures.

  9. Explain the advantages and disadvantages of the different types of HIE consent models.

    a. No consent

    b. Opt-out

    c. Opt-out with exceptions

    d. Opt-in

    e. Opt-in with restrictions

  10. Analyze the issues and challenges encountered when securing provider and consumer acceptance of HIE.

  11. Describe the difference between population and public health.

  12. Discuss the use of HIEs in relationship to Accountable Care Organizations.

REFERENCES

Adler-Milstein, J., S.C. Lin, and A.K. Jha. 2016. The number of health information exchange efforts is declining, leaving the viability of broad clinical data exchange uncertain. *Health Affairs* 35(7):1278–1285. doi: 10.1377/hlthaff.2015.1439.

AHIMA. 2014. *Pocket Glossary for Health Information Management and Technology.* 4th ed. Chicago: AHIMA Press.

Beckjord, E., R. Rechis, S. Nutt, L. Shulman, and B. Hesse. 2011. What do people affected by cancer think about electronic health information exchange? Results from the 2010 LIVESTRONG Electronic Health Information Exchange Survey and the 2008 Health Information National Trends Survey. *Journal of Oncology Practice* 7(4): 237–241. doi:10.1200/JOP.2011.000324.

Centers for Disease Control and Prevention (CDC). 2015. Ebola (Ebola Virus). https://www
    .cdc.gov/vhf/ebola/pdf/ebola-factsheet.pdf.

Centers for Medicare and Medicaid Services. 2015a. CMS Fact Sheet: EHR Incentive
    Programs in 2015 and Beyond. https://www.cms.gov/Newsroom/MediaRelease
    Database/Fact-sheets/2015-Fact-sheets-items/2015-10-06-2.html.

Centers for Medicare and Medicaid Services. 2015b. EHR Incentive Programs: 2015 to
    2017 (Modified Stage 2) Overview. https://www.cms.gov/Regulations-and-Guidance
    /Legislation/EHRIncentivePrograms/Downloads/2015_EHR2015_2017.pdf.

Centers for Medicare and Medicaid Services. 2015c. EHR Incentive Programs in 2015
    through 2017: Health Information Exchange. https://www.cms.gov/Regulations
    -and-Guidance/Legislation/EHRIncentivePrograms/Downloads/2016_Health
    InformationExchange.pdf.

Centers for Medicare and Medicaid Services. 2015d. *Data Segmentation*. https://www
    .healthit.gov/providers-professionals/data-segmentation-overview.

Centers for Medicare and Medicaid Services. 2015e. *Enabling Privacy: Data Segmentation*.
    https://www.healthit.gov/providers-professionals/ds4p-initiative.

Centers for Medicare and Medicaid Services, 2012. Electronic Health Record Incentive
    Program—Stage 2; Health Information Technology: Standards, Implementation
    Specifications, and Certification Criteria for Electronic Health Record Technology,
    2014 ed.; Revisions to the Permanent Certification Program for Health Information
    Technology; Final Rules. Code of Federal Regulations. http://www.gpo.gov/fdsys
    /pkg/FR-2012-09-04/pdf/2012-21050.pdf.

Department of Health and Human Services. 2010. Health Information Technology:
    Initial Set of Standards, Implementation Specification and Certification Criteria for
    Electronic Health Record Technology. Code of Federal Regulations. http://edocket
    .access.gpo.gov/2010/pdf/2010-17210.pdf.

Department of Health and Human Services, Centers for Medicare and Medicaid Services,
    Medicare Program. 2011. Medicare Shared Savings Program: Accountable Care
    Organizations, Final Rule. http://www.gpo.gov/fdsys/pkg/FR-2011-11-02/pdf
    /2011-27461.pdf.

Dhopeshwarkar, R.V., L.M. Kern, H.C. O'Donnell, A.M. Edwards, and R. Kaushal. 2012.
    Health care consumers' preferences around health information exchange. *Annals of
    Family Medicine* 10(5):428–434.

Dimitropoulos, L., V. Patel, S. Scheffler, and S. Posnack. 2011. Public attitudes toward
    health information exchange: Perceived benefits and concerns. *American Journal of
    Managed Care* 17:SP111–116.

Fine, A.M., B.Y. Reis, L.E. Nigrovic, D.A. Goldmann, T.N. LaPorte, K.L. Olson, and K.D.
    Mandl. 2010. Use of population health data to refine diagnostic decision-making
    for pertussis. *Journal of the American Medical Informatics Association* 17(1):85–90.
    doi:10.1197/jamia.M3061.

Friedman, D.J., and R.G. Parrish. 2010. The population health record: Concepts,
    definition, design, and implementation. *Journal of the American Medical Informatics
    Association* 17(4):359–366. doi:10.1136/jamia.2009.001578.

Frisse, M.E., K.B. Johnson, H. Nian, C.L. Davison, C.S. Gadd, K.M. Unertl, P.A. Turri, and Q. Chen. 2012. The financial impact of health information exchange on emergency department care. *Journal of the American Medical Informatics Association* 19(3):328–333. doi:10.1136/amiajnl-2011-000394.

Gadd, C.S., Y.X. Ho, C.M. Cala, D. Blakemore, Q. Chen, M.E. Frisse, and K.B. Johnson. 2011. User perspectives on the usability of a regional health information exchange. *Journal of the American Medical Informatics Association* 18(5):711–716. doi:10.1136/amiajnl-2011-000281.

Gourevitch, M.N., T. Cannell, J.I. Boufford, and C. Summers. 2012. The challenge of attribution: Responsibility for population health in the context of accountable care. *American Journal of Public Health* 102(S3):S322–S324. doi:10.2105/AJPH.2011.300642.

Gray, P. 2011. Consent Options for HIE in Texas. Houston, Texas: Texas Health Services Authority. http://hietexas.org/resources/policy-guidance.

HL7.org. 2015, October. *FHIR Overview.* https://www.hl7.org/fhir/overview.html.

Haas, S.A. 2016. Developing Staffing Models to Support Population Health Management and Quality Outcomes in Ambulatory Care Settings. *Nursing Economics* 34(3):126–133.

Hardcastle, L., K. Record, P. Jacobson, and L. Gostin. 2011. Improving the population's health: The Affordable Care Act and the importance of integration. *Journal of Law, Medicine and Ethics* 39(3):317–327. doi:10.1111/j.1748-720X.2011.00602.x.

HcPro. 2016. Providers preparing for MIPS. *Doctor's Office* 35(7):1–5.

Healtheway Inc. 2012. Home. http://healthewayinc.org/.

Herwehe, J, W. Wilbright, A. Abrams, S. Bergson, J. Foxhood, M. Kaiser, L. Smith, K. Xiao, A. Zapata, and M. Magnus. 2012. Implementation of an innovative, integrated electronic medical record (EMR) and public health information exchange for HIV/AIDS. *Journal of the American Medical Informatics Association* 19(3):448–452.

Hess, J. 2011. The brave, new world of HIEs. *Healthcare Financial Management* 65(2):44–48.

Hincapie, A.L., T.L. Warholak, A.C. Murcko, M. Slack, and D.C. Malone. 2011. Physicians' opinions of a health information exchange. *Journal of the American Medical Informatics Association* 18(1):60–65. doi:10.1136/jamia.2010.006502.

ICare. 2016. Integrated Care Collaboration. http://icc-centex.org/.

Joshi, J. 2011. Clinical value-add for health information exchange (HIE). *Internet Journal of Medical Informatics* 6(1):1.

Khurshid, A., M.L. Diana, and R. Jain. 2015. Health information exchange readiness for demonstrating return on investment and quality of care. *Perspectives in Health Information Management*.12(Fall): 1–15.

Kim, J., Robert L. Ohsfeldt, Larry D. Gamm, Tiffany A. Radcliff, Luoha Jiane. 2016. Hospital characteristics are associated with readiness. *The Journal of Rural Health* (9):1–9. doi: 10.1111/jrh.12193.

Kyounghae, K., J.S. Choi, C. Eunsuk, C.L. Nieman, J. Jin Hui, F.R. Lin, L.N. Gitlin, and H. Hae-Ra. 2016. Effects of community-based health worker interventions to improve chronic disease management and care among vulnerable populations: a systematic review. *American Journal of Public Health* 106(4):e3–e28. doi: 10.2105 /AJPH.2015.302987.

McCann, E. 2014. Landmark year ahead for HIE. Healthcare IT News. http://www.health careitnews.com/news/landmark-year-ahead-hie.

Office of the National Coordinator, DHHS 2012. Consumer Engagement in Health Information Exchange. https://www.healthit.gov/sites/default/files/consumer _mediated_exchange.pdf.

Office of the National Coordinator, DHHS. 2016a. HealthIT.hhs.gov: HIE Bright Spots— Lab Exchange. https://www.healthit.gov/sites/default/files/lab_exchange_bright _spots_synthesis_final_09302013.pdf.

Office of the National Coordinator, DHHS. 2016b. HealthIT.gov. https://www.healthit .gov/.

Office of the National Coordinator, DHHS. 2013. HealthIT.hhs.gov: State Health Information Exchange Program. https://www.healthit.gov/policy-researchers-implementers/state -health-information-exchange.

Patel, V., R. Dhopeshwarkar, A. Edwards, Y. Barrón, J. Sparenborg, and R. Kaushal. 2012. Consumer support for health information exchange and personal health records: A regional health information organization survey. *Journal of Medical Systems* 36(3):1043–1052. doi:10.1007/s10916-010-9566-0.

Penfield, S.L., K.M. Anderson, M. Edmunds, and M. Belanger. 2009. Toward health information liquidity: Realization of better, more efficient care from the free flow of health information. Booz Allen Hamilton. https://www.boozallen.com/content/dam /boozallen/media/file/Toward_Health_Information_Liquidity.pdf.

Pevnick, J., M. Claver, A. Dobalian, S. Asch, H. Stutman, A. Tomines, and P. Fu. 2012. Provider stakeholders' perceived benefit from a nascent health information exchange: A qualitative analysis. *Journal of Medical Systems* 36(2):601–613. doi:10.1007/s10916- 010-9524-x.

Reider,.J. 2015. Agency for healthcare research and quality. The risks of absent interoperability: medication-induced hemolysis in a patient with a known allergy. https://psnet.ahrq.gov/webmm/case/359/the-risks-of-absent-interoperability -medication-induced-hemolysis-in-a-patient-with-a-known-allergy.

Shapiro, J., F. Mostashari, G. Hripcsak, N. Soulakis, and G. Kuperman. 2011. Using health information exchange to improve public health. *American Journal of Public Health* 101(4):616–623. doi:10.2105/AJPH.2008.158980.

Tsai, J., and R. Rosenheck. 2012. Use of the internet and an online personal health record system by US veterans: comparison of Veterans Affairs mental health service users and other veterans nationally. Journal of the American Medical Informatics Association 19 (6):1089-1094. doi: 10.1136/amiajnl-2012-000971.

US Government. 2009. *American Recovery and Reinvestment Act of 2009.* http://frwebgate .access.gpo.gov/cgi-bin/getdoc.cgi?dbname=111_cong_bills&docid=f:h1enr.pdf.

Vest, J., L. Gamm, R. Ohsfeldt, H. Zhao, and J. Jasperson. 2012. Factors associated with health information exchange system usage in a safety-net ambulatory care clinic setting. *Journal of Medical Systems* 36(4):2455–2461. doi:10.1007/s10916-011-9712-3.

Vest, J., and J. Jasperson. 2012. How are health professionals using health information exchange systems? Measuring usage for evaluation and system improvement. *Journal of Medical Systems* 36(5):3195–3204. doi:10.1007/s10916-011-9810-2.

Vest, J.R., and L.D. Gamm. 2010. Health information exchange: Persistent challenges and new strategies. *Journal of the American Medical Informatics Association* 17(3):288–294. doi:10.1136/jamia.2010.003673.

Yeager, D. 2016. The Challenges of Population Health Management. *For the Record (Great Valley Publishing Company, Inc.)* 28(2):22–25.

ADDITIONAL RESOURCES

Adler-Milstein, J, D.W. Bates, and A.K. Jha. 2011. A survey of health information exchange organizations in the United States: Implications for meaningful use. *Annals of Internal Medicine* 154(10):666–671.

Adler-Milstein, J., D.W. Bates, and A.K. Jha. 2009. U.S. regional health information organizations: Progress and challenges. *Health Affairs* 28(2):483–492. doi:10.1377/hlthaff.28.2.483.

AHIMA. 2016, April. *Three Keys to Simplifying Interoperability in Healthcare.* http://journal.ahima.org/2016/04/15/three-keys-to-simplifying-interoperability-in-healthcare-sponsored/.

Council of State and Territorial Epidemiologists. 2012. *List of Nationally Notifiable Conditions.* www.cste.org/resource/resmgr/PDFs/CSTENotifiableConditionListA.pdf.

Frisse, M.E. 2010. Health information exchange in Memphis: Impact on the physician-patient relationship. *Journal of Law, Medicine and Ethics* 38(1):50–57. doi:10.1111/j.1748-720X.2010.00465.x. https://www.illinois.gov/sites/ilhie/Documents/Consent%20Options%20for%20HIE%20Texas_June2011.pdf.

Office of the National Coordinator, DHHS. 2013 (January). *Can you use texting to communicate health information, even if it is to another provider or professional?* https://www.healthit.gov/providers-professionals/faqs/can-you-use-texting-communicate-health-information-even-if-it-another-p.

Using Healthcare Data and Information

- Explain the different secondary uses of healthcare data and information
- Distinguish between unstructured data and structured data
- Delineate how natural language processing is used to support secondary uses of healthcare data and information
- Relate the opportunities and challenges encountered when using unstructured data for secondary uses
- Identify and compare the major data sets, classification systems, clinical terminologies, and other standards utilized for secondary data use
- Articulate big data utilization in healthcare

KEY TERMS

Big data

Classification system

Clinical phenotyping

Comparable and consistent

Healthcare code sets

Healthcare Common Procedure Coding System (HCPCS)

International Classification of Diseases, 10th revision, Clinical Modification (ICD-10-CM)

International Classification of Diseases, 10th revision, Procedure Coding System (ICD-10-PCS)

Linearization

Logical Observation Identifiers Names and Codes (LOINC)

Mortality

Natural language processing (NLP)

Ontology

Population health

Primary data use
Public health
RxNorm
Secondary data use
SNOMED CT

Structured data
Terminology
Unstructured data
Vocabulary

There are two main ways to utilize healthcare data. The most common is the **primary data use** for treatment or care of the patient. The data are compiled as the care is being provided such as in an outpatient visit to a physician or physical therapist or during an inpatient stay in a hospital. These data include the information that is compiled for assessment (report of physical exam, lab and x-ray results, vital signs) or treatment (physician orders, documentation of operative procedures, medication records). This is the clinical information that is used for care at the time provided and for subsequent medical care of the patient. The other use is the **secondary data use**. Secondary use of health data is the "non-direct care use of personal health information (PHI)" (Safran et al. 2007).

Although the patient record is used as the data source for patient care, secondary data uses are not possible without data collection. The formats for the data in an electronic system are many, can vary by type and the source of the data, and must be understood to assure quality and integrity for use for the secondary purposes. This chapter begins by discussing uses of primary and secondary data and natural language processing and continues with unstructured and structured data entry, the data standards, and the use of secondary data now and in future possibilities.

⊙ Primary and Secondary Uses of Healthcare Data

Public health reporting, reimbursement, and quality improvement are purposes for collecting healthcare data. Less known are purposes such as provider certification or accreditation; disease management; determining best practices or clinical guidelines; detecting financial fraud; monitoring patient compliance; and identifying candidates for clinical trials or using electronic health record (EHR) data for clinical trials. In fact, one of the phrases often heard is "collect once, use many" to describe healthcare data that are collected for patient care purposes and then used to meet a myriad of additional requirements. Organizations describe "big data" to convey the message that the widespread implementation of health information technology (HIT) has resulted in extraordinarily large and detailed databases being made available for secondary data use.

⊙ Natural Language Processing (or Understanding)

Natural language processing (NLP) (or natural language understanding [NLU]) "is a technology that converts human language (structured or unstructured) into data that can be translated then manipulated by computer systems; branch of artificial intelligence" (AHIMA 2014, 101). Within the field of computer or information science, an **ontology** is a common vocabulary organized by meaning, allowing for an understanding of the structure of descriptive information that facilitates a specific topic or domain (AHIMA 2014, 108).

NLP is a branch of artificial intelligence that uses computer algorithms and statistical probabilities to convert human free text into computer-readable forms and formats. The NLP processor or software receives the language and, if necessary, parses or separates it to help with the understanding. NLP programs have codified language structure and can often use the context of the word or sentence to help with the understanding. NLP has been in existence for a long time, only recently being refined to the point where it can be widely incorporated into everyday use and applications. Anyone who has used a smart phone with voice recognition assistance is using NLP. The more technical details of NLP are beyond the scope of this text; however, informaticists should be aware of the current uses and utility of NLP in healthcare.

A major use of NLP in healthcare is to support high-quality patient care. For example, NLP was used to identify methicillin-resistant *Staphylococcus aureus* in Veterans Affairs Medical Centers (Jones et al. 2012). Microbiology data, including free text, for a 20-year period was stored in the Veterans Affairs' system called VistA, which is an electronic health record system. Specifically, because the microbiology free text data was not stored in sentences and paragraphs, it was necessary to develop rules to infer semantic meaning and relationships (Jones et al. 2012). Using these rules, data on organisms and susceptibilities were extracted from the free text for analysis.

Another use of NLP is developing algorithms to determine tumor status from MRI reports at levels comparable to humans (Cheng et al. 2010). Tumor status data stored in unstructured radiology reports' free text fields were extracted using NLP and compared the tumor status determinations, important for disease progression monitoring, that were made by humans who evaluated the same reports. Results indicated good accuracy between the groups (Cheng et al. 2010). NLP processing methods developed in these and other studies will assist clinicians and researchers in cases where the needed data come from multiple, nonstandard, sources.

A related clinical use of NLP is for the discovery of point-of-care data. Previous research has revealed that clinicians have many questions each day that require knowledge-based answers (Ely 2004). Indeed, the provision of evidence-based support is one of the major tasks of today's EHRs. One resource used by clinicians seeking health-related knowledge is MEDLINE, the index of medical literature citations created and maintained by the National Library of Medicine. However, while MEDLINE might be an authoritative source of medical information, it is not easily used when clinicians are in a hurry providing patient care.

Researchers are also using NLP for biosurveillance purposes within hospitals as well as across geographic regions or countries. A NLP tool was used to examine electronic emergency department (ED) patient records in an effort to identify patients who might carry community-acquired infections, thus posing an infection risk to other patients in the hospital (Gerbier et al. 2011). Other researchers focused on the ability of NLP to improve public health biosurveillance by identifying potential flu cases from encounter notes as opposed to the traditional chief complaint structured data fields (Elkin et al. 2012). This type of use of NLP is important to continued improvement in the timeliness of tracking diseases and providing adequate care as patients present for care.

NLP can also provide support in the administrative realms of healthcare, specifically for assigning the International Classification of Disease (ICD) and Current Procedural Terminology (CPT) codes required for payment for services. Studied for decades with varying degrees of success (Stanfill et al. 2010), computer-assisted coding (CAC) is experiencing widespread adoption in the United States for use with ICD-10-CM/PCS and other more detailed standards for the effective use of EHRs (Hartman et al. 2012).

In the past, unstructured data was considered to be more difficult to use, but companies such as Nuance are working to utilize NLP for clinical documentation (Nuance 2016). Healthcare is just beginning to develop methods and procedures to use it accurately and appropriately; however, it is important to continue to allow and even encourage the use of unstructured data in healthcare. Unstructured data provides detail. When providers are forced to use structured data over unstructured data they are forced to make their clinical documentation fit into preconceived categories. Once this occurs the detail around the clinical event is lost forever. It can never be regained. Healthcare must develop methods and processes to convert unstructured data to structured data for secondary use purposes. Table 11.1 compares structured and unstructured data.

Table 11.1. Comparison of structured and unstructured data

Structured data	Unstructured data
Definition: Discrete facts and figures that can be encoded and processed by a computer.	Definition: Textual objects and images that can be stored in a computer but not processed by a computer.
Examples: • Data entered into templates • Coded data (for example, ICD, CPT, SNOMED) whether coded by a person or encoded by the computer • Bar codes, radio frequency identification data (RFID)	Examples: • Narrative notes • Print files • Video and voice files • Scanned images of documents • Pictures • Bar codes • Medical device data

Source: Adapted from Amatayakul 2016, 20

⊙ Unstructured Data

Unstructured data are free text or string data that are not in a database or another kind of data structure as defined by AHIMA (AHIMA 2014, 149). Unstructured data are nonbinary, human-readable data, which does not mean that there is no organization to the data, just that the data are not structured with specific data elements, allowable values, and so on. Unstructured data might be organized into data fields or text boxes such as the history of present illness portion of a History and Physical or the Progress Note for the physician's hospital visit or it might be a Procedure Note. However, this organization only conveys very general meaning and is usually only relevant regarding the type of documentation one can expect to find. Inferring meaning and effective interoperability from native, unstructured data is difficult. Unstructured data require more complex processing before use as secondary data, but they provide a rich store of patient information. Indeed, unstructured data are often preferred because they enable providers to document details and nuances that are usually not available with structured data. In healthcare documentation, unstructured data includes most provider notes during a course of care, the history of an illness, the description of a procedure, or any situation where the number of different permutations is almost infinite.

Given the difficulties associated with unstructured data two questions come to mind:

1. Why would one choose to use unstructured data?
2. If one uses unstructured data, how can it be used most effectively?

The short answer to the first question is that unstructured data contain the detail, in fact, the nuance, which is the "art" of medicine. The answer to the second question is the effective implementation of natural language processing. Unstructured data can be further classified by whether or not they are textual or nontextual.

Textual Data

Textual unstructured data are based on text such as e-mails and other free-form entries or documents. There is a wealth of this type of data but reading and analyzing them is overwhelming. They require integration to be usable, especially for analysis. Advances are being made with initiative to integrate software in to existing systems (such as email) that would provide help with analyzing textual data. However, the barriers are a significant reliance on IT for help with this software, a loss of contextual considerations, and the data standardization inherent in the process of integrating the software results in a loss of details and that can lead to a weaker analysis of the textual data.

Nontextual Data

Nontextual data are unstructured data that are not text based. With the advancement of technological capabilities these continue to increase in kind and complexity. Speech recognition technology takes the spoken word such as a physician dictating a discharge summary and translates this to text using a word translation database. **Public health** deals with the health of people in geopolitical regions such as countries or states (AHIMA, 2014 122). **Population health** refers to collecting and using health care data for public health purposes such as reporting diseases (AHIMA 2014, 116). Biometric data, such as fingerprints, photos, and heel prints, were stored and utilized for personal identification as part of an effort to link health facility use to population health data (Odei-Lartey et al. 2016). Results indicated biometric data provided good accuracy for identifying patients during healthcare visits.

Nontextual data can be digitized images. Picture Archiving and Communications Systems (PACS) stored digitized medical images, like ultrasound or radiology images, and electronically transfer the medical image data in a Digital Image and Communications in Medicine (DICOM) format. According to one study, PACS are highly integrated with dictation and radiology systems, but not well integrated with electronic medical records, which is concerning for value-based healthcare reimbursement systems (Forsberg et al. 2016).

Bar code data and Radio Frequency Identification Data (RFID) have many healthcare uses. In a time study, special RFID-enabled vital sign tools were distributed to patients, and their vital signs were automatically transmitted to an EMR (Kimura et al. 2016). Results indicated this technology reduced the time for nurses to take vital signs. RFID technology, in the form of RFID readers and RFID tags, has been integrated with clinical error management systems (Pourasghar 2016). To evaluate RFID device usage for drug administration, patients were given RFID tags, nurses wore bracelets with RFID tags, drug packages were barcoded. Physicians' orders and drug information were entered into a database (Pourasghar 2016). RFID readers were used to scan nurse's bracelets, drug packages and patient's bracelets at the time of drug administration. The system was able to provide voice signals when medication errors occurred when the doctor's orders did not match the intended drug administration (for example, wrong drug, patient, or time). The RFID system functioned well to detect potential medication errors (Pourasghar 2016). Other examples are digital signature technology and automatic identification technologies to include bar codes, intelligent character recognition (ICR) and optical character recognition (OCR). In OCR where there is translation of analog or printed or typed text to machine-editable text, the application is mainly with the printed text from the claims form (Kohn 2009).

Check Your Understanding 11.1

Answer the following questions.

1. Natural language processing is used for which of the following?
   a. Tracking diseases and biosurveillance purposes
   b. Developing algorithms in support of high-quality patient care
   c. Providing knowledge-based answers for clinicians
   d. All of the above are uses of NLP

2. Primary data use is required for which of the following?
   a. Direct patient care
   b. Public health reporting
   c. Provider certification or accreditation
   d. Monitoring patient compliance

3. Which type of data provide details?
   a. Natural language processing
   b. Unstructured data
   c. Primary use data
   d. Secondary data

4. Which is not an example of the secondary use(s) of data?
   a. For accreditation purposes
   b. Determining best practices
   c. Quality improvement activities
   d. Review by a consulting physician

Match the terms with the appropriate descriptions.

   a. Use of PHI for other than direct care
   b. Turns speech or text into computable data
   c. Common vocabulary organized by meaning that allows for understanding

5. _____ Ontology

6. _____ Natural language processing

7. _____ Secondary data use

Indicate whether each of the following is true or false.

8. Unstructured data are generally more difficult to use than structured data.

9. Physician progress notes would be considered structural data.

10. Data gained from speech recognition technology would be considered non-textual.

⊙ Coded and Structured Data

Structured data, also called discrete data, are binary, machine-readable data in discrete fields, with limitations on what can be entered into the field (Sandefer 2016, 364). Whether these data are in the form of specific, allowable text entries or numerical representations, they are preferred for the majority of secondary data uses. In and of itself, the use of structured data does not translate to automatic usability. Structured data come in many different flavors and formats, some of which rise to the level of standards; others do not. Because healthcare is a very complex business, there are many concepts and ideas that must be accessed, combined, manipulated, and shared. Healthcare information systems use vocabularies, terminologies, and classification systems. A **vocabulary** is a dictionary of terms; that is, words and phrases with their meanings. A **terminology** is a set of terms representing a system of concepts, usually around a specific domain such as healthcare. Finally, a **classification system** arranges or organizes like or related entities (Giannangelo 2015, 4). This section will explore code sets, classification systems, clinical terminologies, as well as other data set standards important to health informatics and the interoperability of health information. The discussion of value sets can be found in chapter 5.

Healthcare Code Sets

Healthcare code sets are defined as "any set of codes used for encoding data elements, such as tables of terms, medical concepts, medical diagnostic codes, or medical procedure codes" (US Congress 1996). This very broad definition encompasses a wide array of different data types from demographics such as race, ethnicity, state, and country to very detailed clinical data elements such as clinical findings, procedures, or laboratory results. It is important for the array of code sets to be standardized so that data can be easily shared between organizations.

The Office of the National Coordinator (ONC) in the Department of Health and Human Services (HHS) is advised on HIT standards (including code sets) development and adoption by a federal advisory committee (FACA) known as "the HIT Standards Committee." One subgroup of the HIT Standards Committee is the Vocabulary Task Force, with the specific charge to "identify gaps, issues and needs for clinical and administrative vocabulary solutions within the scope of the HIT Standards Committee; to develop recommendations to the HIT Standards Committee for methods, actions, and/or programs to mitigate, manage, or solve these vocabulary concerns" (ONC, HHS 2013). The recommendations made by the HIT Standards Committee and its subgroups, if adopted, are ultimately included in the meaningful use EHR certification criteria. The remainder of this chapter will describe many of the different code sets that have been adopted or are under consideration for adoption by the HIT Standards Committee.

Classification Systems

Classification systems have a wide range of uses in healthcare, including the collection and reporting of public health data; the design and administration of healthcare reimbursement systems; and the development and use of quality measures and other performance measures.

International Classification of Diseases

The standard classification system for epidemiology, population health, and clinical systems in the United States, and many other nations, is the International Classification of Diseases (ICD) (WHO 2016). The ICD system is used by clinicians, researchers, insurance companies, and other agencies to classify diseases and health conditions using data extracted from health records, death certificates, and other treatment and vital documents (WHO 2016). Once the diseases are classified, the data can be stored and transmitted electronically for coding, billing, reimbursement, quality management, and research. Additionally, the WHO receives ICD data from many countries that they aggregate to compile mortality and morbidity statistics (WHO 2016). Thus, ICD is used for health trend analysis globally.

Mandatory reporting of death statistics is another use of ICD data. In fact, the ICD system was originally developed by the World Health Organization (WHO) for **mortality** reporting, that is, for reporting the cause of death on death certificates

(CDC 2016). The mortality data are stored in the National Vital Statistics System and are used to present the characteristics of those dying in the United States, determine life expectancy, and compare mortality trends with other countries. For example, in the United States in 2014 the life expectancy was 78.8 years, and the number of deaths was 2,626,418 (CDC 2016). Currently, the 10th version of ICD is in use, with an 11th version available in 2018.

ICD-10-CM

On October 1, 2015, the United States began using the 10th edition, *International Classification of Diseases, Tenth Revision, Clinical Modification* (**ICD-10-CM**) for reporting diagnoses, inpatient procedures and services in all healthcare settings, and deaths (AHIMA 2014, 81). Similarly, the *International Classification of Diseases, Tenth Revision, Procedure Coding System* (**ICD-10-PCS**) provides codes for all procedures performed on inpatients (AHIMA 2014, 81). Using ICD-10-CM/PCS enables greater comparability between the United States and other countries and within the United States between mortality and morbidity codes.

ICD-10-CM includes a total of 21 chapters (see table 11.2); and a maximum of seven digits (see figure 11.1); the inclusion of alpha characters as the initial digit for all codes and as a seventh digit code extension when applicable; and the use of a placeholder X when necessary. Within ICD-10-CM, factors influencing health status and external causes are listed in the main classification; the sense organs and nervous system disorders are separated; injuries are grouped by body part; the excludes notes have been moved to the beginning of each chapter; and postoperative complications are in the procedure-specific body system chapters.

Figure 11.1. Format of ICD-10-CM

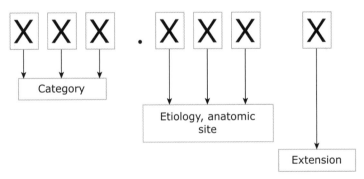

Table 11.2. ICD-10-CM chapter titles

CHAPTER	TITLE	CATEGORIES
1	Certain infectious and parasitic diseases	A00–B99
2	Neoplasms	C00–D49

(Continued)

Table 11.2. ICD-10-CM chapter titles (*Continued*)

CHAPTER	TITLE	CATEGORIES
3	Diseases of the blood and blood-forming organs and certain disorders involving the immune mechanism	D50–D89
4	Endocrine, nutritional and metabolic diseases	E00–E89
5	Mental and behavioral disorders	F01–F99
6	Diseases of the nervous system	G00–G99
7	Diseases of the eye and adnexa	H00–H59
8	Diseases of the ear and mastoid process	H60–H95
9	Diseases of the circulatory system	I00–I99
10	Diseases of the respiratory system	J00–J99
11	Diseases of the digestive system	K00–K94
12	Diseases of the skin and subcutaneous tissue	L00–L99
13	Diseases of the musculoskeletal system and connective tissue	M00–M99
14	Diseases of the genitourinary system	N00–N99
15	Pregnancy, childbirth and the puerperium	O00–O9A
16	Certain conditions originating in the perinatal period	P00–P96
17	Congenital malformations, deformations and chromosomal abnormalities	Q00–Q99
18	Symptoms, signs and abnormal clinical and laboratory findings, not elsewhere classified	R00–R99
19	Injury, poisoning and certain other consequences of external causes	S00–T88
20	External causes of morbidity	V01–Y99
21	Factors influencing health status and contact with health services	Z00–Z99

Source: CDC 2013b

The move to ICD-10-CM was a huge transition for the United States. When compared to earlier versions, ICD-10 is more specific and granular. However, this increased specificity requires more precise documentation to ensure that medical record coders can accurately assign the correct codes. After the transition, clinical documentation specialists were finding gaps in documentation that made it difficult to accurately assign ICD-10 codes (Tompkins 2016). Problem areas where coders need greater documentation specific are laterality (which side of the body), location, drug and substance abuse, and disease manifestations type, acuity, and stage (Tompkins 2016). Physician education and increased physician engagement are needed.

CMS contracted with 3M Health Information Systems to develop ICD-10-PCS, a procedural coding system for inpatient procedure reporting in the United States. ICD-10-PCS has a seven-character alphanumeric structure, with each character having many different possible values, as the letters and numbers are mixed throughout the

Table 11.3. Sections of ICD-10-PCS

Section	Title
0	Medical and Surgical
1	Obstetrics
2	Placement
3	Administration
4	Measurement and Monitoring
5	Extracorporeal Assistance and Performance
6	Extracorporeal Therapies
7	Osteopathic
8	Other Procedures
9	Chiropractic
B	Imaging
C	Nuclear Medicine
D	Radiation Oncology
F	Physical Rehabilitation and Diagnostic Audiology
G	Mental Health
H	Substance Abuse Treatment

Source: CMS 2016

Figure 11.2. Meaning of characters for medical and surgical procedures

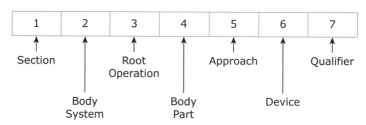

code. The first character can either be alpha or numeric. The digits 0–9 and the letters A–H, J–N, and P–Z are used. Letters O and I are omitted to avoid confusion with 0 and 1. Figure 11.2 shows the meaning of each of the seven characters from section to body system to root (or main) operation to body part to approach to device to qualifier. The different sections of ICD-10-PCS can be found in table 11.3.

To assist during the transition from ICD-9 to ICD-10-CM, the Centers for Medicare and Medicaid collaborated with the CDC to generate General Equivalency Mappings (GEMs) for translating ICD-9-CM codes into ICD-10-CM/PCS codes (Bowmen et al. 2016). The GEMs users includes payers, programmers, researchers, and informatics professionals. GEMs are useful for retrospective data analysis and long-term studies involving data collected from both classification systems (Bowmen et al. 2016).

ICD-11

The present revision process of the ICD, the 11th, is under way at the World Health Organization in Geneva. ICD-11 promises substantial improvements over historical rendering, embracing a tripartite structure of

1. An ontological core in partnership with the Systemized Nomenclature of Medicine (SNOMED).

2. A foundation layer of richly interlinked concepts with explicit preferred terms, fully specified terms, synonyms, definitions, and detailed attributes.

3. Several linearizations deriving from the Foundation Layer that will resemble the traditional mutually exclusive and exhaustive coding structure of historical ICD tabular versions. A **linearization** is "a subset of the ICD-11 foundation component, that is

   o fit for a particular purpose: reporting mortality, morbidity, or other uses
   o jointly exhaustive of the ICD universe (foundation component)
   o composed of entities that are mutually exclusive of each other
   o each entity is given a single parent" (WHO 2013)

The most important linearization will be the standard derivative used for morbidity coding in hospitals and clinical care. A proper and much smaller subset of this linearization will be used for mortality coding. Distinct from these will be specific linearizations for primary care, low-resource delivery environments in developing countries, and various specialty derivatives such as neurology, cancer, or psychiatry. Finally, the historical pattern of nations creating their own national modifications, such as the American ICD-10-CM (where the CM is the US Clinical Modification), can correspondingly be accommodated by nations invoking their own derivatives from the Foundation Layer of ICD-11, the advantage being that because all linearizations derive from the Foundation Layer, establishing linkages and mapping between and among virtually all linearizations—morbidity, mortality, specialty, primary care, or national derivations—can be achieved by mapping through the Foundation Layer in a hub and spoke model, rather than creating "point to point" mappings among the permutations.

An additional feature of ICD-11 will be its use of postcoordination for many attributes in order to avoid the excessive repetition evident in ICD-10-CM for many injury patterns. For example, each injury has a separate code for initial encounter, subsequent encounter, and sequela. Postcoordination means that the terms with modifiers are created as they are needed rather than the developers of the classification trying to conceive of all possible permutations for inclusion in the classification. Parameters such as severity, stage, detailed anatomy, acuity, or topography (for example, laterality, anterior, distal, and so on), could be rendered using postcoordination rather than creating hundreds of precoordinated terms for each of the combinations on such dimensions. Nevertheless, to maintain longitudinal continuity with historical versions of ICDs, the ICD-11 mortality linearization will retain the approximate level of precoordination evident in ICD-10.

The developers of ICD-11 recognize that postcoordination opens the possibility for multiple ways to code the same concept, for example, postcoordinating a disease and severity when a precoordinated version of disease by severity might exist. To avoid violating the requirement that a statistical classification must have mutually exclusive categories (to avoid counting the same things twice or separately in different categories), ICD-11 introduces a body of "sanctioning rules" that are intended be computationally executed, not manually practiced, because there will likely be many thousands of such rules. An example of such a sanctioning rule might be mapping a postcoordinated expression of renal failure and a severity code to its corresponding precoordinated version.

An interesting speculation, as one proposal to obviate a proliferation of national modifications, is to consider that some modes of precoordination would be required or prohibited as a set of restrictions, for example the United States might require the postcoordination of laterality where appropriate. Building on the notion that national modifications of ICD may become simply various linearizations derived from the Foundation Layer of ICD-11, a country's transition to ICD-11 can be facilitated by rendering their current system—such as ICD-10-CM in the United States—as a linearization of the ICD-11 Foundation Layer (this is technically straightforward), and simply evolving that linearization to become incrementally closer to the standard ICD-11 Morbidity Linearization over time. This provides a nondisruptive pathway for graceful adoption of the new revision without the abrupt transformation witnessed around ICD-10-CM adoption in the United States today.

Clinical Terminologies

It is implausible that a single terminology or classification can or should function as the only reference set for all the complexities of clinical information. Laboratory or genomic data are not well suited to representation in any version of the ICD, even the ever-versatile ICD-11. Thus, many purpose-specific terminologies are widely used today. The more common terminologies used are presented here.

Healthcare Common Procedure Coding System

The **Healthcare Common Procedure Coding System (HCPCS)** consists of two levels or systems. Level I is the CPT, a large, well-curated catalog of clinical and surgical procedures maintained by the American Medical Association as a proprietary and copyrighted resource. Its primary purpose is to enable the classification of resource categories for reimbursement, though it has levels of detail and granularity that support its reuse for secondary analyses such as quality improvement or comparative effectiveness research. Although comprehensive, it is lacking for coherent overall structure, hierarchy, or conceptual organization, rendering its facile adoption for secondary use sometimes challenging.

Level II of the HCPCS is maintained by CMS. CMS creates and administers the Level II HCPCS codes as alphanumeric identifiers for products, supplies, and services not included in CPT. The codes consist of a leading alpha character followed by four numbers. They are used primarily for claims processing.

SNOMED CT

The Systemized Nomenclature of Medicine developed by the College of American Pathologists merged with the Clinical Terms (CT) vocabulary from the United Kingdom to create SNOMED CT. **SNOMED CT** is a logically organized and massive terminology, mostly ordered by a formal description logic, which permits SNOMED CT to benefit from the classifying reasons developed by computer science and the fields of formal ontology and logic. Each entry in SNOMED CT contains a concept identifier, a description that helps define the concept and relationships or attributes for the entry (IHTSDO 2013). It has highly detailed and granular characterization of diseases, findings, symptoms, anatomies, manifestations, and many related axes. It is the largest, most complex, and comprehensive terminology about clinical medicine (NLM 2016). Architecturally, it is intended for representing hierarchies and relationships between concepts (Giannangelo 2015, 122). It can be used to record smoking status and to update smoking status changes (Giannangelo 2015, 124). Figure 11.3 is an illustration of the multiple granularities available in SNOMED CT.

SNOMED CT use in the United States is growing because SNOMED CT is specified as an acceptable standard for several meaningful use requirements for entering structured data into electronic health records. Examples include representing patient problem lists, symptoms, and procedures (ONC 2013). It is also recommended, in meaningful use criteria, for encoding lab, diagnostic, encounter, substance, family health, and medical device data (Giannangelo 2015,

Figure 11.3.   Multiple levels of granularity in SNOMED CT

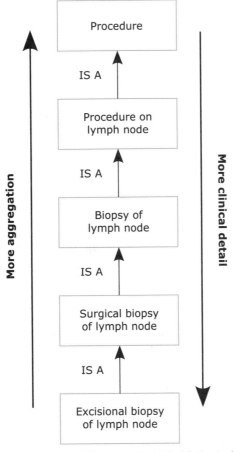

Source: Figure reprinted by kind permission of the International Health Terminology Standards Development Organization http://www.ihtsdo.org. 2013

123). SNOMED CT is more easily understood if patient context data are entered into the system along with the data used for generating the SNOMED CT codes (Nandigam and Topaz 2016). However, this is time consuming for physicians. An alternative is to define a commonly used subset of SNOMED CT codes for a given setting and have providers select the subset codes that match the patient's problems (Nandigam and Topaz 2016). In fact, the National Library of Medicine has mapping guidelines for SNOMED CT and ICD-10-CM codes that can assist informatics specialists who are designing electronic systems (NLM 2016).

LOINC

Logical Object Identifiers Names and Codes (LOINC) comprise a dictionary of laboratory codes and clinical test descriptors, originated by Regenstrief Institute and funded by federal support grants as a public resource for the common good. It is publicly usable and used worldwide without any fees or licenses. Laboratory codes are synthesized from a six-part naming model: analyze/component (for example, sodium), property (for example, concentration), timing (for example, a moment or integrated over a defined period), sample type (for example, blood serum), scale (for example, quantitative), and optionally method. LOINC has two sections, lab and clinical codes (Palkie 2016, 156). Clinical codes examples are vital signs, EKG and cardiac echocardiogram (Palkie 2016, 156). Variations on this six-part model are also used for clinical measurements (for example, blood pressure) and clinical scales or survey instruments (for example, the Glasgow Coma Scale). Selected examples from the LOINC tables are found in figure 11.4.

LOINC was originally adopted for Health Level 7 (HL7) clinical messages, because most labs use proprietary test codes and an exchange standard for lab results was needed. LOINC is now endorsed as the preferred coding for laboratory data, and drug label section headers (Palkie 2016, 156) as specified by the meaningful use regulations for the US HHS (ONC 2013). Use of LOINC facilitates data exchange and interoperability between EHRs and lab systems. However, given the structure and complexity of LOINC lab codes, converting a lab system's proprietary codes into LOINC codes is a substantial undertaking, because additional information will need to be captured for the six-part model. After the model data are entered into the local systems, the local lab result codes can be mapped to LOINC codes by using Regenstrief LOINC Mapping Assistant, a desktop program (Giannangelo 2015, 171). LOINC is adopted by the Veterans Affairs and the Consolidated Health Informatics initiative (Palkie 2016, 156).

RxNORM

Another standard for electronic data exchange is **RxNorm,** a standardized nomenclature for clinical drugs created and curated by the National Library of Medicine (NLM 2016). RxNorm is the meaningful use recommendation for pharmaceutical names and codes in the United States. To be certified EHRs must satisfy the e-prescribing medications vocabulary standard, which can be accomplished with RxNorm codes (NIST 2016). Additionally, it is used in pharmacies and drug interaction software such as First Databank and MediSpan (NLM 2016). RxNorm is a relatively sophisticated database that enumerates "orderable drugs" such as Chewable Amoxicillin Tablet, 250 mg, and links these to their component medicines (Amoxicillin), trade name variations, and active ingredients.

Data in RxNorm are standardized from names found in many other drug nomenclatures, which facilitates interoperability. A typical listing for a drug contains the ingredients, strength, actions, and dosage forms (NLM 2016). Linkages within the system can present the drug's generic and brand names, as well as the active ingredients (Palkie 2016, 157). For example, RxNorm includes the Veteran's Health Administration National Drug File—Reference Terminology used for coding drug actions and usages. The US Food and Drug Administration's free Adverse Event Reporting System (FAERS) data for drug names can be mapped to RxNorm codes (Banda et al. 2016). In a study on mining patterns of drug interactions from the FAERS system that focused on early detection of drug interactions, RxNorm was used to map drugs under study to their generic names (Ibrahim et al. 2016).

Figure 11.4.   Selected examples from LOINC Tables

LOINC #	Long Common Name	CLASS	Class Override
6019-4	Almond IgE Ab [Units/volume] in Serum	Allergy	Allergy
6020-2	Alternaria alternata IgE Ab [Units/volume] in Serum	Allergy	Allergy
19000-9	Vancomycin [Susceptibility]	ABXBACT	Antibacterial susceptibility
7059-9	Vancomycin [Susceptibility] by Gradient strip (E-test)	ABXBACT	Antibacterial susceptibility
38483-4	Creatinine [Mass/volume] in Blood	Chem	Chem
2160-0	Creatinine [Mass/volume] in Serum or Plasma	Chem	Chem
35591-7	Creatinine renal clearance predicted by Cockcroft-Gault formula	Chem	Chem

Source: This material contains content from LOINC® (http://loinc.org). The LOINC table, LOINC codes, and LOINC panels and forms file are copyright © 1995–2016, Regenstrief Institute, Inc. and the Logical Observation Identifiers Names and Codes (LOINC) Committee and available at no cost under the license at http://loinc.org /terms-of-use.

Other Data and Information Uses

This section has emphasized terminology, vocabularies, and classifications, though illustrated only a few. Additionally, there are information model and messaging standards that provide syntax to complement the raw semantics of controlled terms, or put another way, the context for the words. A detailed discussion of these standards is beyond the scope of this chapter, but includes simple structures such as HL7 Version 2 bar-delimited ASCII strings as well as the more elegant Consolidated Clinical Data Architecture specification more recently emergent from HL7 and destined for meaningful use health information exchange (HIE). This section describes other emerging data and information uses.

Perhaps the most promising initiative presently under way is the Clinical Information Modeling Initiative (CIMI), which is an international initiative that is unifying the midlevel modeling of healthcare data structures for representing clinical observations such as blood pressure measurements (Blobel 2014). One goal is to facilitate seamless data exchange of medical records and decision support tools by providing a reference model for informatics developers to use that can be translated in Unified Metalanguage (UML), which is commonly used existing modeling language (Blobel 2014).

Clinical information modeling tools (CIMTs) are applications and software that facilitate the creation of clinical information modeling (CIM) definitions and the subsequent system implementation (Moreno-Conde et al. 2015). For example, domain experts and information technologists would collaborate to define clinical data models for EHRs, which are used to write the software components that are tested and implemented. One study explored the level of consensus of the essential requirements for clinical information modeling tools by interviewing experts and synthesizing existing literature. Essential requirements included supporting semantic interoperability of EHRs, importing and exporting data in XML, supporting version management, and collaborating when creating CIMs (Moreno-Conde et al. 2015). As the healthcare industry continues to develop its ability to effectively exchange data, the standards will likewise evolve.

Metadata

In order to use data and information appropriately, it is important to understand metadata. Metadata are

> descriptive data that characterize other data to create a clearer understanding of their meaning and to achieve greater reliability and quality of information. Metadata consist of both indexing terms and attributes. Data about data: for example, creation date, date sent, date received, last access date, last modification date (AHIMA 2014, 96).

Metadata are essential for a full understanding of the underlying data. For example, without metadata such as the creation or modification date, it may be impossible to determine which version of ICD-10-CM was used for coding a record. This is essential to ensure the code is interpreted correctly. Other metadata such as the access date are important for legal reasons such as ensuring no breach of confidentiality has occurred. Finally, metadata can simply help explain the data or information by defining the data element or specifying the length of the field or providing the values that are allowed to be entered in the field. Metadata about the data can even change over time. For example, a healthcare organization may have specified metadata related to its EHR data; however, if the EHR data are transmitted a new metadata field could be added to indicate the healthcare organization as the source of the data. Metadata are one of those hidden, necessary tools for effective use of data and information.

Check Your Understanding 11.2

Answer the following questions.

1. Which of the following is utilized in the United States for reporting the cause of death on death certificates?
   a. ICD-10-CM
   b. SNOMED CT
   c. LOINC
   d. RxNORM

2. Which of the following have a wide range of uses in healthcare, including the development and use of quality and performance measures?
   a. Code sets
   b. Classification systems
   c. Clinical terminologies
   d. Data set standards

3. Which is not a benefit that ICD-10-CM/PCS codes provide?
   a. More comparability
   b. Additional detail
   c. Factors influencing health
   d. Require more specific documentation to assign the codes

4. Which of the following would be considered metadata?
   a. ICD-10-CM codes
   b. Source of the data
   c. Trend analysis
   d. Data of admission

5. A dictionary of terms is:
   a. Vocabulary
   b. Terminology
   c. Classification system
   d. Code set

Indicate whether each of the following is true or false.

6. ICD-11 is currently in development and includes plans for graceful evolution from ICD-10.

7. Data without metadata are just as easy to understand as data with metadata.

8. SNOMED CT is a detailed clinical terminology with over 310,000 unique concepts.

9. There is a finite number of codes in ICD-10-CM/PCS.

◉ Secondary Data Uses of the Future

Historically, the primary and only use of clinical data was for care providers to document the progress and details of a specific patient for their own records and to share with partnering healthcare providers. However, in this era of increasingly coordinated, cooperative, and preventive care, the use of clinical findings and outcomes across large numbers of patients may emerge to be the more important use of information from a societal perspective. Broadly labeled "secondary use," these practices involve data quality metrics, population-based guideline application, best evidence discovery, adverse event detection, comparative effectiveness analyses, and clinical and outcomes research of many varieties including clinical trials and observational epidemiology. Perhaps the single most important modality of secondary use is the identification of patients for whom a particular rule or guideline should "fire," commonly called clinical decision support. Thus aggregated patient information analyses and monitoring can improve the quality of care for an individual patient, by predicting and avoiding drug–drug or drug–disease interactions, inappropriate tests or treatments, or overlooked results and implications.

Big Data

One of the concepts that is evolving in the present and for the foreseeable future is "big data." **Big data** are defined as "high-volume, high-velocity and high-variety information assets that demand cost-effective, innovative forms of information processing for enhanced insight and decision making" (Gartner 2013). The first differentiator for big data is the sheer size of the databases. Large hospital systems are accumulating terabytes of data every year, with Accountable Care Organizations and others wanting to combine the databases to be able to utilize the richness of all of the data. The CMS databases from 1965 to present would qualify as big data. The second issue is the speed with which the data needs to and does move around the system. This will continue to accelerate as HIE organizations become more prevalent and are more widely used. The third characteristic of big data is the variety of the data. The industry is beginning to seek ways to combine individually identifiable patient record information with genomic data, staffing data, or other types of data, which adds to the complexity of the data. In particular, it may be difficult to find tools that can handle such a wide variety of data. Big data are and will continue to be a focus for health informatics professionals.

Central to any secondary use is the principle of transforming heterogeneous clinical data into **comparable and consistent** representations. Comparable and consistent data has been normalized or transformed so that they conform to the designated standards. Absent such transformation, clinical data are not comparable and cannot contribute to the myriad benefits of secondary uses. An example of data normalization is the use of NLP coupled with controlled terminologies to transform unstructured information into structured and semantically consistent forms that can sustain inferencing. More sophisticated forms include the practice of high-throughput **clinical phenotyping** from electronic medical records using validated phenotyping algorithms to identify patients for a particular study. Clinical phenotyping involves determining which observable characteristics are applicable for a given subset of patients (SHARP-C Project 2013). For example, researchers need to be able to identify patients and their relevant characteristics for inclusion or exclusion for numerators or denominators of quality metrics, inclusion criteria for clinical trials, appropriateness for a clinical decision support rule, or selection for a research cohort to further understand best practices and outcomes. Meaningful use is bringing the United States closer to achieving comparable and consistent clinical data among practitioners, though most would agree that we have some distance yet to go.

Data mining performed on large databases provides valuable information. For example, the National Institutes of Health's Undiagnosed Disease Program (UDP) contains medical and genetic sequencing (AHIMA 2016a). These data were collected from examining and testing patient volunteers who have diseases that have not currently been able to be diagnosed. Human phenotype data (for example, height or eye color) is stored for each patient. Data mining, in conjunction with machine learning, was used to analyze and reanalyze the data in order to determine over time what was the patient's diagnosis (AHIMA 2016a).

Case Study: Patient Tracking with RFID

This case study illustrates the need for interoperability in healthcare systems with respect to tracking patients' locations and orders within the hospital. RFID technology in the form of a bar-coded patient wristband and the presence of an EMR to read that data could have prevented the errors in this study.

An elderly woman with leukemia and diabetes presented on the oncology unit for a scheduled treatment. As she was not in distress, the day nurse asked her to wait in the lounge while her room was prepared. When the shift changed, the patient was taken by the evening nurse to her room. The evening nurse said she would come by later to finish the check-in process.

Although the patient was actually checked in later by the evening nurse, she did not call the admitting doctor assuming that the day nurse had done so. As a result, the patient had no admitting orders on the chart; thus no meal was ordered. The patient prepared for bed, and took her own insulin, but did not have anything to eat, which she assumed was part of the treatment plan. In the morning, the patient was unresponsive due to severely low blood sugar levels. The patient suffered a prolonged hospital stay and delayed chemotherapy.

The use of patient bracelets with RFID codes embedded in them and an EHR with an RFID reader would have reduced the likelihood of this occurrence. The patient's admission bracelet information could have been scanned into the EHR, which would have alerted the staff to the lack of patient orders, and further indicated the diabetic condition. Additional glucose monitoring at the bedside could have sounded alerts to notify clinicians of the patient's low blood sugar. Moreover, as a best practice, nurses should check all patient charts for orders at a minimum once a shift, and definitely on admission. Physicians should have staff assigned to making rounds on patients with overnight stays for treatment.

(Source: Adapted from Vogelsmeier and Despins 2016)

Chapter 11 Review Exercises

Match the term to the correct definition.

- **a.** Clinical phenotyping
- **b.** Healthcare code sets
- **c.** Morbidity
- **d.** Ontology
- **e.** Secondary data use
- **f.** Structured data
- **g.** Terminology
- **h.** Unstructured data

1. _____ Use of data for nondirect care purposes
2. _____ Nonbinary, human readable
3. _____ Discrete, machine readable
4. _____ Set of terms representing a system of concepts
5. _____ Set of codes used for encoding data elements
6. _____ Involves determining which observable characteristics are applicable
7. _____ Common vocabulary organized by meaning to allow for understanding of the structure of descriptive information
8. _____ Disease or conditions for which treatment is sought

Discussion.

9. Explain what big data are and how they are used.
10. Discuss the importance and uses of SNOMED CT.

REFERENCES

AHIMA. 2014. *Pocket Glossary for Health Information Management and Technology.* 4th ed. Chicago: AHIMA Press.

AHIMA. 2016a. Big data mining assists in undiagnosed disease database. *Journal of AHIMA* 87(1):8.

Amatayakul, M. 2016. *Health IT and EHRs.* Chicago: AHIMA Press.

Banda, J.M., Lee Evans, Rami S. Vanguri, Nicholas P. Tatonetti, Patrick B. Ryan, Nigam H. Shah. 2016, March. Data descriptor: A curated and standardized adverse drug event resource to accelerate drug safety research. *Science Data* 3. doi: 10.1186 /s13326-016-0048-2.

Blobel, B., W. Goossen, and M. Brochhausen. 2014. Clinical modeling—A critical analysis. *International Journal of Medical Informatics* 83(1):57–69. doi: 10.1016 /j.ijmedinf.2013.09.003.

Bowman, S., Rhonda Butler, Kathy Giannangelo, Nelly Leon-Chisen, Rita Schichilone. 2016. Putting the ICD-10-CM/PCS GEMs into practice (Updated). *Journal of AHIMA* 87(1):48–53.

Cheng, L.T., E.J. Zheng, G.K. Savova, and B.J. Erickson. 2010. Discerning tumor status from unstructured MRI reports—Completeness of information in existing reports and utility of automated natural language processing. *Journal of Digital Imaging: The Official Journal of the Society for Computer Applications in Radiology* 23(2):119–132.

Elkin, P.L., D.A. Froehling, D.L. Wahner-Roedler, S.H. Brown, and K.R. Bailey. 2012. Comparison of natural language processing biosurveillance methods for identifying influenza from encounter notes. *Annals of Internal Medicine* 156(1 Pt 1):11–18.

Ely, J.W. 2004. Answering physicians' clinical questions: Obstacles and potential solutions. *Journal of the American Medical Informatics Association* 12(2):217–224. doi:10.1197/jamia.M1608.

Forsberg, D., B. Rosipko, J.L. Sunshine, and P.R. Ros. 2016. State of integration between PACS and other IT systems: A national survey of academic radiology departments. *Journal of American College of Radiologists* 13(7):812–818 e2. doi: 10.1016/j.jacr.2016.01.018.

Gartner Inc. 2013. Big Data Definition. *IT Glossary.* http://www.gartner.com/it-glossary/big-data/.

Gerbier, S., O. Yarovaya, Q. Gicquel, A.L. Millet, V. Smaldore, V. Pagliaroli, S. Darmoni, and M.-H. Metzger. 2011. Evaluation of natural language processing from emergency department computerized medical records for intra-hospital syndromic surveillance. *BMC Medical Informatics and Decision Making* 11:50.

Giannangelo, K. 2015. *Healthcare Code Sets, Clinical Terminologies, and Classification Systems.* 3rd ed. Chicago: AHIMA.

Hartman, K., S.C. Phillips, and L. Sornberger. 2012. Computer-assisted coding at the Cleveland Clinic: A strategic solution. Addressing clinical documentation improvement, ICD-10-CM/PCS implementation, and more. *Journal of AHIMA* 83(7):24–28.

Ibrahim, H., Amr Saad, Amany Abdo, and Eldin A. Sharaf. 2016. Mining association patterns of drug-interactions using post marketing FDA's spontaneous reporting data. *Journal of Biomedical Informatics* 60:294–308. doi: 10.1016/j.jbi.2016.02.009.

International Health Terminology Standards Development Organization. 2013. SNOMED-CT User Guide. http://ihtsdo.org/fileadmin/user_upload/doc/.

Jones, M., S.L. Duvall, J. Spuhl, M.H. Samore, C. Nielson, and M. Rubin. 2012. Identification of methicillin-resistant *Staphylococcus aureus* within the nation's Veterans Affairs Medical Centers using natural language processing. *BMC Medical Informatics and Decision Making* 12:34.

Kimura, E., M. Nakai, and K. Ishihara. 2016. Evaluation of efficiency improvement in vital documentation using RFID devices. *Nursing Informatics* 225:1042.

Kohn, D. 2009. How information technology supports virtual HIM department. *Journal of AHIMA* 80(3). Web extra.

Moreno-Conde, A., F. Jódar-Sánchez, and D. Kalra. 2015. Requirements for clinical information modelling tools. *International Journal of Medical Informatics* 84(7):524–536. doi: 10.1016/j.ijmedinf.2015.03.005.

Nandigam, H., and Maxim Topaz. 2016. Mapping Systematized Nomenclature of Medicine–Clinical Terms (SNOMED CT) to International Classification of Diseases, Tenth Revision, Clinical Modification (ICD-10-CM): Lessons learned from applying the National Library of Medicines' Mappings. *Perspectives in Health Information Management* (Summer):1–10.

National Institute of Standards and Technology (NIST). 2016. Standards and Testing FAQs. http://healthcare.nist.gov/use_testing/faq.html.

National Library of Medicine, National Institutes of Health. 2016. *SNOMED CT to ICD-10-CM*. https://www.nlm.nih.gov/research/umls/mapping_projects/snomedct _to_icd10cm.html.

Nuance. 2016. *Natural Language Understanding*. http://www.nuance.com/for-business /natural-language-understanding/index.htm.

Odei-Lartey, E. O., D. Boateng, S. Danso, A. Kwarteng, L. Abokyi, S. Amenga-Etego, S. Gyaase, K. P. Asante, and S. Owusu-Agyei. 2016. The application of a biometric identification technique for linking community and hospital data in rural Ghana. *Global Health Action* 9:29854. doi: 10.3402/gha.v9.29854.

Office of the National Coordinator, HHS. 2013. Vocabulary Task Force. http://www .healthit.gov/policy-researchers-implementers/vocabulary-task-force.

Palkie, B. 2016. Clinical Classifications, Vocabularies, Terminologies, and Standards. Chapter 5 in *Health Information Management: Concepts, Principles, and Practice*, 5th ed. Edited by Oachs, P. and A. Watters. Chicago: AHIMA.

Pourasghar F., T. J. S., Yarifard Khadijeh. 2016. Design and Development of a Clinical Risk Management Tool Using Radio Frequency Identification (RFID). Acta Informatica Medica 24 (2):111–115. doi: 10.5455/aim.2016.24.111-115.

Safran, C., M. Bloomrosen, W.E. Hammond, S. Labkoff, S. Markel-Fox, P.C. Tang, and D.E. Detmer. 2007. Toward a national framework for the secondary use of health data: An American Medical Informatics Association white paper. *Journal of the American Medical Informatics Association* 14(1):1–9. doi:10.1197/jamia.M2273.

Sandefer, R.H. 2016. Health Information Technologies. Chapter 12 in *Health Information Management: Concepts, Principles, and Practice*, 5th ed. Edited by Oachs, P. and A. Watters. Chicago: AHIMA.

SHARP-C Project. 2013. Division of Informatics. http://informatics.mayo.edu/sharp /index.php/HTP_Research.

Stanfill, M.H., M. Williams, S.H. Fenton, R.A. Jenders, and W.R. Hersh. 2010. A systematic literature review of automated clinical coding and classification systems. *Journal of the American Medical Informatics Association* 17(6):646–651. doi:10.1136 /jamia.2009.001024.

Tompkins Diop, K. 2016. ICD-10 Opens documentation gaps. *Journal of AHIMA* 87(3):54–55.

US Congress. 1996. *Health Insurance Portability and Accountability Act of 1996*. http://aspe .hhs.gov/admnsimp/pl104191.htm#1171.

Vogelsmeier, A., and L. Despins. 2016. Agency for Healthcare Research and Quality. A Room without Orders. https://psnet.ahrq.gov/webmm/case/365/a-room-without-orders.

World Health Organization. 2016. Classifications. http://www.who.int/classifications/icd/en/.

World Health Organization. 2013. International Classification of Diseases. http://www .who.int/classifications/icd/en/.

World Health Organization. 2013. The International Classification of Diseases, 11th Revision. www.who.int/classifications/icd11/.

ADDITIONAL RESOURCES

AHIMA. 2016b. Survey: ICD-10-CM/PCS has reduced coding productivity. *Journal of AHIMA* 87(1):9.

American Medical Association. 2013. Current procedural terminology. https://www.ama-assn .org/about-us/current-procedural-terminology-cpt-editorial-panel.

Averill, R.F., R. L. Mullin, B.A. Steinbeck, N.L. Goldfield, M.T. Grant, and R. R. Butler. 2016. Development of the ICD-10 Procedure Coding System (ICD-10-PCS).

Bielby, J.A. 2016. Continuing on the intriguing ICD-10 journey. *Journal of AHIMA* 87(5):50–52.

Bowman, S. 2008. Why ICD-10 is worth the trouble. *Journal of AHIMA* 79(3):24–29.

Centers for Disease Control and Prevention. 2016. *Mortality Data*. http://www.cdc.gov /nchs/nvss/deaths.htm.

Centers for Disease Control and Prevention. 2013a. *ICD—ICD-9-CM—Coordination and Maintenance Committee*. http://www.cdc.gov/nchs/icd/icd9cm_maintenance.htm.

Centers for Disease Control and Prevention. 2013b. International Classification of Diseases, 10th rev, Clinical Modification (ICD-10-CM). http://www.cdc.gov/nchs /icd/icd10cm.htm.

Centers for Medical and Medicaid Services. 2016. *ICD-10-PCS*. https://www.cms.gov /Medicare/Coding/ICD10/downloads/pcs_final_report2012.pdf.

Department of Health and Human Services. 2012. Administrative Simplification: Adoption of a Standard for a Unique Health Plan Identifier; Addition to the National Provider Identifier Requirements; and a Change to the Compliance Date for the International Classification of Diseases, 10th ed. Final Rule. *Federal Register*. https://www.federalregister.gov/documents/2012/09/05/2012-21238 /administrative-simplification-adoption-of-a-standard-for-a-unique-health-plan -identifier-addition-to.

Health Level Seven International. 2013. http://www.hl7.org/.

Health Story Project. 2013. http://www.healthstory.com/.

HIMAGINE. 2015. *The Landscape of Health Information Management*. http://info .himaginesolutions.com/hubfs/Content/2015_HIM_Benchmark_Report.pdf.

Logical Observation Identifiers Names and Codes (LOINC®). 2016. http://loinc.org/.

Mayo Clinic Informatics: CIMI. 2013. http://informatics.mayo.edu/CIMI/index.php /Main_Page.

National Library of Medicine, National Institutes of Health. 2016. RxNorm. https:// www.nlm.nih.gov/research/umls/rxnorm/.

Ramanathan, T., C. Schmidt, A. Menon, D. Pepin, M. Penn. 2015. Issue Brief, Federal Public Health Laws Supporting Data Use and Sharing. https://www.cdc.gov/phlp /docs/datasharing-laws.pdf.

Chapter

12

Privacy for Health Information

Learning Objectives

- Interpret the HIPAA Privacy Rule and regulations
- Identify protected health information
- Distinguish uses and disclosures of PHI
- Relate administrative requirements for covered entities
- Comply with the HIPAA privacy, security, and breach audit requirements
- Address legal considerations other than HIPAA

KEY TERMS

Access
Accounting of disclosures
Administrative Simplification
American Recovery and Reinvestment
    Act (ARRA)
Business associate (BA)
Business associate agreement (BAA)
Covered entity
Deidentified health information
Designated record set
E-discovery
Electronic media
Electronic protected health information
    (ePHI)

Health Information Technology for
    Economic and Clinical Health
    (HITECH) Act
Health Insurance Portability and
    Accountability Act of 1996 (HIPAA)
Health plan
Healthcare clearinghouse
Healthcare provider
Legal hold
Limited data set
Minimum necessary
Mitigation
Notice of Privacy Practices (NPP)
Office for Civil Rights

Operations	Transaction
Payment	Treatment
Pre-empt	Valid authorization
Protected health information (PHI)	Workforce

Throughout history, consumers of healthcare have been concerned about the privacy of their health information. In general, most American citizens understand that the communications between a patient and his or her physician are confidential. However, beyond this, most citizens would probably agree they have little understanding about their rights to access their health information and, furthermore, who else has a legal right to the information and how it may be used. State laws, which vary significantly, have provided some privacy protections, but nuances exist that challenge both patients and the healthcare professionals who provide treatment. Coupled with the need for federal privacy standards and greater efficiencies in the US healthcare system, industry leaders have worked on solutions to these salient challenges for decades.

In an effort to improve the efficiency and effectiveness of the nation's healthcare system, the **Health Insurance Portability and Accountability Act of 1996 (HIPAA)** was enacted by the US Congress and signed into law by President Bill Clinton (HIPAA 1996). HIPAA is a complex federal law that addresses the provision of continuity of health coverage, the control of fraud and abuse in healthcare, the reduction of healthcare costs, and the security and **administrative simplification** that includes (1) adopting standards for transaction and code sets used to exchange health data, (2) standard identifiers for health plans, providers, employees, and individuals used in standard transactions, and (3) protection of the security and privacy of PHI (45 CFR 160, 162 164 2015). For the purposes of this chapter, the focus is on the Administrative Simplification section of Title II, and even more specifically, the privacy and security of health information. HIPAA was updated in 2009 with the passage of American Recovery and Reinvestment Act (ARRA), which included the Health Information Technology for Economic and Clinical Health (HITECH) legislation, the issuance of the 2013 HIPAA Omnibus Rule, and the guidance for patient access to their health information issued in 2016. All will be addressed in this chapter.

⊙ HIPAA Privacy Rule

The **Office for Civil Rights** of the Department of Health and Human Services has been given responsibility for the oversight and enforcement of the HIPAA regulations. As stated in the Office for Civil Rights (OCR) Privacy Rule Summary:

> A major goal of the HIPAA Privacy Rule is to assure that individuals' health information is properly protected while allowing the flow of health information needed to provide and promote high quality health care and to protect the public's health and well-being. The Rule strikes

a balance that permits important uses of information, while protecting the privacy of people who seek care and healing. Given that the health care marketplace is diverse, the Rule is designed to be flexible and comprehensive to cover the variety of uses and disclosures that need to be addressed (OCR 2003).

Since the Privacy Rule was originally issued there have been many changes in the healthcare industry as well as technology so that the HIPAA Privacy Rule now includes regulations to update the HIPAA Breach Notification Rule; to modify the HIPAA Privacy Rule to include the provisions of section 105 of Title I of the Genetic Information Nondiscrimination Act (GINA) of 2008; and to try to increase the workability of the HIPAA regulations for covered entities and business associates (BAs) (OCR 2013).

⊙ Focus of HIPAA Privacy Regulations

The Administrative Simplification provisions within HIPAA focus on the adoption of standards for the electronic transmission of financial and administrative transactions, national identifiers, privacy, and security. With the expectation of reducing costs and administrative burdens, Congress also recognized that advances in electronic technology could erode the privacy of a person's health information. Taking this into consideration, Congress incorporated into HIPAA legislation mandates for the adoption of federal privacy protections for individually identifiable health information. The HIPAA Privacy Regulations address the use and disclosure of **protected health information (PHI),** which is defined as "individually identifiable health information that is transmitted by electronic media, maintained in electronic media, or transmitted or maintained in any other form or medium" (45 CFR 160.103). The US Department of Health and Human Services (HHS) published the final HIPAA Privacy Rule in December 2000, which was later modified in August 2002 (OCR 2003). Health plans, healthcare clearinghouses, and healthcare providers had to comply with the HIPAA Privacy Rule by April 14, 2003, with the exception of small health plans, which were given an additional year.

In the years that followed enactment of HIPAA, some privacy advocates criticized the federal legislation as a "paper tiger" (Belfort 2010). Examples of criticisms were that privacy and security rules do not apply to many organizations that routinely handle large amounts of health information and the potential sanctions are not sufficiently severe except in rare cases of criminal conduct (Belfort 2010). Congress responded to these issues with the passage of the **Health Information Technology for Economic and Clinical Health (HITECH) Act**, which was enacted as part of the **American Recovery and Reinvestment Act (ARRA)** of 2009. The HITECH Act strengthened enforcement of the rules promulgated under HIPAA. This chapter covers federal legislation on privacy of health information originally enacted under HIPAA and subsequently expanded and strengthened with the passage of the HITECH Act, with the issuance of the HIPAA Omnibus Rule in 2013, and the "Individuals' Right Under HIPAA to Access Their Health Information" (CFR 164.524).

⊙ Basics of the HIPAA Privacy Regulations

Although the HIPAA privacy regulations are only one part of the original law, they are very complex, especially after the various expansions and clarifications. In order to fully understand them, it is important to understand the definitions and other foundations upon which the regulations are built.

Covered Entities and Workforce

All of the various HIPAA privacy regulations apply to covered entities and all BAs of covered entities. A **covered entity** is a healthcare provider, health plan, or healthcare clearinghouse that transmits health information in electronic form in connection with healthcare transactions (OCR 2003). Under HIPAA, a **healthcare provider** is any person or organization who furnishes, bills, or is paid for healthcare in the normal course of business (45 CFR 160.103 2013). Healthcare providers include persons such as doctors, dentists, nurses, and therapists as well as entities such as hospitals, clinics, urgent care centers, pharmacies, and institutions (OCR 2003) who provide and bill for services. A **health plan** is an individual or group plan that provides, or pays the cost of, medical care (45 CFR 160.103 2013). Examples of health plans include group health plans, health insurance issuers, health maintenance organizations (HMO), Medicare Part A or Part B, and the Medicaid program. A **healthcare clearinghouse** is defined by HIPAA as "a public or private entity, including a billing service, repricing company, community health management information system, or community health information system, and 'value-added' networks and switches, which do either of the following functions:

1. Processes or facilitates the processing of health information received from another entity in a nonstandard format or containing nonstandard data content into standard data elements or a standard transaction.

2. Receives a standard transaction from another entity and processes or facilitates the processing of health information into nonstandard format or nonstandard data content for the receiving entity" (OCR 2003).

When applying HIPAA, covered entities must also consider members of their workforce who may not be limited only to employees. The Privacy Rule defines **workforce** as "employees, volunteers, trainees, and other persons whose conduct, in the performance of work for a covered entity (CE) or BA, is under the direct control of such covered entity or business associate, whether or not they are paid by the covered entity or business associate" (OCR 2013). An example of nonpaid workforce would be a health information technology (HIT) or health information management (HIM) student who is completing a professional practice experience in the hospital setting.

Healthcare Transactions

The HIPAA law amended by HITECH delineates the meaning of healthcare transactions. **Transaction** means "the transmission of information between two

Table 12.1.   Healthcare transactions

1	Healthcare claims or equivalent encounter information
2	Healthcare payment and remittance advice
3	Coordination of benefits
4	Healthcare claim status
5	Enrollment and disenrollment in a health plan
6	Eligibility for a health plan
7	Health plan premium payments
8	Referral certification and authorization
9	First report of injury
10	Health claims attachments
11	Other transactions the Secretary may prescribe by regulation

Source: AHIMA 2014

parties to carry out financial or administrative activities related to healthcare" (OCR 2003). This definition applies to transmissions of electronic health information. Table 12.1 provides a list of healthcare information transactions affected by HIPAA.

Business Associates

The term "business associate" has a very specific meaning for covered entities when complying with HIPAA. **Business associates (BAs)** essentially are all entities that are not members of the workforce but are providing a service or performing a task on behalf of a CE with the expectation or possibility that they will have access to PHI. The full definition can be found in Figure 12.1. Examples of typical BAs of the health information department are an outsourced medical transcription company and coding or reimbursement consultants. The individuals performing these functions are not members of the facility's workforce but they use or disclose health information to perform their respective duties on behalf of the CE. The newly expanded definition explicitly includes health information organizations that will be involved in exchanging information electronically. The new definition also carries the BA obligation out to BA subcontractors so that everyone or anyone handling PHI on behalf of a CE should consider themselves a BA.

Once a person or organization is identified as a business associate, the CE must initiate a **business associate agreement (BAA)** that meets all of the HIPAA requirements, including the most recent. Covered entities should utilize the help of legal counsel to ensure that the BAA clearly documents the requirements of

Figure 12.1. Definition of HIPAA business associate

Business associate:

1. Except as provided in paragraph (4) of this definition, business associate means, with respect to a covered entity, a person who:

   i. On behalf of such covered entity or of an organized health care arrangement (as defined in this section) in which the covered entity participates, but other than in the capacity of a member of the workforce of such covered entity or arrangement, creates, receives, maintains, or transmits protected health information for a function or activity regulated by this subchapter, including claims processing or administration, data analysis, processing or administration, utilization review, quality assurance, patient safety activities listed at 42 CFR 3.20, billing, benefit management, practice management, and repricing; or

   ii. Provides, other than in the capacity of a member of the workforce of such covered entity, legal, actuarial, accounting, consulting, data aggregation (as defined in § 164.501 of this subchapter), management, administrative, accreditation, or financial services to or for such covered entity, or to or for an organized health care arrangement in which the covered entity participates, where the provision of the service involves the disclosure of protected health information from such covered entity or arrangement, or from another business associate of such covered entity or arrangement, to the person.

2. A covered entity may be a business associate of another covered entity.

3. *Business associate* includes:

   i. A Health Information Organization, E-prescribing Gateway, or other person that provides data transmission services with respect to protected health information to a covered entity and that requires access on a routine basis to such protected health information.

Source: 45 CFR 160.103

the BA "to implement administrative, physical, and technical safeguards that reasonably and appropriately protect the confidentiality, integrity, and availability of the PHI that it creates, receives, maintains, or transmits on behalf of the covered entity" (45 CFR 164.308(b)(1) and 164.314). As amended by HITECH, "a contract between the covered entity and a business associate must establish the permitted and required uses and disclosures of protected health information by the business associate" (HHS 2013) and provide specific content requirements of the agreement. The contract may not authorize the business associate to use or further disclose the information in a manner that would violate the requirements of HIPAA, and requires termination of the contract if the covered entity or business associate are aware of noncompliant activities of the other (45 CFR 164.504 2013). Other areas to be addressed in the agreement include the role of agents or subcontractors who are provided PHI; safeguards to protect the PHI; procedures for the reporting of security incidents of which it becomes aware; and authority of the covered entity to terminate the contract if the BA violates a material term of the contract. With an acceptable BAA in place, covered entities may lawfully disclose PHI to BAs to perform services for the covered entity.

Before HITECH came into force, BAs who failed to properly protect patient information were liable to the covered entities via their BAA, but they did not face governmental penalties. The HITECH Act expands HIPAA data privacy and security requirements to include the BAs of covered entities. Under the HITECH Act, a person or organization identified as a BA is now directly subject to the following HIPAA privacy requirements:

- Impermissible uses and disclosures
- Failure to provide breach notification to the CE
- Failure to provide access to a copy of electronic PHI either to the CE or individual
- Failure to disclose PHI to the Secretary as required to investigate or determine the BAs compliance
- Failure to provide an accounting of disclosures (OCR 2013)

Check Your Understanding 12.1

Indicate whether each of the following is true or false.

1. The Privacy Rule is the name given to the 1996 HIPAA law, its regulations, the HITECH Act, and other related regulations.
2. If a business associate contracts with another party for services and they have access to PHI, they are not subject to HIPAA.
3. The only covered entities, as defined by HIPAA, are healthcare providers, health plans, and healthcare clearinghouses.
4. Only persons who are paid by the covered entity are considered to be members of the workforce.
5. Business associates must comply with all provisions of the Privacy Rule.

Match the term with the correct definition.

  a. Business associate
  b. Covered entity
  c. Healthcare clearinghouse
  d. Protected health information
  e. Transaction

6. _____ Individually identifiable health information

7. _____ Entity that processes or facilitates the processing of health information received from another facility or receives a standard transaction from another entity for processing

8. _____ Provider, health plan, or healthcare clearinghouse that transmits health information electronically in connection with transactions

9. _____ Transmission of information between two parties for financial or administrative healthcare activities

10. _____ Providing a service or task on behalf of a covered entity

⊙ Protected Health Information

To better understand the HIPAA Privacy Rule and the goal of ensuring individuals' protection of health information, it is important to examine the meaning of protected health information (PHI) because this fundamental term is used throughout much of the legislation. As mentioned earlier in the chapter, PHI is defined as "individually identifiable health information that is transmitted by electronic media, maintained in electronic media, or transmitted or maintained in any other form or medium" (45 CFR 160.103). A three-part test to determine whether or not information meets the definition of PHI is as follows:

1. The information must either identify the person or provide a reasonable basis to believe the person could be identified from the information given.

2. The information must relate to one's past, present, or future physical or mental health condition; the provision of healthcare; or payment for the provision of healthcare.

3. The information must be held or transmitted by a CE or its BA (Brodnik et al. 2012, 220–221).

Furthermore, the Privacy Rule provides guidance on what is not PHI and specifically addresses personnel and educational records. Health information noted in education records covered by the Family Educational Rights and Privacy Act (FERPA), 20 USC 1232g, and employment records held by a CE in its role as employer are exempt from the rule (OCR 2013). As an example, employee physical examination reports contained within personnel files would not be subject to the Privacy Rule (Brodnik et al. 2012).

Another point to consider when interpreting the Privacy Rule is that the information must be "created or received" by a CE. Therefore, information that a patient communicates to his or her doctor is covered, but information that is created or received by another party other than a CE is not protected under HIPAA. An example of this would be a patient disclosing health information to a family member or friends. In this instance, HIPAA does not prevent the family or friends from disclosing the health information to others (Sullivan 2004).

Deidentification of Protected Health Information (PHI)

The Privacy Rule does not restrict the use or disclosure of **deidentified health information**. In the Privacy Rule summary, HHS explains that

> deidentified health information neither identifies nor provides a reasonable basis to identify an individual. There are two ways to deidentify information; either: (1) a formal determination by a qualified statistician; or (2) the removal of specified identifiers of the individual and of the individual's relatives, household members, and employers is required, and is adequate only if the covered entity has no actual knowledge that the remaining information could be used to identify the individual (164.514(a) 2013).

45 CFR 164.514(b) provides a distinct list of data elements that a CE can remove to ensure that a patient's information is deidentified. The 18 data elements are listed in table 12.2. Some examples of where deidentified health information is useful are research, decision support, and education in health professions.

In November 2012 the HHS OCR released guidance to ensure the deidentification of PHI meets the intent of the HIPAA Privacy Rule. Figure 12.2 is a graphic depicting the two acceptable methods. The first method requires an expert to use statistical or scientific methods to ensure there is a very small probability of any identification of the individuals. The second method requires that the 18 data elements listed in table 12.2 be removed. However, the second method also requires that there be no actual knowledge that the residual data can identify an individual (OCR 2012). For example, if the data were deidentified by the second method, yet

Figure 12.2.   Two methods of HIPAA privacy rule deidentification

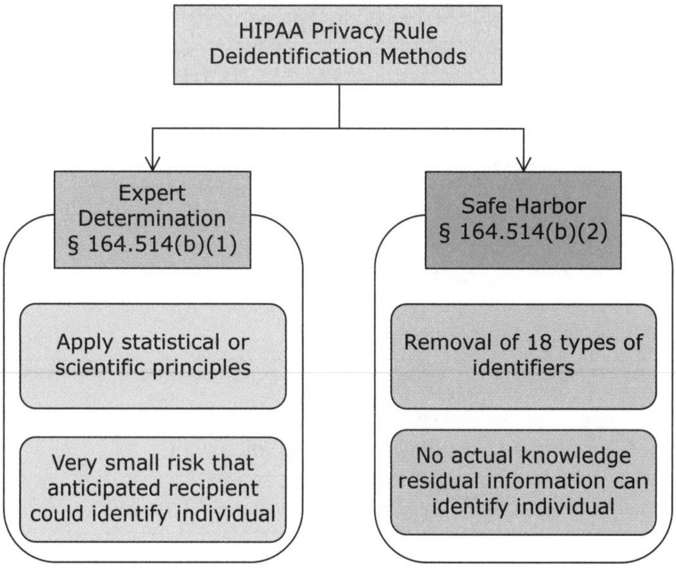

Source: OCR 2012

Table 12.2.   Requirements for deidentification of PHI

	To meet the intent of HIPAA requirements the following identifiers of the individual or of relatives, employers, or household members of the individual, must be removed:
1	Names
2	All geographic subdivisions smaller than a State, including street address, city, county, precinct, zip code, and their equivalent geocodes, except for the initial three digits of a zip code if, according to the current publicly available data from the Bureau of the Census: (1) The geographic unit formed by combining all zip codes with the same three initial digits contains more than 20,000 people; and (2) The initial three digits of a zip code for all such geographic units containing 20,000 or fewer people is changed to 000
3	All elements of dates (except year) for dates directly related to an individual, including birth date, admission date, discharge date, date of death; and all ages over 89 and all elements of dates (including year) indicative of such age, except that such ages and elements may be aggregated into a single category of age 90 or older
4	Telephone numbers
5	Fax numbers
6	Electronic mail addresses
7	Social security numbers
8	Medical record numbers
9	Health plan beneficiary numbers
10	Account numbers
11	Certificate/license numbers
12	Vehicle identifiers and serial numbers, including license plate numbers
13	Device identifiers and serial numbers
14	Web Universal Resource Locators (URLs)
15	Internet Protocol (IP) address numbers
16	Biometric identifiers, including finger and voice prints
17	Full face photographic images and any comparable images
18	Any other unique identifying number, characteristic, or code except a code used for Reidentification purposes

Source: 45 CFR 164.514(b) 2013

retained a rare diagnosis code for a very small population of people, it is possible the person might be able to be recognized so the data would not be "deidentified" according to HIPAA.

Reidentification

A covered entity is allowed to have a policy and procedure in place for reidentifying information that had been previously deidentified. A code or other means of record identification can be used provided that the code is not derived from information about the individual and cannot be translated in some manner to identify the individual. Furthermore, the CE cannot use or disclose the code for any other purpose and must not divulge the mechanism for reidentification (45 CFR 164.514).

Electronic Protected Health Information (ePHI)

In looking at the privacy and security of patient health information, **electronic protected health information (ePHI)** must be considered. The term ePHI refers to "individually identifiable health information that is transmitted by electronic media or maintained in electronic media" (45 CFR 160.103). The HIPAA Security Rule, discussed in detail in chapter 13 is a key law written to protect ePHI and to provide guidance for how electronic health information can be accessed appropriately (Brodnik et al. 2012).

HIPAA sets forth clear definitions of **electronic media,** which is helpful for interpreting the intent of the legislation. Electronic media is defined as

1. Electronic storage material on which data is or may be recorded electronically, including, for example, devices in computers (hard drives) and any removable/transportable digital memory medium, such as magnetic tape or disk, optical disk, or digital memory card;

2. Transmission media used to exchange information already in electronic storage media. Transmission media include, for example, the Internet, extranet or intranet, leased lines, dial-up lines, private networks, and the physical movement of removable/transportable electronic storage media. Certain transmissions, including of paper, via facsimile, and of voice, via telephone, are not considered to be transmissions via electronic media if the information being exchanged did not exist in electronic form immediately before the transmission (OCR 2013).

These definitions are with the privacy and security rule reinforcing that any PHI that is electronically stored or electronically stored information that is then transmitted must be protected from inappropriate access.

⊙ Uses and Disclosures of PHI

It is important to distinguish between the concepts of use and disclosure as emphasized in the HIPAA Privacy Rule:

⊙ "Use means, with respect to individually identifiable health information, the sharing, employment, application, utilization, examination, or analysis of such information within an entity that maintains such information" (45 CFR 160.103).

⊙ "Disclosure means the release, transfer, provision of access to, or divulging in any other manner of information outside the entity holding the information" (OCR 2013).

This section will examine uses and disclosures covered by HIPAA as well as those that are permitted by the legislation.

Individual Rights Regarding Access to PHI

45 CFR 164.524 addresses an individual's right of **access** to "inspect and obtain a copy of protected health information about the individual in a designated record set, for as long as the protected health information is maintained in the designated record set." Furthermore, 45 CFR 164.501 defines the **designated record set** as the "medical records and billing records about the individual and the enrollment, payment, claims adjudication, and case or medical management record systems and used for the CE to make decisions about the individual." Exceptions to the right to access include psychotherapy notes; that compiled in reasonable anticipation of a civil, criminal, or administrative action or proceeding; PHI subject to the Clinical Laboratory Improvements Amendments of 1988, 42 USC § 263a; and PHI that are exempt from the Clinical Laboratory Improvements Amendments of 1988, pursuant to 42 CFR 493.3(a)(2) (45 CFR 164.524). When a request is received for access to PHI, the CE must respond in a timely manner for both paper and electronic records. The individual has the right to specify the form and format for the covered entity to provide access to their PHI, if it can be readily producible as requested or a copy can be provided in another form and format agreed on by both parties. If a paper copy is requested, the information should be provided in paper whether original is in paper or electronic. When the request is for an electronic copy of a paper record, the CE is required to provide an electronic copy if it can be readily producible in that format such as scanning the paper record into an electronic format. If an electronic copy of electronically stored information is requested, the CE is required to provide access if this can be accomplished in a reasonable manner and in an agreed on alternative electronic format (CFR 164.524).

Grounds for Denying an Individual's Access to PHI

The right to access regulation, 45 CFR 164.524, includes requirements for denying an individual access to PHI. Grounds for denial are unreviewable (denial without providing an opportunity to review or appeal the denial) or reviewable (may deny access but individual must be given right to have denials reviewed). Unreviewable grounds for denial include psychotherapy notes, correctional institutions or providers acting under the direction of a correctional institution, in some research studies, PHI obtained from someone other than a provider under promise of confidentiality, or PHI contained in records subject to the Federal Privacy Act. In these situations, a CE may deny an individual access. Health professionals are urged to read and examine the law carefully, as well as consult with their legal counsel, before denying access.

Uses and Disclosures Permitted by HIPAA

A CE is permitted, but not required, to use and disclose PHI without an individual's authorization for access to the individual or representative for the individual following the 2013 HIPAA Omnibus Rule. The Omnibus Rule covers other instances where use and disclosure can be done without authorization, treatment, payment, and healthcare operations (TPO). **Treatment** is the "provision, coordination, or management of health care and related services by one or more health care providers, including coordination or management of health care by a health care provider with a third party; consultation between health care provider relating to a patient or the referral of a patient for health care from one health care provider to another" (AHIMA 2014, 147). An example of treatment would be the freedom of healthcare providers from two separate organizations involved in an individual's care to discuss an individual's diagnosis, treatment, and prognosis.

Payment are "activities undertaken by a health plan to obtain premiums or to determine or fulfill its responsibility for coverage and provision of benefits under the health plan; or a health care provider or health plan to obtain or provide reimbursement for the provision of health care" (AHIMA 2014, 113). Billing, claims management and collection, utilization review, and reviewing healthcare services for medical necessity, coverage, or to justify charge are examples of payment activities.

Healthcare **operations** are "certain administrative, financial, legal, and quality improvement activities of a covered entity that are necessary to run its business and to support the core functions of treatment and payment" (45 CFR 164.506). Examples of operations include quality assessment and improvement activities, competency assurance activities, conducting or arranging for medical reviews, audits, or legal services; specified insurance functions such as underwriting, enrollment, and premium rating; business planning, development, management, and administration and business management and general administrative activities of the entity (Sullivan 2004).

Opportunity to Agree or Object

There must be a balance between the patient's right to control the use and disclosure of their health information but for it to still be available when and where needed. There are situations where the patients can indicate whether or not their information may be used or disclosed. Providers need the patient information for the treatment, payment, and operations and the patient cannot restrict this use. Instances where they can control the use include their name being included in the facility directory from which it might be given out to visitors, clergy, and those who contact the facility to see if they are a patient there. What patient information can be disclosed, and to whom (family, relatives, friends, or others), is identified by the individual (OCR 2013).

Incidental Use and Disclosure

There is a potential risk for an individual's health information to be disclosed incidentally due to established practices in healthcare communications and various environments. An example of this is in the emergency department where a patient or family member overhears a discussion between providers regarding the patient in the next treatment room. A use or disclosure of this nature is permitted as long as the CE has adopted reasonable safeguards as required by the HIPAA Privacy Rule. Reasonable safeguards include speaking quietly when discussing a patient's condition with family members in a public area such as a waiting room and avoiding the use of patient names in public places. In addition, proactive measures such as training and posting signs to remind employees to protect patient confidentiality are also reasonable safeguards (OCR 2003).

Public Interest and Benefit Activities

The Privacy Rule permits use and disclosure of patient information as it relates to national priority issues where there are important uses of health information outside the context of direct patient care and treatment. Twelve public interest purposes are identified in the Privacy Law and must be reported when required by law, for public health activities, serious threats to health or safety, and research. All 12 public interest purposes are identified and explained with special conditions or limitations in the Privacy Law 42 CFR 164.512 as special conditions or limitations may apply. The public interest purposes are:

- ⊙ Required by law: statute, regulation, court orders
- ⊙ Public health activities: for preventing or controlling disease, subject to FDA regulation, cases of communicable disease, and work-related illness or injury and surveillance
- ⊙ Victims of abuse, neglect, or domestic violence when necessary
- ⊙ Health oversight activities: for legally authorized activities including audits and investigations related to the healthcare system and governmental benefit programs
- ⊙ Judicial and administrative proceedings: with appropriate notice to the individual or protective order provided
- ⊙ Law enforcement purposes: with conditions that must be met for the disclosure
- ⊙ Decedents: for identifying or determining cause of death
- ⊙ Cadaveric organ, eye, or tissue donation: to facilitate the donation and transplantation
- ⊙ Research: when privacy rule definition is met and in specific instances
- ⊙ Serious threat to health or safety: to prevent or lessen a serious imminent threat to person or public
- ⊙ Essential government functions: those authorized by law for proper execution of a military mission or conducting intelligence and national security activities
- ⊙ Worker's compensation: as allowed by applicable laws (42 CFR 164.512)

Limited Data Set

A **limited data set** is "PHI that excludes direct identifiers of the individual and the individual's relatives, employers, or household members but still does not deidentify the information" (AHIMA 2014). Limited data sets may be used for research, public health, or healthcare operations provided that the recipient of the data set enters into a data use agreement that requires the recipient to safeguard the information.

Authorized Uses and Disclosures

As a general rule, a **valid authorization** must be obtained by the CE for the disclosure of PHI unless the PHI is for TPO or other allowable uses as stated in the Privacy Rule. The 2013 Final rule updated the Privacy Rule and included items that afforded more protections to PHI while expanding individuals' rights to control and access their health information. The changes included requiring a reasonable cost-based allowable fee for patients to obtain a copy of their records, provided in a format desired, and streamlining the request process where a signature is not required and the reason for use may not be required in some instances. Valid authorization must contain the following:

1. A description of the protected health information to be used or disclosed;

2. The person authorized to make the use or disclosure;

3. The person to whom the covered entity may make the requested use or disclosure;

4. Expiration date; and

5. In some cases, the purpose for the use or disclosure of the information (HHS 2016a).

Other core elements that may be in a valid authorization are a statement of right to revoke; a statement regarding the possibility of redisclosure; a statement specifying that treatment, payment, enrollment, and eligibility for benefits cannot be denied when the individual declines to sign an authorization; and a copy of the signed authorization if provided to the individual when authorization for the use and disclosure is sought by the covered entity. One purpose of the authorization is to ensure that the CE and the individual fully understand the confidential relationship boundaries and what information is to be disclosed.

Denial of Access

Access to PHI may be denied with the right, in some cases, for the denial to be reviewed by a licensed professional who was not a part of the original determination of the request. Certain limited explicit situations are considered to be unreviewable, which means that the denial remains with no further review of the request. These situations are requests:

- For psychotherapy notes or information compiled for potential legal proceedings.
- By an inmate for a copy of PHI where the covered entity is a correctional institution, or provider acting at direction of the institution, and the copy would jeopardize the health, safety, security, custody, or rehabilitation of the inmate or other inmates, or safety of correctional officers, employees, or others at the institution or responsible for transporting the inmate. The inmate retains the right to inspect the PHI.

⊙ That are in a designated record set part of a research study still in progress that includes treatment (for example, clinical trial) provided the consent to participate in the study required the individual to agree to a temporary suspension of access. The right of access is reinstated when the study is completed.

⊙ For PHI in records protected by the Privacy Act such as those under the control of a federal agency, if the denial is consistent with the Privacy Act requirements.

⊙ Where the requested information was obtained by someone other than a healthcare provider such as a family member of the individual who was assured confidentiality, and the source of the information would reasonably be revealed if access granted (OCR 2013).

Right to Authorize Access to PHI

The person who consented to the treatment, typically an adult patient who is mentally and physically competent, can also authorize access to the PHI. Other parties who can authorize access include

⊙ A parent, guardian, or custodian of a minor patient under 18 years of age

⊙ A parent, guardian, or custodian of an incompetent patient

⊙ Legal healthcare representative

⊙ Power of attorney for healthcare

⊙ Personal representative or executor or administrator of a deceased patient's estate

The other parties mentioned here are considered to be the personal representative for the patient and are authorized to make healthcare decisions.

Authorization for Psychotherapy Notes

An authorization is required for psychotherapy notes with the exception of carrying out the following treatment, payment, or healthcare operations listed in 45 CFR 164.508(a)(2):

⊙ Use by the originator of the psychotherapy notes for treatment;

⊙ Use or disclosure by the covered entity for its own training and to defend itself in a legal action or other proceeding brought by the individual, for HHS investigations or to determine compliance, to avert threats to public safety, to an oversight agency and for lawful activities of a coroner or medical examiner (HHS 2013).

Psychotherapy and other types of records, including those related to substance abuse, mental health, and other sensitive conditions, may be subject to either federal or state regulations above and beyond the HIPAA regulations.

Minimum Necessary Requirement

To be in compliance with HIPAA, a covered entity must have policies and procedures in place that limit the protected information to be disclose only to the amount necessary to achieve the purpose of the disclosure, the **minimum necessary**. This requires reasonable efforts to see, disclose, and request only the minimum amount of protected health information needed to accomplish the intended purpose of the use, disclosure, or request (45 CFR 164.502(b)).

Exceptions to the minimum necessary requirement are:

- ⊙ Disclosures to or requests by a healthcare provider for treatment
- ⊙ Uses or disclosures made to the individual
- ⊙ Uses or disclosures made pursuant to an authorization
- ⊙ Disclosures made to HHS for complaint investigation, compliance review or enforcement
- ⊙ Uses or disclosures required by law
- ⊙ Uses or disclosures required for compliance with other applicable requirements of HIPAA Transactions Rule or other HIPAA Administrative Simplification Rules (45 CFR 164.502)

The minimum necessary information provided should be enough to address the intended purpose of the request but should also limit unnecessary or inappropriate information from being provided. The requirement was written with the minimum necessary words to allow it to be flexible to cover the many various circumstances associated with the request. The intent of updates to the HIPAA law was to provide more protection for the PHI while granting a greater level of control to the individual. This is in great contrast to the "any and all information" requests that were received in the past.

Check Your Understanding 12.2

Indicate whether each of the following is true or false.

1. In order to be compliant with HIPAA, all releases of PHI require a signed authorization to be legal.
2. Patients have an unconditional right to access their health information.
3. Appropriately deidentified health information is not subject to the HIPAA regulations.
4. If a patient revokes their authorization for releasing information, the covered entity or business associate can no longer rely on that authorization for releasing PHI.
5. The minimum necessary standard presumes that all information in a record needs to be included when any information is requested.

Match each term to the correct definition.

- a. Deidentified information
- b. Designated record set
- c. Healthcare operations
- d. Limited data set
- e. Minimum necessary
- f. e-Protected health information

6. _____ Individually identifiable health information that is transmitted by electronic media or maintained in electronic media

7. _____ Used for many activities by the CE for such things as quality assessment, competency assurance, medical reviews, certain insurance functions, and business administration and planning

8. _____ Medical records maintained by or for a provider for treatment, enrollment, and payment

9. _____ Neither identifies nor has a reasonable basis to identify

10. _____ That which is reasonably necessary to achieve the purpose of disclosure

11. _____ PHI where specific direct identifiers of individuals, relatives and employers have been removed

⊙ Other Legal Considerations

Prior to HIPAA many privacy protection regulations were at the state level. There were inconsistencies in these regulations between states and many states did not have any regulations. HIPAA, specifically the Privacy Law, provides a primary source of regulations for securing the privacy of protected health information and HIPAA. Changes made with the enactment of HITECH and the 2013 Ombudsman Act updated and refined portions of HIPAA. The 2013 final rule improved an individual's privacy protections, provided new rights for access to PHI, and gave the government greater capacity to enforce the law. Other considerations to consider for PHI are covered briefly here.

Pre-emption of State Law

Laws regarding privacy standards are at the federal level (HIPAA) and many states have privacy regulations as well. When there is a law at both levels, one of the laws must **pre-empt** or take precedence over the other law. State laws that are contrary to the Privacy Rule are generally pre-empted by the federal requirements, which means that the federal requirements will apply (45 CFR 160.202). As addressed in the HIPAA regulations, state law will prevail if it meets one or more of the following purposes:

1. Relates to the privacy of individually identifiable health information and provides greater privacy protections or privacy rights with respect to such information,

2. Provides for the reporting of disease or injury, child abuse, birth, or death, or for public health surveillance, investigation, or intervention, or

3. Requires certain health plan reporting, such as for management or financial audits (45 CFR 160.203)

In short, as with most things related to the HIPAA Privacy Rule, whether the state or federal law has precedence is complex and must be considered on a case-by-case basis with a different decision applicable in each state. For example, a state law requires that psychologists obtain a consent from new patients for disclosure of information whereas HIPAA does not. In this case the state law prevails because it provides more protection for the PHI.

e-Discovery

Traditionally, patient medical records documented much-needed information to support the medical care provided to the patient. Much more information is captured with electronic systems about the record itself, not just the healthcare data related to the care provided. This type of information is referred to as metadata and is the descriptive data that explains other data. In the context of the EHR metadata can include the dates for the day the data was created, sent, or received or last accessed or modified. **E-discovery** refers to the Federal Rules of Civil Procedures and Uniform Rules Relating to Discovery of Electronically Stored Information. These rules address electronic information that is not usually considered a part of the legal EHR of a facility and is subject to motion for compulsory discovery. Audit trails, the source code of the program, metadata, and other electronic information are all electronically stored information and subject to discovery (AHIMA 2014).

Preparation for response to requests is paramount. Requests are increasing for health records along with the associated metadata. Preparation for these kind of requests include becoming as familiar with the EHR system as possible to identify when documented EHR events actually occurred, what is and is not accessible, and policies and procedures related to the creation, utilization, maintenance, retention, and destruction of the information (Dimick 2007). Revision of the information management plan including the schedules for storage, retention, and destruction to address items specific to e-discovery should be done. A number of policies and procedures will need to be updated or developed to support the information management plan. A legal hold policy, procedures, and employee training are important aspects of preparing for the eventual receipt of a request for the record and related metadata. A **legal hold** is "a communication issued because of current or anticipated litigation, audit, government investigation, or other such matters that suspend the normal disposition or processing of records" (AHIMA 2014, 87). A legal hold for a paper health record can be locking it in a drawer to be preserved from alteration, changes, and such that are of concern when the record may be requested for legal purposes. With the EHR, there may be multiple systems, accessible to many authorized users, plus the metadata and other information that can be maintained in the EHR system so there needs to be a means of freezing or preserving the record from potential alterations or destruction of the health record itself plus the metadata. This process will involve communication with IT with a hold, freeze, preservation, or similar kind of notice and they will then complete the steps necessary to preserve the record at a specific point in time.

Case Study: Litigation and Metadata

A malpractice lawsuit was filed against a hospital in 2002 questioning the competency of a surgeon for performing the surgery that was done, which left the patient with a severe permanent complication. In reviewing the records obtained through e-discovery, issues in the anesthesia record were noted that changed the focus of the lawsuit to the anesthesiologist rather than the surgeon. There were 90 minutes where no vital signs were recorded and the anesthesiologist documented his presence for the entirety of the surgery (7 hours) just minutes after the beginning of the surgery. This information was found due to the presence of time stamps embedded in the system. Although the anesthesiologist was present for the total time of the surgery, he recorded his surgery notes for the whole time at the beginning of the surgery, instead of as the events occurred. The complication suffered by the patient was not likely to have been caused or affected by the shortcomings identified in the data. Because it was known that the metadata could be used to discredit the anesthesiologist, the hospital settled the case with the patient prior to the case being heard in court (Dimick 2007).

This case illustrates how having the metadata available for consideration in litigation can change the focus of a whole case. The original claim of malpractice against the hospital for incompetence by the surgeon was going to be difficult to prove due to the diminished state of the patient before surgery followed by a lengthy procedure. It was found that there were issues of documentation during the surgical procedure that were discovered with review of the metadata. This changed the focus of the case from the surgeon to the anesthesiologist and even though his documentation issues did not cause the patient's complication, this information was enough to discredit his competency and the case was settled by the hospital. The care provided was good but the issue with the timing of the documentation cast doubt on the quality.

⊙ Administrative Requirements for Covered Entities

There are several administrative requirements that must be met to be in compliance with HIPAA and the HITECH Act. These requirements include policies and procedures to comply with the HIPAA Privacy Rule, notices of privacy practice, data safeguards, mitigation protocol, designation of a privacy officer, workforce training, and accounting of disclosures.

Notice of Privacy Practices

The **Notice of Privacy Practices (NPP)** is an essential statement by a healthcare organization that informs individuals of the uses and disclosures of patient-identifiable health information that may be made by the organization, as well as the individual's rights and the organizations legal duties with respect to that information (AHIMA 2014). The NPP is an important tool to help patients understand their rights. Many models of NPP are available at the Health IT website for facilities to refer to when preparing their own but care should be taken to assure the final NPP is specific to that organization (HealthIT 2016).

Safeguards

Covered entities are required to ensure appropriate administrative, technical, and physical safeguards to protect the privacy of PHI (45 CFR 164.530(c)). Reasonable safeguards for paper records include isolating and locking file cabinets or record storage rooms. Safeguards for EHRs include passwords, firewalls, and workstation cubicles.

Mitigation

To the extent realistic, covered entities must mitigate known harmful effects due to use or disclosure of protected health information (45 CFR 164.530). **Mitigation** is the process of moderating the severity and potential harmful effects to an organization from wrongful use and disclosure. The protocol establishes a plan for potential courses of action which may include such steps as extending an apology, disciplining the responsible party, updating procedures, and gestures of good public relations (AHIMA 2014, 97).

Training

Training in HIPAA policies and procedures regarding PHI is required for all workforce members to carry out their job functions appropriately. The training should be ongoing and documented for each employee.

Privacy Official

Per 45 CFR 164.530(a)(1), a CE must designate a person to be responsible for developing and implementing privacy policies and procedures. This may be a full-time position or can be a responsibility added to another's job duties. There must also be a contact person or office responsible for receiving complaints.

Accounting of Disclosures: HIPAA and HITECH

HIPAA was written to provide individuals with a right to an **accounting of disclosures** regarding PHI. Disclosure is defined as "the release, transfer, provision of access to, or divulging in any other manner of information outside the entity holding the information" (45 CFR 164.501). The request for an accounting of disclosures is allowed within the six-year period prior to the individual's request. Exceptions to the accounting of disclosures rule are

1. For treatment, payment, or healthcare operations
2. PHI given to individual
3. Incidental or otherwise permitted or required
4. Pursuant to an authorization
5. For use in a facility directory
6. To meet national security or intelligence purposes
7. To correctional institutions or law enforcement officials

8. Disclosure made as part of a limited data set

9. Disclosure that occurred before the HIPAA privacy compliance date (45 CFR 164.528(a)(1))

Information that must be included in the accounting report is the date of disclosure, name and address of the entity or person who received the information, and a brief statement of the purpose of the disclosure or, in lieu of such statement, a copy of a written request for disclosure (45 CFR 164.528(b)). The time to respond to a request for accounting is 60 days and may be extended once by no more than 30 days. A CE cannot charge a fee for the first accounting request by an individual. For each subsequent request, a reasonable, cost-based fee may be charged. Documentation regarding accounting of disclosures must be kept for six years (45 CFR 164.528(d)).

The HITECH Act of 2009 provided individuals new rights regarding the accounting of disclosures as listed here.

⊙ Disclosure to carry out treatment, payment, and healthcare operations no longer exempt if disclosure is made through an EHR.

⊙ Period accounting of disclosure requirement shortened to three years prior to the request.

⊙ When a BA makes a disclosure via an EHR for purposes of treatment, payment, and healthcare operations on behalf of the CE, either be included in the report on disclosure by the CE, or for the CE to provide requestor with a list of all BAs in the requested time period (this is later changed in the requirements).

⊙ Regulations governing information is collected about the disclosures taking into account the interests of the individual versus the administrative burden on the provider of the accounting.

⊙ Requirements for an accounting of disclosures issued in an accounting of disclosures regulation and included in EHR certification criteria.

⊙ Compliance date requirements specifying EHRs acquired by "CEs after January 1, 2009, is January 1, 2011, or the date that it acquires an EHR, whichever is later. For CEs that acquired EHRs prior to January 1, 2009, the effective date is January 1, 2014. The state authorized the Secretary to extend both of these compliance deadlines to no later than 2013 and 2016, respectively " (HHS 2011)

⊙ Breach Notification Audit Program

National standards for the privacy and security of PHI were established with HIPAA. Breach notification requirements were added by the HITECH Act to provide increased transparency for those whose information could be at risk. Periodic audits related to compliance by the BAs and CEs became a required activity to be conducted by the HHS Office for Civil Rights (OCR). Phase 1 of the program involved implementation of a pilot program for the assessment of implemented controls and processes followed by a comprehensive evaluation review of the pilot program. Phase 2 of the program went into effect in 2016 for the next phase of audits to analyze implemented policies and procedures of designated standards and specifications of CEs and BAs.

Breach Audit Protocol

The reviews for Phase 2 will be based on an updated audit protocol that reflects the 2013 Omnibus Final Rule. An example of the audit protocol for one section to be audited is shown in table 12.3.

The audit program is important for meeting compliance requirements and provides means to assess compliance activities that are being carried out by the covered entities and business associates. The audits also provide information on the processes of how they are meeting compliance, discover issues that may not have been recognized through the investigation of breach complaints, and aid in the development of best practices all of which will improve the CEs and BAs with compliancy in the future.

⊙ Individual Rights Regarding Health Information

AHIMA is committed to the advocacy and protection of consumers with regard to their health information. The *AHIMA Consumer Health Information Bill of Rights* provides a model for protecting health information principles as shown in figure 12.3.

⊙ Genetic Information

Genetic testing has become almost commonplace in healthcare. However, genetic information is not always understood, even by healthcare professionals. Because of the complexities of the information, as well as the potential consequences, Genetic Information Nondiscrimination Act (GINA) was passed in 2008. GINA prohibits discrimination based on genetic information by health insurers related to eligibility, coverage, underwriting, or premium-setting decisions (Brodnik et al. 2012). Employers, employment agencies, labor organizations, and others are also prohibited from using genetic information for making employment decisions

Figure 12.3.   AHIMA Consumer Health Information Bill of Rights

An individual has the right to:

1. Look at their health information and/or get a paper or electronic copy of it
2. Accurate and complete health information
3. Ask for changes to their health information
4. Know how their health information is used or shared and who receives it
5. Ask for limitations on the use and release of their health information
6. Expect their health information to be private and secure
7. Be informed about privacy and security breaches of their health information
8. File a complaint or report a violation regarding their health information

Source: AHIMA 2015

Table 12.3.   Audit protocol for HIPAA Section 164.502(i)

Audit type	Section	Key activity	Established performance criteria	Audit inquiry	Required/ addressable
Privacy	§164. 502(i)	Uses and disclosures consistent with notice	§164.502(i) Standard: Uses and disclosures consistent with notice: A covered entity that is required by §164.520 to have a notice may not use or disclose protected health information in a manner inconsistent with such notice. A covered entity that is required by §164.520(b)(1)(iii) to include a specific statement in its notice if it intends to engage in an activity listed in §164.520(b) (1)(iii)(A)–(C) may not use or disclose protected health information for such activities, unless the required statement is included in the notice.	Are uses and disclosures made by the covered entity consistent with its notice of privacy practices?

Inquire of management whether uses and disclosures of PHI are consistent with the entity's notice of privacy practices.

Obtain and review policies and procedures regarding uses and disclosures.

Evaluate whether the uses and disclosures of PHI are consistent with the entity's notice of privacy practices. | |

Source: HHS 2016b

(Brodnik et al. 2012, 344–345). This law has now been included in the 2013 HIPAA Omnibus amendments related to GINA to further define the terms health plan, underwriting purposes, and genetic information. Continued diligence in protecting the health information of consumers' genetic testing technologies is required as the uses for genetic information continue to evolve.

Chapter 12 Review Exercises

Answer the following questions.

1. State laws can pre-empt HIPAA:
    a. If the state law was written first, before HIPAA
    b. At the discretion of the facility and written in hospital policy
    c. If they are more stringent than HIPAA
    d. Never; HIPAA always prevails

2. An accounting of disclosures must be maintained in which of the following situations:
    a. Identifiable health information for use in the facility's internal operations
    b. Patient identifiable information released to external entities
    c. In both of the above situations
    d. Neither of these situations

3. Which of the following will not allow state law to prevail over HIPAA law?
    a. Necessary to prevent fraud and abuse related to payments
    b. Purpose is to regulate manufacture, registration, and distribution of controlled substances
    c. Where it provides means for the reporting of diseases, injury, child abuse, birth, or death
    d. When state laws are contrary to the Privacy Rule

4. Data safeguards, mitigation protocol, and designation of a privacy offer are:
    a. Physical safeguards
    b. Administrative requirements
    c. Policies and procedures
    d. At the discretion of the facility

5. E-discovery is:
    a. Making a request for copies of the EHR
    b. A legal discovery
    c. Related to electronically stored information
    d. Requesting for copies of requested information be provided electronically

6. Genetic information can be used:
    a. For insurance coverage decisions
    b. For employment consideration
    c. As a part of a patient's PHI
    d. To establish insurance rates

7. The primary focus of phase 2 of the breach audit protocol is:
   a. Compliance
   b. Monitoring notices of privacy practices
   c. Assessing controls and processes
   d. Reviewing policies and procedures

Discussion.

8. Briefly explain what is the intent of the breach notification audit program.

9. Explain the differences between the use and disclosure of PHI.

10. Discuss the intent of the HIPAA Privacy Rule.

REFERENCES

42 CFR 164.512: Privacy Law. 2013.

42 CFR 493.3(a)(2): Laboratory requirements. 2013.

45 CFR 160.103: Definitions. 2013.

45 CFR 160.202: Definitions. 2013.

45 CFR 160.203: General rule and exceptions. 2013.

45 CFR 162.103. Definitions. 2015.

45 CFR 164.308(b)(1): Administrative safeguards. 2013.

45 CFR 164.501: Definitions. 2013.

45 CFR 164.502: Uses and disclosures of protected health information: General rules. 2013.

45 CFR 164.502(b): Uses and disclosures of protected health information: General rules. 2013.

45 CFR 164.504: Uses and disclosures: Organizational requirements. 2013.

45 CFR 164.506: Uses and disclosures for treatment, payment and operations: General rules. 2013.

45 CFR 164.508: Uses and disclosures for which an authorization is required. 2013.

45 CFR 164.508(a)(2): Uses and disclosures for which an authorization is required. 2013.

45 CFR 164.514(b): Implementation specifications. 2013.

45 CFR 164.524: Access of individuals to protected health information. 2013.

45 CFR 164.528(a)(1): Accounting of disclosures of protected health information. 2013.

45 CFR 164.528(b): Accounting of disclosures of protected health information. 2013.

45 CFR 164.528(d): Accounting of disclosures of protected health information. 2013.

45 CFR 164.530(a)(1): Administrative requirements. 2013.

45 CFR 164.530(c): Administrative requirements. 2013.

45 CFR 164.530(f): Standard: Mitigation. 2013.

AHIMA. 2015. *Consumer Health Information Bill of Rights.* http://bok.ahima.org/Pdf View?oid=107674.

AHIMA. 2014. *Pocket Glossary of Health Information Management and Technology*. 4th ed. Chicago: AHIMA.

Belfort, R. 2010. *HITECH Raises the Stakes on HIPAA Compliance*. https://www.manatt.com/insights/newsletters/health-update/client-alert-%c2%a0hitech-raises-the-stakes-on-hipaa-co.

Brodnik, M., L. Rinehart-Thompson, and R. Reynolds. 2012. *Fundamentals of Law for Health Informatics and Information Management*, 2nd ed. Chicago: AHIMA.

Department of Health and Human Services. 2016a. *Individuals' Right under HIPAA to Access their Health Information 45* CFR § 164.524. Health Information Privacy. http://www.hhs.gov/hipaa/for-professionals/privacy/guidance/access/index.htmlHIPAA Administrative Simplification Statute and Rules. http://www.hhs.gov/ocr/privacy/hipaa/administrative/index.html.

Department of Health and Human Services. 2016b. *HIPAA Privacy, Security, and Breach Notification Audit Program*. http://www.hhs.gov/hipaa/for-professionals/compliance-enforcement/audit/protocol/index.html.

Department of Health and Human Services. 2013. *Uses and Disclosures for Treatment, Payment, and Health Care Operations*. http://www.hhs.gov/hipaa/for-professionals/privacy/guidance/disclosures-treatment-payment-health-care-operations/index.html.

Department of Health and Human Services. 2011. HIPAA Privacy Rule accounting of disclosures under the Health Information Technology for Economic and Clinical Health Act. *Federal Register* 76(104):31426–31449.

Dimick, C. 2007. e-Discovery: preparing for the coming rise in electronic discovery requests. *Journal of AHIMA* 78:24–29.

Health Insurance Portability and Accountability Act of 1996. Public Law 104-191.

Health IT. 2016. *Model Notices of Privacy Practices*. Privacy and Security. https://www.healthit.gov/providers-professionals/model-notices-privacy-practices.

HIPAA Privacy Rule, Part 160, 2007. http://www.access.gpo.gov/nara/cfr/waisidx_07/45cfr160_07.html.

Office for Civil Rights, Department of Health and Human Services. 2013. Modifications to the HIPAA privacy, security, enforcement, and breach notification rules under the health information technology for economic and clinical health act and the genetic information nondiscrimination act; other modifications to the HIPAA rules. *Federal Register* 78(17):5566–5702.

Office for Civil Rights, Department of Health and Human Services. 2012. *Guidance Regarding Methods for De-identification of Protected Health Information in Accordance with the Health Insurance Portability and Accountability Act (HIPAA) Privacy Rule*. http://www.hhs.gov/ocr/privacy/hipaa/understanding/coveridentities/De-identification/hhs_deid_guidance.pdf.

Office for Civil Rights, Department of Health and Human Services. 2003. *Summary of the HIPAA Privacy Rule*. http://www.hhs.gov/ocr/privacy/hipaa/understanding/summary/privacysummary.pdf.

Sullivan, J. 2004. *HIPAA: A Practical Guide to the Privacy and Security of Health Data*. Hartford: American Bar Association.

ADDITIONAL RESOURCES

45 CFR 164.508(b)(2): Uses and disclosures for which an authorization is required. 2013.

45 CFR 164.510: Uses and disclosures requiring an opportunity for the individual to agree or to object. 2013.

45 CFR 164.514: Other requirements relating to uses and disclosures of protected health information. 2013.

45 CFR 164.514(b)(2): Other requirements relating to uses and disclosures of protected health information. 2013.

Breach Notification Rule 2009. http://www.hhs.gov/ocr/privacy/hipaa/administrative /breachnotificationrule/index.html.

Brocato, L., S. Emery, and J. McDavid. 2011. Keeping compliant: Managing rising risk in physician practices. *Journal of AHIMA* 82(11):32–35.

Centers for Medicare and Medicaid Services (CMS), Office of E-Health Standards and Services (OESS). 2008. *HIPAA Compliance Review Analysis and Summary of Results.* http://www.hhs.gov/ocr/privacy/hipaa/enforcement/cmscompliancerev08.pdf.

Department of Health and Human Services, Office for Civil Rights. 2003. *Protected Health Information.* http://www.hhs.gov/ocr/privacy/hipaa/understanding/training/udmn .pdf.

Guidance on Risk Analysis Requirements under the HIPAA Security Rule. 2010. http://www .hhs.gov/ocr/privacy/hipaa/administrative/securityrule/rafinalguidancepdf.pdf.

Heubusch, K. 2011. Access report: OCR tries subtraction through addition in accounting of disclosure rule. *Journal of AHIMA* 82(7):38–39.

HIPAA Compliance Review Analysis and Summary of Results. 2008. http://www.hhs.gov /ocr/privacy/hipaa/enforcement/cmscompliancerev08.pdf.

Ouellette, P. 20014. HIPAA Privacy Rule: Permitted PHI uses and disclosures. *Health IT Security.* http://healthitsecurity.com/news/hipaa-privacy-rule-permitted-phi-uses -and-disclosures.

Recent Changes to HIPAA—the HITECH Act. 2009. http://www.lifespanrecycling.com /site/content/articles/RecentChangestoHIPAA-theHITECHAct.pdf.

13

Security for Health Information

Learning Objectives

- Interpret the HIPAA Security Rule
- Apply security risk analysis activities
- Analyze HIPAA Security Risk Safeguards
- Articulate the importance of confidentiality, integrity, and availability in regard to the HIPAA Security Rule
- Relate HIPAA Security Rule penalties and enforcement process
- Explain how HITECH modifies the HIPAA Security Rule
- Summarize medical identity theft and the potential impacts
- Develop plans for disaster preparedness

KEY TERMS

Addressable implementation
   specifications
Administrative safeguards
Availability
Breach
Break the glass
Business continuity planning (BCP)
Business impact analysis
Civil penalties
Cold site
Confidentiality
Criminal penalties
Disaster recovery planning (DRP)

Encryption
Health Information Technology for
   Economic and Clinical Health
   (HITECH) Act
HIPAA Enforcement Rule
Hot site
Integrity
Medical identify theft
Office for Civil Rights (OCR)
Physical safeguards
Recovery point objective (RPO)
Recovery time objective (RTO)
Red flags

Required implementation specifications
Risk
Sanctions policy
Security incident
Security Risk Analysis

Technical safeguards
Threat
Vulnerability
Warm site

Although there are many similarities between the Privacy and Security Rules, there are also notable differentiations. Where the HIPAA Privacy Rule protects all "individually identifiable health information" (45 CFR 160.103), in any form or media, whether electronic, paper, or oral, the Security Rule is singularly concerned with electronic protected health information (ePHI). The Security Rule covers all ePHI created, received, maintained, or transmitted by an organization (OCR 2010). This chapter will introduce specific guidelines to assure compliance with the security of the electronic health information. The enforcement of the guidelines will be covered as well as guidelines for handling breaches if they occur. HIPAA requires that the patient identifiable health information is protected and that the PHI is available as needed for the delivery of care. Consequently, protection against medical identify theft and disasters are two considerations for a facility to ensure that they will be able to have the correct information available in a timely manner to support patient care.

⊙ Security Rule

The Security Rule is grounded in the same reasonable language as its Privacy Rule counterpart. The required standards include required and addressable implementation specifications intended to provide covered entities (CEs) and business associates (BAs) with flexible, scalable, technology-neutral solutions and alternatives for complying with the standards. **Required implementation specifications** are not optional, but must be implemented in conformance with the regulation. The term addressable implementation specification does not imply that the specification is optional. **Addressable implementation specifications** should be implemented unless an organization determines that the specification is not reasonable and appropriate. If this is the case, then the organization must document why it is not reasonable and appropriate and adopt an equivalent measure if it is reasonable and appropriate to do so (45 CFR 164.306(d)(3)).

In addition to the extensive language in the Rule intended to secure ePHI, a **security incident** is defined as "the attempted or successful unauthorized access, use, disclosure, modification, or destruction of information or interference with system operations in an information system" (45 CFR 164.304). This definition is important as it serves as the method by which to evaluate reported Security Rule violations.

The foundational basis of a CE's and BA's information security program rests on its identification and management of potential risks to ePHI. The Security Rule outlines a broad set of regulations that include administrative, technical, and physical safeguards intended to ensure confidentiality, integrity, and availability of ePHI. Even in the best of situations, risk can turn into reality. For this reason, the Security Enforcement Rule outlines penalties and enforcement for violations of the Rule. Building on HIPAA, the **Health Information Technology for Economic and Clinical Health (HITECH) Act** outlines breach notification requirements and starts to lay the groundwork for additional protections as healthcare continues to move toward an integrated health information exchange environment.

Security Risk Analysis

The HIPAA Security Rule requires full evaluation of the methods, operational practices, and policies used by the CE to secure ePHI (45 CFR 164.302–318). CEs' and BAs' obligations in regard to risk analysis are outlined in 45 CFR 164.308(a)(1)(ii)(A). The **Security Risk Analysis** process provides CEs and BAs with the structural framework upon which to build their HIPAA Security Plan. CEs and BAs are required to conduct a Security Risk Analysis "to evaluate risks and vulnerabilities in their environment and to implement reasonable and appropriate measures to protect against reasonably anticipated threats or hazards to the security or integrity of the e-PHI" (OCR 2010).

The value of a risk analysis stems from its uniqueness to the specific organization in which it is conducted. Every organization is different and every risk analysis should reflect the unique and complex interrelationships between a multitude of systems, processes, and policies that in combination result in that specific organization's HIPAA Security Plan. For this very reason, the Security Rule is not prescriptive in requiring any specific method or approach for conducting the risk assessment. The Risk Analysis Final Guidance Document spells out some essential questions organizations should consider during the risk analysis process (OCR 2010). These questions arise from the National Institute of Standards and Technology (NIST) Special Publication (SP) 800-66 and include the following:

- ⊙ Have you identified the ePHI within your organization? This includes ePHI that you create, receive, maintain, or transmit.
- ⊙ What are the external sources of ePHI? For example, do vendors or consultants create, receive, maintain, or transmit ePHI?
- ⊙ What are the human, natural, and environmental threats to information systems that contain ePHI?(NIST SP 800-66 2008).

Vulnerabilities

The ultimate goal of the risk analysis process is to guide organizations in the decisions made and actions taken to comply with the Security Rule's standards and addressable or required implementation specifications. Although necessary to put the risk analysis discussion in context, the concepts of **vulnerability**, threats, and risks are not expressly defined in the Security Rule. The Risk Analysis Guidance Document again refers to the NIST SP 800-66 document to frame the risk analysis discussion. Vulnerability is defined as an inherent weakness or absence of a safeguard that could be exploited by a threat (AHIMA 2014, 152). Vulnerabilities are grouped into either technical or nontechnical categories. Technical vulnerabilities reflect inappropriate information systems that potentially provide the means for assault, harm, or unauthorized corruption.. Nontechnical vulnerabilities are demonstrated by such things as policy and procedure weaknesses.

Threats

A **threat** is the potential for exploitation of a vulnerability or potential danger to a computer, network, or data (AHIMA 2014, 145). Threats are grouped into three categories: natural, human, and environmental. Natural threats are often weather related and include tornados, floods, and the like. Human threats are broad in nature and can be intentional or unintentional. Access to information by unauthorized individuals is a good example of a human threat because this can occur through intentional actions of the user, or can result from an accidental key entry error that exposes information to an unauthorized user. Environmental threats center on power failure or chemical or other environmental agents with the potential to damage electronic data.

Risks

Risk is the probability of incurring injury or loss, the probable amount of loss foreseen by an insurer in issuing a contract, or a formal insurance term denoting liability to compensate individuals for injuries sustained in a healthcare facility (AHIMA 2014, 131).

Securing ePHI can be very costly and time consuming. It may not be possible to eliminate some threats and in those cases organizations must determine the extent of effort needed to reduce and mitigate the remaining risk. Figure 13.1 represents a

Figure 13.1.   The risk impact/probability chart

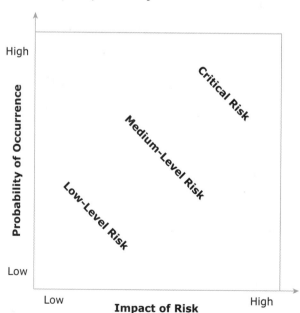

Source: Reproduced with permission from MindTools.com.

typical project management tool used to assist in the evaluation of the likelihood and impact of risks. As one can see from this illustration, when there is a low probability of the occurrence of a risk and the impact of the potential risk is low, the risk would then be considered to be a low-level risk. Conversely, if the probability of the risk is high along with a high impact due to the risk, the risk would then be considered critical.

Risk Analysis Methods

The Security Rule intentionally leaves the methods for conducting the required risk analysis to the discretion of the entity. Regardless of the methods selected for conducting and documenting the risk analysis, the Security Rule does mandate several elements that must be included in the analysis:

- Define scope of the risk analysis
- Identify means of data collection
- Identify and document potential threats and vulnerabilities
- Assess current security measures
- Determine the likelihood of threat occurrence
- Determine the potential impact of threat occurrence
- Determine the level of risk
- Finalize documentation
- Perform periodic review and updates to the risk assessment (45 CFR 164.308(a)(1))

Even though these elements must be included, they are to be considered a guide and a communication of the expectations. A healthcare facility should first consider its own characteristics and environment before proceeding with a risk analysis. Once this has been completed the healthcare facility can then determine the best way to conduct a risk analysis specific to itself and its situation while maintaining compliance with the mandated elements.

⊙ HIPAA Security Rule Safeguards

The Security Rule outlines a variety of safeguards necessary to ensure appropriate management and protection of ePHI. Working in concert, administrative, physical, and technical safeguards can produce the intended outcome of preserving the confidentiality, integrity, and availability of ePHI. Although the intent and approach of each of these forms of safeguards vary greatly from one another, each form of safeguard is necessary.

Administrative Safeguard Standards

Administrative safeguards are administrative actions and policies and procedures to manage the selection, development, implementation, and maintenance of security measures to protect ePHI and manage the conduct of the CE's or BA's workforce in relation to the protection of that information (AHIMA 2014, 4; 45 CFR 164.304 2013).

Security Management Process Standard

The administrative safeguards comprise over half of all the safeguards included in the Security Rule. Many believe the administrative safeguards are the most difficult to address as they rely heavily on human involvement to ensure compliance with the safeguards. The first standard in the administrative safeguards section of the Security Rule is the security management process, which is found at 45 CFR 164.308(a)(1). This broad standard has four required implementation specifications that include the previously discussed risk analysis, a required risk management element, a required sanctions policy, and a required information systems activity review element. The risk management implementation specification picks up where risk analysis left off and outlines how the identified risks will be managed. Two critical factors in the risk management process include communication of security processes and leadership involvement with risk mitigation.

The **sanctions policy** must outline how cases of noncompliance will be addressed within the organization knowing that even with a strong risk management plan, the potential for noncompliance (either intentional or nonintentional) still exists. Some of the components of sanctions policy are a discussion of the significance of noncompliance, examples of noncompliance, and a sliding scale of discipline based on the severity of the act of noncompliance.

The implementation specification requires CEs to "implement procedures to regularly review records of information system activity, such as audit logs, access reports, and security incident tracking reports" (CMS 2007a). Today's information systems have the ability to track and record a multitude of user activities, but unless specific measures are enacted by the organization to review these tracking progeny, security violations could go unnoticed. This implementation specification advises CEs to consider not only the technical abilities of their systems to create audit logs and reports, but also to address the nontechnical use of these tools through policy and procedures.

Security Officer

Assigned security responsibility is the second administrative safeguard standard detailed in 45 CFR 164.308(a)(2). This standard requires CEs to "identify the security official who is responsible for the development and implementation of the policies and procedures required by this subpart [the Security Rule] for the entity" (45 CFR 164.308(a)(2)). CEs must establish who in their organization is responsible for compliance with the Security Rule requirements. This position is similar in scope and responsibility to that of the privacy officer required by the HIPAA Privacy Rule. CEs may (but are not required to) appoint the same individual to fill the role of both the privacy and the security officer.

Workforce Security Standard

Workforce security (45 CFR 164.308(a)(3)) is the third administrative safeguard standard and has three associated addressable implementation specifications. This standard requires the organization to ensure that those with a legitimate need to access information are able to do so while at the same time ensuring that those workforce members who do not have a legitimate need to that information are prevented from gaining access.

The first implementation specification for this standard is authorization and supervision, which speaks to the unique needs of an organization based on size, function, and structure and spells out how each organization must determine each workforce member's level of access. The second implementation specification, workforce clearance procedures, states that CEs must "implement procedures to determine that the access of a workforce member to electronic protected health information is appropriate" (45 CFR 164.308(a)(3). The third implementation specification in this section is termination procedures, which challenges CEs to implement appropriate methods to ensure workforce members access privileges are removed when they terminate employment (willingly or unwillingly). This implementation specification also outlines the need to ensure changes in employee scope and function be addressed by policy and procedures that facilitate timely revisions to access level as indicated by position changes.

The workforce of an organization poses a particular risk in regard to security due to the ability of employees to access PHI and the innate nature of people's desire to know. Organizations address this risk with new employee orientation, policies and procedures, employee handbooks, continuing education, and monitoring and follow up. Although all of these are carried out in healthcare organizations, there continue to be instances of violations of the Security Rule.

The examples of data breaches listed here are just a few examples of the kinds of breaches that are commonly made by employees working in a healthcare facility:

⊙ An employee may have inappropriately accessed the health records of over 5,000 patients as determined by an internal audit. Compromised information included demographics such as insurance and Social Security numbers and treatment information. There was no indication that the information was disclosed or used. The employee was terminated per hospital policy.

⊙ Patient information (name, address, phone number, and birth date) was taken by a former employee when leaving employment from the facility. The affected patients were notified.

⊙ A health system employee accessed patient records inconsistent with her job functions using the information to file claims with other employees' health insurance companies. Compromised information included name, birth date, driver's license number, insurance information, clinical information and potentially Social Security numbers. Affected individuals were notified and the employee was terminated.

⊙ 14 employees of a clinic inappropriately accessed a patient's records as oftentimes done with celebrity or well-known patients. All employees were investigated to determine their role and level of participation in accessing the information and all disciplined with some terminated from employment.

- ⊙ A vendor's employee may have accessed patient information unrelated to job duties.

- ⊙ A hospital employee being investigated for identity theft was found to have hospital documents with patient information in his home (*Becker's Health IT and CIO Review* 2015 and 2016).

These information breaches are just a few examples of the many ways that many members of the workforce are a leading cause of PHI breaches. They have access to the EHR systems to meet the obligations of their job but that does not give them the right to access information on all patients and certainly not to use the PHI for personal gain. The workforce security safeguard is a crucial component for achieving compliance with the Security Rule.

Information Access Management Standard

The fourth administrative safeguard standard is the information access management standard (45 CFR 164.308(a)(4)). This standard works in tandem with 45 CFR 164.308(a)(3) to uphold the basic security tenet of restricting access to only those who need it to perform their jobs. However, this standard specifically calls out a required implementation specification for isolating healthcare clearinghouse functions to ensure that clearinghouses that are part of a larger organization have their own policies and procedures to segregate ePHI access from unauthorized access by the larger organization.

Two addressable implementation specifications for access authorization and access establishment and modification are also included in the information access management standard. In terms of access authorization, the previous workforce security standards established workforce member rights to access information; the access authorization implementation specification addresses the policies and procedures for granting access to ePHI. Parallels are also drawn between the workforce security implementation specifications and the authorization and access establishment and modification implementation specification. This implementation specification is "Implement policies and procedures that, based upon the entity's access authorization policies, establish, document, review, and modify a user's right of access to a workstation, transaction, program, or process" (45 CFR 164.308(a)(4)).

Security Awareness and Training Standard

The fifth administrative safeguard standard requires CEs to "implement a security awareness and training program for all members of its workforce (including management)" (45 CFR 164.308(a)(5)). Four addressable implementation specifications support this standard and provide ample flexibility for CEs to meet both the intent and spirit of this standard. This standard requires all existing workforce members to receive security training and periodic retraining as indicated by changing conditions and training for new staff.

Security reminders, protection from malicious software, log-in monitoring, and password management are the four addressable implementation specifications. Each of these addressable implementation specifications have a single requirement (if reasonable and appropriate for the CE), but the CE may choose from many options to meet the requirement. For instance, in the security reminder implementation specification, the requirement mandates the CE to implement periodic security updates. The organization can use print, electronic, or face-to-face reminders as the way to achieve this mandate. Security awareness and training specific to a workforce member's role in protecting the CE's information assets from potential damage resulting from malicious software is addressable. Monitoring system log-ins is used to help detect and prevent unauthorized access to information and includes such techniques as locking out users who enter their log-in name incorrectly more than once. In the password protection implementation specification, CEs must have appropriate policies and procedures in place to create, change, and safeguard passwords.

Security Incident Procedures Standard

The security incident procedures standard states that CEs must "implement policies and procedures to address security incidents" (45 CFR 164.308(a)(6)). The numerous preceding standards are all foundational supports that enable the achievement of this standard. Response and reporting is the single required implementation specification that states CEs must "identify and respond to suspected or known security incidents; mitigate, to the extent practicable, harmful effects of security incidents that are known to the covered entity; and document security incidents and their outcomes" (45 CFR 164.308(a)(6)). Among others, some examples of security incidents include such things as lost or stolen passwords, information system virus attacks, and theft of electronic media storage devices.

Contingency Plan Standard

The contingency plan standard is central to being able to ensure availability of data. This standard requires CEs to "establish (and implement as needed) policies and procedures for responding to an emergency or other occurrence (for example, fire, vandalism, system failure, and natural disaster) that damages systems that contain electronic protected health information" (45 CFR 164.308(a)(7)).

This standard is supported by three required and two addressable implementation specifications. The required data backup plan implementation specification requires CEs to "establish and implement procedures to create and maintain retrievable exact copies of electronic protected health information" (45 CFR 164.308 (a)(7)). To meet this implementation specification, organizations have to document what data needs to be backed up, and must understand the sources of all of that data. The disaster recovery plan implementation specification is also required and mandates CEs to "establish (and implement as needed) procedures to restore any loss of data" (45 CFR 164.308 (a)(7)). For the development of such a plan, a facility must determine the potential means of loss for their specific facility and location. Fire, water, and system destruction losses might be common among most organizations but loss due to tornadoes and hurricanes would be more specific to the geographic area. The required emergency mode operation plan implementation specification demands that CEs "establish (and implement as needed) procedures to enable continuation of critical business processes for protection of the security of electronic protected health information while operating in emergency mode" (45 CFR 164.308(a)(7)). Prior to developing these procedures, the critical business processes must be identified as a first step before the procedures can be developed.

Testing and revisions procedures are the first of the two addressable implementation specifications in this section. Where this implementation specification is reasonable and appropriate for a CE it must "implement procedures for periodic testing and revision of contingency plans" (45 CFR 164.308(a)(7)). This implementation specification applies to data backup plans, disaster recovery plans, and emergency mode operations. Many factors may influence the frequency and comprehensiveness of the testing and revisions procedures. Some of these factors include the organization's size as well as the availability of financial and human resources. Application and data criticality analysis is the second addressable implementation specification falling under this standard. When this implementation specification is deemed reasonable and appropriate for the specific CE, then it must "assess the relative criticality of specific applications and data in support of other contingency plan components" (45 CFR 164.308(a)(7)). In essence, this specification compels organizations to truly understand the value of their systems and to balance recovery and management efforts to the criticality level of each system in the organization. Procedures must also be in place for assessing the systems as new ones are added or any other changes made in the normal operations of the systems.

Evaluation Standard

The eighth standard of the administrative safeguards is referred to as the "evaluation" standard (45 CFR 164.308(a)(8)). This standard is singular in requirement and has no supporting implementation specifications. It requires CEs to

> perform a periodic technical and nontechnical evaluation, based initially upon the standards implemented under this rule and subsequently, in response to environmental or operations changes affecting the security of electronic protected health information, that establishes the extent to which an entity's security policies and procedures meet the requirements of this subpart of the Security Rule (45 CFR 164.308(a)(8)).

The constant advances in technology and the growing use of new technologies are just two reasons demonstrating the need for this standard. An ongoing evaluation process is most likely to meet the spirit of this regulation, but the complexity of integrated health information technology often limits such an approach. The evaluation standard recognizes the limitations organizations may face in using an ongoing evaluation tool and supports alternative approaches provided they meet the intent of this standard.

Business Associate Contracts and Other Arrangements Standard

45 CFR 164.308(b)(1) is the final standard in the administrative safeguards section of the Security Rule; it addresses BAs. By definition, a business associate is, according

to the HIPAA Privacy Rule, (1) an individual (or group) who is not a member of a CE's workforce but who helps the CE in the performance of various functions involving the use or disclosure of individually identifiable health information, or (2) a person or organization other than a member of a CE's workforce that performs functions or activities on behalf of or affecting a CE that involve the use or disclosure of individually identifiable health information (AHIMA 2014).

In January 2013 a final omnibus rule went into effect to provide greater protections for patient information than were in the original Health Insurance Portability and Accountability Act (HIPAA) of 1996 (OCR 2016a). The changes were, in part, to address items from the American Recovery and Reinvestment Act (ARRA) of 2009 and the Genetic Information Nondiscrimination Act (GINA) of 2008. One of the four final rules was to "make business associates of covered entities directly liable for compliance with certain of the HIPAA Privacy and Security Rules' requirements" (OCR 2016a). The final rule modified business associates to include health information organizations (HIO), e-prescribing gateways, and other persons who facilitate data transmissions, as well as vendors of personal health records.

Specific items that were addressed included that BAs must

- Follow the Security Rule for ePHI.
- Have business associate agreements (BAAs) with their subcontractors who must also follow the security rule for ePHI. CEs do not have BAAs with these subcontractors.
- Obtain authorization prior to marketing (AHIMA 2013).

There is much implied under the first item regarding following the Security Rule. This means that the BA must follow all of the requirements of the rule just as the CEs do. They will need to have their security procedures in place, assess them, have BAAs with their subcontractors, and report breaches or potential breaches of information, to name a few of their new responsibilities.

Check Your Understanding 13.1

Answer the following questions.

1. An inherent weakness or absence of a safeguard that could be exploited by a threat is a
   a. Security incident
   b. Breach
   c. Vulnerability
   d. Threat

2. The Security Rule safeguards are to address:
   a. All ePHI
   b. All patient records, paper and electronic
   c. The records being exchanged electronically
   d. Workforce working with patient records

3. Which one of the following is an administrative safeguard action?
   a. Facility access control
   b. Documentation retention guidelines
   c. Maintenance record
   d. Media reuse

4. The data backup plan requires that organizations
   a. Know what data needs to be backed up and sources of that data
   b. Create nightly data backup procedures
   c. Utilize off-site storage
   d. Act in accordance with the contingency plan

5. Which of the following is not a requirement of risk analysis?
   a. A full evaluation of the methods
   b. A full evaluation of the operational practices
   c. A full evaluation of the policies
   d. A full evaluation of the standard process

Indicate whether each of the following is true or false.

6. The Security Rule specifies the methods for conducting the required risk analysis.

7. The required implementation specification for the security incident procedures standard is response and reporting.

8. Addressable implementation specifications are optional for the facility to implement.

9. In a security risk analysis, the entity does not have to be concerned with the external sources of ePHI.

Physical Safeguards Standards

The Security Rule defines **physical safeguards** as "physical measures, policies, and procedures to protect a covered entity's electronic information systems and related buildings and equipment, from natural and environmental hazards, and unauthorized intrusion" (45 CFR 164.310; CMS 2007b). These standards are far reaching as they require CEs to consider all physical access to the organization's ePHI. Like the administrative safeguards standards, the physical safeguards standards also have addressable and required implementation specifications. Where a CE deems an implementation specification to be reasonable and appropriate for their organization, they must then fulfill the addressable or required specifications.

Facility Access Control Standard

The facility access control standard requires CEs to "Implement policies and procedures to limit physical access to its electronic housed, information systems and the facility or facilities in which they are housed, while ensuring that properly authorized access is allowed" (45 CFR 164.310(a)(1)). Important to this discussion is an understanding of what the term facility means. For the purposes of the Security Rule, the definition of facility is "the physical premises and the interior and exterior of a building" (45 CFR 164.310(a)(1)). The four addressable implementation specifications for this section of the Rule are: contingency operations, security plan, access control and validation procedures, and maintenance records.

The contingency operation addressable implementation specification requires CEs to "establish (and implement as needed) procedures that allow facility access in support of restoration of lost data under the disaster recovery plan and emergency mode operations plan in the event of an emergency" (45 CFR 164.310(a) (1)). Contingency operations are complex and will vary from organization to organization with the intent being that CEs have the flexibility to determine the best approach for their given situation.

The facility security plan is the second addressable implementation specification under this standard. The intent of this implementation specification is that the facility security plan is to document the use of access controls. The CE is required to "implement policies and procedures to safeguard the facility and the equipment therein from unauthorized physical access, tampering, and theft" (45 CFR 164.310(a)(1)). To meet this implementation specification, organizations should consider methods such as lock and key controls, security tagging equipment, using video cameras for surveillance, monitoring identification badges, and the use of human workforce to perform facility security checks.

The third addressable implementation specification associated with this standard is access controls and validation procedures. This specification indicates that CEs must "implement procedures to control and validate a person's access to facilities based on their role or function, including visitor control, and control of access to software programs for testing or revision" (45 CFR 164.310(a)(1)). The characteristics of the CE (that is, size) may influence some of the decisions made in regard to this specification. For example, in large facilities badge access may be visually confirmed for every workforce member every day. In smaller organizations where the staff is small, identification badge access confirmation may not be a daily activity since, presumably, everyone knows the workforce members by face. In addition to workforce members, CEs must evaluate practices to control and limit visitor access to information. This implementation specification requires CEs to document the rationale for how they reach their security decisions.

Maintenance records are the final implementation specification in this section. This specification states that CEs must "implement policies and procedures to document repairs and modifications to the physical components of a facility which are related to security (for example, hardware, walls, doors and locks)" (45 CFR 164.310(a)(1)). Again, environmental (facility size, location, and so on) factors may influence how an organization makes it decisions for this specification. Manual logs may be appropriate in some cases and more sophisticated controls may be appropriate in other cases.

Workstation Use Standard

The workstation use standard stands alone without additional implementation specifications. To meet this standard, the CE must

> Implement policies and procedures that specify the proper functions to be performed, the manner in which those functions are to be performed, and the physical attributes of the surroundings of a specific workstation or class of workstation that can access electronic protected health information (45 CFR 164.310(b)).

An important note is that this standard applies not only to workstations located physically in the facility. It applies at a much broader level to workforce members using workstations off-site to complete their work activities. At a minimum, any safeguards that are required in the office must also be required off-site. An example of this kind of safeguard are time-outs or log-outs that break the system connection if the workstation remains idle for a specified period of time.

Workstation Security Standard

The workstation security standard requires CEs to "implement physical safeguards for all workstations that access electronic protected health information, to restrict access to authorized users" (45 CFR 164.310(c)). This standard differs from the previous workstation use standard that addresses policies and procedures for how workstations should be used and protected. The workstation security standard addresses how workstations are to be physically protected from unauthorized access.

Device and Media Controls Standard

The device and media controls standard states that CEs are to "implement policies and procedures that govern the receipt and removal of hardware and electronic media that contain electronic protected health information, into and out of a facility, and the movement of these items within the facility" (45 CFR 164.310(d)(1)). The Security Rule defines electronic media as "electronic storage material on which data is or may be recorded electronically, including, for example, devices in computers (hard drives) and any removable/transportable digital memory medium, such as magnetic tape or disk, optical disk, or digital memory card or transmission media used to exchange information already in electronic storage media" (45 CFR 160.103).

A major consideration for organizations trying to meet this standard is the need to understand what all of their information resources are and where they all lie. This often leads to the need for establishing an effective method for inventorying systems. Not only do organizations need to document their existing and new systems, they must also track movement of components of each system as well as track system and system component obsolescence and replacement. Two addressable and two required implementation specifications support this standard. The two addressable specifications are accountability and data backup and storage. The required specifications are disposal and media reuse.

The required disposal implementation specification states that CEs must "implement policies and procedures to address the final disposition of electronic protected health information, and/or the hardware or electronic media on which it is stored" (45 CFR 164.310(d)(1)). There are multiple methods that can be used to make ePHI unusable or unreadable. The Security Rule specifically mentions degaussing as one of those methods, but stops short of requiring degaussing as the preferred method for rendering data unreadable or unusable when a CE wishes to dispose of electronic media that contains ePHI.

The required media reuse implementation specification states that CEs must "implement procedures for removal of electronic protected health information from electronic media before the media are made available for re-use" (45 CFR 164.310(d)(1)). This implementation specification is applicable to both internal and external reuse of media scenarios and requires organizations to develop policies and procedures to address media reuse.

The addressable accountability implementation specification states that the CE must "maintain a record of the movements of hardware and electronic media and any person responsible therefore" (45 CFR 164.310(d)(1)). This implementation specification presents a growing challenge in many healthcare organizations where mobile technology is increasing in use, increasing in cost, increasing in data storage, and decreasing in size. The decreasing size factor creates an increased risk due to the opportunity for concealment and theft. The flipside to this discussion is the value it offers in terms of convenience to the user. Like so many concepts addressed by HIPAA, organizations must devise methods to ensure an appropriate balance of protection and access or use. This addressable implementation specification speaks again to the need for inventorying and tracking of electronic media.

Data backup and storage is the final addressable implementation specification for this standard. Under this implementation specification the CE must "create a retrievable, exact copy of electronic protected health information, when needed, before movement of equipment" (45 CFR 164.310(d)(1)). This implementation specification parallels the data backup plan for the contingency plan standard in the administrative safeguards section of the Rule. As such, both components of the rule are often fulfilled with a combined policy and procedure that meets the requirements of both sections.

⊙ Technical Safeguards Standards

As technological advances occur they often bring with them new security challenges. The conundrum of duality of interests again presents itself here. Advancing technology leads to great opportunity, but at the same time increases organizational risk. Balancing these two facets to capitalize on the benefits and reduce the risks is often at the center of both the HIPAA Privacy and Security Rules.

The Security Rule defines **technical safeguards** as "the technology and the policy and procedures for its use that protect electronic protected health information and control access to it" (45 CFR 164.308). In keeping with the flexibility, scalability, and technological neutrality concepts of meeting the Security Rule requirements,

CEs must determine which security measures and technologies are reasonable and appropriate for implementation in its organization (CMS 2007c).

Access Control Standard

The access control standard directs CEs to "implement technical policies and procedures for electronic information systems that maintain electronic protected health information to allow access only to those persons or software programs that have been granted access rights as specified in §164.308(a)(4) [information access management]" (45 CFR 164.312 (a)(1)). Of importance here is the concept that access controls should be appropriate for the role and function of the workforce member. Two required and two addressable implementation specifications are included in this standard.

The required unique user identification implementation specification states that CEs must "assign a unique name and/or number for identifying and tracking user identity" (45 CFR 164.312(a)(1)). Unique identification methods allow for the user's actions to be monitored and serve as the method of enforcing accountability of user actions.

The second required implementation specification is referred to as the emergency access procedure. This specification states that CEs must "establish (and implement as needed) procedures for obtaining necessary electronic protected health information during an emergency" (45 CFR 164.312(a)(1)). This description, at face value, conveys the import of ensuring availability of information as needed to perform one's role in emergency situations. From a technology standpoint, many systems have a "**break the glass**" method that allows users to access data that they may not otherwise be allowed to access. The users are alerted in advance that their actions are being monitored giving them an opportunity to halt their actions, if inappropriate.

Automatic log-off is the first addressable implementation specification, which states that CEs must "implement electronic procedures that terminate an electronic session after a predetermined time of inactivity" (45 CFR 164.312(a)(1)). This concept is probably not foreign to readers as it is commonly used in many types of information systems, healthcare and otherwise.

Encryption and decryption is the final addressable implementation specification. Where this implementation specification is a reasonable and appropriate safeguard for a CE, the CE must "implement a mechanism to encrypt and decrypt electronic protected health information" (45 CFR 164.312(a)(1)). **Encryption** is a technical method that reduces access and viewing of ePHI by unauthorized users. Encryption is defined as "the process of transforming text into an unintelligible string of characters that can be transmitted via communications media with a high degree of security and then decrypted when it reaches a secure destination" (AHIMA 2014, 55).

Audit Control Standard

The audit control standard is singular in focus and requires CEs to "implement hardware, software, and/or procedural mechanisms that record and examine activity in information systems that contain or use electronic protected health information" (45 CFR 164.312(b)). This standard recognizes that regardless of the controls put into place to prevent unauthorized access, there must be a way to track and record user activities in the system. Such tracking can be used to monitor intentional and unintentional actions taken by users to access ePHI.

Integrity Standard

The integrity standard is supported by one addressable implementation specification. The integrity standard states that CEs must "implement policies and procedures to protect electronic protected health information from improper alteration or destruction" (45 CFR 164.312(c)(1)). This standard is intended to ensure data integrity, which is defined as the extent to which healthcare data are complete, accurate, consistent, and timely; it is a security principle that keeps information from being modified or otherwise corrupted either maliciously or accidentally (AHIMA 2012, 120). Ultimately, data integrity supports high-quality clinical care and the effect of compromised data integrity can be significant. For these reasons, organizations must take steps to ensure data are not improperly altered or destroyed. The addressable implementation specification mechanisms to authenticate ePHI requires CEs to "implement electronic mechanisms to corroborate that electronic protected health information has not been altered or destroyed in an unauthorized manner" (45 CFR 164.312(c)(1)).

Person or Entity Authentication Standard

The person or entity authentication standard requires CEs to "implement procedures to verify that a person or entity seeking access to electronic protected health information is the one claimed" (45 CFR 164.312(d)). Simply put, this standard seeks to ensure that organizations put methods in place to verify that users are who they claim they are. Passwords, smart cards, tokens, fobs, and biometrics are some of the many methods used in healthcare settings to confirm user identity.

Transmission Security

The transmission security standard recognizes the potential risk involved with data in transit and requires CEs to "implement technical security measures to guard against unauthorized access to electronic protected health information that is being transmitted over an electronic communications network" (45 CFR 164.312(e)(1)). Two addressable implementation specifications are associated with this standard. The integrity controls implementation specification directs CEs to "implement security measures to ensure that electronically transmitted electronic protected health information is not improperly modified without detection until disposed of" (45 CFR 164.312(e)(1)). Specifically covered in this implementation specification is the assurance that ePHI is not improperly modified during transmission. The encryption addressable implementation specification states that CEs must "implement a mechanism to encrypt electronic protected health information whenever deemed appropriate" (45 CFR 164.312(e)(1)). Encryption converts the original message into encoded or unreadable text. When decrypted, the message returns to its original state and can be read by the recipient. Senders and receivers must use compatible technology tools in order to encrypt and decrypt messages.

To meet the requirements for transmission security, transmitted ePHI that has been inappropriately altered is detected and destroyed, and ePHI is encrypted where necessary. The following are a few examples of how ePHI can be inappropriately made available to unauthorized individuals:

⊙ A missing unencrypted flash drive containing patient information was missing from a hospital

⊙ A breach at a multifacility clinic was reported when it was discovered that an employee created an unencrypted, nonpassword protected patient list on the employee's own personal laptop to help with her job of cataloging records.

⊙ Information was compromised for 700 members of a health plan when an e-mail including PHI was inadvertently sent to an incorrect e-mail address. Functionality for encryption or destruction was not a part of the system (*Becker's Health IT and CIO Review* 2015).

The potential for breaches with transmission of PHI are wide and varied. In addition to the technical requirements to protect against this kind of breach, policies, procedures, and employee education are very important.

⊙ Confidentiality, Integrity, and Availability

The HIPAA Security Rule seeks to uphold confidentiality, integrity, and availability of data. The previously discussed administrative, physical, and technical safeguards also require and recommend methods to ensure confidentiality, integrity, and availability of data.

Confidentiality

Confidentiality is "a legal and ethical concept that establishes the healthcare provider's responsibility for protecting health records and other personal and private information from unauthorized use or disclosure" (AHIMA 2014, 34). In the context of the Security Rule, confidentiality means that ePHI is accessible only by authorized people and processes.

Integrity

Maintaining data integrity is central to the Security Rule. Under the Rule, **integrity** means that ePHI is not altered or destroyed in an unauthorized manner. With continuing advancements in technology and electronic data management come additional legal obligations for ensuring data integrity. In addition to Security Rule requirements, concepts such as e-discovery that implore organizations to establish and follow methods to ensure integrity are becoming commonplace in healthcare organizations.

Availability

Equally as important as protecting ePHI from unauthorized users is the concept of ensuring that it can be accessed as needed by authorized users. **Availability** refers to "the property that data or information is accessible and useable upon demand by an authorized person" (CFR 45 164.304 2013). This requirement almost seems contradictory in the discussion of protecting information from inappropriate access but the patient information must be able to be available for treatment and other vital uses of the information. Encompassed in the concept of availability are many of the previously discussed safeguards such as the data backup and storage specification.

⊙ Penalties and Enforcement

Penalties and enforcement were addressed in the original HIPAA bill but have changed over time. The determination of penalties is complex depending on the kind of violation; whether it was an inadvertent release of information, neglectful, or done knowingly; whether it was a primary or subsequent violation; and whether there was negligence in correcting known policies and procedures that led to violations. The history of the enforcement is complex due to the numerous changes of the agencies responsible; however, the duplication of efforts has been recognized and responsibility streamlined as a result.

The Office for Civil Rights

The **Office for Civil Rights (OCR)** is currently the enforcement agency for the HIPAA Privacy and Security Rule. Since April 14, 2003, the Privacy Rule has been enforced by the OCR. The Security Rule was enforced by the Centers for Medicare and Medicaid Services (CMS) from its effective date of April 20, 2005, through July 26, 2009. Since that time, the Security Rule has been enforced by the OCR as well. Although the Privacy and Security Rules were enforced by separate enforcement agencies, lack of clarity and duplication of efforts were noted. For these reasons, the OCR became the single enforcement agency for both Rules. The OCR must investigate all reported violations and appropriately initiate investigations for cause in absence of a reported violation.

Civil Penalties

The Privacy and Security Rules both outline various penalties for violations. **Civil penalties** are generally fines or money damages used to sanction violators. The Final Rule for HIPAA modified civil penalty enforcement language in both the Privacy and Security Rules by outlining a tiered structure of enforcement guidelines. The tiered method specifies a minimum to maximum penalty range based on the specific category of violation. The four main categories of civil violations escalate in nature and start at the bottom rung with violations where the individual did not know (or through reasonable diligence would not have known) that he or she violated HIPAA and range to the fourth and final category, which is reserved for those who violate HIPAA through willful neglect and do not correct the violation pattern. The civil money penalties prior to February 18, 2009, were restricted penalties of not more than $100 per violation, or not in excess of $25,000 for identical violations during a calendar year.

The amount of civil money penalties imposed on or after February 18, 2009, are subject to the limitations in table 13.1.

Table 13.1.   Overview of penalties

Intent	Minimum per incident	Annual cap for all violations
Did not know or could not have known	$100–$50,000	$1.5 million
Reasonable cause and not willful neglect	$1,000–$50,000	$1.5 million
Willful neglect, but corrected within 30 days	$10,000–$50,000	$1.5 million
Willful neglect and not corrected within 30 days	$50,000	$1.5 million

Source: HHS 2015b

Criminal Penalties

If the OCR reviews a complaint and determines that it qualifies as a criminal violation the case is referred to the Department of Justice (DOJ). In 2005, the DOJ clarified that criminal violation enforcement is applicable to both individuals and CEs. When **criminal penalties** are appropriate, the OCR works in conjunction with the DOJ to pursue possible violators. Criminal penalties can be imprisonment of 1 to 10 years and/or a fine plus possible restitution of moneys received. When the breach of PHI is found to be a HIPAA violation, the criminal violations vary by cause beginning with (1) reasonable cause or possibly being unaware of the violation and continuing with (2) acquiring PHI by false pretenses, and (3) obtaining the PHI for personal gain or malicious intent, which has the most severe penalties (45 CFR 160.404).

Enforcement Activities to Date

The **HIPAA Enforcement Rule** is found at 45 CFR 160, subparts C, D, and E. This Rule spells out the authority of the OCR as previously described. The complaint process is fully outlined on the OCR website and presents the process from initial complaint through referral, investigation, and resolution. After investigation, resolutions range from the OCR finding no violation to obtaining corrective action to the issuance of formal findings of violation. In addition, reported violations may be found unenforceable due to technical issues such as not filing the complaint within the required time frame, the entity not being considered a CE, or the incident as described not violating the Rules.

Figure 13.2 shows privacy and security rule enforcement results for 2014. This chart reflects first the total number of resolutions for the year for all reported events and then the results for those that were actually investigated. Of note, there were 1,516 Privacy Rule cases resolved by the OCR in 2003 with this number continuing to rise almost every year. In 2013 when OCR became the enforcement agency for the Security Rule as well, the number of cases increased significantly with the 17,748 cases in 2014.

Since the April 2003 HIPAA Rule compliance date through May 31, 2016, over 134,246 complaints were filed with the OCR. Five hundred and seventy-five

Figure 13.2.   Enforcement results for privacy and security rules, 2014

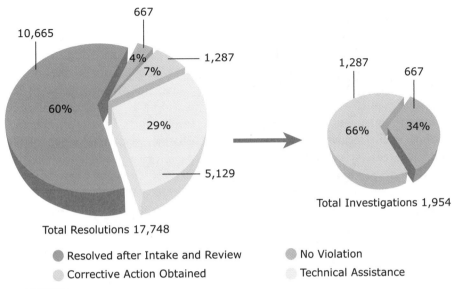

Total Resolutions 17,748

● Resolved after Intake and Review   ● No Violation
○ Corrective Action Obtained   ○ Technical Assistance

Source: HHS 2016

complaints (less than 0.5 percent) were referred by OCR to the DOJ for cases involving the knowing disclosure or obtaining information in violation of the rules resolved. The remaining 128,872 (96 percent) of the complaints were resolved as outlined:

- ⊙ 24,241 (18.8 percent) required changes in privacy practices and corrective actions by or providing technical assistance to CEs and their BAs
- ⊙ 11,018 (8.5 percent) no violation occurred following investigations
- ⊙ 13,748 (10.7 percent) early intervention with technical assistance by OCR to CEs, BAs and individuals exercising their rights as stated in the Privacy Rule, with no need for investigation
- ⊙ 79,865 (62 percent) determination made in the rest of these remaining cases that complaint was not eligible for case enforcement. These cases included those where OCR lacks jurisdiction under HIPAA or the complaint was untimely or withdrawn. (HHS 2016a)

From April 2003 through May 31, 2016, the complaints investigated were from many different types of entities with the most common listed in order of frequency: private practices, general hospitals, outpatient facilities, pharmacies, and health plans. The most investigated compliance issues listed in order of highest to lowest are:

- ⊙ Impermissible uses and disclosures of PHI
- ⊙ Lack of safeguards of PHI
- ⊙ Lack of access by patients to their PHI
- ⊙ Use or disclosure of more than the minimum necessary
- ⊙ Lack of administrative safeguards of ePHI (HHS 2016a)

Security Rule enforcement activities have been less structured than their privacy rule counterparts. This may be partly due to the methods by which security violations are found. Security violations are more insulated within the organization and may not be found without external review. For this reason, the OCR initiated compliance reviews in 2008. CMS initiated these reviews based on complaints filed against the entities, identification of potential Security Rule violations through the media, or recommendations from HHS and OCR (HIPAA Compliance Review Analysis 2008). With transitioning of enforcement activities to the OCR in 2009, more routine complaint reporting is anticipated due to increased efforts to educate consumers about how to file security complaints. Since OCR began reporting its Security Rule enforcement results in October 2009, approximately 940 complaints have been received alleging a violation of the Security Rule. Of these complaints, 689 (73 percent) have been closed following investigation and appropriate corrective action. At the last reporting, OCR still had 316 open complaints and compliance reviews (HHS 2016a).

The following case study is an example of an issue with HIPAA Privacy and Security Rules. An outcome of this case was a resolution agreement. A resolution agreement is a contract between HHS and the covered entity outlining obligations to be met, such as the development of policies and procedures or required staff training, plus the required reporting to HHS for a specified period of time.

Case Study: HIPAA Privacy and Security Rule Violation

In violation of HIPAA Privacy and Security Rules, two entities within a healthcare system, home health services and hospice services, had several instances over about a seven-month period where backup tapes, optical disks, and laptops were left unattended and eventually lost or stolen. All of the devices contained unencrypted ePHI on over 386,000 patients. The healthcare organization responded to state notification laws and to the HHS with over 30 complaints submitted as a result of this. Working together OCR and CMS focused the investigation on the organization's failure to implement policies and procedures to safeguard this information. The HHS entered into a Resolution Agreement with the organization to settle the violation. It was agreed that the CE would pay a $100,000 resolution amount (due to cooperation, this resolution amount was in lieu of a civil monetary penalty that could have been much more) and implement a robust Corrective Action Plan. This plan included revising policies and procedures for physical and technical safeguards (encryption), governing off-site transport and storage of the electronic media that contained PHI, training workforce on the safeguards, conducting routine audits and site visits of facilities within the organization, and submitting the required compliance reports to HHS for three years (HHS 2008).

This case is an example of a situation where a resolution agreement is suitable. In the majority of compliance issues investigated there is one facility with one type of breach involved and one major corrective action imposed. In this case there were two different entities with several different types of data storage devices involved. There were several different corrective actions including a payment to be made and a comprehensive corrective action plan with numerous items to be accomplished over a period of time. The required compliance reports assured compliance and accountability.

Breach Notification

In January 2013 the Final Rule on breach notifications went into effect. The Final Rule is based on the original HIPAA rules and supplants an interim final rule published in 2009. It fulfills provisions of the HITECH Act and strengthens privacy and security protection of PHI. The Final Rule increased the patient's privacy protection, provides patients with new rights regarding their health information, and increases the ability for enforcement of the law to protect PHI (HHS 2013).

The rule requires CEs and BAs to report breaches of "unsecured protected health information. Unsecured protected health information is protected health information that has not been rendered unusable, unreadable, or indecipherable to unauthorized individuals through the use of a technology or methodology" (ARRA 2009). Protecting health information from the unauthorized use is accomplished by utilizing methods that will make it unusable, unreadable, or indecipherable (HHS 2016b). The National Institute for Standards and Technology of the US Department of Commerce (NIST) has issued a series of special publications that address encryption of data at rest and in motion as well as destruction of both electronic and nonelectronic media. These special publications are numbered in the 800 series and can be located at the NIST website (NIST 2016).

A **breach** is defined under the 2013 final rule as "the acquisition, access, use, or disclosure of protected health information in a manner not permitted which compromises the security or privacy of the protected health information" (45 CFR 164.402). Reporting requirements mandate notification to the individual whose information was breached, and in the case of breaches of more than 500 individuals' information, to the media and secretary of HHS. Three exceptions to this definition exist with the first being when a workforce member unintentionally acquires, uses, or discloses PHI while acting under the authority of a CE or BA. The second exception is applicable when an authorized workforce member inadvertently discloses protected health information to another authorized workforce member within the same CE or BA setting. The final exception is applicable when the CE or BA who made an inadvertent disclosure has reason to believe that the recipient of the PHI would not have been able to retain the information. For example, if the provider called a patient with a common name to discuss laboratory results they might dial the wrong phone number. Although they might discuss "John Smith's" lab results, as long as no hard copy results were sent to the wrong patient, it is reasonable to believe that the wrong John Smith could not keep the information.

Risk Assessment

Covered entities and business associates must have procedures in place to conduct a risk analysis. This is done to assess the potential risks and areas of vulnerability to the security of the protected health information just as is required for the privacy aspect of HIPAA. It is important to identify and correct those things that might threaten the confidentiality, integrity, and availability of the information. Failure to conduct such an audit could be detrimental in the event of an audit or investigation of a complaint.

Check Your Understanding 13.2

Answer the following questions.

1. Inventorying systems does not include
   a. Existing and new systems
   b. Movement of components of each system
   c. Tracking system and system component obsolescence
   d. Training records for employees to be able to use the systems

2. The technology and the policies and procedures for its use that protect electronic protected health information and control access to it is
   a. Administrative safeguards
   b. Technical safeguards
   c. Physical safeguards
   d. Integrity controls

3. The integrity standard protects
   a. From unauthorized access
   b. From unauthorized use
   c. From improper transmission of data
   d. From improper alteration or destruction

4. Which of the following is not a resolution to HIPAA violations?
   a. No violation found
   b. Obtaining corrective action
   c. Issuance of formal findings of violation
   d. No investigation required

5. What has been the most common complaint investigated for potential HIPAA violations?
   a. Lack of safeguards for PHI
   b. Lack of access by patients to their PHI
   c. Impermissible uses and disclosures of PHI
   d. Lack of administrative safeguards for PHI

Indicate whether each of the following is true or false.

6. Small mobile devices are at greater risk due to the potential for concealment and theft.

7. When encrypted information is decrypted, it is in a different format than the original state.

8. Maintaining access to ePHI is less important than the protection of ePHI.

9. The difference between the levels of civil penalties has to do with whether the CE knew or should have known that a violation occurred.

10. CEs are not held to same level of accountability as BAs for breach notification.

⊙ Medical Identity Theft

Health information serves many functions, the most important of which is patient care. However, health information serves many other functions. The legal considerations for health information extend beyond privacy, security, and the legal electronic health record (EHR). The legal considerations now include the responsibility of providers to protect against medical identity theft, consider legal liability related to medical malpractice in light of EHR use, and incorporate disaster planning and preparedness. The first two issues are relatively new and the third requires new and different ways of thinking, but they are vitally important in the evolving world of health information technology and EHRs. This section will discuss the challenges and recommendations for addressing each of these.

Medical Identity Theft

Medical identity theft occurs when personal information (such as name, Social Security number, or Medicare number) is taken without the patient's knowledge to obtain medical care, buy drugs, or submit fake billings to Medicare in the name of the patient. Medical identity theft can disrupt a person's life, damage credit rating, and waste and inappropriately use taxpayer dollars. The damage can also alter treatment or even be life threatening to a victim of identity theft if the wrong information subsequently ends up in the patient's personal health records (HHS 2015b). Figure 13.3 presents the results of surveys reflecting the findings for three different years on what the information was used for when an individual's medical identity was stolen. The findings of these studies illustrate that there are implications for the patient when health records are accessed and modified, credit accounts are created, and credit scores are accessed and changed. There are also consequences for the third-party payers related to their payment for services, drugs, and equipment. There are costs that the facility or provider must bear associated with follow up to resolve claims and receive the appropriate payment. The patient health information must also be rectified so there will be complete and correct information on each patient for continuity of care and to alleviate issues in releasing PHI when information on the wrong person is combined with that of the patient.

Instances that would not be considered identify theft are where health information on the wrong patient was inadvertently put in the incorrect record. When the financial information on a patient is used to purchase nonmedical items and services, this is not considered medical identify theft. The key factors for a situation to be medical identify theft are that a form of a patient's identification is taken without the patient's knowledge and the identification is then used to acquire some sort of medical services.

In addition to the financial implications of medical identity theft, the theft carries the very real possibility that the incorrect information could be used in

Figure 13.3. Reasons for medical identify theft

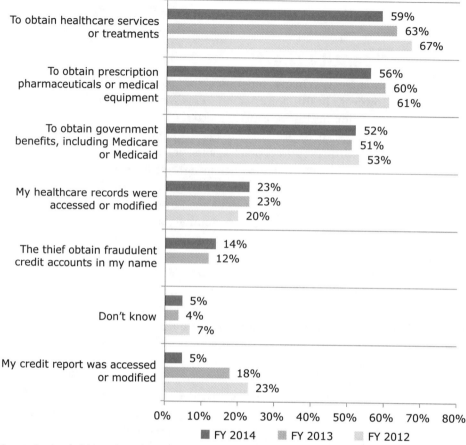

Source: Reprinted with permission from Ponemon Institute©. Sponsored by the Medical Identity Fraud Alliance with support from: Kaiser Permanente, ID Experts, Experian Data Breach Resolution and Identity Finder, LLC.

the delivery of patient care, putting patients at risk. This can occur if critical medical conditions, procedures, medications, allergies, and other information are either omitted from the record or wrongfully included (Brodnik et al. 2012). An example of this would be when a medical report of the perpetrator is filed in the health record of a patient and the report indicates the blood type to be different than that of the victim of the identity theft. This might not be noticed for some time, if ever, because the erroneous report would have the patient's name and other identifying information filed among reports with the same identifying information. Unfortunately, victims of identity theft can find themselves unable to access their records because some providers will refuse to release the records containing another patient's information—even if the other patient broke the law. Figure 13.4 illustrates how medical identity theft can affect an individual from the initial theft to the integrity of the health information.

A study was conducted to determine if patient identity was confirmed during the admission and registration processes, as well as the methods used to establish patient identity at admission and registration (Mancilla and Moczygemba

Figure 13.4.   The cascading effect of medical identity theft

The effects of medical identity theft cascade throughout the healthcare continuum. Beyond being used to submit false claims, false data make their way into oversight agency databases, skewing public health findings. Ultimately, corrupted data in the victim's medical record may place the individual at risk in future treatment.

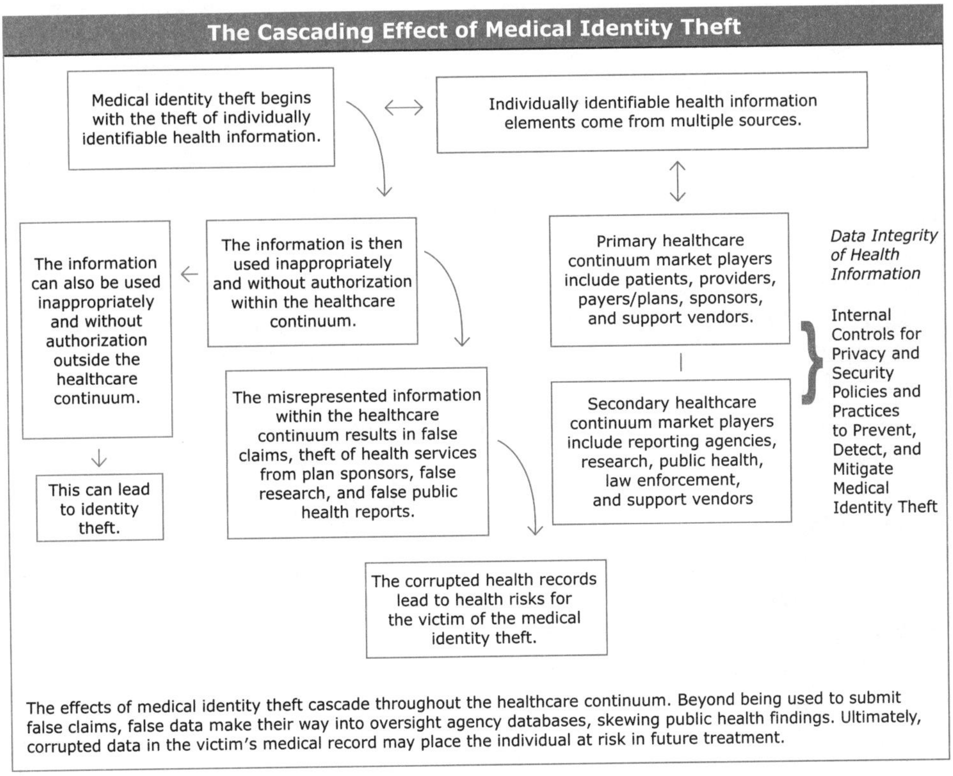

Source: AHIMA 2008

2009). Using a combination of online surveys, telephone interviews, and onsite observation, these HIM researchers learned that the majority (91.9 percent) of healthcare providers established identity with a driver's license, while just over 20 percent of the respondents indicated they were not aware of how their organizations handled exceptions to standard practices (Mancilla and Moczygemba 2009). Other interesting information from the study was that the majority of medical identity theft cases arose in the emergency room, time constraints or demands placed on admissions personnel may result in noncompliance with policies and procedures, biometrics are not widely used, and the widespread use of the Social Security number helps contribute to medical identity theft (Mancilla and Moczygemba 2009). The study concluded that healthcare organizations face multiple regulations from many oversight agencies when attempting to detect and prevent medical identity theft (Mancilla and Moczygemba 2009).

The occurrences and consequences of medical identify theft continue to increase. The 2014 annual study sponsored by Medical Identify Fraud Alliance (MIFA) revealed that there were approximately 500,000 more victims than reflected in the 2013 report. The costs incurred by the victims to correct the misidentification and deal with resulting problems also increased (MIFA 2015). It is more difficult to quantify risks to the affected individuals' healthcare in the form of delayed care, misdiagnosis, and mistreatment but these continue to be a factor in cases of medical identity theft.

Red Flag Rules

In response to increasing identity theft, often used for financial gain, the Federal Trade Commission (FTC), Department of the Treasury, Federal Reserve System, Federal Deposit Insurance Corporation, and the National Credit Union Administration simultaneously issued regulations known as the "Red Flag Rules" in November 2007 (King and Williams 2008). These rules require creditor and financial institutions to implement an Identity Theft Prevention Program (King and Williams 2008). The portion of these rules that apply to healthcare organizations are contained in 16 CFR 681, under the enforcement authority of the FTC (Springer 2009). The **red flags** that are addressed in the rules are the potential patterns, practices, or specific activities indicating the possibility of identity theft (FTC 2013). Examples of red flags include inconsistencies in documents (driver's license and insurance card), documents that appear to be altered, and not having more than one form of ID (insurance card but no other form of ID).

First, healthcare organizations must understand whether they are subject to the Red Flag Rules. Healthcare providers may be subject to the Red Flag Rules if they (1) meet the definition of creditor under the Fair Credit Reporting Act; or (2) use consumer credit reports, subjecting them to the Address Discrepancy Rule (Springer 2009). A healthcare creditor would include any organization that allows for payment on medical services provided to a patient after those services were provided or over a period of installment payments (King and Williams 2008). This includes most healthcare organizations, especially hospitals. Fortunately, the Red Flag Rules include guidelines to assist in the development of an Identity Theft Prevention Program:

1. Identify Covered Accounts: Most patient accounts and billing records qualify as covered accounts because they contain information sufficient to enable identity theft if lost or stolen.

2. Identify Relevant Red Flags: A red flag is a pattern or practice of specific activity that indicates the possible existence of identity theft. Red flags can include alerts, notifications, or other warnings that might be received from consumer report agencies or other service providers; suspicious documents such as identification cards or other documents that are inconsistent or appear to be falsified; other suspicious information such as odd changes of address; or other unusual use of or other suspicious activity related to a given account.

3. Detect Red Flags: Organizations must develop reasonable approaches for detecting potential red flags. This requires that organizations determine what information and documentation will be required of patients. Many now require both an insurance card and a photo identification card such as a driver's license. Additionally, organizations must establish policies and procedures. This is quite important because liability increases if the workforce either cannot or does not follow the policies and procedures. Thus, the policies and procedures should support the detection of red flags in a feasible way.

4. Respond to Red Flags: An adequate response to red flags includes prevention and mitigation via monitoring covered accounts; contacting patients or consumers if needed; changing passwords and security codes; handling accounts carefully; or notifying law enforcement. These responses will, of necessity, be context-dependent and often require judgment on the part of the healthcare organizations. For example, what will the organization do if the patient cannot produce all of the identification required or the identification presented has discrepancies?

5. Oversee the Program: As with all operations, the Identity Theft Prevention Program falls under the purview of the board of directors, trustees, or the designated member of management.

6. Train Employees: The workforce, especially those responsible for creating, maintaining, and administering patient accounts, must be trained in all aspects of identity theft prevention.

7. Oversee Service Provider Arrangements: The healthcare organization must take steps to ensure that any service providers granted access to covered accounts carry out the Identity Theft Prevention Program.

8. Approve the Identity Theft Prevention Program: The board of directors or appropriate committee must review and approve the Identity Theft Prevention Program.

9. Provide Reports and Periodic Updates to the Identity Theft Prevention Program: A written report on the status of the program, service provider arrangements, any significant incidents, and recommendations for any needed changes should be included in the annual report (King and Williams 2008).

Organizations that have already implemented the Red Flag Rules report finding increases in attempted and successful identity theft (Keith 2010). Unfortunately, they report that it is difficult to detect red flags at the time identity theft is being perpetrated though they do try. Some have implemented special designations in their registration pathways so that all employees can identify records of victims, perpetrators, or those with suspicious activity. Yet, most medical identity theft is still detected when the bill is issued (Keith 2010).

Operational Recommendations

The obligations of health informatics and HIM professionals related to medical identity theft fall into three general areas. The first is to urge and educate consumers to adopt preventive measures such as

- Exercising caution when sharing personal and health information with providers
- Monitoring the Explanation of Benefits (EOB) they receive from insurance companies
- Maintaining copies of healthcare records

- Monitoring credit reports and history documents for unexpected medical charges or liens
- Protecting all health insurance and financial information (AHIMA 2008).

The second area is establishing organizational methods to prevent and detect medical identity theft. Some of these methods include

- Conducting and acting upon an information security risk analysis on an annual basis
- Ensuring background checks are performed for employees and BAs when hiring, especially for work in high-risk areas
- Establishing patient identification verification processes that are compliant with the HIPAA Security Rule, but are also feasible for high-throughput areas with significant time demands
- Minimizing the use of Social Security numbers for identification, suppressing it when possible and, when not, displaying only the last four or six digits of the number
- Implementing policies and procedures that safeguard the privacy and security of individually identifiable health information, in compliance with applicable HIPAA and other federal and state regulations
- Creating an alerting and identity theft response plan if any suspicious activity is discovered
- Implementing ongoing staff training programs to ensure all employees with access to identifiable patient information can assist in preventing identity theft (AHIMA 2008).

The third medical identity theft area where HIM professionals have an obligation to assist is related to the data in the patient record and is particularly important. The steps an HIM professional can help with include

- Drafting policies and procedures to ensure victims of medical identity theft are not denied access to their patient records
- Establishing mechanisms to correct inaccurate information in patient records, which includes assisting victims in identifying those who may possess inaccurate records by providing a full accounting of disclosures
- Staying abreast of medical identity theft–related legislation and regulations
- Providing victims of medical identity theft with the checklist of actions and resources that can be found in appendix H. Examples of responses included in the checklist include:
  - Review credit reports, correct them, and place a "Fraud Alert" on them.
  - For stolen passports, contact the US Department of State.
  - Request an accounting of disclosures of medical records.
  - Review health records to assure that information has been corrected prior to seeking healthcare (AHIMA 2008).

Medical identity theft or financial identity theft causes significant problems for consumers, insurers, and providers at a minimum. It is important that all possible steps be taken to both prevent medical identity theft and mitigate or minimize the effects of medical identity theft once it occurs.

⊙ Disaster Preparedness

Health informatics and information management professionals have two very important roles related to disaster preparedness: (1) ensure the protection of the organization's information assets; and (2) ensure the information functions will continue in the event of a natural or man-made disaster affecting the entire organization. These two roles can be separated because the first can occur without the second, but they are related. The first role of protecting the information assets needs to be done in all situations, including those that might not technically be termed a disaster, such as attacks by hackers or technical system failure due to network or software malfunctions. Because this role focuses largely on protecting the information assets, it is largely under the purview of the HIM and IT departments. The second role crosses all departments or functions in the organization and, while HIM and IT are expected to meet the organizational needs, it is extremely collaborative in nature.

Protecting Information Assets

Protection of organizational information assets is a part of the HIPAA Security Rule. Although the technical requirements of the Security Rule seem fairly straightforward, the information security team must prepare thoroughly, thinking outside of the box, envisioning worst-case scenarios or trying to imagine how a technically savvy person could do harm to the organization via the different installed information systems. The NIST has published guides to help organizations, including the federal government, prepare contingency plans for information systems operations. NIST Special Publication 800-34 Rev. 1, Contingency Planning Guide for Federal Information Systems, gives guidance and provides multiple templates for developing disaster plans for information services. NIST Special Publication 800-30, Rev. 1, Guide for Conducting Risk Assessments, can also help with information asset protection planning. These and additional NIST guidance can be found at http://csrc.nist.gov/publications. Several examples of risks follow to illustrate the possibilities.

Significant risks to information systems that might put the organization at risk include hackers attacking computers that control medical equipment and facilities that are on networks with weak security, or significant downtime due to a massive system failure. For example, the heating, ventilation, and air conditioning system for a medical center had been set up to be accessed remotely by an outside company that managed the system (Gupta 2011). Hackers attempted to use this poorly secured computer to gain access to other systems. Upon investigation by law enforcement, it was discovered that the system had been attacked previously more than 10 times (Gupta 2011). In that same vein, another healthcare system experienced a worst-case scenario when the geographic area where their data system was located suffered a massive loss of power (Conn 2012). Because it was not where the organization itself was located, operations in the organization needed to continue unimpeded. Unfortunately, the backup generators only worked for a short time (Conn 2012).

Information technology and health information management personnel must prepare for these and other potential threats to their systems with the initial step of a business impact analysis (BIA). Concepts important to a BIA are the **recovery point objective (RPO)** and the **recovery time objective (RTO)** (Ranajee 2012). RPO represents the length of time that you can operate without a particular application. RTO is the maximum amount of time tolerable for data loss and capture (Ranajee 2012). The goal of the BIA is to identify any gaps in your current recovery capability and to develop a strategy for meeting the identified RTO and RPO. The following steps should be taken and the following questions should be asked:

1. Identify the minimal resources required to maintain business operations. What are essential operations and what is required to keep them running? What might be out of sight downstream that needs to be considered?

2. Determine the business recovery objectives and assumptions. How much downtime and loss of data can each department sustain? How is the data received and processed by each department?

3. Establish order of priority for restoration of business functions. What are the key patient care departments? What are the IT applications that support these critical operations?

4. Estimate the operational, financial, and reputational impact due to loss of data. Although IT and HIM can provide data and information regarding these impacts, it is more appropriate for executives with input from the board of directors or trustees to make the final estimations and decisions (Ranajee 2012). Table 13.2 illustrates a matrix for conducting a **business impact analysis**, which is one method for evaluating and prioritizing the risks to help make decisions to address the risks. This tool is used to identify the risk level to prioritize the potential threats identified.

Table 13.2.   Information security threat analysis quadrant

	Low Risk to Operations	High Risk to Operations
Low probability of occurring	Green	Orange
High probability of occurring	Yellow	Red

The colors used are similar to what is used in a heat map to show temperatures geographically with red representing the hottest, then orange, yellow and green representing the coolest. Items that fall into the red or orange quadrants should be handled first. Those that fall into the yellow and green quadrants should still be addressed but are a lower priority.

Once the BIA and prioritization have been accomplished many decisions remain to be made such as the type and location of backup data facilities. There are usually three different types of facilities:

1. **Hot site**: for critical applications and operations, which can be online within hours. This option is the most expensive.

2. **Warm site**: provides basic infrastructure, but takes time, possibly a week, to activate. Obviously, this is less expensive.

3. **Cold site**: equipment must be brought in, but the site is powered and secure. Much less expensive, but this could take up to a month to operationalize (Ranajee 2012).

Requirements such as HIPAA security regulations, BAAs, and so forth, continue to pertain. Additionally, the backup data center should be located in a low-risk geographic location, that is, not in an earthquake or tornado zone; and should have multiple layers of physical security such as biometrics, mantraps, video monitoring, and so on; expansion capabilities; and an established history of uptime and redundancy (Ranajee 2012).

Protecting the various patient care and other information systems, some of which might not have been considered, such as HVAC systems, is the first step to health information disaster preparedness. These systems can be attacked or compromised in situations that do not necessarily include natural or man-made larger disasters and must be planned for accordingly.

Continuity of Information Services

Hurricanes, tornadoes, flooding, earthquakes, and man-made disasters such as terrorist attacks and shooting sprees cannot, unfortunately, be ignored by health information professionals. Keeping operations going during an external disaster, whether an act of nature or man-made, is required. Although disasters often result in some type of gap in services, a significant failure to plan could be considered negligence in certain circumstances. This section will explore different models and include recommendations for organization-wide information services **disaster recovery planning (DRP)**. For the purposes of this book, DRP for organizational information services is focused upon the recovery of physical disasters, including some elements usually included as a part of **business continuity planning (BCP)**. BCP includes the recovery and use of the technology as in DRP as well as the ability of the organization to continue the processes required for ongoing business operations. Sometimes BCP requires operational procedures in the absence of information technology.

Overview of Disaster Planning

Disaster planning can occur at many different levels, especially in a healthcare organization. It can occur for the entire organization; however, departments can also plan for disaster, as can the entire community, which may be dependent upon that healthcare organization. A 2015 study on preparedness for natural disasters among older US adults emphasized the need for the public health aspect of healthcare organizations and communities to work together in preparation and planning for potential disasters (Al-rousan et al. 2014). In a national survey the study found that the majority of this population 50 years older and above had no emergency plans and no basic supply of food, water, or medical supplies all of which could lead to declining health in the presence of a disaster (Al-rousan et al. 2014). In conjunction with many different levels of planning are the different components of preparedness, planning, response and recovery involved in disaster planning. Figure 13.4 is a graphical representation of how the different levels and different phases may interact.

One of the strategies learned after major disasters in the United States is that the workplace should help its workforce with their individual disaster planning. Given that the disaster plan for any organization often rests with the workforce, the organization may want to ensure that its "essential" personnel have a personal disaster plan in place. For example, if in an earthquake zone, do the different family members know how they are supposed to communicate if an earthquake occurs? If in a hurricane or flood zone has the employee thought through when, where, and how his or her family would evacuate? If power is lost does the employee have a generator or a backup plan? One study reported that persons who feel their family might be at risk would be less likely to report to work (Beaton et al. 2008).

Naturally, healthcare organizations must have a disaster plan; however, within the organization the plans may exist at different levels. In the model included in figure 13.5, hospitals are considered a special case of workplace. Unfortunately, even the best planning does not make hospitals immune from significant problems. Following Hurricane Sandy in 2012 challenges were reported with infrastructure failures related to electricity and communication and with community collaboration over resources to include fuel, transportation, hospitals beds, and public shelters (HHS 2014). Likewise, Mercy Hospital in Joplin, Missouri, was unprepared for the total destruction of their facility during the 2011 tornado (Braun 2012). The bottom line from an organizational perspective on planning is that it is almost impossible to truly envision the worst case unless it is total destruction. Therefore, the planning must be comprehensive and cannot presume continued electricity, operating generators, or other "niceties."

Community-level planning, at the town, city, county, state, or national level, relies heavily on the quality of the planning done at the lower levels, especially for hospitals and healthcare organizations. It is imperative that those doing the planning and carrying out the plan remember that the nature of disasters is dynamic and in flux, requiring constant adjustment and, ultimately, learning from previous disasters (Beaton et al. 2008).

Figure 13.5. Model with disaster planning levels and steps

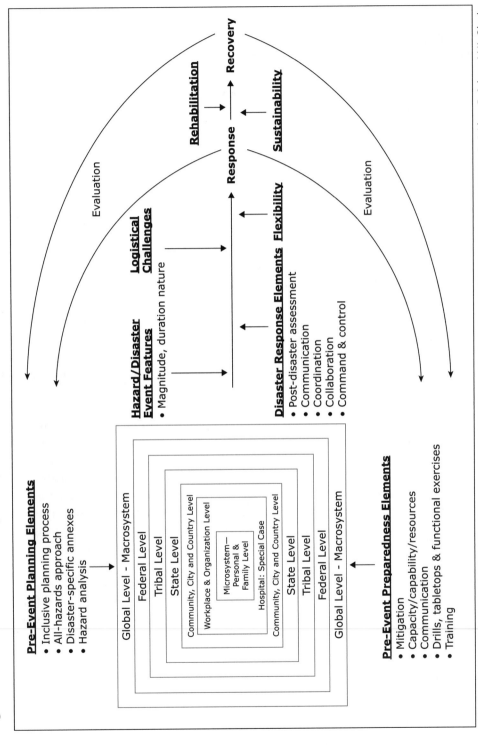

Source: Republished with permission of SAGE Publishing, from (2008), *AAOHN Journal*. Ecological model of disaster management, Beaton, R., Bridges, E., Salazar, M.K., Oberle, M.W., Stergachis, A., Thompson, J., Butterfield, P., 56(11):471-478, copyright 2008; permission conveyed through Copyright Clearance Center, Inc.

Considerations for Disaster Planning

This section will explore the different components of disaster planning, especially related to information system and information process continuity. The four generally accepted components are planning (or mitigation or prevention), preparedness, response, and recovery (Beaton et al. 2008; Reynolds and Tamanaha 2010; Smith and Macdonald 2006; Gibson et al. 2012). The first two components must be accomplished prior to the disaster, with the third constituting the response to the disaster, and the fourth including an analysis of how well the organization was served during the disaster. Each will be examined in turn.

Planning

Sometimes called planning or mitigation or prevention, the first step in the process is to involve all stakeholders so that understanding, agreement, and consensus can be reached regarding the goals for the disaster plan under development (Beaton et al. 2008). In the hospital this would include the executives, but also the frontline workers and key representative from all business units or functional areas. A good place to start is with the goal of the disaster plan. The BIA is an excellent tool for understanding what is needed to achieve the goals. For example, continuing full operations with admissions still being accepted is quite a different goal than the orderly shutdown of operations. Neither is better or worse than the other but will be dependent upon the mission or business focus of the healthcare organization. Generally, acute-care hospitals with emergency rooms must usually continue operations, while a clinic or specialty hospital might be able to discontinue clinical operations.

The second step for the planning process is to conduct a risk assessment or hazard vulnerability assessment (HVA) (Herzig 2010). This involves identifying persons, situations, or events that pose a particular danger or are particularly vulnerable (Beaton et al. 2008). For example, newborns and the elderly are more vulnerable to environmental changes or extremes. Thus, it would be important to consider the needs of special populations such as these in the disaster plan.

These two steps are really the prework for the disaster plan, ensuring that all of the necessary parties are involved and special situations that might change the plan are identified.

Preparedness

The next step is preparedness. This largely entails determining how the different risks that have been identified will be handled. Risks can be removed, reduced, assigned, or accepted (Nelson 2008). The preparedness component includes

1. Developing the plan
2. Organizing to carry out the plan
3. Training
4. Acquiring equipment
5. Testing or disaster drills

6. Evaluating

7. Improving

The development of the plan requires significant input from information technology or systems because the success of the healthcare organization's disaster plan will be dependent upon communication during the disaster. The plan should be concise, well-written, easy to read, use generic job titles instead of names, and define the command structure and responsibilities (Herzig 2010).

There are recommendations to include in the organization of the plan that have been learned and shared by organizations that have survived other disasters. First and foremost is the importance of communication. Specifically, many organizations will have a telephone tree in place for contacting employees in case of emergency. However, those who have tried to communicate via telephone have found that it often does not work. Fortunately, texting often does work because it requires much less bandwidth than maintaining an open line for a call (Herzig 2010; Harrison et al. 2008). In one disaster report, a flood severely displaced staff. The organization put information including emergency contact information on its website; however, this had not been a part of the communication plan so people did not know to check there (Anon 2011). Another important part of the plan organization is to ensure that roles and responsibilities are clear. Everyone should understand at least their initial tasks when disaster strikes (Beaton et al. 2008).

Training is a very essential part of preparedness. As was shared in the previous paragraph, staff had not been trained for the ultimate communication method rendering it somewhat ineffective. One reference maintains that all staff should know

- Where the disaster plan is located
- Which staff members are essential and should be contacted
- Emergency contact details for all staff members
- Evacuation procedures for their department or work location
- The location of any disaster records in the hospital
- How to access any electronic lists of patient details that exist (Smith and Macdonald 2006)

Equipment acquisition for preparedness can include everything including determining where, when, and how a hot backup of the EHR will operate; ensuring that adequate emergency documents are available in selected storage sites; ensuring solar-powered batteries are purchased and available for cell phones or other communication devices if necessary; and ensuring adequate water and food is available for patients and essential staff in an emergency (Beaton et al. 2008). Because these decisions for additional equipment or supply acquisition may involve considerable expense they are usually made at the executive or above level.

Healthcare facilities are required to conduct training, disaster drills, and other exercises to maintain their accreditation (Beaton et al. 2008). These exercises and drills often reveal weaknesses or other deficiencies that can then be addressed in the disaster plan. Any backup systems or remote storage or anything not used day-to-day should be tested to ensure it works as planned.

Ongoing evaluation of the disaster plan is essential. At a minimum the plan should be reviewed annually or sooner if significant changes to operations or information systems are made. Changes, including new clinical processes or equipment, are easy to implement without consideration given to disaster preparedness. Of course, the main reason for evaluation is to continue to improve the disaster plan and preparedness.

Although organizations must go through the planning and preparedness components, they do it in the hopes that they will never have to experience the next two, response and recovery.

Response and Recovery

Activation of the disaster plan can be chaotic due to the nature of the disaster that has occurred but a comprehensive plan and adequate training will expedite the response. When a disaster actually occurs, it is more than likely it is not exactly as anticipated and planned for in a number of ways such as intensity, destruction and collateral damages, disruption of services, and number and types of patients. For example, a plan for a tornado would include the potential for large numbers of injured to be treated at the hospital but it is not known who these might be. The medical needs of those injured from an elementary school would be quite different than those of the injured from a long-term care facility. A situation such as this would require a quick analysis of the circumstances to determine what adjustments are required to carry out the plan. Flexibility, ingenuity, and rapid decision making are required to address the needs as presented. An example of adjusting to meet the needs in a disaster as they unfolded is related to the 2013 tornado in Moore, Oklahoma. The storm arose so fast, there was little warning. It was classified as F-5 with winds over 200 mph and up to two miles wide, with more than 240,000 structures damaged or destroyed including two elementary schools and the only hospital in the community (NIST 2014). Tornadoes are of high risk in this geographic area and significant planning and preparation is done to prepare for them, however the intensity and type of destruction could not have been anticipated nor the fact that the hospital would be a part of the destruction. Other healthcare facilities in the area had to quickly be engaged to accommodate the number of injured that included a large number of elementary school children and communication plan established to communicate with their parents. Following the initial response phase immediately after the tornado, preparation began to be able to provide long-term safety and appropriate care for the residents without a hospital in the immediate area. Having a disaster plan was important for this event to facilitate the response to such an occurrence but this tornado is a prime example of when flexibility, ingenuity, and problem solving is vital when an actual disaster occurs.

Once past the response crisis, it is important to use recovery to learn from the experience. It is also important to pay attention to the psychosocial effects of a disaster on the workforce. Once the adrenaline and worst of the crisis passes people can experience posttraumatic stress or depression as they learn how to cope with changed circumstances, sometimes in both their personal and their work lives.

Chapter 13 Review Exercises

Answer the following questions.

1. Which of the following is not considered to be identity theft?
   a. Using information accessed in a patient chart to receive medical care
   b. Information inadvertently put in wrong patient's chart
   c. Medical care solicited using insurance information obtained from another's insurance card
   d. Using patient identification information to buy drugs

2. For a situation to be considered medical identity theft, which of the following factors must be present?
   a. Patient's identification is taken without the patient's knowledge
   b. Used to acquire medical services
   c. Patient consents to use of PHI for billing
   d. All of the above
   e. a and b only

3. Red flags can include:
   a. Original unaltered documents (insurance card, driver's license)
   b. Inconsistent address or other information on documents
   c. Two forms of valid ID
   d. Consistent birthdates on all documents

4. Which organization(s) issued the regulations for Red Flag Rules for healthcare?
   a. Federal Trade Commission
   b. Department of Treasury
   c. Federal Reserve System
   d. HHS

5. One method for evaluating and prioritizing risks related to the protection of organizational information is:
   a. Business impact analysis
   b. Recovery point objective
   c. Recovery time objective
   d. Disaster preparedness

6. University Hospital needs to decide what type of backup data facility they need for data backup. Because their main priority for the backup data facility is a site that can bring their critical applications and operations online within hours, their best choice for a backup facility is a
   a. Hot site
   b. Warm site
   c. Lukewarm site
   d. Cold site

7. Which of the following is not a required element of a security risk safeguard?
   a. The means of data collection for the organization
   b. Documentation of potential threats
   c. Assessment of the current security measures
   d. A Contingency plan

Discussion.

8. Other than the fact that it occurs in a healthcare facility, medical identity theft is identical to financial identity theft.

9. Discuss the process for a security risk analysis.

10. What would you consider in preparing a comprehensive disaster plan?

REFERENCES

45 CFR 160.103 Definitions 2013.

45 CFR 160.404: Amount of a civil money penalty. 2013.

45 CFR 164.302: Applicability. 2013.

45 CFR 164.304: Definitions. 2013.

45 CFR 164.306: Security standards: General rules.

45 CFR 164.308(a): Administrative safeguards. 2013.

45 CFR 164.308(a)(1): Administrative safeguards. 2013.

45 CFR 164.308(a)(1)(ii)(A).Administrative safeguards: Risk analysis. 2013.

45 CFR 164.308(a)(2): Administrative safeguards. 2013.

45 CFR 164.308(a)(3): Administrative safeguards. 2013.

45 CFR 164.308(a)(4): Administrative safeguards. 2013.

45 CFR 164.308(a)(5): Administrative safeguards. 2013.

45 CFR 164.308(a)(6): Administrative safeguards. 2013.

45 CFR 164.308(a)(7): Administrative safeguards. 2013.

45 CFR 164.308(a)(8): Administrative safeguards. 2013.

45 CFR 164.308(b)(1): Administrative safeguards. 2013.

45 CFR 164.310: Physical safeguards. 2013.

45 CFR 164.310(a)(1): Physical safeguards. 2013.

45 CFR 164.310(b): Physical safeguards. 2013.

45 CFR 164.310(c): Physical safeguards. 2013.

45 CFR 164.310(d)(1): Physical safeguards. 2013.

45 CFR 164.312(a)(1): Technical safeguards. 2013.

45 CFR 164.312(b): Technical safeguards. 2013.

45 CFR 164.312(c)(1): Technical safeguards. 2013.

45 CFR 164.312(d): Technical safeguards. 2013.

45 CFR 164.312(e)(1): Technical safeguards. 2013.

45 CFR 164.014: Organizational Requirements. 2013.

45 CFR 164.016: Policies and procedures and documentation requirements. 2013.

45 CFR 160.18: Compliance date. 2013.

45 CFR 164.402: Definitions. 2013.

AHIMA. 2014. *Pocket Glossary for Health Information Management and Technology*. 4th ed. Chicago: AHIMA Press.

AHIMA. 2013. *Analysis of Modifications to the HIPAA Privacy, Security, Enforcement, and Breach Notification Rules under the Health Information Technology for Economic and Clinical Health Act and the Genetic Information Nondiscrimination Act: Other Modifications to the HIPAA Rules*. http://library.ahima.org/xpedio/groups/public/documents/ahima/bok1_050067.pdf.

AHIMA e-HIM Work Group on Medical Identity Theft. 2008. Mitigating medical identity. *Journal of AHIMA* 79(7):63–69.

Al-rousan, T., L. Rubenstein, and R. Wallace. 2014. Preparedness for natural disasters among older US Adults: A nationwide survey. *American Journal of Public Health* 104(3):506–511.

Anon. 2011. All IRBs should prepare for possible disaster interruptions. *IRB Advisor* 11(11):109–111.

American Recovery and Reinvestment Act of 2009. Public Law 111-5 13402(h)(2) 2009. https://www.gpo.gov/fdsys/pkg/PLAW-111publ5/content-detail.html.

Beaton, R., E. Bridges, M.K. Salazar, M.W. Oberle, A. Stergachis, J. Thompson, and P. Butterfield. 2008. Ecological model of disaster management. *AAOHN Journal* 56(11):471–478.

Becker's Health IT and CIO Review. 2015 and 2016 issues. http://www.beckershospitalreview.com/healthcare-information-technology/19-latest-healthcare-data-breaches.html.

Braun, J. 2012. HIPAA rules stay in place during disaster—Address privacy and security issues in plans. *Hospital Access Management* (August 2):1–2.

Brodnik, M., L. Rinehart-Thompson, and R. Reynolds. 2012. *Fundamentals of Law for Health Informatics and Information Management, Second Edition*. Chicago: AHIMA.

CMS. 2007a. HIPAA Security Series—Security Standards: Administrative Safeguards. https://www.hhs.gov/sites/default/files/ocr/privacy/hipaa/administrative/securityrule/adminsafeguards.pdf.

CMS. 2007b. HIPAA Security Series—Security Standards: Physical Safeguards. https://www.hhs.gov/sites/default/files/ocr/privacy/hipaa/administrative/securityrule/physsafeguards.pdf.

CMS. 2007c. HIPAA Security Series—Security Standards: Technical Safeguards. https://www.hhs.gov/sites/default/files/ocr/privacy/hipaa/administrative/securityrule/techsafeguards.pdf.

Conn, J. 2012. Bracing for a crash. *Modern Healthcare* 42(20):32–33.

Department of Health and Human Services. 2016a. *Enforcement Results by Year.* http://www.hhs.gov/hipaa/for-professionals/compliance-enforcement/data/enforcement-results-by-year/index.html#2014Department.

Department of Health and Human Services. 2016b. *HIPAA Enforcement. Health Information Privacy.* http://www.hhs.gov/hipaa/for-professionals/compliance-enforcement.

Department of Health and Human Services, Office of Inspector General. 2015a. *The Response to Superstorm Sandy Highlights the Importance of Recovery Planning for Child Care Nationwide.*

Department of Health and Human Services, HealthIT. 2015b. *Guide to Privacy and Security of Electronic Health Information.*

Department of Health and Human Services. 2008. *Resolution Agreement. Health Information Privacy.* http://www.hhs.gov/hipaa/for-professionals/compliance-enforcement/examples/providence-health/index.html.

Federal Trade Commission. 2013 *Fighting Identity Theft with the Red Flags Rule: A How-To Guide for Business.* https://www.ftc.gov/tips-advice/business-center/guidance/fighting-identity-theft-red-flags-rule-how-guide-business.

Gibson, P., F. Theadore, and J. Jellison. 2012. The common ground preparedness framework: A comprehensive description of public health emergency preparedness. *American Journal of Public Health* 102(4):633–642. doi:10.2105/AJPH.2011.300546.

Gupta, A. 2011. Hackers, breaches, and other threats to elect. *Health Data Management* 19(9):3.

Harrison, J.P., R.A. Harrison, and M. Smith. 2008. Role of information technology in disaster medical response. *Health Care Manager* 27(4):307–313.

Herzig, T.W, ed. 2010. *Information Security in Healthcare: Managing Risk.* Chicago: HIMSS.

Keith, B. 2010. Catch fraud upfront: Medical identity theft is on the rise: It's time to revamp your processes. *Hospital Access Management* 29(5):49–51.

King, P., and R.L. Williams. 2008. *Red Flag Compliance for Healthcare Providers: Protecting Ourselves and Our Patients from Identity Theft.* Chicago: American Health Lawyers Association and HIMSS.

Mancilla, D., and J. Moczygemba. 2009. Exploring medical identity theft. *Perspectives in Health Information Management* 6:1–11.

Medical Identity Fraud Alliance. 2015. Fifth Annual Study on Medical Identity Theft. http://medidfraud.org/2014-fifth-annual-study-on-medical-identity-theft/.

MindTools. 2013. *The Risk Impact/Probability Chart.* http://www.mindtools.com/pages/article/newPPM_78.htm.

National Institute of Standards and Technology (NIST). 2016. Publications Series 800-66. *An Introductory Resource Guide for Implementing the Health Insurance Portability and Accountability Act.* http://nvlpubs.nist.gov/nistpubs/Legacy/SP/nistspecialpublication800-66r1.pdf.

National Institute of Standards and Technology (NIST). Engineering Laboratory. 2014. *Tornado, Moore, Oklahoma.* http://www.nist.gov/el/disasterstudies/weather/moore_tornado_2013.cfm.

National Institute of Standards and Technology (NIST). 2008. Special Publication 800-66. An *Introductory Resource Guide for Implementing the Health Insurance Portability and Accountability Act (HIPAA) Security Rule*. http://nvlpubs.nist.gov/nistpubs/Legacy/SP/nistspecialpublication800-66r1.pdf.

Nelson, S.B. 2008. Information management during mass casualty events . . . Includes discussion. *Respiratory Care* 53(2):232–238.

Office for Civil Rights. Department of Health and Human Services. 2003. *Summary of HIPAA Security Rule*. https://www.hhs.gov/hipaa/for-professionals/security/laws-regulations/.

Office for Civil Rights. Department of Health and Human Services. 2010. *Guidance on Risk Analysis Requirements under the HIPAA Security Rule*. http:/www.hhs.gov/ocr/privacy/hipaa/administrative/securityrule/rafinalguidancepdf.pdf.

Office for Civil Rights, Department of Health and Human Services. 2013. Modifications to the HIPAA Rules. *Federal Register* 78(17):5566–5702.

Office for Civil Rights, Department of Health and Human Services. 2016a. *Health Information Privacy, Breach Notification Rule*. http://www.hhs.gov/hipaa/for-professionals/breach-notification/index.html.

Office for Civil Rights, Department of Health and Human Services. 2016b. *Enforcement Highlights*. http://www.hhs.gov/ocr/privacy/hipaa/enforcement/highlights/index.html.

Ponemon Institute LLC. 2015. Sponsored by the Medical Identity Fraud Alliance with support from: Kaiser Permanente, ID Experts, Experian Data Breach Resolution and Identity Finder, LLC. Fifth Annual Study on Medical Identity Theft. http://medidfraud.org/wp-content/uploads/2015/02/2014_Medical_ID_Theft_Study1.pdf.

Ranajee, N. 2012. Best practices in healthcare disaster recovery planning. *Health Management Technology* 33(5):22–24.

Reynolds, P., and I. Tamanaha. 2010. Disaster information specialist pilot project: NLM/DIMRC. *Medical Reference Services Quarterly* 29(4):394–404. doi:10.1080/02763869.2010.518929.

Smith, E., and R. Macdonald. 2006. Managing health information during disasters. *Health Information Management Journal* 35(2):8–13.

Springer, R. 2009. Medical identity theft—Red flag and address discrepancy requirements. *Plastic Surgical Nursing* 29(2):131–134. doi:10.1097/01.PSN.0000356874.56338.2c.

ADDITIONAL RESOURCES

Amesh A, M. Watson, N. Boeri, K. Minton, R. Morhard, and E. Toner. 2014. Absorbing citywide patient surge during Hurricane Sandy: A case study in accommodating multiple hospital evacuations. *Annals of Emergency Medicine* https://www.jointcommission.org/assets/1/6/Hurricane_Sandy_Hospital_Evacs_adalja2014.

Belfort, R. 2009. *HITECH raises the stakes on HIPAA compliance*. https://www.manatt.com/insights/newsletters/health-update/client-alert-%c2%a0hitech-raises-the-stakes-on-hipaa-coht.

Brocato, L., S. Emery, and J. McDavid. 2011. Keeping compliant: Managing rising risk in physician practices. *Journal of AHIMA* 82(11):32–35.

Dinh, A. 2008. HIPAA security compliance—What comes next? *Journal of Health Care Compliance* 10(3):37–39.

Health Information Technology for Economic and Clinical Health (HITECH) Act. Public Law 111-5.

Hoffman, S., and A. Podgurski. 2009. E-health hazards: Provider liability and electronic health record systems. *Berkeley Technology Law Journal* 24(4):1523–1582.

Neal, D. 2011. Choosing an electronic health records system: Professional liability considerations. *Innovations in Clinical Neuroscience* 8(6):43.

Rhinehart-Thompson, L.A. 2008. Raising awareness of medical identity theft: For consumers, prevention starts with guarding, monitoring health information. *Journal of AHIMA* 79 (10)74–75, 81.

Schiff, G.D., and D.W. Bates. 2010. Can electronic clinical documentation help prevent diagnostic errors? *New England Journal of Medicine* 362(12):1066–1069. doi:10.1056/NEJMp0911734.

Scott, R.L. 2006. Physicians' reliance on electronic health records. University of Houston.

Sullivan, J. 2004. *HIPAA: A Practical Guide to the Privacy and Security of Health Data.* Chicago: American Bar Association.

US Congress. 2009. Health Information Technology for Economic and Clinical Health (HITECH) Act. *Code of Federal Regulations.* http://edocket.access.gpo.gov/2010/pdf/2010-17210.pdf.

Vigoda, M. 2008. e-Record, e-Liability: Addressing medico-legal issues in electronic records. *Journal of AHIMA/American Health Information Management Association* 79(10):48–52.

Virapongse, A., D.W. Bates, P. Shi, C.A. Jenter, L.A. Volk, K. Kleinman, L. Sato, and S.R. Simon. 2008. Electronic health records and malpractice claims in office practice. *Archives of Internal Medicine* 168(21):2362–2367. doi:10.1001/archinte.168.21.2362.

Legal Health Records

By Kelly McLendon,
RHIA, CHPS

Learning Objectives

- Explain the legal health record for disclosure
- Compare and contrast a paper-based legal health record, a hybrid legal health record, and an electronic legal electronic health record
- Determine the stakeholders and their roles for electronic legal health record definition projects
- Relate the steps involved in defining the legal health record
- Articulate the importance of developing a legal health record policy
- Interpret the attributes that can impact the legal health record definition and e-discovery
- Analyze patient record documentation regulations for correct utilization within legal health record policies and procedures

KEY TERMS

Accounting of disclosures
Any and all records
Audit logging
Data
Designated record set
Disclosure
Document and data nonrepudiation
e-discovery
Federal Rules of Civil Procedure (FRCP)
Federal Rules of Evidence (FRE)
Hybrid health records
Information governance (IG)

Legal health records
Legal hold
Litigation response
Metadata
Protected health information
  (PHI)
Record custodians
Rendition
Spoliation
State Rules of Civil Procedure
State Rules of Evidence
Uniform Rules for e-discovery

The goal of this chapter is to provide readers with a thorough understanding of the concepts surrounding **legal health records** (LHRs), which are a foundational element of informatics. Conceptually, LHRs are the data, documents, reports, and information that comprise the formal business record(s) used during the legal proceedings of any healthcare organization. AHIMA defines the legal health record (LHR) as "documents and data elements that a healthcare provider may include in response to legally permissible requests for patient information" (AHIMA 2014, 87). Informatics is based upon electronic health data and the use of this data within the legal system is guided by the concepts surrounding LHRs. Understanding LHRs requires comprehension of business records used as LHRs, what processes are used by those components, and what physical and electronic systems are used to manage these records.

Although it has been recognized for years that patient safety is positively impacted by the technological advantages of electronic health records (EHRs), there has been fragmented and sporadic migration toward these electronic systems throughout the past two decades. The Health Information Technology for Economic and Clinical Health (HITECH) Act (part of the American Recovery and Reinvestment Act of 2009 [ARRA], also known as the Stimulus Plan) has incentive payment funding for the meaningful use of certified EHRs (ARRA 2009). These tightly focused meaningful use requirements for vendors and providers contributed to migration of most hospitals and many providers of healthcare away from a paper-based to an electronic record system. Although this migration offers unparalleled opportunities for patient safety and care improvement, it also raises risks and challenges to everyone involved with the access, use, and overall management of these records, including those who use the records for legal purposes. Although the incentives for the adoption of EHRs under the meaningful use program will expire, the use of increased or reduced reimbursements through value-based care or risk-based reimbursement will provide the incentive to continue the migration efforts rather than direct monetary incentives.

Another dimension of change that opens realms of opportunity for cost reduction, quality, and effectiveness of care and patient safety are the health information exchanges (HIEs), which are moving information beyond the original, single health record and single provider of care. Ideally, the HIEs and their facilitating infrastructures, the Regional Health Information Organizations (RHIOs) and the Nationwide Health Information Network (NHIN), will provide the framework for fully interoperable healthcare where previous test results, medications, and treatments are available for each new provider's use. Transitions to the many forms of health information exchange are proceeding at different speeds across local, regional, and national levels, and the terms referring to them are constantly evolving. But one commonality has been seen; the potential for impact to legal health record definitions and cataloging. This impact must be assessed with regard to best practices for technologies, authorizations, consents, data transmission, and data storage.

As if these previous changes were not enough, one more development in health informatics must be considered: personal health records (PHRs). PHRs are very different than EHRs or paper-based provider records because the patients, not the providers, store and retain the healthcare data in paper or electronic form. This is important when defining the LHR because the patient's PHR data are often imported into the providers' EHR, where it can then potentially become part of the patients' LHR. Given the move away from paper-based records, it may seem that they have become obsolete and thus do not need to be accounted for when defining the LHR. However, paper records will remain in use for another decade or two, or until the older records gradually age out of the retention time frames when they may be destroyed. A common retention time reflected by common industry best practices indicates the retention period may range from 7 to 25 years, depending upon state, federal, and other rules, regulations, statutes, and typical practices. Therefore, LHR planning must encompass the newly evolving electronic record, the PHR, which may include patient-generated or provided data, and the older paper record for the foreseeable future.

There are few, if any, instances where any type of legal records are called out by name in an EHR standard. As a result of the failure to define LHRs, there is no standard terminology for these records, and the wide audience of record users and creators do not understand exactly what is meant when the term legal health record is used. As a result, there are an increasing number of parties working to create their own definitions of legal health records. Thus the term LHR has become de facto acceptable parlance in the healthcare industry, even without a real standards-based definition. Given that there is legitimacy in the *concept* of LHRs, these concepts will be illustrated and clarified, along with describing the best practices commonly found on the subject from an introductory perspective. There are other publications that explore these concepts in greater depth. This chapter is intended to define the foundations and preliminary elements for the reader in a fashion that creates a good starting point for understanding the issues surrounding LHRs.

⊙ Legal Health Records

Many within the healthcare industry believe that well-recognized health information, including the documentation of care at the point of care and the provision of patient histories for care delivery, are almost exclusively the driving forces for creating and maintaining health records. This tends to be the point of view of the providers of care; one that, while not incorrect, is limited in scope. In reality, there are many more reasons for creating and maintaining sound health records. Health records have many uses, such as continued treatment, payment, healthcare operations, quality management, research, and public health reporting. They are also the starting point for assuring compliance with the myriad of rules, regulations, and laws that guide healthcare delivery in the United States.

There have been objections to the term legal health record because it might indicate that some records are more legal or usable in litigation than others. This is not the intended meaning of the term. Nearly all healthcare records and related electronic data (except those that are privileged or otherwise excluded) are admissible into evidence in court if they are kept according to widely accepted legal practice standards. Rather, the term legal health record is related to a larger conceptual framework. Great care has been taken within this text to avoid confusion and to clarify the use of the word legal including precise definitions such as the *LHR defined for disclosure* as opposed to simply naming the concepts *legal records.* Caution should be exercised with the use of *legal record.* It can be misleading and its use should be avoided or questioned when seen. Modifiers such as "for disclosure" create a more accurate view of the definition and concept. The use of the term *legal health record* or *LHR* in this text is describing the concept surrounding the health record defined for disclosure or its accompanying attributes and not its legal admissibility. It is also worth noting that the LHR for disclosure is distinct from the HIPAA Designated Record Set. Any set of health records that are maintained with individually identifiable information or protected health information (PHI) are a HIPAA Designated Record Set. However, that does not mean the record set will be a part of the LHR for disclosure. For example, the data maintained in EHR feeder systems such as a pharmacy system or laboratory information system, though using PHI, will not usually be included in the LHR for disclosure.

The concepts surrounding LHRs have been coalescing for a period of years and will continue to evolve for the foreseeable future. EHRs and the legal environment are complex. Therefore, judicial decisions, laws, rules, regulations, and precedence will continue to refine the concepts and tenets of this subject. These are not static environments. The pertinent changes stemming from these judicial decisions, laws, rules, and regulations need to be tracked on a continual basis.

Information Governance (IG) is "an organization-wide framework for managing information throughout its lifecycle and supporting the organization's strategy, operations, regulatory, legal, risk, and environmental requirements" (AHIMA 2016). IG includes the governance of both the data and information technology. IG is a subject that is becoming increasingly clarified and utilized to organize enterprise-wide management of data, records, and the systems that contain them. At their core, legal health record principals and methodologies, as described within this chapter, are foundational components of an overarching IG program.

The most common legal processes, and usually the most coherent, are the federal rules, laws, decisions, and guidance issued by the US Supreme Court, especially in reference to **e-discovery** (the discovery of electronic records for legal proceedings). These apply across the United States and often take precedence over other guidance. There is also work from a group called the Uniform Commissioners from which state laws and rules may be derived that are very similar to the **Federal Rules of Civil Procedure (FRCP)** for rules of both civil procedure and evidence. The FRCP, the guidelines that govern the procedures for civil trials, were amended in 2006 to include electronic records and continue to be very important as benchmarks for how electronic data and information can be used in both federal and state courts.

There has been a significant ongoing rise in state laws that provide guidance regarding the **State Rules of Evidence** and **State Rules of Civil Procedure** within each state. For a period of time after the FRCP were introduced the state courts were reticent to adopt the changes for their venues. However, that trend has abated and each state has typically adopted some, if not many, changes to address electronic records related to evidence and in civil procedures. State laws and rules are certainly important to most legal actions and are so widely variable that no single book can account for all of them. Individual state laws and rules should be analyzed for subpoenas, court orders, discovery, and similar legal processes to determine which apply to the venues where records may be admitted into evidence. Vetting LHR strategies and policies and procedures (P&Ps) with legal counsel is a best practice obtaining advice and guidance.

⊙ Setting the Stage for LHRs

Perhaps one of the most important concepts to remember during the discussion of health records is that formal health record management is actually enterprise-wide in nature as opposed to solely departmental. No matter whether they are paper, electronic, or a hybrid mixture of multiple record formats, the basic principles of record management have not changed. The **Federal Rules of Evidence (FRE)** govern what and how electronic records may be used and the roles of record custodianship for purposes of evidence in a trial. In general, record management remains the same as it has been for decades with its basis in statutes and regulations, such as the **FRE,** the FRCP, Medicare regulations, HIPAA, and various state requirements (including civil procedure and rules of evidence). What has changed is a vast expansion of the specific requirements related to use of electronic records in court proceedings as opposed to rules that strictly address requirements of paper records.

Carefully planned and organized work processes that are efficiently executed so that they provide high-quality record keeping are still a requirement for healthcare providers. Now the requirements for managing all the disparate components of information comprising the dozens of types of **data** including dates, numbers, images, symbols, letters, and words that represent basic facts and observations about people, processes, measurements, and conditions have come together to form health records. Thus, while the basic concepts underlying the work needed remain unchanged, the scope and depth of the work have been greatly expanded.

Stakeholders for LHR Definition Projects

In any LHR definition project, the stakeholders and the processes that surround the legal and healthcare processes to manage these records are enterprise-wide and diverse. Any LHR definition project should include stakeholders from as many levels of the organization as possible. Prospective stakeholders need to be vetted to ensure they have the organization's best interest at heart. Recommended stakeholders are listed in table 14.1.

Paper, Electronic, and Hybrid Health Records

Paper health records have prevailed for more than a century, are mostly self-evident in their content and practices, and can be easily described. Paper records permanently record health information through the use of handwriting,

Table 14.1.   Recommended stakeholders

Stakeholder	Role
C-suite and practice managers	In general, the more supporting C-suite (chief executive officer, chief operating officer, chief information officer, and others) and practice manager–type stakeholders brought into the project the better, as they will support development of project materials and strategies that must be institutionalized.
HIM professionals	Lead the LHR definition project as much as possible. The strategies decided upon are typically carried out in large part by HIM staff, who ensure the accessibility, completeness, accuracy, reliability, and archiving of the EHR and paper-based medical record information. HIM staff also typically manage the subpoena disclosure and release-of-information processes for medical records.
Information technology staff	From the CIO to HIM and EHR analysts, IT also has key roles. Management and direct custodians of the various EHR and source systems that feed the EHRs are absolutely crucial to the success of an LHR project. IT staff are responsible for the hardware and software applications that manage electronic records contained within EHR systems. They have invaluable information about the granular level of details on how the software should operate and how it is implemented to work within the organization.
Record custodians	These staff, who are from patient accounts, diagnostic imaging, and physician practice areas, along with secondary custodians such as source system (for example, laboratory, radiology, and transcription) managers, are also valuable to the project. Record or data stewards are titles also related to record custodians; however, their scope of responsibility may be somewhat wider than record custodians.
Privacy, compliance, and security officers; risk managers; and quality managers	All have key roles to play in these projects because the decisions arrived at directly affect their daily work processes. Risk managers are many times an important HIM ally in LHR definition projects as they understand the liabilities and embrace strategies to reduce them.
Clinicians (including physicians, nurses, and ancillary clinical staff)	These staff who develop, create, input, modify, update, and use the data contained inside EHR systems as part of their daily practice bring unique and vital information to the project team. Clinical informatics professionals, especially nursing clinical informaticists, are extremely valuable in guiding legal aspects of documentation procedures that factor into LHR definition and organization projects.
Legal counsel	Whether internal or external, legal counsel and risk managers both play roles in subpoena disclosure, litigation response, and discovery (or e-discovery) processes. Vetting of LHR P&Ps is also required.

transcription, or printouts. They are stored in paper folders or similar hard copy files and are maintained in this form until destruction. At some point in their life cycle, healthcare entities may convert and replace their paper records with archival scanning into electronic document management systems or EHR systems, at which point the paper record becomes a hybrid health record.

There are myriads of federal, state, and other statutes, rules, and regulations that guide what must comprise a health record and, to date, these have largely been promulgated for paper records. Electronic records can and should utilize these requirements, combined with current paper health record documents, to help create the LHR defined for disclosure. Defining EHRs in the sense of what is to be disclosed for legal requests is more difficult than defining disclosure from paper records.

Hybrid health records are increasingly seen as the most common transition points between fully paper and completely electronic records. Transitioning from paper to electronic records is costly, very time consuming, and hugely reliant on vendor applications that may not be as well conceived as their users would like for them to be (as is often discovered during system implementation). Hybrid records may be a mixture of paper and electronic or multiple electronic systems that do not communicate or are not logically architected for record management.

Health **record custodians**, also known as record stewards, are typically a part of an HIM workgroup or an employee of the HIM department. Record custodians have the responsibility for the maintenance, custody, and oversight of the health records and are charged with leading multidisciplinary definition projects for both the HIPAA-required **Designated Record Set** and the LHR. The designated record set is a group of records maintained by or for a covered entity comprised of the medical records and billing records, enrollment, payment, claims adjudication, or medical case management records, which are used in whole or part by or for the covered entity to make decisions about individuals (45 CFR 164.501). Record custodians are also expected to develop proper organization, management, guidelines, and processes related to the use of business records as a protective legal defense tool. Most of the time, this effort is performed in conjunction with other stakeholders such as IT, compliance, and risk management.

Check Your Understanding 14.1

Indicate whether each of the following is true or false.

1. The term legal health record has the same meaning across all settings.
2. Legal health record concepts are a core foundation of Information Governance.
3. State rules of civil procedure and rules of evidence have decreased in importance over time.
4. Incentives for adoption and use of electronic health records will continue even after the HITECH meaningful use incentive program has ended.
5. Maintenance and protection of a healthcare organization's legal health record is solely the responsibility of the record custodian.

6. E-discovery refers to the type of discovery within legal proceedings that utilizes electronic records.

7. The HIPAA Designated Record Set is the same as the legal health record.

8. The most important use of health records is for public health reporting.

⊙ Why Define a Legal Health Record?

LHR definitions provide formal recognition of which record sets, components, data, and documents comprise the official business records denoted as medical or health records. These LHRs may be purely paper, electronic, or a hybrid combination. Creating sound LHR definitions clarifies the roles of all records and their uses and sets foundational policy for record management operations. Note that these definitions must be formal and published in-house. However, definitions will change as documents and data migrate from paper or other electronic systems, so they must be continually reviewed and updated as their constituent record components evolve.

LHR Definition Project Steps

Several high-level activities comprise LHR definition projects. Adequate time should be allocated to define the LHR for an organization. At each step in the process, there are requirements for learning new concepts, researching the literature, and exploring the best practices from others who have solved similar problems. The project team needs to have access to knowledgeable experts and resources to perform these steps. There is much to consider when creating an organization-wide LHR definition project. If the LHR definition project is part of a larger EHR implementation, it is recommended that the LHR project timeline be embedded within the critical path of the organization's overall implementation of an EHR. The following LHR definition steps are based upon common and standard best practices.

Step 1: Determine the LHR Stakeholder Team

The stakeholder team will drive the creation of the LHR documentation, undertake the LHR definition project, and be responsible for its continued maintenance. The record custodian should be in charge or included as a member of the team. In addition to the C-suite stakeholders, HIM professionals, information technology staff, record custodians from related areas, privacy and security officers, risk management, clinicians, and legal counsel should all be included on the team.

In the first step of undertaking an LHR definition, the team should create a process to move the project along according to formal rules adopted by the enterprise. Creating a definition in a small, physicians practice office is usually simple enough. The stakeholders are all nearby and there may be few of them. But in the larger organization with a more complex electronic record environment, it is harder to achieve consensus regarding an LHR definition. Therefore, using formal project methodology is highly recommended. It is up to record custodians, risk management, and legal staff to facilitate the project with carefully selected project team members.

Step 2: Determine Strategy and Plan for the LHR Definition Project, and Get Executive Sponsorship and Empowerment

Project governance and leadership is another important aspect of an LHR project. The executive or senior management must sponsor and empower the team to make the difficult decisions related to the LHR. Often the HIM department primary record custodian manages the LHR definition processes and other times, risk management, compliance, or legal staff may lead the initiative. Regardless of which staff members provide the leadership, it is crucial that LHR definition projects be managed as formal projects, with an explicit strategy and plan, until they are completed. The C-suite or executives are vital to help determine strategies, sign off on them, and help make them operational. These are good reasons to have some powerful stakeholders to get the respect and attention these projects require.

Step 3: Gather LHR-Related knowledge

The next step of the process is to become familiar with existing guidance and resources. The resources listed at the end of this chapter represent guidance on LHRs (McLendon 2012; Glondys and Kadlec 2016). Reading, continuing education, networking, keeping up with American Health Information Management Association (AHIMA) resources, and questioning experts are all excellent learning methods. The mission is to become one of the facility's experts on legal records. Additionally, most healthcare providers should have access to some type of legal counsel, whether it is in-house or external to the organization. Establishing and maintaining that relationship is key. Record custodians need to understand federal, state, and local record retention requirements and evidentiary and civil procedure requirements that are applicable to each organization.

Step 4: Develop a Master Source System Matrix

Regardless of its title, the first deliverable from an LHR definition project should be a master list of all clinical, financial, and administrative EHR systems (referred to as EHR modules under the 2010 meaningful use rules) that manage or contribute to the health record as well as patient accounts and diagnostic imaging records, if they are a focus of the project. This is necessary to identify all the systems that are used and to be able to communicate to the team and others as needed. If there is already such a list from the IT department, it should be examined to confirm either that it is current or that it is necessary to add other systems. IT staff should be involved when starting anew as they manage the hardware platforms and software applications that comprise the EHR systems.

Step 5: Create a Document Matrix of LHR Components

Once an EHR source system matrix is created, the next step is to develop a list of documents, data, and reports that comprise the LHR as defined for disclosure. The matrix of LHR components will vary from organization to organization. A small physician practice may only have a few applications, while a large integrated health system may have thousands of applications. In fact, the larger system may have an application to help manage IT resources, such as applications, which may make maintaining the list of LHR components easier. However it is accomplished, it is essential to know how to create the matrix of LHR components so that the user knows exactly what comprises the LHR.

Step 6: Assess and Catalog EHR Systems for Their LHR Attributes

The next step is to create a form for assessing and cataloging the EHRs' LHR attributes with LHR evaluation criteria, questions to be posed, and a space for recording the answers. Such evaluation criteria will facilitate the assessment of EHR systems for their attributes that may be important during e-discovery. These questions might be related to attributes such as the ease of producing a single, readable electronic record upon request, the ability of the system to segregate sensitive data subject to separate regulations, or the functionality employed when a patient requests an amendment to the EHR. The key to this assessment is not just asking the suggested questions but asking everything necessary to ensure the EHR and its functionalities and limitations related to record management are clearly understood. This cataloging is also a key requirement of information governance.

Step 7: Determine the Need for New and Revised Related Policies and Procedures

It is necessary to create new P&Ps related to the LHR definition project. There may also exist P&Ps that need to be updated, therefore any existing P&Ps may be impacted.

Step 8: Determine the LHR Maintenance Plan

The team should conduct regular reviews and provide updates of related P&Ps to ensure the organization is always in compliance with the latest rules and trends in LHRs. It is also a good idea to utilize actual P&P documents to train workforce members. As IT projects are added or updated, it should also be documented where data is located and how it fits into litigation response, legal hold, and other potential legal responses. The source system matrix should also be updated to include new applications, pertinent data stored therein, and the custodians for each system.

Steps 9 and 10: Create a Presentation (9) and Conduct Education and Training for Appropriate Workforce Members (10)

As many staff as possible should be educated so they will understand and have direction in following defined LHR P&Ps. These educational sessions should include administrative, departmental, nursing, medical, and IT staff. It is crucial to educate not only the project stakeholders but also key members from across the enterprise on the realities and processes used to create highly defensible health records, regardless of the format of the records (McLendon 2010a).

Check Your Understanding 14.2

Indicate whether each of the following is true or false.

1. It is only important for HIM department staff to understand and abide by the LHR policies and procedures.

2. Once the legal health record is defined, the healthcare organization will need to regularly review the policies and procedures.

3. It is not necessary to have organizational legal counsel review and approve the LHR policies and procedures.

4. A matrix of all LHR components is not needed.

5. Appropriate sponsorship of an LHR project is required.

6. Educating appropriate staff and other key stakeholders is essential for successful creation of defensible health records regardless of their format.

7. Cataloging systems and their attributes that contain patient data is not an essential element of a legal health record definition.

8. Keeping current with changing rules and regulations impacting legal record definitions is required to perform the role of record custodian.

⊙ Defining the Components of an LHR

Each organization may have different components that serve to define their LHR. It is not reasonable to expect a solo primary care practitioner to have the same components in their LHR as a tertiary care academic medical center. The problem with failing to define the components adequately is that the organization has little reasonable defense should they receive a request for a component in the absence of a definition. For example, if the clinicians use e-mail to communicate regarding patients and e-mail is not explicitly excluded from the LHR, attorneys can legitimately request any e-mail related to a particular patient's care and the organization will have to produce them. Thus, following the guidance below to define what is and is not included in the LHR is essential.

Creating a Tailored LHR Definition for Disclosure

The first task to be accomplished after the identification of stakeholders and project structure is to request a list of all clinical information EHR systems. These may be referred to as clinical EHR modules or source systems. The list should include the names of the systems as well as additional data fields such as the resident system expert, vendor name, data format, and others listed in table 14.2.

The next task is to create a document matrix, which is a list of all documents and data that comprise the current LHR utilized for routine disclosure. This may actually be a list or simply point to the master document table within an electronic document management system (EDMS). This typically comprises a list of hundreds of documents and can become unwieldy. Therefore, it is recommended that a list of chapters (sometimes known as index tabs) be created of what is included in the

Table 14.2.   Source system matrix

List EHR systems that contain data	Basic e-Discovery Information										
Provider Site Name of System	Application Name from Vendor	Vendor Company Name and Contact Information	Responsible Department	Department Primary Contact / Custodian	IT Primary Contact	List and Description of Data / Documents	Does system contain PHI; Designated Record Set	How to Access Data or Documents	Reasonably Accessible or Not Reasonably Accessible	Time / Cost to Obtain
Main/ EHR	Powerchart	Cerner	Health Information Management	Jill Jones	John Smith	History and Physical; MD Orders	Yes, both	Request via HIM	Dependent upon type of request	10 business days; $80

paper or hybrid health record. A spreadsheet-based matrix can be used to manage these data (see table 14.3). It is a good idea to create a single spreadsheet-based workbook (using Microsoft Excel or a comparable program) and to have these lists of source systems and LHR data and documents on separate worksheets within the workbook.

It is important to keep in mind the reason for creating a document matrix as a part of the LHR definition. The record custodian has the responsibility to determine what business records or components of these records they will release upon legal request and to also determine which records actually fulfill the content of the record request as stated in the request document.

Table 14.3.   Document matrix for documents, data, and reports defined as included in an LHR (with examples)

Facility			
Document Name Data Set Report Name	**EHR or Hybrid**	**Source System**	**Comments**
Approved for LHR and Routine Disclosure			
Advanced Directives	EDM	Paper	
Consents	EDM	Paper	
Emergency Department Report	EDM	ED System	
Continuity of Care Documents	Clinical Repository	HIE, Clinical EHR	
Diagnostic Imaging Reports	PACS	RIS	
EKG & EEG Reports	EDM	Paper	
Laboratory Reports	EDM	Lab	
MAR	Clinical Repository	Medication Mgmt	Different system than the Inpatient EHR
Multidisciplinary Notes	Clinical Repository	Inpatient EHR	
Nursing Documentation	Clinical Repository	Inpatient EHR	

(Continued)

Table 14.3. Document matrix for documents, data, and reports defined as included in an LHR (with examples) (*Continued*)

Facility			
Document Name Data Set Report Name	**EHR or Hybrid**	**Source System**	**Comments**
Operative, Recovery Room, Anesthesia Notes	EDM	Paper	Will be scanned into EDM soon
CPOE—Orders	Clinical Repository	Inpatient EHR	
Problem List	Ambulatory EHR	Ambulatory	
Psychological Assessment Document	Paper	Paper	Soon will be scanned into EDM
Physician Progress Notes	Clinical Repository	Inpatient EHR	
Physician Orders	Clinical Repository	Inpatient & Ambulatory EHR	Can be related to either Inpatient or Ambulatory encounters
Transcription	Paper	Paper	
Patient Billing Documents	Billing System	Billing System	
Remits	Paper	Paper	Soon to be electronically captured
Patient ID Photo and Documents	EDM	EDM	
Use to catalog your documents, data, and reports included in your defined LHR.			

Typically, a document matrix (such as table 14.4) is created in a spreadsheet with details about the documents and data included in the LHR defined for disclosure. Excluded documents and data that are commonly used or filed and stored with LHR components should be listed as well (see table 14.3). Common documents from the previous or current paper-based health record are nearly always included; therefore, paper records are typically a good starting point for populating the matrix.

The organization may already have completed projects that generated lists of documents that could serve as the basis of a document matrix. Such projects include

Table 14.4. Document matrix for documents, data, and reports defined as excluded from an LHR.

Facility			
Document Name Data Set Report Name	EHR or Hybrid	Source System	Comments
Excluded for LHR and Routine Disclosure			
Administrative Documents, Data, or Reports			
Abbreviation Lists			
Audit Logs			
Coding Query Forms			
Derived Data (that is, Accreditation Reports, Best Practice Guidelines, Clinical Paths, Statistical Reports)			
Indexes			
Metadata (that is, not otherwise viewable within medical record documentation reports or printouts)			
Operational Documents, Data, or Reports			
Physician Task Lists			
Privileged Legal Information			
Worksheets			
Use to catalogue your documents, data, and reports excluded from your defined LHR.			

forms redesign projects, especially for an EDMS, or forms-on-demand projects. In other cases, healthcare organizations have found that the HIPAA Designated Record Set (DRS) may be a useful starting point for an LHR defined for disclosure if the DRS has been cataloged. The DRS list of components and documents should be checked for concurrence with the LHR defined for disclosure, as they might be very similar. The formal definition of the DRS should expand well beyond that of the LHR. The DRS applies to any information within a healthcare organization that is used to make a decision about patient care and includes nearly all documentation with any **protected health information (PHI)**. PHI is individually identifiable health data or information, maintained or used by a covered entity (CE) or business associate (BA). This is usually a much wider set than the LHR defined for disclosure, even though the LHR is a subset of the DRS. If already cataloged, the DRS may be a great place to derive documents and data for the document matrix.

The LHR Policy Imperative

Creating an LHR defined for disclosure is important for a healthcare organization. The LHR policy determines what data and information can or should be released pursuant to a request from a third party. Without the LHR policy, a healthcare organization is at risk related to requests for data and information that the organization is not prepared to release. For example, if the organization does not determine how e-mail will be treated, a third-party requester could request any e-mails related to patient care and the organization would have no standing for refusing the request. Typically, this policy is created within an organization's defined template and filed in an appropriate filing system, which increasingly is maintained online for all authorized users to access. In fact, all policies should be accessible and readily usable by the entire authorized workforce. The policies should be used as training tools for regularly scheduled review.

Figure 14.1 shows an example of a few sections of an LHR policy. This policy was created in conjunction with source system and document matrixes. The length and complexity of an LHR policy will depend upon the needs of the healthcare organization.

Litigation Response Policy and Procedures for Record Custodians

The most common meaning of the term disclosure in healthcare is the act of releasing, upon proper authorization, copies of business or health records. Healthcare providers must take great care to recognize any release of information request that may become involved in litigation. **Litigation response** is typically the term used to describe the processes invoked if the potential for lawsuits or litigation is detected. Litigation response is not only triggered by atypical record disclosure requests but by any sign or action that shows a potential for a lawsuit. Litigation response should result in protective measures being taken by the provider to ensure maximum defensive posture, including appropriate responses to subpoenas and court orders, and protecting against **spoliation** (the malicious alteration, concealment, or destruction of evidence, be it in paper or electronic form) or other acts that later can be questioned and even sanctioned by the courts and opposing counsel.

Upon any legal request for disclosure of health information, the appropriate healthcare staff members or contractors will examine the request and determine what is to be disclosed according to predefined policies. A well-defined LHR will assist in appropriately determining exactly which record components are to be disclosed upon routine legal request. If the request is in any way unusual or meets the criteria to invoke litigation response as set by each organization, different procedures must immediately be instituted. Staff training and well-written P&Ps

Figure 14.1. Sections from an LHR policy created in conjunction with source system and document matrixes

SCOPE: All organization workforce members.

PURPOSE:

The business record documenting the delivery of healthcare rendered at **<insert site name>** is defined as the *Legal Health Record* (otherwise referred to as the LHR). This LHR will be disclosed upon routine legal or administrative record disclosure requests, such as subpoenas. Other routine record (PHI) disclosures will also be based on this defined LHR, such as the subset of the HIPAA defined Designated Record Set for individual inspection, copies, amendment of PHI, and other release of information requests. Minimum necessary provisions under HIPAA will apply to all disclosure requests.

This LHR Defined for Disclosure is a hybrid record **(if indeed your record is a hybrid, if not modify this language)** created from the paper medical record and **<insert EHR system(s) name(s)>** documents.

The scope of this policy is for **<insert site name>** HIM managed records. Other **<insert site name>** medical record types (that is, medical practices and certain other Outpatient Services records) are not currently addressed by this policy.

The LHR at **<insert site name>** includes the documentation of healthcare services provided to an individual in all delivery settings by our clinical and professional staff. The LHR consists of individually identifiable data in any medium, collected, processed, stored, displayed, and directly used in documenting healthcare delivery or health status.

The LHR at **<insert site name>** is a hybrid record **<modify as necessary to reflect your environment>** utilizing both paper-based and electronic documents, which are captured both manually and via electronic processes; see the LHR Source System Matrix and Document Matrix worksheet for details of the LHR component documents. Each encounter is maintained under a unit record number and includes subsequent patient visits. Only individuals authorized to do so by hospital or medical staff policies and procedures make entries into the LHR. Standardized formats are used for documenting all care, treatment, and services provided to patients.

The LHR contains sufficient information to identify the patient, support the diagnosis, justify the treatment and services, document the course and results of care, and promote the continuity of care among health providers.

The LHR will include records from *other healthcare providers* as the result of tests and exams when they were utilized for the evaluation of the patient and subsequent treatment.

The Federal Rules for Civil Procedure (FRCP) instituted December 1, 2006, expand the process of discovery and provide guidelines for electronic records

(Continued)

Figure 14.1.   Sections from an LHR policy created in conjunction with source system and document matrixes (*Continued*)

utilized as evidence and this policy is in accordance with the guidance provided by these rules.

It is important to define the location of the documents (in either paper or **<insert EHR system(s) name(s)>**) within the **<insert site name>** Legal Health Record (LHR) for timely access, use, and disclosure as necessary for patient care and other requirements, such as disclosure requests. As **<insert site name>** transitions from a paper-based record to hybrid records, and then to a more complete EHR, the location and management of the **<insert site name>** LHR must be evaluated, monitored, and kept updated for medicolegal purposes.

The Document Matrix will serve as a dynamic tool used to define the LHR components in their present form. As **<insert site name>** implements new EHR systems, the matrix will be reviewed and updated. It will serve as the guideline for the legal location of our medical record from which we disclose protected health information.

Related Materials:

- Source System Matrix
- Document Matrix

are key to maximizing the use of healthcare business records as tools in legal defense. Litigation response is simply a set of procedures that, when instituted, protects the records, whether they are health records, billing records, administrative, or metadata, whenever litigation is involved.

Within the FRCP and **Uniform Rules for e-Discovery** (amendments to the FRCP specifically designed for electronically stored information), once litigation is suspected or known to be occurring, a specific litigation response, including record protection, must be established. The Uniform Rules apply to federal but not state courts. However, they are appropriate guidance to follow since state courts have been generally less proscriptive in these areas, although that is changing as states adopt updated rules of civil procedure and evidence to more adequately address electronic records. State laws and regulations must be considered when creating litigation response policies and procedures.

Creating Litigation Response Policies and Procedures

Typically, the larger and more complex an organization's healthcare delivery system, the more likely it is to have formalized P&Ps to guide actions when litigation is known or suspected. But experience has shown that even these organizations may not have codified their litigation response into clearly defined procedures used to train staff and ensure all parties act accordingly. Failure to have well-defined processes can increase liability and financial risk. All healthcare entities, from the very largest to the smallest, should examine their litigation response P&Ps to prevent potentially costly lapses during legal actions. Litigation response may or may not be the responsibility of a single department or staff member.

Development of litigation response P&Ps starts with documentation of the steps and personnel already performing these tasks. Once the current practices are assessed, formalization into model processes can occur. The best practices guidelines presented in the next section have been drawn from actual practice settings. As always, customize these practices to fit your specific requirements.

Check Your Understanding 14.3

Indicate whether each of the following is true or false.

1. Healthcare providers must be concerned about policies and procedures to guide formal litigation response.

2. There is little need to organize the small amount of data defining legal records into tables or spreadsheets.

3. Litigation response is simply a set of procedures that, when instituted, protects the records.

4. Designated Record Sets (DRS) and Legal Health Record (LHR) definitions and cataloging are closely related.

5. Spoliation is not as much of an issue for electronic records as paper records.

6. When creating policies for legal health record definitions and litigation response only federal, not state rules of evidence and civil procedure need to be addressed.

Match the terms with the appropriate descriptions.

    a. Individually identifiable health information
    b. The processes invoked if the potential for lawsuits or litigation is detected
    c. Federal rules governing how litigation proceeds
    d. The malicious alteration, concealment, or destruction of evidence

7. _____ Spoliation

8. _____ Protected health information

9. _____ Uniform Rules for e-Discovery

10. _____ Litigation response

⊙ EHR System Attributes That Impact LHR Definitions and e-Discovery

It is crucial to understand each installed EHR system, its purpose in the normal course of daily business, and it functionality from a legal process perspective. This functionality will come into play at many points within litigation or routine legal proceedings. This is especially true as related to questions of accuracy, trustworthiness, and reliability.

When responding to a legal request relating to the EHR, there is not a great deal of time to put together lists of all the important system attributes, functionalities, and user experiences within an EHR system that works to create and manage health records. Therefore, it is advisable to catalog these attributes during the LHR definition project. If not performed in advance, the cataloging must be performed during the course of litigation. If performed during litigation, all answers to specific questions in reference to functionality and system record management attributes should be kept on a permanent basis for future reference.

The following functionalities are important to assess and use in practice to demonstrate that important and mandated attributes are met by your EHR system for optimal defensive legal purposes. It is recommended that these questions be logged into spreadsheets for permanent access and future usage.

Audit Logs

Audit logging refers to metadata kept on each transaction or event that occurs within an EHR system. Not all audit logs are the same. There is wide variability between products and vendors. Audit logs are key records that are expected to be producible if required in legal cases involving health records. Audits logs are essential to successfully execute many required operations such as reporting on who accessed and used data within an EHR. Certification of EHR products includes a requirement (45 CFR 170) to have audit logs with a minimum capability to generate an audit log, record the actions of users, and have the ability to be sorted. In order to meet these criteria, the audit log must contain the following for all transactions (or "uses") of an EHR:

- Date
- Time
- Patient identification
- User identification (including name, not just an assigned user number)
- Brief description of the actions taken by the user (for example, create, print, view, update, and so on) (45 CFR 170)

Audit logs should be managed as an important component of the organization's "content" (another term for data), documents, and various electronic record sets. Managing audit logs is an important part of the organization's business records that imposes retention and storage issues. The audit logs should be maintained for a retention period of at least six years for HIPAA and longer if required by other regulations.

Authorship and Authentication of Entries and Electronic Signatures

An author is a person or system who originates or creates information that becomes part of the record. Each author must be granted permission by the healthcare entity to make such entries. Not all users will be granted authorship rights into all areas of the EHR. The individual must have the credentials required by state and federal laws to be granted the right to document observations and facts related to the provision of healthcare services. Through medical staff bylaws and rules and regulations or through documentation guidelines, a provider will indicate the type and frequency of entries to be made in the health record. Often, the bylaws, rules and regulations, or guidelines are based on the documentation requirements published by various government and regulatory agencies.

How clinical documentation and documents are authenticated or electronically signed by the author can have significant ramifications in legal definitions and proceedings. Authentication is a process by which a user (a person or entity) who authored an EHR entry or document is seeking to validate that they are responsible for data contained within it. Authentication can be performed manually with a pen or it can be performed with electronic (and digital) technology. If performed with electronic technology, it is usually called an electronic signature.

Business Continuity

It is important to understand, from an LHR perspective, backups, disaster recovery, and business continuity in the face of routine to catastrophic failures. Determining backups and disaster recovery is a product of performing Security Risk Analysis as required by HIPAA as well as part of meaningful use compliance. There are many guidance documents published by the National Institute of Standards and Technology (NIST 2010; Glondys and Kadlec 2016) to guide the creation of the systems and processes to ensure continuity of business in the face of disaster or any kind of downtime.

Business Rules

The rules and triggers that create work lists, workflows, and other automated processes including clinical decision support alerts and reminders within an EHR are called "business rules" and should be well documented to ensure the best legal defensibility. There can be a large number of these rules. If they are not well documented and are called into e-discovery or court with a limited time frame for production, the organization may find it difficult to put together the details of these rules and their impact on work processes.

Data, Document Management, and Nonrepudiation

The integrity of each piece of data, including any document, must be ensured to maintain highly defensible business records. **Document and data nonrepudiation**, characteristics that defend against charges questioning the integrity of data or documents, delineate the methods by which the data are maintained in an accurate form after their creation, free of unauthorized changes, modifications, updates or similar changes. All EHRs have features to provide for this integrity but with varying combinations of technologies and recommended business processes. How each user organization decides to utilize and continually maintain the highest level of integrity are variables that need to be addressed during each EHR system implementation and operation.

Accuracy, trustworthiness, and reliability are key legal tests of any EHR; however, they are conceptual in nature, defined generally for use in the law but more specifically in each instance based on the needs of the legal proceeding. There are many ways to ensure EHR data accuracy, trustworthiness, and reliability, which include policies and procedures, workforce education, and functions with technology to monitor for potential errors and send alerts for the documenter to consider and make changes if warranted. As EHRs are being developed and implemented, the combination of technological features and means with which the users apply them determine the overall capabilities in these areas.

Retention, Data Permanence, and Migration Plans

Planning for the eventual obsolescence of a technology is often not given a high priority. Record managers need to understand how data would be migrated to ensure compliance with the long retention periods (years to decades) required for EHR systems. There are no standardized guidelines for this type of planning except generally to adopt standards-based sources of EHR data and record management as much as possible. Technology continues to advance and will for decades to come. Migration of data of all kinds needs to be established as systems are expanded and changed. Standards-based technology is essential to continued operational efficiency and integrity of older, but still useful, data and documents. Open formats, such as XML, PDF, and formatted continuity-of-care content such as Clinical Continuity Documents (CCD) and Clinical Continuity Records (CCRs), are already providing some guarantee of portability and permanence and making obsolescence less of an issue. More standards will continue to emerge to address these needs.

Interfaces

Typically, most EHR systems import and export documents and data in some fashion via interfaces. As with most other attributes of EHR systems, there are few mandated standards, although Health Level 7 (HL7) has become ubiquitous for some types of interfaces due to industry adoption rather than a mandate (Health Level Seven International 2007). As for LHR ramifications, there are not many with interfaces directly. It is necessary to catalog the interfaced data or documents for inclusion within the defined LHR and make them a part of the receiving facility's records. Once a record is received and made a part of a legal record set, it becomes a part of the record to be redisclosed upon appropriate request. The receiving facility cannot attest to accuracy, but if used, or even possibly used for care delivery, the record becomes a part of the receiving facility's legal record.

How interfaces are actually executed and reconciled (checked for quality and appropriate placement of data record) is important for record custodians. Their processes should strive to ensure the procedures for managing interfaced data are well thought out and documented so that they do not become problematic during court proceedings.

Legal Hold

There is a concept of **legal hold** in the healthcare environment. The legal hold requires special, tracked handling of patient records to ensure no changes can be made to a record involved in litigation. Common in the paper record environment to substantiate the integrity of the record, this is also very common in the electronic environment even where audit logs are in place as the audit logs typically do not store all data and metadata that may be required for a court case. Audit logs must be secured as previously discussed, but so must all of the data associated with a patient or pertaining to a case as outlined in an order for a legal hold. Any assumption that a record or set of data will be used in a court case may trigger a legal hold, these holds are not necessarily required to be issued by the court to be assumed to be in force. Record managers need to address the use of legal hold for patient records in any information mode or medium. Very often, consultation with legal counsel will be required.

Metadata

Metadata are data about data and are sometimes very hard to quantify. Litigation is highly dependent upon metadata, and metadata are sure to be an issue in e-discovery. Advanced assessment of these characteristics is important to meet short court clocks. Record custodians need to list all reasonably accessible (per FRCP rules) metadata within the source system. They also need to consider the following:

- ⊙ What data elements are kept for each system document, data, or report within the database, not necessarily within the audit log? Are the following included?
    - o Patient or user identification information
    - o User name or user ID
    - o Name or number of computer (dependent upon system capabilities) used to create the data or document
    - o Date and time created, modified, accessed, or printed, and file or network path location
    - o Revision history, if any changes were made to the data
    - o Patient identification number
    - o What data, documents, or reports were created, modified, accessed, or printed

This list indicates the data about the data that are maintained in the system and describes who recorded the data, on what computer, data and time, if changes were made in the date and other similar information. These items could be important in situations where there are concerns the data were altered or if there is a question of who actually recorded the information and other similar issues. These may be related to a quality of care issue or could be paramount in discrediting a witness.

Electronic Health Record Output

Maintaining control of PHI has always been a challenge. In the paper world, records could be copied and even carried out of the facility. These challenges have evolved and increased in the electronic environment. Output can now take the form of printed documents, or electronic documents that can be attached to e-mails, texted, downloaded to portable storage such as flash drives, captured as screenshots, and sent to social media sites, along with other as yet unidentified output mechanisms. It is essential for the organizational health information manager, privacy officer, security officer, and legal counsel to carefully consider the different types of potential output and how those can be controlled. For example, audit logs can track output to a printer. The printed copies could have annotations indicating that they are not full copies of the record. Likewise, many organizations have decided to disable the USB ports on many or all of the computers in the organization to prevent unauthorized downloads of PHI. The goal with controlling output is not to hinder patient care or any authorized access to PHI but rather to prevent any unauthorized release of PHI.

Another intersection of meaningful use and the LHR defined for disclosure is being sure to catalog all mandatory EHR output as a part of the LHR defined for disclosure. Discharge instructions, copies of records including summaries, and HIE data need to be cataloged within the list of document types that are to be disclosed as appropriate. They may be a part of a hybrid record or all contained within a single EHR. It is most important to keep these catalogs current as the EHR system is increasingly widely adopted.

Rendition

Rendition is the act of rendering data into documents, usually in report form. Report writers are the most common form of rendering, but there are others such as the creation of documents for continuity of care based on preprogrammed routines as required by meaningful use. Production of an LHR may be required in paper or other standard formats. It is important to take this into account when creating policies, procedures, and a litigation response plan.

Snapshots and Screen Views

Snapshots of data, or how screens are populated and what they looked like at discrete points in time, are increasingly being asked for in legal proceedings but are rarely provided in a satisfactory manner within EHR systems. Snapshots and screen views are difficult to create due to a lack of vendor capability.

Privacy Attributes

Given that HIPAA has strengthened privacy rules and increased enforcement, the following EHR system attributes take on elevated importance in determining privacy violations and breach notification:

- Does the EHR system create secured or unsecured PHI by HIPAA definition?
- How are patient's requests for access, viewing, and copying accomplished for this source system?
- In what format are electronic copies given to patients upon requests for access to their own records?
- How are patient requests for restrictions that have been accepted by the organization accomplished?
- How are patient amendment requests addressed?

- How is **accounting of disclosures** (AOD) tracked? AOD is a HIPAA requirement to list, upon patient request, all disclosures made outside of the entity holding the information.
- Is the audit log work detailed enough for privacy and access audits?

Monitoring violations and breaches of PHI is vital to identifying when these occur and more importantly identifying the reasons for them so corrections can be made to avert these occurrences in the future.

Version Controls

The LHR must be the record as created during the course of business. In some respects, EHR technology is still evolving. For example, a record may have been printed for an attorney or the software was upgraded and the record as viewed currently is different from the original view of the record. When changes, new data, or documents are added to the EHR, how are the old versions managed? Are they available or overwritten? Each EHR system typically has its own version management and also contains flexibility in implementation.

Check Your Understanding 14.4

Answer the following questions.

1. Which of the following is not an attribute of systems impacting privacy?
   a. Accomplishing patient requested amendments
   b. Applying patient requested and organizationally approved restrictions
   c. Auditing log reviews
   d. Legibility

2. Which of the following is not a key legal test for the EHR?
   a. Legibility
   b. Reliability
   c. Trustworthiness
   d. Accuracy

3. It is important to get data and information out of EHRs. Which of the following is not a consideration for EHR output?
   a. Version controls
   b. Screen snapshots
   c. Audit logs
   d. Payment source

4. Which of the following is not a form of metadata?
   a. Name or number of computer (depending on system capabilities) used to create the data or document
   b. Name that a computer system is typically referred to by users
   c. Revision history, if any changes were made to the data
   d. Date and time created, modified, accessed, or printed, and file or network path location

Indicate whether each of the following is true or false.

5. How data is output from an EHR is a key attribute of a legal health record definition.

6. The formats for electronic copies given to patients upon request is a privacy attribute.

7. Rendition converts documents into data.

⊙ Patient Record Documentation Considerations

All healthcare providers must establish P&Ps to maintain the health record in a way that establishes its validity, preserves its integrity, and facilitates efficient and timely responses to legally permissible requests. Some record management considerations to factor into your LHR P&Ps are included in this section.

Accuracy

Accurate documentation in a health record should reflect the true, correct, and exact description of the care delivered for both content and timing. The accuracy and the completeness of the entries in the health record are the responsibility of the author(s) and are governed by the organization's P&Ps. The P&Ps should include documentation standards based on the regulations, standards, and other sources noted in this chapter. Any decision regarding the inclusion or exclusion of information in the content of the LHR should be noted in the P&P documentation.

Amendments, Corrections, Deletion, and Other Documentation Issues

Providers must have a process in place for handling amendments, corrections, and deletions in health record documentation. Other concerning documentation issues are copy and paste forward, unexpected late entries, and the use of canned text, boilerplates, or other mechanisms that limit documentation. When healthcare providers determine that patient care documentation is inaccurate or incomplete, they must follow the established P&Ps to ensure the integrity of the record.

Patient-Requested Amendments

Healthcare organizations need policies to address how patients and their representatives can request amendments to their health records. An amendment is an alteration of the health information by modification, correction, addition, or deletion (AHIMA 2012a). HIPAA standards require that specific procedures and time frames be followed for processing a patient's request for changes or additions to the patient record. A separate entry, such as a progress note, form, or typed letter, can be used for patient amendment documentation. The amendment should

⊙ Refer back to the information questioned, by type of document or information, and the date and time of the original entry

⊙ Document the information believed to be inaccurate and the information the patient or legal representative believes to be correct

The documentation in question must not be removed from the health record or obliterated in any way. The patient cannot require that the documentation be removed or deleted, and the provider of care is not required to perform record amendments. However, if they do not allow the amendment, they must advise the patient of this and there are complex rules to follow in order to document this refusal.

Corrections

Proper procedures must be followed when correcting documentation problems or mistakes. A correction is a change in the information meant to clarify inaccuracies after the original electronic document has been signed or rendered complete (AHIMA 2012a). The system must have the ability to track corrections or changes to the entry once the entry has been entered or authenticated. An individual viewing the record should see an indicator that a new or additional entry has resulted and should also be able to see the new information. It must be clear to the user that there are additional versions of the data being viewed. Additional information related to error corrections can be found in the AHIMA Practice Brief: Maintaining a Legally Sound Health Record—Paper and Electronic (AHIMA 2005b).

Deletions

Deletion and retraction are closely related concepts, sometimes used synonymously. Both refer to totally eliminating or hiding from view information that was determined to be incorrect or invalid. A deletion is the action of permanently eliminating information that is not tracked in a previous version. A retraction is the action of correcting information that was incorrect, invalid, or made in error, and preventing its display or hiding the entry or documentation from further general views (AHIMA 2014). Any record documentation policies must address the occasional need to delete or retract information from a patient record without a visible record. An example of when this might be utilized is when information is filed or saved to the wrong patient's record. This might happen when two patient names are very similar. Another example might be when the clinician hears the patient say they have an allergy when they do not. The incorrect information needs to be hidden from view so that it is not used for future decision making. At the same time, the audit logs for the system should retain a record of the deletion or retraction and who completed the action. Additionally, it is important that the organizational policies strictly control deletion and retraction functionality, as it should be used sparingly.

Copy and Paste Forward

The technology used to support the EHR can provide many enhancements over the paper record (for example, multiple simultaneous access and audit trails). Technology also presents the potential for weakening the integrity of the information. One such risk occurs with the copy-and-paste-forward functionality present in many operating system and software programs. This functionality allows a user to highlight all or a portion of a document or screen display and then copy and paste the portion into a different or new document, potentially overwriting the original text. How they are implemented and used by the provider is usually a differentiator in system functionality. Regardless of the technology used, there are certain foundational concepts to be addressed about whether data can be copied and pasted. The appropriate use of these functions can support billing compliance and clinical data trustworthiness issues.

Fundamentally, the underlying concern of copy functionality is that it can damage the trustworthiness and integrity of the record for medicolegal purposes (AHIMA 2012b). The aspect of patient care provides a powerful reason for using the copy functionality in a judicious manner. Clinically, patient care may be impacted when copied information that is incorrect, old, and not pertinent to a given patient is used. Inconsistencies can occur due to indiscriminate use of copy functionality such as the copy forward of resolved health conditions and physical findings and symptoms that can confuse other providers and staff. Arbitrary use of the copy functionality that provides documentation not created for a specific patient or a specific episode of care can result in the submission of fraudulent billing (AHIMA 2012b).

When provider copy functionality is used as intended, it can help providers work efficiently while with compliant documentation. The appropriate copy functionality is:

- ⊙ Based on verifiable sources, such as demographic information that does not change over time.
- ⊙ Distinguishable from original information. This would include information identified as nonoriginal as seen with automatic summaries that populate data fields.
- ⊙ Not a part of the record until a reauthentication process is completed and provides documentation to identify the origination source (AHIMA 2012b).

There are many appropriate uses of copy forward functionality such as bringing forward a patient's problem or medication list if it has remained unchanged (AHIMA 2012b).

Late Entries

Late entries occur when a pertinent entry is missed or is not written in a timely manner (AHIMA 2014). When a late entry is documented, it should be clearly identified as a late entry. The author of the entry needs to record the current date and time as well as the date of the event that is the subject of the late entry. The author should also refer to counsel or any sources of information or circumstances surrounding the late entry. The longer the time period between the occurrence of the event and the recording of the late entry, the less reliable the information entered becomes.

Resequencing and Reassignment

The action of resequencing involves moving a notation or document within the same episode of care for the same patient (AHIMA 2014). It does not require tracking or any special action. Reassignment of documentation is defined as moving a document or notation between episodes of care within the record of a single patient (AHIMA 2014). It is recommended that a notation be left at the original location so clinicians can consult the documentation if necessary.

Templates, Boilerplates, Canned Text, and Structured Input

Care must be taken that devices such as templates, boilerplates, canned text, and structured input support clinical care and accurate documentation and are not used simply to expedite the documentation process, which can result in a lack of documentation accuracy. Creation and periodic review of these tools should be based on clinically appropriate, standards-based protocols for common or routine information. Documentation by these methods should require an active choice by the provider of care. When a clinician reviews and authenticates an entry in a patient's health record, the author is indicating that he or she reviewed and completed the documentation and accepts its accuracy as his or her own.

⊙ e-Discovery Overview

There are two main legal processes that custodians of records need to be concerned about related to defined electronic or hybrid LHRs: disclosure and e-discovery. Legal counsel will be concerned with both of these processes as well as more traditional legal process issues such as waivers, timing, and strategies. **Disclosure** is the output and release upon request of appropriate health record documents. E-discovery is the process of discovering what parts of the patient's records may be used for litigation or further legal proceedings and is an opportunity for opposing counsel to obtain relevant information. E-discovery is named to reflect an emphasis on electronic records; however, paper–electronic hybrids may also be included. E-discovery can be required from a single or a mix of EHR systems and may also require hybrid portions.

The FRCP distinguishes between reasonably accessible records and those that are not. This is the key that allows healthcare providers to define exactly what the LHR will consist of that will be released upon typical, appropriate requests.

LHR information derived from organizations' business records is admissible into evidence through an exception to the hearsay rule contained within FRE 803(6) and the Uniform Business and Public Records Act, which most states have adopted. The records must be kept in the normal course of daily business, authenticated, and identified prior to admission into legal proceedings. The legal and regulatory acceptance of electronic records is predicated on these records meeting certain well-established legal requirements. The basic requirement is that records are authentic and can be deemed to be reliable, trustworthy, and accurate. Tests of these requirements show through various means that the electronic record must have been captured at or near the time of the event or transaction and is complete and available for retrieval.

Amended FRCP amendments took effect December 1, 2006, to more consistently conform to the current LHR environment and have continued to evolve over time. These rules in various permutations have been adopted by many, but not all state and local jurisdictions. Adopting them as standards for your facility is prudent. The federal rules continue to mandate formal record custodianship as evidenced by the FRCP for electronic records. The record custodian is charged with the ability to certify exact copies of the original record components; supervise all record inspections by third parties; copy or duplicate records for external release for admission into evidence; and attest to the admissibility, timeliness, and management of the day-to-day record-keeping environment.

Output can be admitted into evidence if it meets the criteria required by the Uniform Photographic Copies of Business and Public Records as Evidence Act (there are both federal and state versions). This act states that a reproduction made by any process that accurately reproduces or forms a durable medium for reproducing the original is as admissible in evidence as the original itself.

The FRCP for e-discovery is responsible for widespread updates and modifications of record management for evidentiary purposes. There are rules addressing legal holds, spoliation, and the e-discovery process, which may take place at the beginning of litigation. Electronic systems must not only securely store data and documents for your defined retention period, but record custodians must also protect them from unauthorized alternation or destruction and be able to secure them from changes during litigation, especially upon court order.

E-discovery is not a "fishing expedition" that grants plaintiffs' counsel the ability to comb through all the patient's records looking for issues to litigate. The concept of **any and all records** can be limited in e-discovery. The term "any and all records" has the expected meaning of all available records. A more focused approach on what is deemed relevant for the case is necessary. Counsels may not agree on these points, and the judge or court officer may be forced to make the determination. Requests stating "any and all records" will be difficult to respond to given the extensive nature of multiple electronic records. If such requests are received, work with your counsel to limit the scope of the request based on relevance to the claim.

Case Study: Patient's Right to Restriction

The HITECH-HIPAA Omnibus Final Rule added complexity to patient restrictions, requiring healthcare providers to restrict disclosures of records if the associated treatment is paid for out-of-pocket by the patient. Because of this, healthcare organizations have had to implement changes in their restrictions policies and procedures. The following case study is how one organization addressed the patients' right to request restrictions on the disclosure of their information.

Watkins Health Services is a large clinic serving the University of Kansas (KU) in Lawrence, Kansas. Although healthcare services are provided to staff and faculty, the vast majority of more than 110,000 annual visits involve KU students. Watkins has nine board-certified physicians, three nurse practitioners, a nursing staff of 15, plus its own pharmacy, physical therapy services, lab, and radiology departments. KU boasts three RHIA-credentialed staff members, a luxury in college health.

The HITECH-HIPAA Final Omnibus Rule's provision giving patients the right to request restrictions on the disclosure of information to a health plan merely codified a practice that had been in place for decades. This is probably true for many college health services that perform third-party billing—and yes, some still do not bill insurance.

At least a couple of times a week, a student will have certain health procedures or lab tests performed, or pick up medications in the pharmacy that he or she prefers not be billed to insurance. KU providers, nurses, lab, and pharmacy personnel are well-versed in advising the student about the "private billing" option. The patient merely has to complete the "Restrictions on Use and Disclosure" form in the business office. Although KU encourages these patients to pay that same day if possible, this is certainly not mandatory. However, it is essential that KU have the correct address for billing these charges so that they can honor a patient's request.

The specific charges are flagged in the system with a private billing transaction code. The restrictions form is sent to the health information management (HIM) department where it is scanned into the electronic health record (EHR) system. The HIM staff will enter an administrative alert in that patient's EHR and registration file indicating this form has been completed and signed.

HIM employees who process requests for disclosure will first look for any administrative alerts. If a restriction alert is there, the employee will review the scanned form and follow it accordingly.

To help spread the word of the private billing option, KU has information about the process on Watkins's business office website. Furthermore, there is an FAQ link on their website that provides students with answers to their frequent questions, such as "Can I pay for certain services without billing my insurance?" Some students also know about the private billing option via word of mouth.

This process works well because all Watkins personnel are well-informed about it and promote it while only business office and HIM staff are actually involved in carrying out the patient's request.

(Source: Adapted from: Beckett, B., K. Downing, J. D. Gillespie, T. Waugh. 2015 Restrictions in Action: Three Case Studies. *Journal of AHIMA* 86 (3): 32–35).

Chapter 14 Review Exercises

Match the terms with the appropriate descriptions.

    a. Spoliation
    b. Corrections
    c. Cut, paste, and copy forward
    d. Deletion or Retraction
    e. Canned text

1. _____ Changes to paper or electronic records after a court ordered legal hold.

2. _____ An example of a time saving method of documentation that has risk to data accuracy.

3. _____ A change in the information meant to clarify inaccuracies after the original electronic document has been signed or rendered complete.

4. _____ Refer to totally eliminating or hiding from view information that was determined to be incorrect or invalid.

5. _____ An action that, if improperly used, can result in billing fraud.

Answer the following questions.

6. Which attributes of record systems are commonly used to create a legal health record definition?
   a. Log-on password methodology
   b. Version controls
   c. Access safeguards
   d. Physical workstation security

7. Which is not an LHR definition step?
   a. List IP addresses of impacted computers
   b. Learn about the changing LHR environment
   c. Identify project stakeholders
   d. Determine impacted policies and procedures for review and updating

8. Why define an organization's LHR?
   a. To reduce the need for legal counsel
   b. For identification of physical security risks
   c. To clarify the roles of all records and their uses
   d. It is required for meaningful use

9. Which of the following is not true regarding legal holds?
   a. May be imposed by a court
   b. May be assumed to be required for any data or document that will be subject to a court case
   c. May prevent spoliation
   d. May be imposed by the patient

Indicate whether each of the following is true or false.

10. e-Discovery rules are being updated in many states.

11. e-Discovery is only of concern to legal counsel and not record managers, custodians, and information governance (IG) stakeholders.

12. Federal Rules of Civil Procedure have been adopted by all states and local jurisdictions to manage the use of electronic records in court processes.

13. Copy and paste forward is appropriate for documenting the findings of a physical examination.

14. LHR definition is a one-time project.

Discussion.

15. What are the differences in the LHR for the paper-based record, the hybrid record, and the EHR?

16. Who are the primary stakeholders in the LHR definition process and why?

17. Why is an LHR policy needed?

REFERENCES

45 CFR 164.501. Uses and disclosures of protected health information: Definitions.

45 CFR 170. Health Information Technology: Initial Set of Standards, Implementation Specifications, and Certification Criteria for Electronic Health Record Technology; Interim Rule.

AHIMA e-HIM Work Group on the Legal Health Record. 2005a. Guidelines for defining the legal health record for disclosure purposes. *Journal of AHIMA* 76(8):64A–G.

AHIMA e-HIM Work Group on Maintaining the Legal EHR. 2005b. Practice brief: Maintaining a legally sound health record—Paper and electronic. *Journal of AHIMA* 76(10):64A–L.

AHIMA. 2012a. *Amendments in the Electronic Health Record Toolkit.* Chicago: AHIMA Press.

AHIMA. 2012b. Copy Functionality Toolkit a Practical Guide: Information Management and Governance of Copy Functions in Electronic Health Record Systems. https://secure.ahima.org/publications/reprint/index.aspx.

AHIMA. 2014. *Pocket Glossary of Health Information Management and Technology.* Chicago. AHIMA Press.

American Recovery and Reinvestment Act (ARRA) of 2009. Public Law 111-5.

Beckett, B., K. Downing, J.D. Gillespie, T. Waugh. 2015. Restrictions in Action: Three Case Studies. *Journal of AHIMA* 86(3): 32–35.

Glondys, B. and L. Kadlec. 2016. EHRs Serving as the Business and Legal Records of Healthcare Organizations (2016 Update). *Journal of AHIMA* 87(5).

Health Level Seven International. HL7 Record Management and Evidentiary Standards. 2007. http://www.hl7.org.

McLendon, K. 2012. Creating a legal health record definition *Journal of AHIMA* 83(1): 46-47.

McLendon, K. 2010a. *The Legal Health Record: Regulations, Policies, and Guidance,* 2nd ed. Chicago: AHIMA Press.

McLendon, K. 2010b. Copy that? Meeting the Meaningful Use objectives for electronic copies, parts 1 and 2. *Journal of AHIMA* 81(4):42–43.

National Institute of Standards and Technology, SP 800-34 Rev. 1. 2010. Contingency Planning Guide for Federal Information Systems (5/2010, including updates as of 11/11/2010), http://nvlpubs.nist.gov/nistpubs/Legacy/SP/nistspecialpublication800-34r1.pdf.

ADDITIONAL RESOURCES

AHIMA. 2011. Fundamentals of the legal health record and designated record set. *Journal of AHIMA*: 82(2).

AHIMA. 2009. e-HIM Workgroup on Best Practices for Electronic Signature, Attestation, and Authentication.

AHIMA e-HIM Work Group: Guidelines for EHR Documentation Practice. 2007. Guidelines for EHR documentation to prevent fraud. *Journal of AHIMA* 78(1):65–68.

AHIMA e-HIM Work Group on e-Discovery. 2006. The new electronic discovery civil rule. *Journal of AHIMA* 77(8):68A–H.

AHIMA EHR Practice Council. 2007. Developing a legal health record policy. *Journal of AHIMA* 78(9):93–97.

AHIMA EHR Practice Council. 2007, October. AHIMA Practice Brief, AHIMA Journal, AHIMA e-HIM Task Force Report.

Burrington-Brown, J. 2007. Legal EHR FAQs. *Journal of AHIMA* 78(9):77, 80.

Butler, M. 2015. Cracking encryption: Despite benefits, technology still not widely used to combat multi-million dollar breaches. *Journal of AHIMA* 86(4):18–23.

California Hospital Association. 2007. State of California Consent Manual.

Dougherty, M. 2005. Practice brief: Understanding the EHR system functional model standard. *Journal of AHIMA* 76(2):64A–D.

Federal Rules of Civil Procedure (FRCP). 2006. Revisions and additions to Rules 16, 26, 33, 34, 37, and 45, as well as Form 35; effective Dec. 1, 2006.

Federal Rules of Civil Procedure (FRCP). 2006. Rule 17, Appendix A, chapter 2.

Federal Rules of Evidence (FRE). Article VIII, Rule 803(6), Rule 901(a).

Klein, S.R. 2007. Legal perspective: Welcome to the digital age. *Journal of Healthcare Information Management* 21(4). 6–7.

McLean, T.R. 2009. Authenticating EHR metadata. *Journal of AHIMA* 80(2):40–41, 50.

McLendon, K. 2007. Record disclosure and the EHR: Defining and managing the subset of data disclosed upon request. *Journal of AHIMA* 78(2):58–59.

McLendon, K. 2006. LHRs in the electronic record age: What we know so far. AHIMA's 78th National Convention and Exhibit Proceedings.

National Conference of Commissioners on Uniform State Laws. 2007. Uniform Rules Relating to Discovery of Electronically Stored Information.

Reich, K.B. 2007. Developing a litigation response plan. *Journal of AHIMA* 78(9):76–78, 86.

Roach, W.H., R.G. Hoban, and B.M. Broccolo. 2006. *Medical Records and the Law*. Sudbury, MA: Jones & Bartlett.

Sarbanes-Oxley Act of 2002. http://www.soxlaw.com/.

The Society of American Archivists—A Glossary of Archival and Records Terminology. http://www.archivists.org/glossary/index.asp.

Uniform Photographic Copies of Business and Public Records as Evidence Act.

US Government. Drug Enforcement Administration. 2010. Electronic Prescriptions for Controlled Substances; Final Rule. *Federal Register* 75(61):16236–16319.

Consumer Health Informatics

By Juliana J. Brixey, PhD, MPH, MSN, RN, Sue Biedermann, MSHP, RHIA, FAHIMA, and Diane Dolezel, EdD, RHIA, CHDA

Learning Objectives

- Interpret consumer health informatics
- Describe characteristics of the online health information consumer
- Compare past, current, and potential consumer health informatics technology
- Discuss ubiquitous computing
- Characterize the differences between validity and reliability
- Explain privacy and security issues for online health information

KEY TERMS

Blue Button
Computer literate consumer
Digital immigrant
Digital native
e-Health literacy
Health
Health literacy
Informatics
Literacy
Mobile device

Numerical or computational literacy
Online diagnoser
Patient-Generated Health Data (PGHD)
Patient portal
Personal health record (PHR)
Reliability
Social media
Technologically literate
Validity
Visual literacy

It is important that consumers be engaged in their own care to support their healthcare providers in maintaining the best healthcare possible. Getting consumers involved in their healthcare and the healthcare of their loved ones is one focus of the Office of the National Coordinator for Health Information Technology (ONC 2013). The widespread use of computers and the Internet have made this an achievable goal for most healthcare consumers. A 2015 Pew survey of Internet users revealed that 84 percent had searched online for health information within the past year. Demographic information on nonadopters (16 percent) revealed them to be less educated and less affluent seniors 65 years of age and older with racial, ethnic, and community differences. Specifically, African Americans and Hispanics and those living in rural populations were less likely to use the Internet (Pew 2015). As the number of nonusers continues to increase, so does the number of **online diagnosers** who use the Internet to determine a diagnosis or identify a medical condition (Fox and Duggan 2013a, 2–6). This is not surprising because today the general public can search for health information anytime and anywhere using a variety of computers and wireless **mobile devices** such as tablet computers and smart phones.

A **patient portal** is "an information system that allows a patient to log in to obtain information, register, and perform other functions." (AHIMA 2014, 112). As part of Meaningful Use Stage 2, Advanced Clinical Processes, clinicians are expected to provide patients with secure access to information in their electronic health record (EHR) via a patient portal, as well as exchange secure e-mail with them (CMS 2016a). The processes in Stage 2 rely on the Stage 1 requirements for Data Capture and Sharing. Additionally, Stage 3 Improved Outcomes requirements use the data capture from Stage 2. Thus, providers must continue to be compliant with previous stages due to the functions advancing at each stage. This chapter will provide an overview to consumer health informatics focusing on the use of technology and information to empower the consumer to achieve better health.

⊙ Consumer Health Informatics: A Standardized Definition?

Definitions are inherently important in the discussion of any domain. Failure to have a standardized definition results in ambiguity, uncertainty, and an overall lack of precision regarding the examination, analysis, evaluation, discussion, or consideration of consumer health information (CHI). For example, CHI combines three concepts: consumers, health, and informatics.

A general definition is provided for each concept before reviewing definitions of CHI.

- ⊙ A **consumer** is defined as a person who purchases goods and services for personal use.
- ⊙ **Health** is defined as the state of being free from illness or injury.
- ⊙ **Informatics** is defined as the study of collecting, organizing, storing, and using electronic information (Oxford 2016).

The previous definitions provide the underpinnings of a universal definition for CHI. However, a review of the literature indicates a lack of consensus in defining CHI. As CHI was emerging, the US Government Accountability Office Accounting and Information Management Division (GAO) defined CHI as "the union of health care content with the speed and ease of technology" (GAO 1996). CHI was later defined as a branch of medical informatics that "analyzes consumers' needs for information, studies and implements methods of making information accessible to consumers, and models and integrates consumers' preferences into medical information systems" (Eysenbach 2000, 1713).

The Agency for Healthcare Research and Quality (AHRQ) defines CHI applications

> as any electronic tool, technology, or system that is: 1) primarily designed to interact with health information users or consumers (anyone who seeks or uses health care information for nonprofessional work) and 2) interacts directly with the consumer who provides personal health information to the CHI system and receives personalized health information from the tool application or system; and 3) is one in which the data, information, recommendations or other benefits provided to the consumer, may be used with a healthcare professional, but is not dependent on a healthcare professional (AHRQ 2012).

The American Medical Informatics Association (AMIA) Consumer Health Informatics Working Group (CHIWG) defines CHI as

> the field devoted to informatics from multiple consumer or patient views. These include patient-focused informatics, health literacy and consumer education. The focus is on information structures and processes that empower consumers to manage their own health—for example health information literacy, consumer-friendly language, personal health records, and Internet-based strategies and resources. The shift in this view of informatics analyses consumers' needs for information; studies and implements methods for making information accessible to consumers; and models and integrates consumers' preferences into health information systems. Consumer informatics stands at the crossroads of other disciplines, such as nursing informatics, public health, health promotion, health education, library science, and communication science (AMIA 2012).

Analysis of the definitions on consumer health information are depicted in a mindmap (figure 15.1), which is a tool used to organize thoughts and ideas on a specific topic or idea. A review of various definitions of consumer health informatics was done looking for keywords and phrases and grouping these by whether or not they were explicit or implicit and by categories and then the more specific information. Both explicit and implicit themes were revealed in this mindmap. The left side of the diagram reflects the process for analyzing the explicit themes, which are concepts that can be clearly expressed and included identifying major categories to be considered. In the mindmap shown the major categories identified for this

Figure 15.1.   Mindmap of analyzing definition of consumer health information

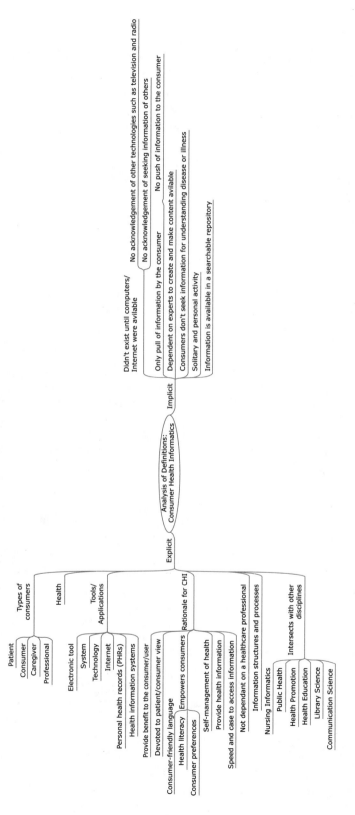

analysis are types of consumers, tools/applications, rationale, nondependency on healthcare professionals, information structures and processes, and intersection with other disciplines. The next step is naming more specific identifiers for each of these categories as seen for types of consumers to be patients, consumers, caregivers, and professionals. The process for analyzing the implicit theme, illustrated on the right side of the mindmap, involves identifying aspects that are not as readily apparent and may come from brainstorming in addition to the review of definitions. The explicit themes that emerged in the analysis of various definitions of consumer health informatics include:

- Types of consumers
- The term health as opposed to disease or illness
- Tools and applications
- Rationale for CHI
- Nondependency on a healthcare professional for health information
- Information on structures and processes
- Intersection with other disciplines

The following include implicit themes that emerge from the definitions:

- Did not exist until computers/Internet were available
- Only pull of information by the consumer
- Dependent on experts to create and make content available
  - Consumers do not seek information for understanding disease or illness
  - Solitary and personal activity
  - Information that is available in a searchable repository

These diverse definitions hinder the examination, analysis, evaluation, discussion, and consideration of CHI. It is imperative that all stakeholders (consumers, clinicians, informaticists, health educators, and developers of consumer health information products) work together to formulate a standard definition.

Literacy: A Fundamental Skill

In order to access and use health information effectively, an individual must possess different literacy skills. **Literacy** is broadly defined as "the ability to read and write" (Oxford 2016) or "using printed and written information to function in society, to achieve one's goals, and to develop one's knowledge and potential" (Kirsch et al. 2002, 2). An individual is considered to be **computer literate** if he or she has the knowledge and skills to use computers and is familiar with the operation of computers (Oxford 2016). Health literacy was introduced as a concept in the mid-1970s. **Health literacy** is defined as "the degree to which individuals have the capacity to obtain, process, and understand basic health information and services needed to make appropriate health decisions" (Ratzan and Parker 2000, 2). Health literacy can make a difference in patient care, especially when a consumer can effectively communicate their health history, such as signs and symptoms, previous treatment, and procedures to providers, understands enough to question instructions, and know when they and their support system lack the capabilities to adhere to treatment recommendations. Visual and numerical literacy should be considered as part of health literacy. **Visual literacy** is defined as the "ability to understand graphs or other visual information" (NNLM 2012). For example, the consumer may need to understand a graph trend line of laboratory results. Whereas **numerical or computational literacy** is defined as the "ability to calculate or reason numerically" (NNLM 2012). An example of the need for this can be found in an understanding of body mass index calculations or calculating drug dosing or the application of a sliding-scale dosage based on blood tests for diabetes.

Today, an individual must have **e-Health literacy** skills, which entails "the ability to seek, find, understand, and appraise health information from electronic sources and apply the knowledge gained to addressing or solving a health problem" (Norman and Skinner 2006). Given the reliance on the Internet for health information and knowledge, this skill is especially important for a patient to be informed and engaged in their care. They must have the ability to review and discriminate among all of the information found in searches to assure reliability and trustworthiness. Additionally, an individual must be computer and **technologically literate** with the ability to use computers and understand the technology involved. Although consumer informatics may not totally rely on computers, the use of computers has made health information much more accessible to consumers with a continuing utilization of this technology. It is reasonable to expect that new literacies will be required as new technologies are introduced.

Lower literacy skills can be attributed to such factors as English as a second language; years of education completed; ethnicity or race; physical, mental, and health conditions; and age over 65. Millions of people have low health literacy and struggle to understand and take actions based on health information, and even people with strong literacy skills may have trouble obtaining, understanding, and using health information (Nielsen-Bohlman et al. 2004, 1–2). The health system is a complicated system for many consumers from the medical perspective with the complex protocols of diagnostics and treatment for conditions and the challenge of navigating provider billing procedures and third-party payer plans and requirements.

Low health literacy can result in:

⊙ Medication errors

⊙ Low rates of treatment compliance due to poor communication between providers and patients

⊙ Reduced use of preventive services and unnecessary emergency room visits

⊙ Ineffective management of chronic conditions, due to inadequate self-care skills

⊙ Longer hospital stays and increased hospital readmissions

⊙ Poor responsiveness to public health emergencies, and

⊙ Higher mortality (CHCS 2013)

For example, medication errors with prescribed drugs can become complicated with incorrect dosages and look-alike pills. For the uninformed there can be issues with the instructions for taking the medications, inability to understand the information provided with the prescription, or not knowing how to access additional information. There is agreement among healthcare professionals that many people lack the skills to find, read, listen to, analyze, understand, and use health information and access health services (Baur 2012). Because of this and similar findings, the national government initiative known as Healthy People 2020 includes a goal to improve health literacy skills for all citizens (Healthy People 2020 2012). The task of health informaticists is to minimize the barriers of understanding and technology for consumers. As an example, instead of using terms such as myocardial infarction, the words heart attack should be used. Likewise, the use of codes and other tools (which help with automatic processing and even bill payment) should be translated for consumers into understandable words. The idea is to make health information more accessible to persons who have not spent many years studying in the healthcare field. In this way, consumers will be empowered to assist healthcare providers who are trying to improve and maintain their health.

It was an expectation of the Office of the National Coordinator for Health Information Technology (ONC) that the use of health IT would support patients to become more engaged and informed regarding their health (Mostashari 2012). Outcomes have shown the increased emphasis on patient engagement has resulted in decreased number of hospital stays, reduced morbidity and mortality rates, and increased patient compliance in treatment of chronic diseases and, consequently, quality of life. These outcomes have reduced costs while maintaining, even improving, quality of care (Kimball et al. 2015).

Digital Immigrant or Digital Native

It is important to understand as much as possible about the health information consumer when designing and providing online health information. For example, is the health information consumer a **digital immigrant** or a **digital native**? A digital native is a person who has only known a world of digital toys and tools (Prensky 2001). In contrast, a digital immigrant is an individual who lived before the advent of the digital age but has adapted more or less to the digital age. This is important because the majority of healthcare is used in two phases of life. In the first phase, parents of young children, many of whom are now digital natives, will use technology to seek or track the care of their children. This can be for a variety of purposes, including tasks such as providing the school with a list of immunizations. In the second phase of life, older citizens, including their adult children and caregivers, use technology to manage their care as they age. The technology and computer literacy of the digital native and the digital immigrant will be different, as will their preferred types of applications and communication creating a digital divide. The **digital divide** refers to that gap between those with and those without convenient Internet access which results in differences in the amount and types of information that can be accessed by the user. The prevalence of smart phones has increased access to the Internet for many users, narrowing the divide.

⊙ Characteristics of the Online Health Consumer

The Pew Research Center conducts periodic surveys of adults living in the United States to learn how people use the Internet to locate health information. From the findings:

- ⊙ 87 percent of US adults use the Internet;
- ⊙ Of those Internet users, 72 percent say they have searched online for health information in the past year;
- ⊙ 50 percent of US adults have searched the Internet for health information in the past year in an effort to determine their own medical condition or that of another individual;
- ⊙ 77 percent of those seeking online health information used a search engine;
- ⊙ 13 percent began at a specialized health information site;
- ⊙ 85 percent of US adults own a cell phone;
- ⊙ 58 percent of US adults own a smartphone;
- ⊙ 31 percent of cell phone users and 52 percent of smartphone owners used their phones to conduct a search for health information;
- ⊙ 19 percent of smartphone users have downloaded a health app;
- ⊙ 7 in 10 US adults have followed a **leading health indicator,** health issues that serve as measures of the nation's health (ODPHP 2016), and of those 34 percent share their records; and
- ⊙ 3–4 percent have shared as a posting their experience with healthcare professionals or treatments (Pew Research Center 2016).

The findings provide important information about online health information consumers. Because a majority of those who are connected have used the Internet to search for health information, it seems to follow that this is a good option when trying to disseminate health information. For example, whether or not the consumer has some college education appears to impact whether or not they will use the Internet to search for health information. The findings also provide insight into the technologies consumers are using to search the Internet.

Health Topics of Interest for the Online Health Information Consumer

It is important to know what health topics online health consumers are exploring. The Pew Survey group began researching consumer behaviors related to online health behaviors in the early 2000s. During 15 years of study, they noted similar results regarding consumers' online searches and the kinds of health information they sought. A comprehensive 2014 study reported in the *Journal of Medical Internet*

Research compiled data for a number of variables related to searches and search topics (Lee et al. 2014). Table 15.1 depicts the kind of information consumers search for and why and when they are most likely to do this.

Table 15.1.　What, why, and when: consumers research for health information

What	Why	When
Medicines or medical devices—includes side effects, and indications for the product	To be more informed	Following a consultation with a health professional
Medical conditions	To clarify/verify information discussed during consultation	Before a consultation with a health professional
Lifestyle information (e.g., information on diets and exercise)	Because the Internet is accessible	When required
Information about individual health professionals, medical clinics and hospitals (e.g., appropriate specialties for particular conditions)	Emotional support, e.g., to read about experiences of others with the same condition(s)	Before and after consultation
Natural products	Out of interest	
Information about disease-specific associations	Disagreement with points made by a health professional	
Medical glossary	To seek alternative/ additional treatment options	
	Insufficient information provided during a consultation	
	Urgency to know	
	To take charge of one's life	
	Self-management of a perceived minor condition, e.g., common cold	

(Continued)

Table 15.1. What, why, and when: consumers research for health information (*Continued*)

What	Why	When
	Limited time during consultation	
	To have written information to read	
	Infrequency of interaction with health professional	

Source: First published in the *Journal of Medical Internet Research* at http://www.jmir.org/2014/12/e262. Lee, H., A. Kreshnik, J. Hughes, and L. Emmerton. 2014. Dr Google and the Consumer: A Qualitative Study Exploring the Navigational Needs and Online Health Information-Seeking Behaviors. *Journal of Medical Internet Research* 16(12):e262.

A 2012 study conducted by PEW revealed that the information mostly frequently accessed by consumers was: specific disease or medical problem (55%), medical treatment or procedures (43%), weight control or loss (27%) and health insurance (25%) (PEW 2013). These study findings validate the need for a variety of kinds of timely and easily accessible information to promote the consumer in being an active participant in their own or a family member's healthcare.

It is essential that the information provider know the reasonable life span of the information, as well as when to update or retract their information. For example, consumers are seeking online health information about time-sensitive topics such as recalls. This time-sensitive information requires the availability of dynamically updated online factual content. In contrast, complex or chronic health conditions do not require minute-to-minute updates but incremental changes as new information becomes available.

Getting Connected to the Internet for the Online Health Information Consumer

Online health consumers require Internet access. The online dial-up services of the 1990s have largely been replaced by broadband and wireless services. A 2016 report based on census data indicates that 75 percent of households had high-speed Internet access and only 1 percent had dial-up access (census.gov 2016). Reliable data is not available on the number who use handheld devices, such as phones with Internet functionality, as their primary source of Internet activity. But that form of Internet access is the means for many to access the Internet and for what seems to be a different demographic with lower income and less education, who used handheld devices more due to owning only a handheld and not both a handheld and home computer, as seen in other groups.

Check Your Understanding 15.1

Answer the following questions.

1. What is an important concept of health literacy?
   a. Having an interpreter available
   b. Visual literacy
   c. Knowledge of medical terminology
   d. Having the capacity to understand basic health information

2. What specific actions that exhibit health literacy by a patient can make a difference in the outcomes of care?
   a. A family member relates symptoms of the patient to the provider.
   b. The patient questions the instructions given by a provider.
   c. The patient chart is used to determine previous procedure done.
   d. A caregiver is provided instructions for administration of medications.

Indicate whether each of the following is true or false.

3. In the design of an online application, it is important to know if the user is a digital immigrant or digital native.

4. The increased use of smart phones has no effect on the digital divide.

5. A recall of a medication is an example of time-sensitive information that could be found on a consumer health information site.

6. The digital divide is synonymous with digital immigrant.

⊙ Consumer Health Informatics Technology

The availability of CHI has been dependent on the endlessly evolving information technology. The current technology-enabled tools making health information available to consumers include

- ⊙ Online self-help books for use on e-readers, computers
- ⊙ Online health articles or sites
- ⊙ Bulletin boards and online discussion groups
- ⊙ Automated appointment reminders
- ⊙ Automated systems for learning more about health conditions
- ⊙ Wearable sensors, such as glucose monitors
- ⊙ Social media sites such as Facebook and Twitter
- ⊙ Smart phone apps
- ⊙ Internet of Things

There are a wide variety of interactive systems where health information consumers can communicate with other individuals using e-mail, bulletin boards, online discussion groups, and social media. The communication is not limited to healthcare professionals but includes self-help groups.

Initial technologies may seem antiquated in comparison to the myriad of technologies that today's health information consumers can choose from. Increasingly sophisticated technologies are becoming available to deliver health information to the consumers and to their healthcare providers. A study on improving hospital patient recovery time assessed patients who had elective cardiac surgery and who were provided postoperatively with a Fitbit to record when they began walking and how many steps they took each day. The results revealed that the earlier in their recovery and the more walking done, the shorter the length of stay in the hospital (Information Week 2013). As indicated in this study, technology is expected to continue evolving, with more and more ways for consumers to monitor their health and the health of their loved ones.

⊙ Social Media

Social media cannot be discussed without a definition of Web 2.0 as the two concepts are often used as synonyms. A definition of Web 2.0 is:

> The network as platform, spanning all connected devices; Web 2.0 applications are those that make the most of the intrinsic advantages of that platform: delivering software as a continually-updated service that gets better the more people use it, consuming and remixing data from multiple sources, including individual users, while providing their own data and services in a form that allows remixing by others, creating network effects through an architecture of participation (O'Reilly 2005).

Similarly, social media is described as "websites and applications that enable users to create and share content or to participate in social networking" (Oxford 2016). The difference between the two definitions has to do with web-based sharing with Web 2.0 encompassing much more than social media. Common examples of social media technologies include:

- ⊙ Blogs
- ⊙ Microblogs
- ⊙ Photo sharing
- ⊙ Social bookmarking
- ⊙ Forums
- ⊙ Video sharing
- ⊙ Social gaming
- ⊙ Virtual worlds
- ⊙ Knowledge and information aggregation
- ⊙ Professional networking

Social media share the common attributes of:

- ⊙ A user account
- ⊙ A profile page

- Friends, followers, groups
- Hashtags
- News feeds
- Personalization
- Notifications
- Information updating, saving, or posting
- Like buttons
- Comment sections
- Review, ratings, or voting systems (Nations 2016)

Social media inspires user-generated content but also supports the sharing of collected content including information within the user's social network (Beattie 2011). A social network is comprised of relationships with people identified as friends or followers. Unmistakably for both Web 2.0 and social media is user involvement and engagement with others of similar interests in a social network on the Internet.

Although the use of social media has been embraced by some industries, healthcare organizations and healthcare professionals have been hesitant to use the technologies. The reluctance rests with concerns related to poor quality of information, damage to professional image, breaches of patient privacy, violation of the patient–healthcare professional boundary, licensing issues, and legal issues (Ventola, 2014). Avoidance of any of the aforementioned issues is paramount to healthcare organizations and professionals. Failure to adequately protect PHI can result in a breach requiring the healthcare organization to follow HIPAA breach notification procedures.

Nonetheless, some healthcare organizations have enthusiastically adopted social media. For patients, social media can be a source of education and information and a means of networking and receiving support within a group. Physicians participate in social media sites for information through publications and recordings, and communicate with peers on diseases, treatments, and other patient issues. Healthcare organizations can use it for engagement with the community, providing information and news and patient education (House 2013). Social media is inexpensive, with unlimited access, flexibility, and ease of use.

Ubiquitous Computing of Online Health Information

Patients no longer have to schedule an appointment with a physician to ask a question about a disease or how to stay healthy. Today, consumers have access to anytime, anywhere information using the Internet. Indeed, there are a plethora of websites on the Internet to choose from depending on the consumer's need. These include free-standing websites designed to serve consumers, healthcare provider and professional association websites, health insurance company websites, and federal, state, and local governmental websites. This abundance of websites indicates that consumers want, and many stakeholders are ready to provide, ubiquitous access to health information.

For example, the WebMD homepage immediately engages the consumer with a wide variety of health, wellness, and disease-oriented content. A selection of health and illness content is available without creating a user account. The website offers the consumer the option of creating a free-of-charge secure account. Consumers who are account holders can create a personalized weight loss plan, track vaccines, or join a community that specializes in a specific health topic (WebMD 2016). There are many similar websites, such as Sharecare—proof of the potential commercial success for these technologies in healthcare.

Healthcare organizations and hospitals are also making information available to consumers. For example, the Mayo Clinic (Mayo Clinic n.d.) launched its social media outreach on May 5, 2011, for patients, caregivers, and consumers. The Mayo Clinic website is a comprehensive patient care site for accessing online health information and communication services that provides resources for a healthy lifestyle, the ability to make appointments, and access to other information that can be utilized to support the patient and their family. Health information is available for symptoms, diseases and conditions, tests, and drugs. The website offers such applications as discussion boards, webinars, and blogs. It provides access to perform a search and contains links to sites by state, as well as a patient app designed to actively engage people in managing their health. The app includes appointment information for scheduled times and resources to request new appointments and see test results, medication list, visit notes, messages, and maps and directions.

Medical libraries provide health information to consumers. For example, MedlinePlus from the US National Library of Medicine (NLM) and the National Institutes of Health (NIH) maintain numerous online information websites to provide consumers with reliable and up-to-date information (NIH n.d.b; NLM 2012b). According to MedLine Plus, consumers can find easy-to-understand information on more than 975 diseases, as well as prescription and nonprescription drugs, along with links to clinical trials and the option to engage in interactive tutorials (NLM 2012b). Additionally, consumers can view videos to learn more about anatomy in addition to surgical procedures. The website provides health information in Spanish. It is updated daily to provide the most current information to consumers. Unlike many commercial sites, the government-sponsored website is free of advertising.

In addition, medical libraries such as The Texas Medical Center (TMC) Library provide on-site services to consumers by making two touch-screen computers available. Librarians are available to help the consumer search and retrieve health information. The library provides a number of training opportunities such as the free delivery of health information via mail, e-mail, or fax; the use of local and national consumer health databases; and in-depth health topics. Also, the library helps consumers find health information through the provision of recommending national and local websites. Additionally, the library makes information available at the TMC International Visitor's Lounge in the International Terminal of Bush Intercontinental Airport. Furthermore, the library supports consumer health outreach in Houston and the surrounding counties (TMC 2012). Likewise, the George J. Farha Library of Health Sciences located at the University of Kansas

Medical School–Wichita makes health information available to consumers (University of Kansas Medical School–Wichita 2015). The website directs consumers to reputable online resources.

A number of disease societies such as the American Cancer Society (ACS) and American Diabetes Association (ADA) have made health information available to consumers. For example, on the ACS website, consumers can learn more about cancer from the provided online health resources and statistics as well as learning more about volunteer efforts, campaigns, potential to participate in research trials, and contact information for local organizations (ACS 2016). Similarly, the ADA provides consumers with information regarding the types of diabetes alongside tips for healthy eating and exercise (ADA 2012), both of which are a very important aspect of the overall health of an individual.

A host of other organizations are making health information available to consumers. This list includes retail pharmacies (Walgreens, CVS), health insurance companies (Blue Cross Blue Shield, UnitedHealth Group), online news services (CNNHealth, Fox News), and grocery stores. These websites provide health information about healthy eating, health risk assessment, surgeries and procedures, tools and trackers, women's health, immunizations, medication resources, weight management, stress management, and guidelines for drug disposal. In the workplace, employers provide health promotion information to their employees (Texas State University n.d.; Nestlé 2012). Additionally, the Centers for Disease Control and Prevention has a website with information that employers can use to make CHI available to their workers (CDC 2012).

The proliferation of mobile technology is an influencing force in how consumers access health information. The consumer can access the health information on their mobile devices (a smart phone or tablet computer). Along with the new technology is the explosion of health applications, more commonly called apps. These apps can help consumers maintain a personal health record (PHR), track their weight, record progress in health and wellness programs, and monitor their heart rate. More sophisticated apps continue to be developed as seen with Fitbit for cardiorespiratory monitoring. Consumers can expect increased opportunities to become more engaged and responsible for their healthcare and providers will have more knowledge of their patients' conditions as seen with diabetic monitoring apps.

It should not be overlooked that consumers are seeking online health information from social networking sites such as Facebook, Twitter, Instagram, Pinterest, and Snapchat. These sites are social media types used primarily to post messages, photos, videos, and links to share with friends and contacts. Videos can be shared on YouTube. Visitors to Second Life's 3-D virtual worlds can create their own user content. They can also learn about health, pregnancy and childbirth, cancer, or experience what it is like for the schizophrenic patient to hear voices by visiting virtual clinics and hospitals. In general, any consumer can search for health information created by both healthcare professionals and nonprofessionals. Last, it is important to carefully evaluate the information from social networking sites.

Indeed, healthcare information is becoming ubiquitous. Consumers have moved from an environment where health information was sparse and difficult to retrieve to a situation of information overload due to the unlimited access and availability of health and wellness resources. Furthermore, CHI is not just accessible using desktop computing but is now available ubiquitously using mobile devices such as smart phones and tablet computers. This requires health information consumers to become educated and to evaluate the quality of information they are accessing.

Check Your Understanding 15.2

Answer the following questions.

1. Which of the following is not an attribute of social media?
    a. User account
    b. Hashtags
    c. Groups
    d. Validated information

2. Which of the following results in a reluctance to use social media in healthcare?
    a. Potential for breaches of privacy of PHI
    b. High-quality of information
    c. Setting qualifications for those who can participate
    d. Information protected from unauthorized users

Indicate whether each of the following is true or false.

3. Government-sponsored libraries for consumers access to disease information are the only reliable healthcare websites.

4. Patient access anytime, anywhere is an advantage of the availability of information found on the Internet.

5. Information maintained on smart phone applications has no relationship to the PHR.

◉ Personal Health Records

A **personal health record (PHR)** is "an electronic or paper health record maintained and updated by an individual for himself or herself; a tool that individuals can use to collect, track, and share past and current information about their health or the health of someone in their care" (AHIMA 2014, 114). PHRs have been promoted as one method to improve health for patients and reduce the costs of healthcare (Hillestad et al. 2005). However, the use of personal health records on a large scale has not occurred and the Meaningful Use Stage 2 requirements include portals to the EHR data versus a PHR-type capability (CMS 2016b). One objective of the Meaningful Use Stage 3 requirements beginning in 2018 is patient electronic access for viewing, downloading, and transmitting their PHI. Timely access and the capability of the patient to use an application of their choice from the providers certified software are required to meet this objective (CMS 2016a). PHRs remain an important consumer tool to enable patients' ability to manage their own health and health information and increase patient engagement.

The PHR can be a paper record, or health information stored on a smart card, USB drive, CD, or computer software such as Apple HealthKit. Apple HealthKit collects data from health and fitness apps like Fitbit and provides easy access to information via a dashboard of data and allows access to others at individual's discretion (Apple 2016). The electronic PHR (ePHR) can be a stand-alone record or tethered to an EHR maintained by a health facility, such as a hospital or health insurance organization or a system such as the US Department of Veterans Affairs, explored in the discussion of the Blue Button functionality below. The PHR is not in common usage, which brings up the question of what are the barriers to the adoption of PHRs? A systematic literature study conducted in 2015 identified the most commonly stated barriers to PHR implementation to be:

- Risk of security and confidentiality, potential for breaches
- Physicians question the quality, accuracy, and integrity of patient-reported data
- Costs and who would bear the costs. Costs to the providers include those for the technology and licensing fees, time for checking records, and increased workload to maintain.
- Health literacy of individuals seeking information and concern for their inability to completely understand the information
- Computer literacy and difficulties for individuals to navigate systems (Vance et al. 2015)

A study of patients who participated in the pilot of My HealtheVet, the personal health record of the US Department of Veterans Affair, examined the patient's experience reading their health information online (Woods et al. 2013). The overall results of the study were positive with three themes emerging to reflect what they perceived to be benefits of having this access. Challenges were identified by a few patients or family members and comprised a fourth theme. The benefits were:

- A positive effect on their communication with providers and the health system.
- Enhanced knowledge of their health with improved self-care.
- Facilitation of increased participation in the quality of their care indicating follow-up on abnormal test results and in decision making on seeking care.

The challenges revolved around the initial stress at seeing the information. Some related this as a discomfort with the language that was used or perceived errors or inconsistencies in the information. Difficulty using the technology was expressed by a few but this was during a pilot phase of the program. It was also noted that a few comments were made that they had not seen or heard this information before and some preferred not knowing this level of information. Overall, the results were predominantly positive for patients to have and use this access to their PHI but there was a perceived need for providers to use new means of communication with their patients.

Disparities in access to health information when it is tied to computer technology is also an issue for the increased use of PHRs and web portals. Patients in underserved areas or without high-speed Internet access, such as with a computer at home or via a smart phone, may find themselves unable to take advantage of the latest health information technology advances. A study in Northern California of a group of over 14,000 diabetes patients, with demographic characteristics similar to the overall population in Northern California, found that older patients were less likely to use the site and found a pervasive racial and educational disparity in use of the computer portal. The study expressed a fear that "those most at risk for poor diabetes outcomes may fall further behind as health systems increasingly rely on the Internet and limit current modes of access and communications" (Sarakar et al. 2011). Thus, although it is good to develop new uses of technology and information technology to help patients, it is important for health information professionals to consider how those who do not possess the latest technology can also improve and maintain their health using information from more traditional means.

Some of the benefits of using electronic PHRs relate to the interoperability of having an electronic PHR tethered to the electronic medical record. Project Health Design is a national program, funded by grants from foundations, designed to stimulate the development of new tools for personal health management by using the PHR (Brennan et al. 2007). The plan is to create a set of prototype applications to support interoperable resources for managing health challenges. If successful, the future of the PHR is bright and vibrant. PHRs have been noted to be "fragmented, non-scalable, without data standards, shared terminologies or common architectures" (Brennan et al. 2007). The usability in the design of applications was felt to be important for full realization of the benefits for healthcare and making the PHRs more usable in the management of chronic diseases.

The idea that the use of personal health records will play a key role in enabling the electronic health environment is becoming more common. The PHR has the possibility of creating a more balanced and complete view of the patient, especially when the consumer has multiple physicians or is unable to care for themselves. The patient is referred to as a consumer, rather than as a patient, to reflect this mind change and to underscore the fact that health records are no longer the sole property of the physician or hospital.

The verdict on the uses and usability of PHRs is far from final; however, especially for patients who suffer from a chronic disease or have multiple providers, they can prove to be very helpful. The American Health Information Management Association (AHIMA) and the AHIMA Foundation maintain the MyPHR.com website, providing an overview of PHRs, as well as guidance on how to initiate a PHR for consumers and their loved ones (AHIMA 2016). As consumers become increasingly tech-savvy and as the population continues to age, understanding and managing personal health information will become ever more important.

There have continued to be advances in technology, new regulatory requirements for patient access to their information, and an increased consumer need and interest for more and complete information so that they can be more in charge of their information. Consumers now have access through portals for test results and other health information and to be able to communicate with their providers and new means of control of their own health is available through mobile devices and applications (Butler 2015). Related to this is the concept of **patient-generated health data (PGHD),** which are "health-related data created, recorded, or gathered by the or from patients (or family members or other caregivers) to help address a health concern" (HealthIT 2016). PGHD differs from data compiled by practitioners in the clinical setting in that the patients are responsible for capturing the data and they also are the ones to determine how it is to be shared or used.

Patients provide their health information to the healthcare professionals as a part of seeking treatment whether it was recorded or not. How the information is captured, transmitted, and stored, however, is evolving. The PGHD consists of health history or similar information recorded by the patient by way of a portal, the biometric data generated from home health monitoring equipment, or assorted kinds of lifestyle information as is obtained from fitness devices or that which has been recorded on mobile device apps such as weight management or diabetes monitoring (AHIMA Work Group 2015). Support for incorporating the PHGD into the patient's EHR seems to be increasing with the continued focus on patient engagement and value-based care, a plan where payment for care is related to the quality and efficiency of care (AHIMA 2014, 151) and its potential use in meaningful use. Including PGHD into the EHR has legal implications, specifically when considering the defined legal health record, risks of using the information, and all of the record management and information management considerations (AHIMA Workgroup 2015).

⦿ Blue Button: Access to Health Information

On August 2, 2010, President Barack Obama stated, "For the first time ever, veterans will be able to go to the VA website, click a simple **Blue Button** and download or print your personal health records so you have them and can share with your doctor outside of the VA" (Obama 2010). An individual has the legal right to access their own health information. This right is made easier through the Blue Button initiative. The idea for the Blue Button began at the Markle Consumer Engagement Workgroup meeting in January 2010 (Nazi 2010). Agreement at the meeting was to place a big button on existing patient portals in order to give patients access to their health information. The intent of the initiative is to make access to personal health information easier for veterans, uniformed service members, and Medicare beneficiaries. The Blue Button initiative was formally launched in October 2010 (Chopra et al. 2010). Other federal agencies and companies are encouraging their members to use Blue Button to securely access and download their health information. Accessible information includes current medications, drug allergies, treatments, and laboratory results. Claims information can be retrieved electronically using Blue Button. The information is available to print or save. The information is saved as an ASCII text file and displays as an organized report.

Changes that have occurred with the Blue Button Initiative 2012 include the scaling of it to provide secure electronic access to health data for more Americans, a Blue Button Connector website was developed to aid individuals in finding their health data, and a national campaign was launched to provide education on using personal health data in making better medical decisions. The Precision Medicine Initiative was launched, which is a research effort for vast improvements to improve health and treatments. The Blue Button is an integral part of this initiative (Precision Medicine Initiative 2016).

Each agency administers Blue Button with its own rules. To use the Blue Button for Medicare data, beneficiaries must register at Medicare.gov. Veterans can use their My HealtheVet record, which they sign up for at their local VA facility, and click the Blue Button to save or print information from their health record. In addition, veterans can use the VA Continuity of Care Document (VA CCD). This is a summary of essential health and medical care information in an XML format for easier exchange of health information between healthcare organizations and clinicians (US Department of Veterans Affairs [VA] 2013).

From this initiative, many patients can now securely access, save, print, and exchange their health information with providers and healthcare organizations. Ultimately, using the Blue Button will not only actively engage the patient in their healthcare but will improve the quality and safety of care. Although not exactly a PHR as described above because it only contains the information from the agency or provider sponsoring the Blue Button, this application does effectively expand access to health information for a large number of citizens.

⊙ Patient Portal

For centuries, patients and consumers have had little access to their personal health information (PHI). Moreover, PHI was chronicled in inaccessible paper records with each physician or hospital siloing the information. Patients and consumers lacked a portal into the information. However, change is under way as patients are conclusively achieving access to their PHI. This is partially due to the Health Insurance Portability and Accountability Act of 1996 (HIPAA) and Meaningful Use requirements for patient engagement in concurrence with the widespread implementation of electronic health records.

HIPAA mandates that individuals have some voice over their PHI such as access, amendment, accounting of disclosure, restriction requests, and confidential communication (Rinehart-Thompson, 2013, 61). Fundamentally, the individual has the right of access to review and acquire a copy of their PHI within a health record. However, in certain defined circumstances an individual may be denied access to their PHI (Rinehart-Thompson, 2013, 61). Full details about denial are described in the HIPAA Privacy Rule (45 CFR Part 160).

Beginning with Meaningful Use Stage 1 with continuation in Stage 2 (CMS. gov 2016a) eligible providers as well as eligible hospitals are directed to provide patients with electronic access to their health information as mentioned earlier in this chapter. One means for providing this access could be the use of a patient portal.

A patient portal is generally integrated with an EHR. Features and functionalities of a patient portal include:

- Record of healthcare visits
- Discharge summaries
- Medication
- Immunizations
- Allergies
- Laboratory results
- Secure e-mail exchange with healthcare providers
- Prescription refill requests
- Scheduling of appointments
- Verification of benefits and coverage
- Update contact information
- Make payments
- Download and complete forms
- Access education materials

Centers for Medicare and Medicaid Services (CMS) are acting to guarantee that patients have access to their PHI. Meaningful Use Stage 2 Advanced Clinical Processes requires the patient have electronic access to more patient-controlled data, which provides patients the ability to view online, download, and transmit their health information within specified time frames both for eligible providers and for hospitals. Stage 3 Improved Outcomes, requires access to self-managed tools and access to data through patient-centered HIEs.

⊙ Validity and Reliability of Online Health Information

Validity and reliability of online resources are a constant concern for those retrieving information from the Internet. **Validity** is defined as "1. The extent to which data correspond to the actual state of affairs or that an instrument measures what it purports to measure. 2. A term referring to a test's ability to accurately and consistently measure what it purports to measure" (AHIMA 2014, 151). **Reliability** is defined as "A measure of consistency of data items based on their reproducibility and an estimation of their error of measurement" (AHIMA 2014, 128).

What is more, healthcare professionals and researchers continue to question the validity and reliability of online information (Hendrick et al. 2012). Concerns about the reliability of health information on the Internet were addressed in 1995 when Health on the Net Foundation (HON), an international, nongovernmental organization, was launched (Health on the Net Foundation 2013). Based on dialogue with webmasters and information providers, the initial version of the HON Code of Conduct (HONcode) for medical and health websites was published in 1996. The code was revised in 1997 and the principles of the code have remained unchanged since that time. Updates are made periodically in policies and guideline information to support the principles in the current environment. The HONcode principles are grounded in the following tenets:

- Authoritative—qualifications of the authors
- Complementarily—information should support, not replace, the doctor–patient relationship
- Privacy—respect the privacy and confidentiality of data submitted to the site by the visitor
- Attribution—cite sources of published information, date medical and health pages
- Justifiability—back up claims relating to benefits and performance
- Transparency—accessible presentation, accurate e-mail address
- Financial disclosure—identify funding sources
- Advertising policy—clearly distinguish advertising from editorial content (HON 2014)

Website certification is offered free of charge with a membership fee required for continued recertification. HON conducts a thorough investigation of the website to ensure the web developers adhere to ethical standards in the presentation of information and the readers can determine the source and intent of the data they are reading. If approved an HON code seal is placed on the website.

Consumers should consider learning more about how to determine the validity and reliability of online health information from such trusted sources as

- MedlinePlus Guide to Healthy Web Surfing (NLM 2015)
- Finding Reliable Health Information Online (National Human Genome Research Institute 2015)
- Evaluating Health Information (NLM 2016b)
- MedlinePlus Quality Guidelines (NLM 2016c)
- Medical Library Association List of 100 Websites You Can Trust (CAPHIS 2015)

The advice offered to consumers of online health information by NIH and NLM is to critically scrutinize online information (NIH 2012; NIH 2016; NLM 2016c). Furthermore, NIH recommends the use of current, unbiased evidence-based information. To a certain extent, consumers accessing health information online should use the information to become more educated about their health, while exercising caution and consulting with quality healthcare providers to ensure the information is valid.

⊙ Privacy and Security

The online health information consumer should expect the privacy and security of any disclosed personally identifiable health information to be maintained. Reputable online health information websites should include a hyperlink to a privacy policy statement. The hyperlink is typically located near the bottom of the webpage. For example, NIHSeniorHealth and MedlinePlus provide information about privacy to the online health consumer regarding the following information:

- ⊙ Type of information collected
- ⊙ Cookies
- ⊙ Personally identifiable information (PII)
- ⊙ Links to other sites
- ⊙ Security
- ⊙ Third-party websites and applications
  - o AddThis
  - o Go.USA.gov and Bit.ly
  - o Facebook
  - o GovDelivery
  - o iTunes App Store
  - o Twitter (NIH 2012; NLM 2012b)

Presently, new challenges for managing privacy and security issues have arisen related to mobile and online health information. Per the Office of Consumer eHealth, "regulations such as HIPAA and HITECH provide some parameters for privacy guidance in this changing environment, and as health information technology evolves, additional initiatives can build on and complement those protections" (Ricciardi 2012). The ONC, primarily through its Office of the Chief Privacy Officer, has initiated the following projects to study privacy and security issues related to mobile and online health information:

- ⊙ Mobile Devices Roundtable: Safeguarding Health Information
- ⊙ mHealth Privacy and Security Consumer Research
- ⊙ Survey on Privacy, Security of Medical Records
- ⊙ Model Privacy Notice for Consumers for Personal Health Records (PHRs) (ONC 2013)

The privacy and security of personal identifiable information collected by a website or other technology must be guaranteed to the health information consumer. The ONC and the HHS OCR continue to make efforts to meet the challenges of privacy and security introduced by new technology.

Case Study: Patient Engagement

Providers are interested in developing long-term patient engagement strategies as well as meeting the objectives of Stage 2 and Stage 3 meaningful use. In their HIT advisory role, RECs can assist providers in their efforts by helping develop strategies and suggesting tools to meet challenges. The benefits to the patient can be improved quality of care and health and reduced costs.

(Continued)

An Iowa REC determined there was a need to show providers the value of increasing patient engagement to counter the perception that there was already an established relationship between patients and providers and new engagement activities would just mean more work for providers. The REC developed a pilot project for data exchange with the VA Blue Button veteran's health data. A goal of this project was to ensure the incorporation of the Blue Button data to non-VA providers to increase engagement by enabling patients to be involved with their data and making it available to others and to support their transition in care. Four critical access hospitals and associated clinics participated in the project for the data exchange. Outcomes reported so far are that the exchange is taking place with the VA planning to expand this activity and use on a national basis. The project has been valuable in demonstrating the value of PHI exchange for the continuity of patient care. Next steps in the project are to evaluate the data being gathered to determine if there is improvement of the quality of healthcare (HealthIT 2014).

This is an example of using something that is already in place, the Blue Button data, and determining ways to use this information in other settings in an expeditious manner. The value of the support of the REC was also important to the project with their experience in data exchange and because providers did not initially recognize the value of the exchange.

Chapter 15 Review Exercises

Answer the following questions.

1. Which of the following organizations is focused on increasing consumer involvement in their healthcare?
   a. Office of the National Coordinator for Health Information Technology
   b. Agency for Healthcare Research and Quality
   c. Centers for Disease Control and Prevention
   d. American National Standards Institute

2. Nonadopters who have not looked online for health information within the past year tend to
   a. Be more affluent
   b. Have no differences among age groups
   c. Be of African American and Hispanic descent in low income areas
   d. Have more education

3. What term describes the ability of consumers to obtain, process, and understand healthcare information for the purpose of decision making?
   a. Health informatics
   b. Numeric Literacy
   c. Visual Literacy
   d. Health literacy

4. What are skills related to calculating insulin dosages or understanding body mass index values?
   a. Health informatics
   b. Numeric literacy
   c. Visual literacy
   d. Health literacy

5. What types of health information are not available to consumers via a search on the Internet?
   a. Medicine or medical device information
   b. Medical conditions
   c. Lifestyle tips
   d. Past medical history

6. Social media is enabled by Web 2.0, which refers to
   a. An electronic data exchange standard
   b. A consumer healthcare website
   c. A consumer application that is downloaded
   d. A platform of connected devices that deliver software

Discussion.

7. What is the main difference between validity and reliability?

8. Provide examples of ubiquitous computing and its advantages.

9. What is a personal health record?

10. What is the difference between a personal health record and a patient portal?

REFERENCES

Agency for Healthcare Research and Quality (AHRQ). 2012. Consumer health IT applications. http://healthit.ahrq.gov/portal/server.pt?open=514&objID=5554&mode=2&holderDisplayURL=http://wcipubcontent/publish/communities/k_o/knowledge_library/key_topics/consumer_health_it/consumer_health_it_applications.html.

AHIMA Workgroup. 2015. Including patient-generated health data in electronic health records. *Journal of AHIMA* 86(2):54–57.

American Cancer Society (ACS). 2016. Resources. http://www.cancer.org/.

American Diabetes Association (ADA). 2012. Diabetes Basics. http://www.diabetes.org/diabetes-basics/.

AHIMA. 2016. myPHR. https://www.myphr.com/.

AHIMA. 2014. *Pocket Glossary for Health Information Management and Technology*, 4th ed. Chicago, IL: AHIMA.

American Medical Informatics Association Consumer Health Informatics Working Group. 2012. Consumer health informatics. http://www.amia.org/applications-informatics/consumer-health-informatics.

Apple. 2016. *Health: An innovative new way to use your health and fitness information.* http://www.apple.com/ios/health/.

Baur, C. 2012. Health literacy around the world [Web log]. http://blogs.cdc.gov/healthliteracy/2012/09/28/health-literacy-around-the-world/.

Beattie, A. 2011, 29 November. What is the difference between social media and Web 2.0? https://www.techopedia.com/2/27884/internet/social-media/what-is-the-difference-between-social-media-and-web-20.

Brennan, P.F., S. Downs, and D. Kenron. 2007. Project health design: Stimulating the next generation of personal health records. *AMIA Annual Symposium Proceedings 2007.* http://www.ncbi.nlm.nih.gov/pmc/articles/PMC2655909/.

Butler, M. 2015. Mastering the inbox information era: Patient-Generated data and mobile health are changing the management of health information. *Journal of AHIMA* 86(9):18-21.

CAPHIS. 2015. Top 100 List: Health Websites You Can Trust. http://caphis.mlanet.org/consumer/.

Center for Healthcare Strategies, Inc. (CHCS). 2013. Fact Sheet #1. What Is Health Literacy? http://www.chcs.org/media/CHCS_Health_Literacy_Fact_Sheets_2013.pdf.

Centers for Disease Control (CDC), National Institute for Occupational Safety and Health. 2012. Total worker health. http://www.cdc.gov/niosh/TWH/totalhealth.html.

Centers for Medicare and Medicaid (CMS). 2015. Medicare and Medicaid Programs; Electronic Health Record Incentive Program-Stage 3 and Modifications to Meaningful Use in 2015 Through 2017. *Federal Register.* https://www.federalregister.gov/articles/2015/10/16/2015-25595/medicare-and-medicaid-programs-electronic-health-record-incentive-program-stage-3-and-modifications.

Centers for Medicare and Medicaid (CMS). 2014. Patient electronic access tipsheet. https://www.cms.gov/Regulations-and-Guidance/Legislation/EHRIncentivePrograms/Downloads/PatientElecAccTipsheet_06182014-.pdf.

Centers for Medicare and Medicaid (CMS). 2016a. EHR Incentive Programs in 2015 through 2017 Patient Electronic Access. https://www.cms.gov/.

Center for Medicare and Medicaid (CMS). 2016b Regulations-and-Guidance/Legislation/EHRIncentivePrograms/Downloads/2016_PatientElectronicAccess.pdf.

Centers for Medicare and Medicaid (CMS). 2016b. Electronic Health Records (EHR) Incentive Program. https://www.cms.gov/Regulations-and-Guidance/Legislation/EHRIncentivePrograms/index.html?redirect=/ehrincentiveprograms.

Chopra, A., T. Park, and P.L. Levin. 2010. *Blue Button' provides access to downloadable personal health data* [Web log]. http://www.whitehouse.gov/blog/2010/10/07/blue-button-provides-access-downloadable-personal-health-data.

Eysenbach, G. 2000. Consumer health informatics. *BMJ* 320(7251):1713-1716.

Fox, S., and M. Duggan. 2013a. Health Online 2013. Pew Research Center. http://www.pewinternet.org/2013/01/15/health-online-2013/.

Fox, S., and M. Duggan. 2013b. *Pew Internet: Health*. http://pewinternet.org /Commentary/2011/November/Pew-Internet-Health.aspx.

Health on the Net Foundation (HON). 2013. *Health on the Net Foundation*. http://www .hon.ch/HONcode/Patients/Conduct.html.

HealthIT.gov. 2016b. Patient-Generated Health Data. https://www.healthit.gov/policy -researchers-implementers/patient-generated-health-data.

HealthIT.gov. 2014. Education and Outreach Case Study: Helping Providers Engage Patients. https://www.healthit.gov/sites/default/files/recservicelinecasestudy _helpingprovidersengagepatients.pdf.

Healthy People 2020. 2012. Health Communication and Health Information Technology. http://healthypeople.gov/2020/topicsobjectives2020/overview.aspx?topicid=18.

Hendrick, P.A., O.H. Ahmed, S.S. Bankier, S.A. Crawford, C.R. Ryder, L.J. Welsh, and A.G. Schneiders. 2012. Acute low back pain information online: An evaluation of quality, content accuracy and readability or related websites. *Manual Therapy*. 17(40):318–324.

Hillestad, R., J. Bigelow, A. Bower, F. Girosi, R. Meili, R. Scoville, and R. Taylor. 2005. Can electronic medical record systems transform healthcare? Potential health benefits, savings, and costs. *Health Affairs* 24(5):1103–1117.

House, M. 2013. *The use of social media in healthcare: organizational, clinical, and patient perspectives*. http://www.ncbi.nlm.nih.gov/pubmed/23388291/.

Information Week. 2013. Fitbit gadget could improve hospital care. http://www .informationweek.com/mobile/fitbit-gadget-could-improve-hospital-care/d/d -id/1111478.

Kimball, A., K. Corey., J. Kvedar. 2015. Engaging Patients to Decrease Costs and Improve Outcomes.*Medical Economics* e-news. http://medicaleconomics.modernmedicine.com /medical-economics/news/engaging-patients-decrease-costs-and-improve-outcomes.

Kirsch, I.S., A. Jungeblut, L. Jenkins, and A. Kolstad. 2002. *Adult literacy in America: A first look at the findings of the National Adult Literacy Survey*, 3rd ed. http://nces.ed.gov /pubs93/93275.pdf.

Lee, H., A. Kreshnik, J. Hughes, and L. Emmerton. 2014. Dr Google and the consumer: A qualitative study exploring the navigational needs and online health information- seeking behaviors. *Journal of Medical Internet Research*: 16(12): e262.

Mayo Clinic. n.d. Mayo Clinic Center for Social Media. https://socialmedia.mayoclinic .org/.

Mostashari, F. 2012, January 25. Health IT taking flight—What is in store for the year ahead [Web log comment]. http://www.healthit.gov/buzz-blog/from-the-onc-desk /healthit-year-ahead/.

National Human Genome Research Institute. 2015. Finding Reliable Health Information Online. http://www.genome.gov/11008303.

National Institutes of Health (NIH). n.d.b. Health and Wellness Resources. http://www .nih.gov/health/wellness/.

National Institutes of Health (NIH). 2012. Senior Health. http://nihseniorhealth.gov /privacy.html.

National Library of Medicine (NLM). 2016a. MedlinePlus Statistics. https://www.nlm .nih.gov/medlineplus/usestatistics.html.

National Library of Medicine (NLM). 2016b. Evaluating Health Information. https:// www.nlm.nih.gov/medlineplus/evaluatinghealthinformation.html.

National Library of Medicine (NLM). 2016c. MedlinePlus Quality Guidelines. http:// www.nlm.nih.gov/medlineplus/criteria.html.

National Library of Medicine (NLM). 2015. MedlinePlus Guide to Healthy Web Surfing. https://medlineplus.gov/healthywebsurfing.html.

National Library of Medicine (NLM). 2012b. MedlinePlus. http://www.nlm.nih.gov /medlineplus/aboutmedlineplus.html.

National Network of Libraries of Medicine (NNLM). 2012. Health Literacy. http://nnlm .gov/outreach/consumer/hlthlit.html.

Nations, D. 2016. What Is Social Media? Explaining the Big Trend. http://webtrends .about.com/od/web20/a/social-media.htm.

Nestlé. 2012. Employee Health and Wellness. http://www.nestle.com/csv/ourpeople /employeehealthandwellness/Pages/employeehealthandwellness.aspx.

Nielsen-Bohlman, L., A.M. Panzer, and D.A. Kindig. 2004. *Health Literacy: A Prescription to End Confusion.* Washington, DC: The National Academies Press.

Norman, C.D., and H.A. Skinner. 2006. eHealth Literacy: Essential skills for consumer health in a networked world. *Journal of Medical Internet Research* 8(2):e9. doi:10.2196 /jmir.8.2. e9.

Obama, B.H. Speech to the Disabled Veterans of America, August 2, 2010. White House. https://www.whitehouse.gov/the-press-office/remarks-president-disabled-veterans -america-conference-atlanta-georgia.

Office of Disease Prevention and Health Promotion (ODPHP). 2016. Leading Health Indicators. https://www.healthypeople.gov/2020/leading-health-indicators/LHI -Infographic-Gallery.

Office of the National Coordinator (ONC) for Health Information Technology. 2013. www .healthit.gov.

O'Reilly, T. 2005. Web 2.0: Compact Definition? http://radar.oreilly.com/2005/10/web -20-compact-definition.html.

Oxford English Dictionary. 2016. http://oxforddictionaries.com.

Pew Internet and American Life Project. 2013. Health Online. http://www.pewinternet .org/files/old-media/Files/Reports/PIP_HealthOnline.pdf.

Pew Research Center. (2015). *American Internet Access: Percent of Adults 2000–2015* http:// www.pewinternet.org/2015/06/26/americans-internet-access-2000-2015.

Prensky, M. 2001. Digital natives, digital immigrants. *On the Horizon* 9(5):1-6. http:// www.marcprensky.com/writing/Prensky%20-%20Digital%20Natives,%20Digital%20 Immigrants%20-%20Part1.pdf.

Ratzan, S.C., and R.M. Parker. 2000. Introduction. In *National Library of Medicine Current Bibliographies in Medicine: Health Literacy.* NLM Pub. No. CBM 2000-1. Edited by

C.R. Selden, M. Zorn, S.C. Ratzan, and R.M. Parker. Bethesda, MD: National Institutes of Health, US Department of Health and Human Services.

Ricciardi, L. 2012, March 15. Protecting Privacy of Health Information and Building Trust as Mobile and Online Health Evolve [Web log]. http://www.healthit.gov /buzz-blog/from-the-onc-desk/privacy-of-health-information/.

Rinehart-Thompson, L.A. (2013). *Introduction to Health Information Privacy and Security*. Chicago, IL: AHIMA.

Sarakar, U., A. Karter, J. Liu, N. Adler, R. Nguyen, A. Lopez, and D. Schillinger. 2011. Social disparities in internet patient portal use in diabetes: Evidence that the digital divide extends beyond access. *JAMIA* 18(3):318–321.

Texas Medical Center (TMC) Library. 2012. Consumer Health Resources: General Information. http://libguides.library.tmc.edu/consumer.

Texas State University. n.d. Wellness Program. http://www.hhp.txstate.edu/Total -Wellness.html.

Woods, S., E. Schwartz, A. Tuepker, N. Press, K. Nazi, C. Turvey, and W. Nichol. 2013. Patient experiences with full electronic access to health records and clinical notes through the My HealtheVet personal health record pilot: Qualitative study. *Journal Medical Internet Research*. http://www.ncbi.nlm.nih.gov/pmc/articles/PMC3636169/.

United States Census Bureau. 2016. Computer and Internet Access in the United States. *Data*. http://census.gov/data/tables/2012/demo/computer-internet/computer -use-2012.html.

US Government Accountability Office (GAO) Accounting and Information Management Division. 1996. *Consumer health informatics: Emerging issues*. Washington, DC: US Government.

United Health Group. n.d. *Innovation*. http://www.unitedhealthgroup.com/About /Modernization/KeyIssues/HealthIT.aspx.

Vance, B., and B. Tomblin, J. Studeny, and A. Coustasse. 2015, March. Benefits and barriers for adoption of personal health records. *Marshall Digital Scholar*. http://mds .marshall.edu/cgi/viewcontent.cgi?article=1135&context=mgmt_faculty.

Ventola, C.L. 2014. Social media and health care professionals: Benefits, risks, and best practices. *Pharmacy and Therapeutics* 39(7):491–520. http://www.ncbi.nlm.nih.gov /pmc/articles/PMC4103576/.

WebMD. 2016. WebMD Homepage. http://www.webmd.com/.

ADDITIONAL RESOURCES

Aichner, T., and Jacob, F. 2015. Measuring the degree of corporate social media. *International Journal of Market Research* 57(2):257–275.

API. 2016. *In techopedia*. https://www.techopedia.com/definition/24407/application -programming-interface-api.

Ball, M. J., C. Smith, and R.S. Bakalaar. 2007. Personal health records: Empowering consumers. *Journal of Healthcare Information Management,* 21(1):76–86. http://www.ncbi.nlm.nih.gov/pubmed/17299929.

Blue Cross Blue Shield of Texas. 2012. *Health and wellness.* https://connect.bcbstx.com/health-and-wellness/b/weblog.

Calabretta, N. 2002. Consumer-driven, patient-centered healthcare in the age of electronic information. *Journal of the Medical Library Association* 90(1):32–37.

Celebrating the 5 Year Anniversary of Blue Button and Open Health Data. 2015 https://www.whitehouse.gov/blog/2015/10/01/celebrating-5-year-anniversary-blue-button-open-health-data.

Centers for Medicare and Medicaid (CMS). 2015. CMS Fact Sheet: EHR Incentive Programs in 2015 and Beyond. https://www.cms.gov/Newsroom/MediaReleaseDatabase/Fact-sheets/2015-Fact-sheets-items/2015-10-06-2.html.

Cline, R.J., and K.M. Haynes. 2001. Consumer health information seeking on the Internet: The state of the art. *Health Education Research 16*:671–692.

CNN. 2012. CNNHealth. http://www.cnn.com/HEALTH.

CVS 2012. Health Center Information. http://health.cvs.com/GetContent.aspx?token=f75979d3-9c7c-4b16-af56-3e122a3f19e3.

Detmer, D., M. Bloomrosen, B. Raymond, and P. Tang. 2008. Integrated personal health records: Transformative tools for consumer-centric care. *BMC Medical Informatics and Decision Making* 8:45. doi: 10.1186/1472-6947-8-45.

Do, N.V., R. Barnhill, K.A. Heermann-Do, K.L. Salman, and R.W. Gimbel. 2011. The military health system's personal health record with Microsoft HealthVault and Google Health. *JAMIA* 18(2):188–124.

Dykes Library 2012. *Patient Health Information.* http://www.kumed.com/patient-visitor/patient-guide.

Federal Register. 2015, 16 October. Medicare and Medicaid programs; *Electronic health record incentive program-Stage 3 and modifications to Meaningful Use in 2015 through 2017.*

Ferguson, T. 1996. *Health Online.* Reading, MA: Addision-Wesley Publishing Company.

File, T., and C. Ryan. 2013. *Computer and Internet Use in the United States: 2013.* http://www.census.gov/content/dam/Census/library/publications/2014/acs/acs-28.pdf.

Fox News. 2012. Fox News Health. http://www.foxnews.com/health/index.html.

Fox, S. 2011, May 12. The Social Life of Health Information. Pew Internet and American Life Project. http://pewinternet.org/Reports/2011/Social-Life-of-Health-Info.aspx.

Fox, S. 2006, October 29. Online Health Search. Pew Internet and American Life Project. http://www.pewinternet.org/Reports/2006/Online-Health-Search-2006.aspx.

Fox, S., and D. Fallows. 2003, July 16. Internet Health Resources. Pew Internet and American Life Project. http://www.pewinternet.org/files/old-media//Files/Reports/2003/PIP_Health_Report_July_2003.pdf.pdf.

Fox, S., and S. Jones. 2009, June. The Social Life of Health Information. Pew Internet and American Life Project. http://www.pewinternet.org/Reports/2009/8-The-Social -Life-of-Health-Information.aspx.

Fox, S., and L. Rainie. 2000, November 26. The Online Healthcare Revolution: How the Web Helps Americans Take Better Care of Themselves. http://www.pewinternet .org/files/old-media/Files/Reports/2000/PIP_Health_Report.pdf.pdf.

Fricton, J.R., and D. Davies. 2008. Personal health records to improve health information exchange and patient safety. In *Advances in Patient Safety: New Directions and Alternative Approaches: Vol. 4. Technology and Medication Safety.* Series edited by K. Henriksen, J. Battles, M. Keyes, and M. Grady. http://www.ncbi.nlm.nih.gov /books/NBK43760/.

Funding Universe. 2013. *WebMD Corporation History.* http://www.fundinguniverse.com /company-histories/webmd-corporation-history/.

Gamire, E. and G. Pearson, eds. 2006. *Tech Tally: Approaches to Assessing Technological Literacy.* Washington, DC: The National Academies Press.

Greenhalgh, T., S. Hinder, K. Stramer, T. Bratan, and J. Russell. 2010. Adoption, non-adoption, and abandonment of a personal electronic health record: Case study of HealthSpace. *BMJ* 341:c5814: doi: 10.1136/bmj.c5814.

Gustafson, D.H., F.M. McTavish, W. Stengle, D. Ballard, E. Jones, K. Julesberg, H. McDowell, G. Landucci, and R. Hawkins. 2005. Reducing the digital divide for low-income women with breast cancer: A feasibility study of a population-based intervention. *Journal Health Communications* 10 (Suppl 1):173-193.

Hassol, A., J. Walker, D. Kidder, K. Rokita, D. Young, S. Pierdon, D. Deitz, S. Kuck, and E. Ortiz. 2004. Patient experiences and attitudes about access to a patient electronic health care record and linked web messaging. *JAMIA* 11(6):505–513.

HealthIT.gov. 2016. *What is a patient portal?* https://www.healthit.gov/providers -professionals/faqs/what-patient-portal.

Horan, T.A., N.E. Botts, and R.J. Burkhard. 2010. A multidimensional view of personal health systems for underserved populations. *Journal of Medical Internet Research* 12(3):e32. doi: 10.2196/jmir.1355.

Houston, T.K., B.L. Chang, S. Brown, and R. Kukafka. 2001. Consumer health informatics: A consensus description and commentary from the American Medical Association Members. *Proceedings of the American Medical Association Symposium 2001,* 269–273.

Impicciatore, P., C. Pandolfini, N. Casella, and M. Bonit. 1997. Reliability of health information for the public on the world wide web: Systematic survey of advice on managing fever in children at home. *BMJ* 314:1875–1881. http://www.bmj.com /content/314/7098/1875.

Kaelber, D., and E.C. Pan. 2008. The value of personal health record (PHR) systems. In *AMIA Annual Symposium Proceedings,* vol. 2008, 343. American Medical Informatics Association.

Kahn, J.S., J.F. Hilton, T. Van Nunnery, S. Leasure, K.M. Bryant, C.B. Hare, and D.H. Thom. 2010. Personal health records in a public hospital: Experience at the

HIV/AIDS clinic at San Francisco General Hospital. *Journal of the American Medical Informatics Association* 17(2):224–228. doi: 10.1197/jamia.M3200corr1.

Keckley, P. H., and Hoffman, M. 2010. *Issue brief: Social networks in health care: Communication, collaboration, and insights.* https://www.ucsf.edu/sites/default/files /legacy_files/US_CHS_2010SocialNetworks_070710.pdf.

Ko, H., T. Turner, C. Jones, and C. Hill. 2010. Patient-held medical records for patients with chronic disease: A systematic review. *Quality Safety Health Care* 19(5):e41. doi: 10.1136/qshc.2009.037531.

Kristen A., C. Corey and J. Kvedar. 2015. Engaging patients to decrease costs and improve outcomes. *Modern Medicine.* http://medicaleconomics.modernmedicine.com/medical -economics/news/engaging-patients-decrease-costs-and-improve-outcomes.

Markle Foundation. 2003. *Americans want benefits of personal health records.* http://www .markle.org/publications/950-americans-want-benefits-personal-health-records.

MHADegree.org. 2016. *Top 50 Most Social Media Friendly Hospitals for 2013.* http:// mhadegree.org/top-50-most-social-media-friendly-hospitals-2013/.

Montelius, E., B. Astrand, B. Hovstadius, and G. Petersson. 2008. Individuals appreciate having their medication record on the web: A survey of attitudes to a national pharmacy register. *Journal of Medical Internet Research* 10(4). e35. doi: 10.2196 /jmir.1022.

National Institutes of Health (NIH). n.d.a. Health information. http://health.nih.gov/.

National Library of Medicine (NLM). 2012a. NLM privacy policy. http://www.nlm.nih .gov/medlineplus/privacy.html.

Nazi, K.L. 2010, December 8. *VA's Blue Button: Empowering people with their data* [Web log]. http://www.blogs.va.gov/VAntage/866/vas-blue-button-empowering-people -with-their-data/.

Patientslikeme. 2012. http://www.patientslikeme.com/about.

Pletneva, N., S. Cruchet, M.A. Simmonet, M. Kajiwara, and C. Boyer. 2011. Results of the 10 HON survey on health and medical Internet use. *Stud Health Technol Inform* 169:73–77.

The Precision Medicine Initiative. 2016. https://www.whitehouse.gov/precision-medicine.

Quick, D. 2012, October 12. Smart Bra Acts as an Early Warning System for Breast Cancer. http://www.gizmag.com/bse-bra-breast-cancer-monitoring/24529/.

Robinson, T.N., L. Patrick, T.R. Eng, and D. Gustafson. 1998. An evidence-based approach to interactive health communication: A challenge to medicine in the information age. *Journal of the American Medical Association* 280:1264–1269.

Saenz, A. 2009, May 12. Smart Toilets: Doctors in Your Bathroom. http://singularityhub .com/2009/05/12/smart-toilets-doctors-in-your-bathroom/.

Safeway. 2012. Healthy living. http://www.safeway.com/ShopStores/Wellness-Center .page?#iframetop.

Seidman, J. 2011. The role of health literacy in health information technology. In *Innovations in Health Literacy: Workshop Summary.* Edited by C. Vancheri (Rappoteur), 23–26. Washington, DC: The National Academies Press.

Sharecare. n.d. http://www.sharecare.com/.

Stat My Web. 2012. Webmd.com. http://www.statmyweb.com/site/webmd.com.

Sunderman, C.L., and L. Goodwin. 2008. *Personal Health Records in the Aging U.S. Population: An Analysis of the Benefits and Issues.* Unpublished manuscript. https://www.researchgate.net/publication/228395484_Personal_Health_Records_in_the_Aging_US_Population_An_Analysis_of_the_Benefits_and_Issues.

Tang, P.C., J. Ash, D.W. Bates, J.M. Overhage, and D.A. Sands. 2006. Personal health records: Definitions, benefits, and strategies for overcoming barriers to adoption. *JAMIA* 13:121–126.

Technopedia. 2016. Technopedia Dictionary. Technopedia.com.

Tenforde, M., A. Jain, and J. Hickner. 2011. The value of personal health records for chronic disease management: What do we know? *Family Medicine* 43(5):351–354. https://www.ncbi.nlm.nih.gov/pubmed/21557106.

Top 20 Social Networks for Doctors. 2014, October 7. http://upcity.com/blog/top-20-social-networks-for-doctors/.

University of Kansas Medical School–Wichita. 2015. Consumer Health. http://wichita.kumc.edu/farha-library/subject-links/consumer-health.html.

US Department of Veterans Affairs. 2013. *New VA Blue Buttons features for 2013*: VA Notes, and CCD and more. http://www.va.gov/bluebutton/.

Wagner, P.J., S.M. Howard, D.R. Bentley, Y. Seol, and P. Sodoma. 2010. Incorporating patient perspectives into the personal health record: Implications for care and caring. *Perspectives in Health Information Management* 7:1e. http://www.ncbi.nlm.nih.gov/pmc/articles/PMC2966356/.

Walgreens. 2012. Health information. http://www.walgreens.com/health/health_info.jsp?tab=Health+Info.

WebMD. n.d. *Investor relations.* http://investor.shareholder.com/wbmd/faq.cfm.

Wiljer, D., S. Urowitz, E. Apatu, C. DeLenardo, G. Eysenbach, T. Harth, and K.J. Leonard. 2008. Patient accessible electronic health records: Exploring recommendations for successful implementation strategies. *Journal of Internet Medical Research* 10(4): e34. doi: 10.2196/jmir.1061.

Wiltry, M.J., W.R. Doucette, J.M. Daly, T.L. Barcedy, and E.A. Chrischilles. 2010. Family physician perceptions of personal health records. *Perspective in Health Information Management.* 7:1d.

Chapter 16

Trends and Emerging Technologies

KEY TERMS

Accountable care organizations (ACOs)
Archival system
Artificial intelligence (AI)
Backup
Central Authority Platform (CAP)
Clinical decision support
Cloud Computing
Data consolidation
Disease management
e-health
Evidence-based medicine (EBM)
Functional genomics
Genetic Information and Nondiscrimination Act (GINA)

Genome
Genomics
Health Information Exchange (HIE)
Meaningful use
mHealth
Patient-centered medical home (PCMH)
Point-of-care testing (POCT)
Precision medicine
Predictive modeling
Quality improvement (QI)
Regional Extension Centers (RECs)
Seamless care or care coordination
Telehealth
Telemedicine

Mentioned in a number of different ways throughout this book, health informatics involves utilizing technology along with health information to affect change, which could be in quality of care or increased use and understanding of informatics data. Currently, a typical health informatics scenario involves using EHR technology in conjunction with information from the patient's health record to capture more data than ever possible within the facility and through exchange of data with external entities. Additionally, the increased usage of health informatics technologies is driving the development of new statistical and data presentation software. Much has been accomplished with the increased utilization of EHRs but the full potential has yet to be recognized. This chapter introduces a few of the possible and future trends in technology, education, employment, and genomics.

⊙ Current and Emerging Trends and Terms

Many examples exist relating how informatics can be utilized to improve patient outcomes and facilitate efficient delivery of healthcare services. Informatics provides expanded provider access to a patient's past health information and timelier reporting of lab and other diagnostic test results critical to patient diagnosis and treatment. It impacts the computerized physician order entry (CPOE) systems that provide information to the physician for decision making when prescribing, which reduces the time needed to determine which medications to order and this results in the patient getting medications faster with fewer potential medication errors (for example, wrong medication, dosage, or frequency to be taken). Informatics increases patient engagement through patient portals that provide access to the patient's health record and additional materials. Topics presented throughout this text reflect on the current status and future possibilities of various aspects of health informatics. These include EHR advances (chapter 3), expanded use of databases (chapter 5), benefits to research and data analysis (chapter 7), the information exchange (chapter 10), expanded uses of information (chapter 11), and the benefits to consumer health (chapter 15).

Although the benefits and advances in health informatics are vast and well understood, there are still areas of concern. Patient privacy and confidentiality pose significant challenges due to the increased use of technology and data exchange as well as the many new uses of these data for decision making, planning, and policy making. Another issue of concern to many includes the cost-effectiveness of developing and implementing systems. The benefits of fully functional electronic health information systems include improvements in the quality and convenience of patient care, improved accuracy of diagnosis and health outcomes, better care coordination, increased patient participation, and increases in efficiencies and cost savings (HealthIT 2015). Questions remain regarding whether the cost benefit should be a consideration when there are such significant positive benefits for patient care. Consumerism will continue to be a factor as patients and providers become accustomed to having access to more information. It is becoming more of an expectation that decisions be based on appropriate data to promote optimal results in the provision and planning of healthcare and in the strategic planning and policy making for the future.

Redefining the Health Informatics Domain

Information is used pervasively throughout healthcare. Specific domains for consideration in formal educational programs are covered in the section on education, which follows. What seems to be paramount to the identity of the health informatics educational domain is establishing the knowledge content to adequately define what informatics is and what it does. A comprehension of hardware and software capabilities are of prime importance. Also important is the standardization of commonly accepted elements of data, languages, and vocabularies. A key component of data analytics is to be able to use the information generated to move from raw data to making conclusions and decisions. The functions presented here are not meant to be all-inclusive but rather a sampling of areas that will be impacted by the influence of health informatics.

Emerging Technology

Advances and new uses for technology in healthcare are ongoing and will continue to be developed. Newer technology ranges from wearables to digital networks. Examples of recently developed technology include:

- Digital diagnostic tools that provide access where it might not otherwise be available. For example, Neurotrack is a computer-based Alzheimer's test measuring eye movement, which might indicate early onset Alzheimer's disease.

- Ultrafast scans that can capture an image of one beat of the heart. Patients who experience a very fast heart rate are typically denied a scan because of their fast heart rate.

- Cloud storage of data, which facilitates access from multiple locations and provides a valuable offsite backup.

- Wearables, which are a technology worn by the patient, are commonly used for tracking fitness levels. Some patients with Parkinson's disease are utilizing wearable devices to determine characteristics of the disease.

- Patient empowerment, which includes correct and dependable medical information will be assessable to the patient providing them the opportunity to play a lead role in healthcare.

Numerous varied technologies are on the horizon for implementation and future development. The examples given here illustrate the variety of the potential new technologies and if known, the status of development of the technology is provided (Mesko 2016a and 2016b):

- **Real-time data** where checking, monitoring, and recording vital signs or other measures is important for healthcare and intervention when needed. This would require a sensor that recognizes such things as chewing movements, coughing, smoking, and talking which would then record the data (for example, when too much is eaten or when some one is smoking). These reports can then be reviewed by medical providers in real time. This technology could be used in individual organs as well to provide real-time data on how they are functioning.

- **Artificial intelligence (AI)** is high-level information technologies used in developing machines that imitate human qualities such as learning and reasoning (AHIMA 2014). Cognitive systems translate information into knowledge for use in better decision-making. For example, IBM Watson provides assistance to physicians in making decisions but does not substitute for human involvement. The strength of Watson is the capability to read 40 million documents in 15 seconds and then suggest the most appropriate therapy (IBM 2017). Similar applications mine data of medical records to provide better and faster service or predict which medications will work in a given situation. Most of these applications are in the initial phases of deployment and are used with select facilities.

- **Gamifying** is "the process of adding games or gamelike elements to something (as a task) so as to encourage participation" (Mirriam-Webster 2010). This can be a motivation for patients to be more compliant with the need to communicate information and providers to track certain activities. One example of gamification in healthcare is an application called Mango Health. This application encourages patients to take medications by rewarding them with points each time they take their medication resulting in monetary prizes, such as a gift card or a donation to a charity (Mango Health 2016).

- **Holographic data input** where screens and keyboards can be projected on the wall or on a table for ease and accessibility in the clinical setting. The data are stored exclusively in a cloud with only a small projector needed to see the data.

- **Multifunctional radiology** is projected to have the ability to detect many symptoms, biomarkers, and medical problems at one time and is predicted to include imaging techniques and personalized diagnostics with interventions in real-time.

- **In silico clinical trials** allow small microchips to be used as models of human cells, organs, or systems for simulation testing rather than the long and expensive traditional clinical trials. A current application of this technology, referred to as human organs-on-chips, uses stem cells to mimic organs using a series of devices (Wyss Institute 2016). Predictions are that the clinical trial process will be changed significantly and completely replace animal testing.

- **Genomics and the Human Genome Project** substantiated the concept of personalized medicine with tailored therapy and tailored drugs. There are already evidence-based medicine applications in existence such as the use of genetic information to determine dosages of medication in heart patients resulting in a decreased hospitalization rate. With the increased emphasis on personalized medicine, there will be new opportunities for doing bedside DNA analysis.

- **Digestibles or sensors** that function like a thin e-skin to transmit information. These sensors measure and transmit to the cloud a variety of health parameters such and blood biomarkers and neurological symptoms in addition to vital signs. Alerts will be sent when an occurrence of a medical event occurs and can even call the ambulance when needed.

⊙ **Real-time diagnostics** can process results as the information is received. For example, the iKnife can analyze tissue through chemical profiling of tissue in real-time without having to send a specimen to the lab for testing and wait for the results. The iKnife is being used at a hospital in London and is in trials for breast, colon, and ovarian cancer (Huffington Post 2016).

Emerging Applications

There are numerous applications for patients, consumers, physicians, and other providers. These applications benefit consumers and healthcare providers by making medical information and disease treatment accessible to the public. There are also engaging tools that inform the general public about the challenges in the field of public health. For example, CDC provides consumers with a free epidemiology application called Solve the Outbreak that casts the user in the role of disease detective, also called an Epidemic Intelligence Service agent, which examines clues and makes decisions about realistic disease outbreak scenarios (CDC 2016). One question for the user to ponder might be, do you ask for a quarantine or for more diagnostic tests? Points are earned for correct decisions as the player advances to harder scenarios. It is beneficial to know that these kinds of applications are possible and understanding the data required to develop them.

For physicians, there are numerous CDC applications available on various diseases with current up-to-date information (CDC 2016). For example, FastStats provides topic-specific facts on diseases and conditions, family life, life stages, populations, and injuries, to name a few. Another example is Tickborne Diseases, which provides tick identification photos and treatment summaries (CDC 2016). These applications can help physicians by putting diagnostic and patient teaching information at their fingertips.

Expanding Methods of Storage

Health information originates in different data types to include paper charts and other documents, such as electronically-generated EHRs and reports, images, and written notes and is increasing at an exponential rate. Even electronic means of storing digital data have space limitations and maintaining the privacy and security of the patient information while meeting the HIPAA required availability of the information remains an issue. There is no best solution to solving the challenge of maintaining adequate and secure means of storing health information.

One initial consideration in storing information is whether to backup or archive. A **backup** is a copy made of the software and data that can be utilized if the primary sources becomes compromised (AHIMA 2014, 15). The backup provides long-term retention and preservation of the data. An **archival system** or database provides a historical copy saved at a particular point in time and used later to recover and restore the information in a database (AHIMA 2014, 11). A Picture Archival and Communication Systems (PACS) is a convenient and economical means of acquiring, storing, retrieving, and displaying images originating from multiple sources.

Another means of storing information, which is becoming more prevalent in healthcare, is cloud computing. The definition of **cloud computing** is "a model for enabling ubiquitous, convenient, on-demand network access to a shared pool of configurable computing resources (for example, networks, servers, storage, applications, and services) that can be rapidly provisioned and released with minimal management effort or service provider interaction" (NIST 2011). Organizations are turning to the cloud to reduce costs to the organization due to less expense for hardware and software, accessibility of the information from multiple locations and devices, and ability to meet disaster recovery needs. Data stored in the cloud are secured with data encryption and other security measures which addresses the ongoing issue of information security.

Data consolidation is a process for bringing together and summarizing large amounts of data and data from multiple sources. Due to the many mergers of healthcare entities and the coordination of care across larger populations and geographic areas, the need for data consolidation has increased. To an extent, EHRs have the capability to consolidate structured data to facilitate the large-scale consolidation processes needed for healthcare mergers. Going forward, there will be greater focus on consolidating the unstructured data present in EHRs and other data stores.

The sheer amount of genetic data generated creates unique situations and challenges in terms of the short amount of time for its creation, complex genomic data sets, and possible data management solutions that would not have applications to other large complex data sets. Several methods for maintaining the data are being used to reduce the size of the genome sequences. It should be recognized first that the genome sequence for individuals is similar with approximately 99 percent of the sequence identical for everyone .(Alzu'bi et al. 2014). It is therefore redundant to store thousands of these sequences in a database. A method for doing this is to record one reference genome and then record differences of the other genomes with this reference or a variation of these two means. It was reported that in one situation, the resulting data set was 750 times smaller when reduced. Another approach is to use a two component distributed information system. In this arrangement an application server manages primarily the metadata and the other component is a data storage system with web interface links to databases where various genomic data sets are maintained (Alzu'bi et al. 2014). Examples of the databases can be found at the National Center for Biotechnology Information (NCBI) website (NCBI 2016).

Expanding Services Geographically

A great deal of health information has been compiled for use across large geographic areas for quite some time with public health monitoring across states and countries, sharing data external to where it was generated, for the support of telehealth and for all that is encompassed by the term e-health. Much of this was done without the use of technological capabilities that continue to be developed and some of these activities only became possible or changed in scope with the use of the technology. The advances in technology have resulted in an increased amount of data available and enhanced the timely access of the data. This has consequently increased potential uses of and the demand for the data.

Public Health

The focus of public health is the health of populations typically in areas such as counties or states. There is a need for swift access to health-related information when critical decisions must be made in situations such as responding to a multistate outbreak of listeriosis linked to a company's use of raw milk or the identification of the increased incidence of viral hepatitis, a communicable disease. A lack of appropriate information can mean that insufficient data are available for the correct conclusions to be drawn regarding health needs for regions, countries, and the world.

Public health programs and services are complex and diverse. Digital information management systems have the capability to facilitate communication among those involved and offer multiple information access points. The Health Resources and Services Administration (HRSA) works to assure that patients have access to personal and public health services essential for access to quality care, that best practices are utilized, and that disparities in care are eliminated (HHS 2016a). Table 16.1 is a strategic plan that communicates the priorities of HRSA related to public health. The performance measures indicate the data that will be obtained to monitor and measure the success of these initiatives. These initiatives should be used by informatics specialists to design performance measures for digital information management systems and mobile applications that eliminate disparities and increase accessibility.

Health Information Exchange

Health information exchange (HIE) is the electronic exchange of health information between providers and others with the same level of interoperability, such as labs and pharmacies (AHIMA 2014, 68). HIE organizations can play a key role in public health by being responsible for oversight of the information. As the HIE efforts continue, policies and systems to support the data needs of public health will continue to evolve. One specific example of the role of informatics in public health is the development of optimal IT-supported surveillance systems for cancer care and management. An example of a large population-based registry used for surveillance of cancer is the National Cancer Institute's (NCI) Surveillance, Epidemiology, and End Results (SEER) program. Information in this registry incudes incidence of new cancer cases, survival rates, and prevalence (the number of people living with cancer at a given time) and is collected from specific population areas to include 28 percent of the population Future initiatives for surveillance programs include garnering support for more information sharing and allowing the use of deidentified information for research studies. The role of health informatics is to support HIEs so that the data can be transformed into information that can then build our public health knowledge base (ACS 2014).

Table 16.1.   2016–2018 Public health strategic plan with performance measures

Mission-critical goals	Performance Measures Used to Review Performance and Progress
Goal 1: Improve access to quality healthcare and services	**Access** • Number of patients served by health centers • Percentage of eligible persons diagnosed with HIV served by the Ryan White HIV/AIDS Program • Number of unique individuals receiving direct services through the Federal Office of Rural Health Policy Outreach grants • Number of participants served by the Maternal, Infant, and Early Childhood Home Visiting Program **Quality** • Percentage of patients served regardless of age, with an HIV viral load less than 200 copies per milliliter at last HIV viral load test during the measurement year • Percentage of health centers meeting or exceeding Healthy People 2020 goals on selected quality measures • Percentage of Home Visiting participants who received appropriate screening for: (a) depression, (b) interpersonal violence, (c) developmental delay **Outreach and Enrollment** • Number of assists provided by trained assisters working on behalf of health centers to support individuals with actual or potential enrollment and reenrollment in health insurance available through marketplace-qualified health plans and/or through Medicaid or CHIP
Goal 2: Strengthen the health workforce	• Field strength of the National Health Service Corps through scholarship and loan repayment agreements • Percentage of individuals supported by the Bureau of Health Workforce who completed a primary care training program and are currently employed in underserved areas • Percentage of trainees in Bureau of Health Workforce–supported health professions training programs who receive training in medically underserved communities • Percentage of trainees in Bureau of Health Workforce programs who are underrepresented minorities and/or from disadvantaged backgrounds
Goal 3: Build healthy communities	• Number of pregnant women and children served by the Maternal and Child Health Block Grant • Percentage of low birth weight births among Healthy Start program participants • Percentage of health centers providing: (a) oral health, (b) behavioral health, and (c) specific preventive health services • Percentage of donated kidneys used for transplantation

Mission-critical goals	Performance Measures Used to Review Performance and Progress
Goal 4: Improve health equity	• Percentage of (a) health centers and (b) Ryan White programs that have reduced disparities on specific clinical performance measures • Number of blood stem cell transplants facilitated for minority patients by the C.W. Bill Young Cell Transplantation Program
Goal 5: Strengthen HRSA program management and operations	• Percentage of HRSA products and services (for example, funding opportunity announcements (FOAs) correspondence, reports, audits, technical assistance) that meet established quality and timeliness benchmarks • Program customer satisfaction: Percentage of HRSA awardees reporting positively on key indicators • Employee satisfaction: Percentage of HRSA staff reporting positively on key indicators

Source: HRSA March 2016

Benefits of HIEs have been reported to include a reduction in costs related to duplicate tests and operational costs, an improvement of health outcomes and public health surveillance, and an improved linkage of health research and practice (AHRQ 2014). The growth in HIEs has been greater in private rather than in public entities. Predictions to the year 2024 include the continued growth in the privately funded HIEs, larger systems created when HIEs join together, easier implementation as time goes on, and data from the HIEs used more effectively (AHRQ 2014). Challenges continue to be the financial aspect of implementing and maintaining HIEs, workflow considerations, and reluctance of patients to participate due to confidentiality concerns.

Telehealth

Telehealth is a telecommunications system that links healthcare organizations and patients from diverse geographic locations and transmits text and images for (medical) consultation and treatment (AHIMA 2014, 144). **Telemedicine** is a similar term that refers specifically to the professional services provided to a patient through an interactive telecommunication system by a practitioner at a distant site (AHIMA 2014, 144). The use of telehealth to deliver health services is expanding due to technological advances and cost pressures for delivery of services to the patient, whether or not the service is reimbursed by a third-party payer. Examples of telehealth services include monitoring and reporting of vital signs and oxygen levels, teleradiology with results transmitted electronically to another site for diagnosis, videoconferencing with physicians and nurse practitioners, and online eye exams.

A 2016 HIMSS survey showed "continued confidence with a slight uptick in telemedicine solutions/services adoption from 57.7 percent in 2015 to 61.3 percent in 2016" (HIMSS 2016). Indications are that the future is positive for telemedicine with more of the study participants indicating an increase in investment for technology to be used for telemedicine applications and the growth in the number of vendors serving this market. The use of two-way communication with video and webcams between physicians and between physicians and patients is continuing to increase. A goal of organizations to maximize technology usage across departments and the entire enterprise also continues in an effort to meet needs by expanding services and access by patients consistent with changing alternative payment models (HIMSS 2016).

Mobile Health

Mobile health, referred to as **mHealth**, is a form of telehealth where wireless devices and phone technologies are used for the generation, aggregation, and dissemination of health information between patients and providers (HIMSS 2016). This form of telehealth includes apps that are "software programs that run on smartphones and other mobile communication devices. They can also be accessories that attach to a smartphone or other mobile communication devices, or a combination of accessories and software." (FDA 2016). Examples are wearables and sensors, devices for prescription monitoring, and those for engagement and communication. Among the top apps changing healthcare are mHealth apps for "seeing" a physician via video consultation, having prescriptions filled, finding specialists for very specific conditions, and maintaining PHRs, including recording daily metrics (blood pressure, oxygen levels, blood sugar readings, and so on) (*PC Magazine* 2015). Other mHealth apps include prescription services by mail with medications prepacked and dispensed as individual doses, services of a personal health coach for a variety of conditions, plus those used by clinicians in the provision of care. Mobile apps can be a useful tool but should be only a portion of coordinated care for the patient. Care should also be exercised in selecting applications because the use of most have not been validated with data, with little research done to date on their usefulness.

Examples on research outcomes when telemedicine has been used are:

⊙ Ability of rural health facilities to keep and treat rather than transfer pediatric patients

⊙ ED visits replaced with less costly telemedicine office visits with an increased number of visits reported

⊙ Reduced use of healthcare services and improved quality of care with remote monitoring of heart failure patients with implantable defibrillators (American Telemedicine Association 2015)

Case Study: Medication Compliance

Medication noncompliance is a problem that leads to many hospitalizations and readmissions of senior patients. These patients generally take more medications and have more complex medical conditions than others in addition to possible cognitive impairment and other issues facing this age group. A study compiled by the American Telemedicine Association found

- Nonadherence to medicine regime is a factor in about 1 of 10 patient hospital admissions. There can be many factors linked to admissions and readmissions but the medication mismanagement can contribute or exacerbate the patient's condition.
- Senior patients, 65 and over, face the most challenges in medication management.
- Compared to all age groups, seniors take both more prescription and more over-the-counter meds due a higher incidence of chronic conditions.
- More than 50 percent of seniors take at least three prescriptions and about one-third use eight or more medications including prescriptions, nonprescriptions, and/or supplements.
- Many in this age group have difficulty remembering to take their pills.

In this study, patients were divided into two groups. One group used a typical pillbox to sort the meds by the day and time they were to be taken. The patients in the other group were provided with an automatic dosage dispenser with a voice-activated message reminder. It was found that

- The group using the pillboxes missed 30 percent of their doses in a month, and
- The group with the dispenser with the voice-activated reminder had less than a 3 percent missed dosage rate for the same period of time (American Telemedicine Association 2015).

The medical status of patients who were noncompliant with less than 3 percent missed doses should remain more stable with less need for doctor visits and hospitalizations. Chronic conditions like diabetes or hypertension are common examples where medication noncompliance can lead to an exacerbation of the illness and complicate other conditions they are being treated for. Most patients prefer to remain in their home and without such an intervention to increase their compliance with taking their medications, they may have to secure home health services or move to a long-term care facility. Hospital admissions, move to long-term care, or home health are all costlier and against the desires of the individual in most instances.

e-Health

e-Health is a term that refers to the provisioning of healthcare using electronic commerce (Reynolds and Sharp 2016). e-Health encompasses treatment, teaching, research, and public health for healthcare companies and healthcare consumers (Eysenbach 2001). One facet of e-health is the use of the Internet to deliver health information that informs consumers and to provide portals that empower consumers to check their labs and make appointments. e-Health can be used to provide easily accessible educational modules as part of a public health series for health workers. e-Health also benefits healthcare businesses that advertise and sell their products using the Internet (WHO 2016).

e-Health for individual patients provides tools such as resources to learn about a diagnosis, portals to access physician office records and appointment scheduling and reminders. The e-health concept is now expanding more into the health of our communities, which will ultimately positively affect the health of individuals. Data are collected on health status and behaviors and on socioeconomic, environmental, biomedical, and genetic influences. It is also amassed on outcomes, use of resources, financial aspects of costs, and expenditures. This data are stored in a wide variety of databases to include EHRs, registries, and required surveillance and reporting locations. The distribution of clinical data is highly fragmented (NCBI 2010). The potential for e-health applications is significant with the ability to use this data.

Improved Continuity of Care and Increased Efficiency

The concepts of efficiency and continuity of care are not new but the capabilities when utilizing the advances in technology are immense. Coupled with new initiatives described below, the improvements can be transformational in terms of continuity of care and efficiency.

Care Coordination

Another concept conceived to improve healthcare in an efficient cost-effective manner is care coordination, which is "the organization of your treatment across several health care providers" (HealthIT 2016). Medical homes and accountable care organizations (ACOs) are two common ways to coordinate care, which are described in the following sections.

Medical Homes

A **medical home** is a "model or a philosophy of primary care that is patient-centered, comprehensive, team-based, coordinated, accessible, and focused on quality and safety" (PCPCC 2016). Patient-centered encompasses a partnership between the patient and their family and the care providers to assure their needs are addressed, can be involved in the decision making and participate in their care. The provider team is accountable for prevention and treatment of both acute and chronic conditions. The coordination of care refers to the whole healthcare system to include specialized care, services of hospitals, home health, available community services, and supporting services. Timely access to care with reasonable wait times and extended hours, continual access electronically or by phone, and using IT solutions to enhance good communication are all part of accessible care. The commitment to quality and safety rely on providers and staff actively engaged in quality improvement to assure that informed decision making is taking place (PCPCC 2016).

Accountable Care Organizations

A definition of an **accountable care organization (ACO)** is groups of doctors, hospitals, and other healthcare providers, who come together voluntarily to give coordinated high quality care to their Medicare patients with the goal of coordinated care to ensure that patients, especially the chronically ill, get the right care at the right time, while avoiding unnecessary duplication of services and preventing medical errors (CMS 2016a).

ACOs are a payment reform model responsible for not only providing care in instances of illness and injury but also offering the potential to improve quality and promote health and wellness while eliminating waste and improving efficiencies. To be able to do this, those involved with such an organization must have complete patient health information and truly understand the care and services they provide. Often this understanding can only be obtained with data collection and analysis supported by coordinated information technology initiatives. Interoperability and a seamless flow of information are key issues for the ACO to meet its objectives. One change that has been made based on ACO involvement is identifying a key member of the care team, usually a physician, to establish a trust relationship with the patient and to increase patient engagement in their care. Another example is the concerted effort to establish relationships for care coordination with organizations and individuals outside of the ACO who may provide services to the patient such as home health agencies and organizations for specific diseases such as American Cancer Society. When ACOs are functioning appropriately, there are increased funds in the Medicare Shared Savings Program due to decreased costs in the provision of care, decreased number of ED visits, and lower hospital readmission rates. These results indicate improved quality of care along with financial savings.

ACOs must demonstrate that they can provide high-quality care at a savings (CMS 2016a). To facilitate this goal, CMS has a new ACO model called the Next Generation Accountable Care Organization (NGACO). The goal of the NGACO model is to pair ACOs that have programs reflecting best practices that combine provisioning of quality care with cost reductions with ACOs that are seeking to achieve that goal (CMS 2016a).

Quality Improvement

Quality improvement (QI) includes the activities that measure the quality of a service or product through systems or process evaluation and then implements revised processes that result in better healthcare outcomes for patients, based on standards of care (AHIMA 2014, 124). Health records are a primary source document for the QI function to reflect the outcomes of care that have been provided in the organization. To date, the utilization of information technology for QI has been as a tool for problem identification, data collection, data analysis, as well as overall project management. A prevailing thought was that IT could also be used as a method of improvement in the management and use of information created to address an identified specific problem to improve care (Bates et al. 2011, 87–88). Many IT solutions are present today in QI processes such as alert devices, new practices of addressing medications through better use of the EHR, and better means of communication among providers. A process that is expected to be more widely used in the future is **predictive modeling,** which can help data analysts identify patterns in observed data that can help predict the odds of a particular outcome (AHIMA 2014, 117). A related area is **point-of-care testing (POCT)** where diagnostic tests are performed at or near where the patient care is taking place. POCT is done primarily for the convenience and support of the patient. However, it also improves the timeliness of test performance and results generation, which could result in higher quality care because data management systems that eliminate the need for manual data entry or required multientry of the same information (patient hospital number) have the potential to significantly improve the reliability of the data.

Patient-Centered Medical Home

A **patient-centered medical home (PCMH),** also referred to as medical home, is a program to provide comprehensive primary care that partners physicians with the patient and their family to allow better access to healthcare and improved outcomes (AHIMA 2014, 93). It provides a model of the organizational and delivery aspects of how primary care is provided. Five functions identified that are key components to a comprehensive program are listed here (AHRQ 2016):

- ⊙ **Comprehensive care:** Provision of physical and mental healthcare, involves a team of providers. Information is used to document the care provided and to serve as a communication tool among providers and caregivers
- ⊙ **Patient-centered:** Relationship based, orientation to whole person
- ⊙ **Coordinated care:** across entire healthcare system to include hospitals, specialty care, home care, community services
- ⊙ **Accessible services:** Easier accessibility for primary care (quicker appointments, more options for appointment times) and 24/7 access to team member either by phone or electronically
- ⊙ **Quality and safety:** Commitment to quality improvement with evidence-based medicine and clinical support tools to guide the shared decision making

Population Health

The definition of population health has continued to evolve over time. In recent years, a threefold purpose has emerged to include improving individual care, reducing the cost of care, and improving the health of populations. The initiatives supporting the population health are increasing due to the movement toward value-based care. Activities to support population health initiatives are limited due to the lack of vendor provided solutions. The CDC through the Division of Population Health has been charged with managing programs that provide cross-cutting, chronic disease, and health promotion expertise (CDC 2016). This group provides several engaging applications such as the Body and Mind and the Immune Platoon game that encourages exploration of the human body and mind, and the immune system, respectively. There are also food and nutrition, physical activity, and safety applications.

Central Authority Platform

More sophisticated clinical data methods are required to meet the information needs of an organization. A number of coding systems are used to capture data associated with different things. ICD-10-CM and ICD-10-PCS are clinical classification systems and organize data to facilitate retrieval but are not designed for data input or primary documentation. SNOMED CT and RxNorm are clinical terminology systems derived from health informatics and as input systems codify clinical information captured during the course of care. Both systems are used with neither one individually meeting the needs of all situations. Developing interfaces is an option but it is costly and complicated. Another option is implementing a **central authority platform (CAP),** which allows any or all of the classification and terminology coding systems to be used to capture and exchange clinical data (Kohn 2013). It is still a complex system that must have the capability of storing large amounts of data (coded data, metadata, and content). It must have the capability to normalize, catalog, track, and monitor among a host of other functions. There has been moderate success with developing CAPs, although limited to date. The Value Set Authority Center (VSAC) with the National Library of Medicine is the public domain for value sets to support meaningful use.

Preventive Care

The goal of preventive care "is to protect, promote, and maintain health and well-being and to prevent disease, disability and death" (ACPM 2016), whereas treatment involves all of the interventions that occur in response to a disease or condition. With the occurrence of disease there are the consequences to a person's health and well-being in addition to the higher costs associated with treatment as opposed to maintenance of good health. Consistent with the increased capabilities to use information in the provision of care, new initiatives are being introduced that support the focus on preventive care. Several of these are discussed here.

Precision Medicine

Precision medicine has to do with tailoring medical treatments to the individual characteristics of each patient through the ability to identify and classify subpopulations that differ in their susceptibility to a specific treatment (An and Vodovotz 2015). Analysis of big data, such as to seek means for an earlier diagnosis of a specific disease, will be fundamental to the precision medicine process to develop the means for prevention and detection and to maintain a healthy life. One result of this analysis is the detection of gene pattern activity that could lead to a blood test that will quickly and accurately detect the presence of sepsis (a deadly, systemic inflammation). A recent study on the predictors of death in adults age 57 to 85 found that the psychosocial well-being, frailty, and similar factors are better predictors of death rather than using standard measures such as having hypertension or diabetes (Okwerekwu 2016). The resources needed for this type of data analysis are available with the technology, means to do the data analysis, and the patient information but will require innovations.

Research on the IT approach and challenges of data integration of clinical and genomic data in precision medicine was conducted with individuals such as CMIOs, physicians, and biomedical and pathology directors. Twenty-nine percent responded that they were conducting precision medicine within their facility (HIMSS 2016).

Precision medicine is primarily done on-site at large medical centers because of funding, technology, and expertise. The focus of precision medicine has been on cancer although other conditions and diseases are included. The reasons for the high number of facilities focusing on cancer is that it is a genomic disease where learning about and understanding the genetic changes can lead to treatment. Precision medicine funding has been provided primarily to the National Cancer Institute (NCI) for the development of cancer treatment (HIMSS 2016).

Disease Management

Disease management (DM) "emphasizes the provider–patient relationship in the development and execution of the plan of care, prevention strategies using evidence-based guidelines to limit complications and exacerbations, and evaluation based on outcomes that support improved overall health" (AHIMA 2014, 49). Disease management has always been important but electronic health records and advanced means of data analysis have provided much information on which to base patient care decisions. Regional Extension Centers, evidence-based medicine and care coordination are examples of disease management.

Self-management is a means to disease management. Self-management involves providing the patient with education and tools to empower them to manage and improve their own condition and improve their quality of life. This is used primarily in cases of chronic conditions such as diabetes, hypertension, heart disease, cancer, arthritis, asthma, and lung diseases.

A program that has been successful in utilizing such a program and providing data analysis to reflect outcomes is the Stanford Chronic Disease Self-Management Program (CDSMP). The most impressive outcomes of the study are that there was "significant, measurable improvements in the health and quality of life of the adults with chronic conditions" with savings "enough through reductions in healthcare expenditures to pay for itself within the first year" (NCOA 2015).

Regional Extension Centers

The **Regional Extension Centers (RECs)** serve as a support and resource center to assist providers in EHR implementation and HealthIT needs. In an advisory capacity, the RECs "bridge the technology gap" by helping providers navigate the EHR adoption process from vendor selection and workflow analysis to implementation and meaningful use (HHS 2015). The **meaningful use** of information supports the expected outcome of an improvement in the quality of care provided, as well as promoting efficiencies in care delivery. The funding for the development of RECs came from the HITECH Act. REC activities include the enabling of HIE for patient-centered health IT, and patient engagement all while maintaining privacy and security. An example of a program developed that relies heavily on physicians utilizing technology to monitor patients is the Million Hearts Program. This is a national initiative with the goal to prevent one million heart attacks and strokes by 2017 (HHS 2016b). A key component of this initiative is that patient information from the physicians' offices is monitored with appropriate interventions to be taken when certain things are identified. These interventions can be improving patients' access to care, smoking cessation programs, cholesterol management, and promoting a healthy lifestyle and educational resources. The program started in 2012 and in 2016 it was reported by the CDC that approximately 1 in 3 American adults had high blood pressure, a leading cause of heart disease and stroke. A goal of the Million Hearts program is to maintain a control rates of or above the target of 70 percent or above (HHS 2016b).

Clinical Decision Support

The advances and utilization of technology in healthcare have provided many advantages including the ways to improve healthcare. One functionality that relies on the EHR is **clinical decision support (CDS),** which "provides persons involved in care processes with general and person-specific information, intelligently filtered and organized, at appropriate times, to enhance health and health care." Other advantages to CDS are the reduction in number of errors and diverse events (drug administration errors, wrong site surgery and other surgical injuries, patient falls), improved efficiency and costs in providing care, and better provider and patient satisfaction (HHS 2013).

Evidence-Based Medicine

Evidence-based medicine (EBM) is "the conscientious, explicit, judicious and reasonable use of modern, best evidence in making decisions about the care of individual patients" (NIH 2016a). The best evidence to support and aid in making medical care decisions is established by assimilating expertise by clinicians, patient values, and desires with clinically sound, relevant research.

Seamless Care

Although a specific definition of **seamless care** or **care coordination** is difficult to find, words used in an attempt to define it include consistent, coherent, logical, without discontinuities or disparities, and of uniform quality (Hammond 2010, 3–13). One common thought emerging in most discussions of health informatics systems to support seamless care is that much of the information needed is the same data required in direct patient care. The redesign of systems is necessary to make systems more patient-centric where all health data about a patient is aggregated to form a single EHR for the individual patient. Systems for maintaining patient information, even when EHR systems are utilized, many times fail to support continuity of care due to multiple providers, lack of interoperability between systems, lack of standards for systems, and lack of standardized definitions and terminologies. These are issues that are directly related to the lack of optimal utilization of health informatics including the lack of multiple providers, interoperability, and standards. CMS Innovation Center's Comprehensive End Stage Renal Disease (ESRD) Care Model exemplifies seamless care in the current healthcare environment. The participants are referred to as ESRD Seamless Care Organizations (ESCOs). The high cost of treating ESRD patients due primarily to the underlying complications and comorbidities is the primary focus of the program. There are 600,000 patients in the United States receiving regular dialysis treatments with 6.3 percent of Medicare spending of over \$30.0 billion for ESRD patients (CMS 2016b). This model provides an example of how care coordination can improve care and help control costs of care by:

- Implementing continuous data-driven learning
- Improving quality of life and functional status
- Coordinating clinical practices for efficiency and improved quality care
- Standardizing performance metrics and benchmark measures
- Minimizing unnecessary ED visits
- Enhancing and coordinating patient-centered care
- Improving beneficiary access to services
- Reducing dialysis-related complications
- Promoting freedom to seek services and providers of choice (CMS 2016b)

Check Your Understanding 16.1

Answer the following questions.

1. Which of the following is a historical copy saved at a specific point in time?
   a. Back-up copy
   b. The cloud
   c. Archival copy
   d. Master data

2. What is e-health?
   a. A patient portal for patients to access their information.
   b. The relationship of internet and technology to the provision of care.
   c. A term that is synonymous with the EHR
   d. An exchange of data from one provider to another

3. Which one of the following is an example of POCT?
   a. A patient taken to the x-ray department with the report then available in the EHR system.
   b. Previous x-ray reports from other facilities are sent to the hospital to be scanned and are available in the patient's record.
   c. Portable x-ray equipment is taken to the patient's room where the x-ray is taken, with a report later available in the patient's EHR.
   d. A patient is referred to an outpatient radiology center to have an x-ray done at their convenience.

4. Which of the following is the organization created to support physicians with their implementation of the EHR?
   a. Regional extension centers
   b. Accountable care organizations
   c. Health information exchanges
   d. Medicare Shared Savings Programs

5. Accountable care organizations:
   a. Support healthcare reform and implementation of the EHR
   b. Offer care that is consistent and of uniform quality
   c. Are a group providing care at the instance of illness and injury
   d. Are a group of providers with the responsibility for improving health status, efficiencies of care, and experiences for a defined population

6. The process for bringing together and summarizing large amounts of data from multiple sources is:
   a. Data consolidation
   b. Purging
   c. Data manipulation
   d. Developing a data dictionary

7. Tailoring treatment to the medical characteristics of the individual patient is:
   a. Patient-centered medical home
   b. Population health
   c. Precision medicine
   d. Preventive care

8. The challenge for storing genetic data is due to:
   a. No systems available for this purpose
   b. The difficulty in understanding the information
   c. The amount of data generated
   d. The subjective nature of the information

9. Which of the following is HIEs role in public health?
   a. To provide guidance in the user of the information
   b. To process requests for information
   c. There is no role
   d. Oversight of the information

10. What is the difference between telehealth and telemedicine?
    a. Telehealth is more related to the system and telemedicine refers more to the services provided
    b. Telehealth and telemedicine are used interchangeably
    c. Telehealth is related to preventive care and telemedicine has to do with treatment of disease
    d. The services provided are different between telehealth and telemedicine

⊙ Health Informatics Workforce

The field of healthcare informatics continues to progress with the development of new technologies, as new uses for healthcare data are identified and with changing regulations. "The demand for health informatics workers is projected to grow at twice the rate of employment overall, but there is strong evidence that the nation already faces a shortage of qualified workers in this field" (Burning Glass 2014, 1). Educational requirements and workforce aspects will be addressed.

Education

Formal education in health informatics has been available for a number of years either as degree programs or courses within other programs. These programs, especially at the master's degree–level have proliferated over the past few years to coincide with the increased use of the EHR and recognized value of the data now available. The curriculum varies among the programs and continues to change with the continued evolution of the field. Although the definitions of biomedical, clinical, nursing, and healthcare informatics, among others, continue to be debated, commonly accepted definitions of the terms are provided here. Biomedical is related to both biology and medicine (Oxford 2016). A clinical nurse specialist is a licensed registered nurse with graduate preparation at the master's or doctoral level and have expert clinical knowledge and skills in a specialized area of nursing practice (NACS 2016). Healthcare or medical informatics is defined as an interdisciplinary study of the development and application of information technology in the planning, delivery, management and of healthcare services. (HIMSS 2016). What the field should become is of more significance with program curriculum development activities conducted to meet the current demands to develop an informatics workforce as well as the needs of the future.

Educational Programs

The field of health informatics is broad. There are a number of different subject matter areas and different job positions have been created to do the work of informatics. Biomedical and health informatics has been purported to be "the most comprehensive term for all fields concerned with the optimal use of information, often aided by the use of technology to improve individual health, healthcare, public health, and biomedical research" (Hersh 2009, 99). Studies have been conducted to compare the curriculums of a variety of programs across the United States and to compare courses within these curricula.

One extensive study was conducted at the University of North Carolina. The study included a review of courses in a variety of programs and a comparison of programs in public health, nursing, health, medical, and biomedical informatics (Kampov-Polevoi and Hemminger 2011, 195–202). This study was successful at identifying common courses or content areas across the domains of biomedical and health informatics. The more common content areas seen across most all of the programs identified as some kind of informatics program include the computer science core, and courses related to statistics and research methods, management, and topics covering the legal, ethical, and social issues that reflect the interaction of informatics with society (Kampov-Polevoi and Hemminger 2011, 195–202).

A recent review was made of the websites of current health informatics degree programs throughout the United States. The focus and the curricula of these programs continues to be varied. The majority of the degree programs reviewed were at the master's level with program names such as Health Informatics, Health Information and Informatics, Medical Informatics, Bioinformatics, and Nursing Informatics. All of these programs were found to be fairly consistent with the more common content areas noted above, but there were unique differences that provided identity and focus to each individual program. The focus areas that distinguished one program from another are combining aspects of health information with health informatics, applications and use of technology, research focus, incorporation of biomedical informatics courses with medical school courses, policy development, incorporation of engineering with the study of biomedical informatics, and advanced practice for nursing leadership.

Commission on Accreditation for Health Informatics and Information Management Education (CAHIIM) is an accrediting organization whose mission is to serve the public interests by establishing and enforcing quality accreditation standards for health informatics and information management educational programs (CAHIIM 2016). They are the accrediting body for Health Information Management associate's, bachelor's, and master's degree programs, which provide the pathway for eligibility for the RHIT and RHIA certifications. One of the six domains in the curriculum requirements for these programs is Informatics, Analytics, and Data Use (Domain III).

CAHIIM also accredits health informatics programs at the master's degree level. As published by CAHIIM, health informatics (HI) graduate programs focus on information systems, informatics principles, and information technology as applied to the continuum of healthcare delivery. Individual programs offer options for areas of practice or research (CAHIIM 2016).

There are a number of healthcare informatics degree programs in the United States that have been developed independent of the CAHIIM accreditation guidelines. These programs tend to be developed to meet a specific need in the workforce or to meet the interests and expertise of the faculty. The majority of these degree programs are at the master's and doctoral level in biomedical or clinical informatics. In addition to meeting a particular workforce need, other critical goals of these educational programs are to promote research in the healthcare informatics domain to validate the profession and define the body of knowledge, develop best practices, and find new applications in healthcare for the potential outcomes related to the intersection of information and technology.

Certificate programs are short-term, non-degree programs and are typically over a narrow subject area. They can provide new opportunities for employment and are usually developed to meet a specific need in the workforce. There are certificate programs designed to address assorted aspects of health informatics. Some of these are offered by colleges and universities in addition to their degree programs and some are offered by professional associations. Others were developed with funding from the ONC for workforce development. Certifications may be earned by taking an examination by an accrediting or approval agency.

The American Health Information Management Association (AHIMA) offers of a number of credentialing examinations with three that are consistent with the health informatics domains. The Certified Healthcare Technology Specialist (CHTS) credentialing exam is associated with various roles related to the implementation and management of EHR systems. The Certified Health Data Analyst (CHDA) credential supports better use of information. Another certification is the Certified Professional in Health Informatics (CPHI) to recognize the knowledge to be able to provide support for and the ability to utilize health informatics (AHIMA 2016b).

There are other organizations that offer opportunities for certification. The American Medical Informatics Association (AMIA) approved the Advanced Health Informatics Certification (AHIC) in 2016 with the exam to be available within two years. The American Society of Health Informatics Managers offers an exam to earn the Certified Health Informatics Systems Professional (CHISP) credential. The certification exam offered by Health Information and Management Systems Society (HIMSS) is to earn the credential, Certified Professional in Health Information and Management Systems (CPHIMS).

Demand

Reports such as the one mentioned previously indicate a tremendous need for health informatics workers. It is sometimes difficult to determine what the positions are because they can range from data analysts to chief information officers (CIOs) or informatics researchers. The adoption of the EHR and the increased reliance on data and data analytics are given as primary reasons for the high demand for workers with positions at all levels with differences in the required knowledge, skills, and experience. Specific statements regarding the openings are as follows: More than 50,000 health informatics openings are projected from now through 2020–2022. Demand is expected to increase at twice the rate of all healthcare jobs overall along with the fact that there is already a shortage of health informatics workers (Burning Glass 2014). One challenge in filling informatics jobs is that they tend to remain open longer than other types of jobs, indicating the difficulty in filling these positions. One reason it takes so long to fill the positions is that health informatics positions require more varied skill sets in order for the informatics employees to have the ability to remain current with the continued evolution of regulations and the varied needs of big data processing such as increased utilization of the information. Some positions can be considered hybrid requiring skills in more than one discipline that is health information management (HIM) and computer technology or nursing and data analysis. A review of job postings reveals a great deal of diversity in the positions that may be available based on job title. For example, a brief list of some of these may include:

- Business Intelligence Analyst
- CHIO, Physician
- Clinical Information Liaison
- Clinical Information Specialist
- Coding Validator
- Data Analyst
- Data Visualization Specialist
- Health Informatics Director
- Health Informatics Faculty
- Health Informatics Scientist
- Health Information Solutions Coordinator
- Health Information Technician
- Health Informatics Project Manager
- Project Analyst
- Public Health Scientist
- Research Analyst
- Senior Consultant, Population Health
- Senior Research Analyst
- Systems Support
- Systems Support Trainer

Positions and Skills Needed

The diversity of the kinds of health informatics positions results in the possibility that different knowledge and skills are needed for individual jobs. Table 16.2 presents a list of identified informatics-related positions from the AHIMA Career Map (AHIMA CareerMap 2016a). The Career Map illustrates positions by level and is an interactive site where career transition and promotion opportunities can be explored. The AHIMA Career Map site provides additional information about each of the positions listed there to include a description of the job, and the responsibilities and skills required. See table 16.2 for a listing of the positions illustrated at Career Map in the section on Informatics and Data Analysis and the specific skills required for each of these positions. In addition to these job specific skills, a number of skills emerged as important for each of the jobs. These general skills for the informatics/data analysis jobs are: working knowledge of Microsoft

Table 16.2. Informatics and data analysis potential job titles with associated skills required

Position	Specific Skills Required for Position
Chief Clinical Informatics Officer Medical Informatics Officer Related Jobs: Professor Consultant	• Managerial • Technical and professional skills of systems/procedure analysis • Programming and hardware capabilities • Strong skills in performance management, quality and data analytics • Knowledge of EMR Applications Systems • High level of problem-solving skills • Ability to work and communicate effectively with all levels of management, both inside and outside the Information Management division • Experience and judgment to plan and accomplish goals • Ability to work in a dynamic environment
Director of Clinical Informatics Director of Medical Informatics Related jobs: Program Director Consultant	• Organizational skills at the director level • Leadership skills with good clinical, physician, and executive communication • Clinical experience • Formal or informal leader within the facility • Listens carefully to respond appropriately, answer questions, or obtain needed information • Demonstrates flexibility in adjusting to the fluctuating needs • Manages the time and availability of personnel and other resources effectively • Proven experience in troubleshooting and problem solving in a demanding management environment • Thorough working knowledge of the facility processes and personnel.

(Continued)

Table 16.2. Informatics and data analysis potential job titles with associated skills required (*Continued*)

Position	Specific Skills Required for Position
Research and Development Specialist Clinical Research Informatics, Lead Analyst Related Jobs: Chief Learning Officer Professor Program Director	• Experience and knowledge in health IT
Project Manager Related Jobs: Director of Clinical Informatics Business Analyst	• Strong presentation skills • Experience in MMIS or other healthcare claims system(s) IT projects preferred • Skills/experience with Medicaid or Healthcare Delivery Systems preferred • Experience working with SharePoint and other typical project management tools, including Visio, PowerPoint, Word, Access, and Excel
Mapping Specialist Point-of-Care Mapping Specialist Related Jobs: Coding Trainer Coding Manager Consultant Director of Clinical Informatics	• Understand and apply rule-based mapping guidance • Follow established data mapping principles and published best practices • Possess knowledge and/or experience in the source and target systems involved in the map • Demonstrates diversified coding and data management experience with clinical terminologies • Have knowledge of current global healthcare informatics—standards • Mastery of medical terminology and medical science principles • Broad understanding and experience with healthcare vocabularies including the World Health Organizations Family of Classifications • Health informatics training or equivalent experience required • Clinical information system experience desirable • Ability to acquire knowledge and skill in information retrieval for map development and use of mapping tools • Ability to meet required delivery dates
Data Integrity Analyst Data Integrity Officer Related Jobs: Consultant Data Quality Manager	• Must have the ability to analyze healthcare data from conceptualization through presentation of the data • Proficiency with analytical tools (Crystal Reports, Excel) • Knowledge of data analysis methodology • Use of presentation software • Strong communication skills

Position	Specific Skills Required for Position
Informaticist Researcher Applied Health Informatics Researcher Related Jobs: Clinical Informatics Coordinator	• Clear understanding of research design and how to develop accurate and correct questions for surveys and research projects • Ability to work in a team environment and with those familiar with research and those not as familiar is essential • Excellent computer skills and knowledge of databases and software programs available for research is very important • Understanding of medical procedures is critical for designing effective research projects • Knowledge of hospital, state, and federal regulations regarding medical procedures and policies as well as data collection and confidentiality is a must for an informatics researcher
Clinical Informatics Coordinator Clinical Information Systems Coordinator Related Jobs: Director of Clinical Informatics Informaticist Researcher	• Working knowledge of computers and computer systems as well as having hand-on experience working in a clinical setting • Experience working with various groups • Patience to teach computer skills to a wide variety of individuals • Experience with advanced clinical software systems, databases, and other computer software programs developed for hospital or healthcare facilities • Additional training in computer skills and information technology is strongly encouraged
Data Analyst Data Informatics Analyst Related Jobs: Informaticist Researcher Data Integrity Analyst	• ICD mapping • Knowledge of CPT
Content Analyst Related Jobs: Informaticist Researcher Data Architect	• Negotiation • Persuasion • Evaluating requirements to determine impact to resources, schedules, tools, and process

Source: AHIMA Health Information Careers, Career Map 2016a

Suite, detail orientation, independent, excellent interpersonal oral and written communication skills, ability to multitask, problem solver and troubleshooter, critical thinking skills, time management, ability to function in a leadership role, organizational skills, ability to interact with professionals at all levels, and diplomacy and tact.

Check Your Understanding 16.2

Indicate whether each of the following is true or false.

1. All health informatics jobs require a degree in informatics.

2. One reason that healthcare informatics jobs remain open longer than many other posted jobs is the varied skill set that might be required for the job.

3. General skills required across most health informatics positions include a working knowledge of ICD-10 coding, the EHR, and clinical expertise.

4. The AHIMA Career Map can be used to obtain information on some of the emerging positions with required job skills and advancement opportunities.

⊙ Genomics

Genomics is "a branch of biotechnology concerned with the genetic mapping and DNA sequencing of sets of genes or the complete genomes of selected organisms" (Merriam-Webster 2013). Advanced technology high-speed methods are used to organize the results in databases. The data can then be used to support medical and biological studies and developments. A **genome** is all the genetic information present in a given organism. One can readily surmise from these definitions that the foundations of health informatics and genomics are closely related when taking into consideration the definition of health informatics. Health informatics is "the interdisciplinary study of the design, development, adoption, and application of IT-based innovations in healthcare services delivery, management and planning" (Procter 2009).

Genomic Information

Genomics seeks to determine the entire DNA sequence of organisms. Initially genomic studies were done for sequencing and mapping of the genes and storing the data to learn more about the roles and functions of individual genes. Today, new studies for genomics include learning the pattern of genes under certain conditions. This is known as **functional genomics.** A discussion of health informatics and genomics would not be complete without including information on the Human Genome Project, a 13-year project coordinated by the US Department of Energy and the National Institutes of Health that was completed in 2003. Although coordinated by the Human Genome Project, a major partner was the Wellcome Trust (United Kingdom) with contributions from the countries of Japan, France, Germany, China, and others. The goals of the Human Genome Project were to

- ⊙ "Identify all of the approximately 20,500 genes in human DNA
- ⊙ Determine the sequences of the 3 billion chemical base pairs that make up human DNA
- ⊙ Store this information in databases

- ◉ Improve tools for data analysis
- ◉ Transfer related technologies to the private sector, and
- ◉ Address the ethical, legal, and social issues that may arise from the project" (US Department of Energy Genome Programs 2012)

The initial stages related to the goals listed are finished. The data that have been gathered during the course of the project will continue to be analyzed over time. The outcomes and benefits will continue to be realized for many years and in many forms. Involving the private sector with technology licensing and the availability of grant funding made available for research projects has already been initiated. Much of the current biotechnology industry developments and new medical applications have been a result of the outcomes of the study.

Use of Genomic Information

The possibilities for genomics are still just being realized, but findings in the area of molecular medicine reveal that the outcomes could include improved means of diagnosing conditions, learning an individual genetic predisposition for certain conditions, and pharmacogenomics, or personalized medicine, which is the ability to customize drugs based on the genetic makeup of the individual. The primary disadvantages related to genetic information are the misuse of the information and misunderstanding of what the tests do and do not mean. Misuse of the data could constitute discrimination based on a potential medical condition, or inability to get insurance due to a genetic predisposition. Misuse or simple misunderstanding could be a potential parent attempting to use genetic information to determine characteristics their children will inherit. Other misunderstandings can occur when consumers do not understand the interaction between genes. For example, a woman with breast cancer in her family may be genetically tested for breast cancer, while overlooking other types of cancers.

At the time of completion of the Human Genome Project, it was projected that having the information provided by the project would facilitate new discoveries for the next century or more. The following are several examples of how the human genome sequence data are being used:

- ◉ Identification of a signature in tumors of DNA that occurs in five different cancers. It is anticipated that this will spur the development of a blood test for detecting these cancers at an early stage.
- ◉ Identification of a genetic mutation responsible for a rare form of inherited hives induced by vibration (running, clapping, towel drying).
- ◉ An international team of scientists from the 1000 Genomes Project Consortium has created the world's largest catalog of genomic differences among humans, providing researchers with powerful clues to help them establish why some people are susceptible to various diseases.
- ◉ Sequencing and analyzing genomes of healthy individuals to find assumed mutations that would potentially predispose a genetic condition.

⊙ Identification of a key to regulating the immune system is related to the genomic switches of a blood cell.

⊙ Discovery of genomic differences of human papillomavirus (HPV) related head and neck cancers.

⊙ Identification of a genomic signature or biomarker, common in five or more kinds of cancer, which can lead to means of early detection (NIH 2016b).

What might the future hold for health genomics as data analysis and technological advances continue? The postgenomics era (referring to the time following the completion of the Human Genome Project) went from interest for biologists to interest for clinicians as they try to develop new treatments. The biologists study one gene at a time, monogenic diseases, tedious genotyping, the DNA level, focus on sequences and structures. They are interested in decoding the genomes and characteristics or diseases resulting from the different combinations as a separate topic. The clinical interest, involving studying hundreds or thousands of genes simultaneously, complex diseases, high throughput genetic profiling (DNA arrays), DNA, RNA, and proteins, focuses on functional and comparative studies where health informatics includes the clinical plus genetic aspects (Martin-Sanchez et al. 2002, 25–30).

Clinicians are dealing with the issues of the difficulty of being able to quickly evaluate the benefits and potential harm of the rapidly growing genetic tests and family health history tools and the need for data to determine baselines and to track progress. However, along with these issues, there are opportunities for the future in genomics to include:

⊙ "Creating and evaluating scientific evidence to support valid and useful genetic tests and family health history tools

⊙ Developing evidence-based practice recommendations that evaluate the net health benefit of the genetic tests and family health history tools

⊙ Conducting research on how to translate recommendations into practice

⊙ Facilitating the use of valid and useful tests and family health history tools to guide clinical practice, policy and national, state, and local programs to find people who are at risk for disease, make diagnoses and provide interventions

⊙ Monitoring use of genetic tests and family health history in populations, the health outcomes related to their use, and disparities of use and outcomes

⊙ Adding genomic information and clinical decision support tools to electronic health records

⊙ Incorporating health-related genomics to education in primary, secondary, undergraduate, and graduate curricula

⊙ Assuring the privacy and confidentiality of genomic information" (ODPHP 2016)

Now, more than 25 years after the initiation of the Human Genome Project, more than 1,800 disease genes have been discovered, suspected genes of inherited diseases can now be found in days instead of years, there are more than 2,000 genetic tests for conditions to inform patients of genetic risks and to help clinicians with diagnosing disease, and there are more than 350 biotech products in clinical trials (NIH 2015a). Currently being done and foreseen for the future are the creation of targeted interventions for disease, the development of more effective medications, reducing costs of the genetic testing, and focusing on prevention of disease.

Privacy

The issue of the confidential nature of the genetic information in general was addressed with the passage of the **Genetic Information and Nondiscrimination Act (GINA)** in 2008. GINA prohibits employers and health plans from requesting or requiring genomic information or discriminating based on genetic information. In 2013, the HIPAA Privacy Rule was amended to reflect that genetic information is health information and is protected if individually identifiable. All aspects of developing, maintaining, and utilizing health information systems must consider genetic information that may be included in a patient's health record. Policies and procedures and system functionality must assure that this information is protected consistent with GINA and HIPAA.

Genomic data are utilized for clinical care purposes, research, and other uses that are protected by laws and policies. The nature of the genomic data raises the question of the need for additional protections for this data. Selected issues regarding this data are:

- DNA sequence is unique to each individual, except for identical twins, so a DNA sequence cannot be truly anonymized.

- Samples acquired for testing (blood spots of newborns and surgical specimens such as blood and tissue) create concern especially with parents of newborns.

- Populations who can be identified by geographic location, ethnicity, or linguistically, which is common in research studies, have a diminished degree of privacy because of this identification.

- Genetic testing is becoming much more common, almost routine in many settings especially where research is being conducted. This additional information captured on a patient adds a degree of risk for the patient and heightens the possibility for misuse of the data.

- The concern for DNA databases that are routinely maintained on select populations, a common occurrence in law enforcement. Two such databases are CODIS (Combined DNA Index systems), used by the FBI, and NDIS (National DNA Index System), which is created with profiles provided by forensic labs at the local, state, and national levels. Although this information in solving crimes is important, the concern exists for who should be included, how maintained, when to destroy, and maintenance/destructions of the DNA samples themselves. A 5–4 decision of the US Supreme Court ruled that law enforcement may collect samples from suspects who have been arrested for a crime (NIH 2015b).

Figure 16.1.   Federal regulations that protect genetic test information

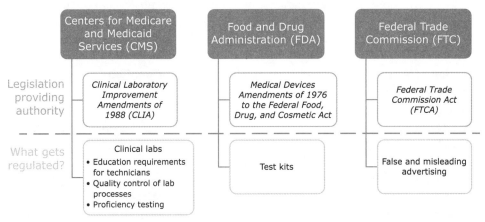

Source: NIH 2016

Ethical Concerns

Ethical issues must be considered with the data generated through health informatics applications. These considerations include the areas of autonomy, beneficence, nonmaleficence, and justice. Genetic information includes data, much more than is generated for the typical provision of care. Genetic testing can be done for diagnostics, to determine the risks for certain diseases and hereditary factors, pharmacogenic testing in drug selection to assess the compatibility between the individual and the drug, prenatal testing for the presence of diseases, and genetic research on the genes' relationship to both health and disease. There are portions of existing regulations for the protection of PHI that protect data generated with genetic testing. These are shown in figure 16.1 and are related to the laboratory testing, test kits, and issues with advertising.

The nature of some genetic information possibly could lead to discrimination by employers or healthcare payers. GINA specifically protects individuals from genetic discrimination in health insurance and employment. The use of human subjects and their information in genetic testing must be protected. There are also social, cultural, and religious influences on the testing and use of the information.

⊙ Cybersecurity

The greatest incidence of breaches of protected health information in 2015 was from hacking (Snell 2016a). For the first part of 2016, the Office for Civil Rights (OCR) data breach reporting tool indicates that the largest events were due to theft, loss, improper disposal, and unauthorized e-mail access or disclosure (Snell 2016a). From June through August 2016, the majority of reported incidents were due to unauthorized access or disclosure, and hacking incidents were a close second with the five largest reported cases of a potential healthcare data breach in these categories (Snell 2016a). The incidents were reported to be from cybersecurity attacks, which includes hacking, or as cases of unauthorized access or disclosure (Snell 2016b). Cybersecurity is "the state of being protected against the criminal or unauthorized use of electronic data, or the measures taken to achieve this" (Cybersecurity 2016).

With health information access, specifically to the EHR system and anywhere else the protected health information is contained, cybersecurity is critical. An executive order was issued in 2013 by President Barack Obama that called for the development of a cybersecurity framework to reduce and manage cybersecurity risks (HealthIT 2016). A number of groups are actively involved in cybersecurity initiatives. NIST developed a Framework for Improving Critical Infrastructure Cybersecurity in support of providing a more secure infrastructure using a set of activities to achieving specific cybersecurity outcomes (NIST 2016). The ONC has been involved with funding initiatives and continues to develop educational resources for healthcare cybersecurity and risk management among other activities (ONC 2016). The ONC recommends for organizations to have an appropriate protection plan in place. The 10 suggestions in this plan are:

- Establish a security culture
- Protect mobile devices
- Maintain good computer habits
- Use a firewall
- Install and maintain antivirus software
- Plan for the unexpected
- Control access to protected health information
- Use strong passwords and change them regularly
- Limit network access
- Control physical access (HealthIT 2016)

These are standard operating procedures that most are familiar with but are the basic requirements for protection from cybersecurity attacks. As a first step, top management must create a culture that supports a secure workplace. They must establish policies and procedures for accessing, analyzing, modifying, storing, transmitting, and sharing data. Today's workplace is collaborative and the workers are mobile. Workers may access data from home or while on travel. They may use their work computers or a personal device such as mobile application on a cell phone. Similarly, data may be entered into business systems from unsecured personal devices or software on the users' personal computer. Failing to establish best practices for protecting PHI is an invitation to hackers. The following are best practices for protecting PHI:

- Ensure mobile devices are equipped with strong authentication and access controls.
  - Ensure laptops have password protection.
  - Enable password protection on handheld devices (if available). Take extra physical control precautions over the device if password protection is not provided.

- Protect wireless transmissions from intrusion.
- Do not transmit unencrypted Protected Health Information (PHI) across public networks (internet, wi-fi).
- Where it is absolutely necessary to commit PHI to a mobile device or remove a device from a secure area, encrypt the data.
- Do not use mobile devices that cannot support encryption.
- Develop and enforce policies specifying the circumstances under which devices may be removed from the facility.
- Take extra care to prevent unauthorized viewing of the PHI displayed on a mobile device (HHS 2010a, 41).
- Use an anti-virus product that provides continuously updated protection against viruses, malware, and other code that can attack computers through web downloads, CDs, email, and flash drives.
- Keep anti-virus software up to date. Most anti-virus software automatically generates reminders about these updates, and many are configurable to allow for automated updating (HHS 2010b, 27)

Chapter 16 Review Exercises

Answer the following questions.

1. Which of the following is all the genetic information present in an organism?
   a. Genomics
   b. Genome
   c. Genetics
   d. Functional genomics

2. What began with the identification of the human genes and led to the development of tools for data analysis?
   a. Genome
   b. Genetics
   c. Human Genome Project
   d. Genomic informatics

3. Which of the following is the postgenomics era?
   a. The time following completion of the Human Genome Project.
   b. The time after a genetic sequence has been determined for an individual.
   c. The time when the EHR system can capture genetic information.
   d. Once a treatment has been developed for a genetically discovered condition.

4. Which is a historical copy of data saved in another country?
   a. Backup
   b. Archival database
   c. Offshore data storage
   d. The cloud

5. Which is an accrediting organization that would access compliance with accreditation standards for a master's of health informatics program?
   a. AHIMA
   b. CAHIIM
   c. HIMSS
   d. AMIA

6. Which federal regulation protects PHI from genetic test kits?
   a. Clinical Lab Improvement Amendments of 1988
   b. Medical Device Amendments of 1976
   c. Federal Trade Commission Act
   d. Genetic Information Nondiscrimination Act

7. Which nationally recognized organization develop a framework for cybersecurity infrastructure?
   a. FDA
   b. FTC
   c. NIST
   d. AHIMA

8. Which of the following is the state of being protected against the criminal and unauthorized use of data?
   a. HIPAA enforcement
   b. Exempt
   c. Cybersecurity
   d. Information Management

9. The confidential nature of genetic information was addressed in all aspects in:
   a. State Privacy laws
   b. GINA
   c. HIPAA
   d. Professional association guidelines

10. Health informatics certificate programs:
    a. Are usually a part of a degree program
    b. Tend to have a narrow, focused area of content
    c. Required for employment
    d. Recognized for comprehensive knowledge of health information

REFERENCES

45 CFR.164, Security and Privacy.

AHIMA. 2016a. Health Information Careers, Career Map. http://www.hicareers.com /CareerMap/.

AHIMA. 2016b. Types of Certifications, Specialty. http://www.ahima.org/certification /exams?tabid=specialty.

AHIMA. 2014. *Pocket Glossary for Health Information Management and Technology.* 4th ed. Chicago, IL: AHIMA Press.

AHRQ. 2016. Defining the PCMH. AHRQ Patient Centered Medical Home Resource Center. https://pcmh.ahrq.gov/.

AHRQ. 2014. AHRQ Health Care Innovation Exchange. Trends in Health Information Exchanges. https://innovations.ahrq.gov/perspectives/trends-health-information -exchanges.

Alzu'bi, A., L. Zhou, and V. Watzlaf. 2014. Personal genomic information management and personalized medicine: Challenges, current solutions, and roles of HIM professionals. *Perspectives in Health Information Management* 11(Spring):1–22.

American Cancer Society (ACS). 2014. Cancer Surveillance Programs in the United States. http://www.cancer.org/cancer/cancerbasics/cancer-surveillance-programs -and-registries-in-the-united-states.

American College of Preventive Medicine. 2016. ACPM.org.

American Telemedicine Association. 2015. Increasing medication compliance in high risk patients by utilizing electronic medication dispensers. http://www.american telemedicine.org.

An, G., and Y. Vodovotz. 2015. What is "Precision Medicine"—and can it work? Elsevier Connect. https://www.elsevier.com/connect/what-is-precision-medicine-and-can-it -work.

Bates D., D. Classen, K. Joynt, J. Lanning, and L. Van Horn. 2011. IT: More than a tool for quality improvement. *Hospital Peer Review* 36(8):87–88.

Burning Glass Careers in Focus. 2014. *Health Informatics 2014: Missed Opportunities? The Labor Market in Health Informatics, 2014.* Burning Glass Technologies 2014 Report. http://burning-glass.com/research/health-informatics-2014/.

Centers for Disease Control and Prevention. 2016. Health care provider/clinician apps. http://www.cdc.gov/mobile/healthcareproviderapps.html.

Center for Medicare and Medicaid Services (CMS). 2016a. Next Generation Accountable Care Organization Model (NGACO Model). https://www.cms.gov/Newsroom /MediaReleaseDatabase/Fact-sheets/2016-Fact-sheets-items/2016-01-11.html.

Center for Medicare and Medicaid Services (CMS)/ 2016b. Comprehensive ESRD Care Model: RFA Fact Sheet. CMS. https://innovation.cms.gov/Files/fact-sheet/cec-py2.pdf.

Commission on the Accreditation of Health Informatics and Information Management Education. 2016. Health Informatics. http://cahiim.org/hi/hi.html.

Cybersecurity. 2016. Oxford English Dictionary Online. Oxford University Press. https://en.oxforddictionaries.com/definition/cybersecurity.

Department of Health and Human Services. 2016a. Health Resources and Services Administration. Strategic Plan 2016–2018. http://www.hrsa.gov/about /strategicplan/index.html.

Department of Health and Human Services. 2016b. About Million Hearts®. http:// millionhearts.hhs.gov/about-million-hearts/index.html.

Department of Health and Human Services. 2013. www.health.it.gov.

Department of Health and Human Services 2010a (Nov. 22). Basic Security for the Small Healthcare Practice. HealthIT Mobile Device Checklist) https://www.healthit.gov /sites/default/files/basic-security-for-the-small-healthcare-practice-checklists.pdf.

Department of Health and Human Services 2010b (Nov. 22). Basic Security for the Small Healthcare Practice. HealthIT Mobile Device Checklist) https://www.healthit.gov /sites/default/files/basic-security-for-the-small-healthcare-practice-checklists.pdf. Eysenbach, G. 2001. What is e-health? *Journal of Medical Internet Research* 3(2).

FDA. 2016. Mobile medical applications. http://www.fda.gov/MedicalDevices/Digital Health/MobileMedicalApplications/default.htm.

Genetic Science Learning Center. 2014. How we study the microbiome. http://learn .genetics.utah.edu/content/microbiome/study/.

Gilpin, Lyndsey. 2014. 10 Technologies changing the future of healthcare. TechRepublic. http://www.techrepublic.com/article/10-technologies-changing-the-future-of -healthcare/.

Hammond, W. 2010. Seamless care: What is it, what is its value; what does it require; when might we get it? In *Seamless Care-Safe Care*. Edited by B. Blobel, E.P. Hvannberg, and V. Gunnarsdottir. Amsterdam, Netherlands: IOS Press. doi:10.3233/978-1-60750-563-1-3.

Health IT. 2016. Privacy and Security. Cybersecurity: A shared responsibility. https:// www.healthit.gov/providers-professionals/cybersecurity-shared-responsibility.

Health IT. 2015. Benefits of Electronic Health Records (EHRs). https://www.healthit .gov/providers-professionals/benefits-electronic-health-records-ehrs.

Hersh W. 2009. A stimulus to define informatics and health information technology. *BMC Medical Informatics and Decision Making* 9:24. http://bmcmedinformdecismak .biomedcentral.com/articles/10.1186/1472-6947-9-24.

HIMSS Analytics. 2016. *Telemedicine Study, 2016.* https://www.healthit.gov/sites/default /files/state_hie_evaluation_stakeholder_discussions.pdf.

HRSA. 2016. Performance measures. http://hrsa.gov/about/strategicplan /performancemeasures.html.

Huffington Post. 2016. The Laser Probe, The iKnife and The Cutting Edge of Surgery. *The Huffington Post.* http://www.huffingtonpost.com/healthline-/the-laser-probe-the -iknif_b_11803814.html.

IBM. 2017. A New Partnership Between Humanity and Technology. https://www.ibm .com/watson/health/.

Intel. 2016, September 21. Using wearable technology to advance Parkinson's research. http://www.healthcareitnews.com/sponsored-content/using-wearable-technology -advance-parkinsons-research.

Kampov-Polevoi, J., and B.M. Hemminger. 2011. A curricula-based comparison of biomedical and health informatics programs in the USA. *Journal of the American Medical Informatics Association* 18(2):195–202.

Kohn, D. 2013. The Case for One Source of Truth: Classification vs. Terminology Systems. http://daksystemsconsulting.com/blog/2013/10/01/the-case-for-one -source-of-truth/.

Mango Health. 2016. About Us. https://www/mangohealth.com/about.html.

Martin-Sanchez, F., V. Maoho, and G. Lopez-Campos. 2002. Integrating genomics into health information systems. *Methods of Information in Medicine* 41(1):25–30.

Merriam-Webster. 2010. Gamification. https://www.merriam-webster.com/dictionary /gamification.

Merriam-Webster. 2013. Genomics. http://www.merriam-webster.com/dictionary /genomics.

Mesko, B. 2016a. 20 Medical Technology Advances: Medicine in the Future – Part I. http://medicalfuturist.com/20-potential-technological-advances-in-the-future-of -medicine-part-i/.

Mesko, B. 2016b. 20 Medical Technology Advances: Medicine in the Future – Part II. http://medicalfuturist.com/20-potential-technological-advances-in-the-future-of -medicine-part-ii/.

National Association of Clinical Nurse Specialists (NACNS). 2016. http://nacns.org /html/cns-faqs1.php.

National Center for Biotechnology Information. 2016. Data and Software. https://www .ncbi.nlm.nih.gov/guide/data-software/.

National Council on Aging. 2015. Chronic Disease Self-Management. https://www.ncoa .org/wp-content/uploads/Chronic-Disease-Fact-Sheet_Final-Sept-2015.pdf.

National Institutes of Health. 2016a. *Current News* Releases. https://www.genome.gov /10000475/current-news-releases/.

National Institutes of Health (NIH). 2016b. National Human Genome Research Institute. Regulation of Genetic Tests. https://www.genome.gov/10002335/regulation-of -genetic-tests/.

National Institutes of Health (NIH). 2015a. All about the Human Genome Project. https://www.genome.gov/10001772/all-about-the--human-genome-project-hgp/.

National Institutes of Health (NIH). 2015b. Privacy in genomics. https://www.genome .gov/27561246/privacy-in-genomics/.

NIST. 2016. Cybersecurity framework. https://www.nist.gov/cyberframework.

Reynolds, R.B. and M. Sharp. 2016. Health Record Content and Documentation. Chapter 4 in *Health Information Management Concepts, Principles and Practice.* Edited by Oachs, P.K. and Watters, A.L. Chicago, IL: AHIMA.

Office of Disease Prevention and Health Professions (ODPHP). 2016. Genomics. HealthPeople.gov. https://www.healthypeople.gov/2020/topics-objectives/topic /genomics.

ONC. 2016. Privacy and security training games. https://www.healthit.gov/providers -professionals/privacy-security-training-games.

Okwerekwu, J. 2016. Overlooked Warning Signs More Accurately Predict Risk of Death. *STAT.* https://www.statnews.com/2016/05/16/health-markers-risk-death/.

PC Magazine. Back Up Your Cloud: How to Download All Your Data. http://www
.pcmag.com/image_popup/0,1871,s=25414&iid=408744,00.asp.

PCPCC (Patient Centered Primary Care Consortium). 2016. Defining the medical home.
https://www.pcpcc.org/about/medical-home.

Procter, R. 2009. (ed.) Definition of health informatics [Internet]. Message to: Virginia
Van Horne. *Health Informatics Journal.* Edinburgh: United Kingdom.

Snell, E. 2016a. Top 5 Healthcare Data Breaches in 2016 Not from Hacking. *Health IT
Security.* http://healthitsecurity.com/news/top-5-healthcare-data-breaches-in-2016
-not-from-hacking.

Snell, E., 2016b. Cybersecurity Attacks Leading Large Health Data Breach Cause. *Health
IT Security.* http://healthitsecurity.com/news/cybersecurity-attacks-leading-large
-health-data-breach-cause.

US Department of Energy Office of Science. 2016. *Human Genome Project Information
Archive 1990-2003, Human Genome Project.* http://web.ornl.gov/sci/techresources
/Human_Genome/index.shtml.

World Health Organization. 2016. Health Topics: eHealth. http://www.who.int/topics
/ehealth/en/.

Wyss Institute at Harvard University. 2016 Human Organs-on-Chips. https://wyss
.harvard.edu/technology/human-organs-on-chips/.

ADDITIONAL RESOURCES

Bird, Julie. 2015. 10 Emerging healthcare trends for 2016. Healthcare. http://www
.fiercehealthcare.com/healthcare/10-emerging-healthcare-trends-for-2016.

Bushko, R. 2009. *Strategy for the Future of Health: Goal Formation and ITicine.* IOS Press.
doi: 10.3233/978-1-60750-050-6-3.

Centers for Disease Control and Prevention. 2016a. Chronic diseases: The leading causes
of death and disability in the United States. http://www.cdc.gov/chronicdisease
/overview/index.htm.

CMS. 2014. Eligible professional meaningful use core measures. https://www.cms.gov
/Regulations-and-Guidance/Legislation/EHRIncentivePrograms/downloads/11
_Clinical_Decision_Support_Rule.pdf.

Cykert, S., and A. Lefebvre. 2011. Regional extension coordinators: Use of practice
support and electronic health records to improve quality and efficiency. *North Carolina
Medical Journal* (72)3:237–239.

Department of Health and Human Services. 2015. Regional Extension Centers. https://
www.healthit.gov/providers-professionals/regional-extension-centers-recs.

Fact Sheet 19: Ethical Issues in Human Genetics and Genomics. 2016. http://www.genetics
.edu.au/Publications-and-Resources/Genetics-Fact-Sheets/FactSheetELSI.

Figlioli, K. 2011. The transformative role of healthcare IT in accountable care. *Healthcare
Financial Management* 65(7):116, 118.

Greens, R. 2009. Informatics and a health care strategy for the future–general directions. In *Strategy for the Future of Health*. Edited by R. Bushko. Amsterdam, Netherlands: IOS Press. doi:10.3233/978-1-60750-00-6-21.

Health IT. 2014. How a screening prompted by clinical decision support saved a patient's life. *Health IT Buzz Case Studies*. https://www.healthit.gov/buzz-blog/ehr-case-studies/screening-prompted-clinical-decision-support-saved-patients-life/.

Healthcare.gov. 2016. Glossary. https://www.healthcare.gov/glossary/care-coordination/.

HIMSS. 2016. mHealth technologies. http://www.himss.org/library/m-health.

HIMSS Analytics. 2016. Precision medicine essentials brief. http://www.himssanalytics.org/research/essentials-brief-2016-precision-medicine-study.

IBM. 2016. *Go beyond artificial intelligence with Watson*. http://www/ibm.com.

Institute of Medicine (US) Roundtable on Value and Science-Driven Health Care. 2010. *Clinical Data as the Basic Staple of Health Learning: Creating and Protecting a Public Good: Workshop Summary*. Washington, DC: National Academy Press. http://www.ncbi.nlm.nih.gov/books/NBK54296/.

Lewandrowski, K., K. Gregory, and D. Macmillan. 2011. Assuring quality in point-of-care testing: Evolution of technologies, informatics, and program management. *Archives of Pathology and Laboratory Medicine* 135(11):1405–1414.

Mell, P. 2010. Updated 2016.. *NIST SP 800-145—The NIST Definition of Cloud Computing*. National Institute of Standards and Technology. https://www.nist.gov/programs-projects/cloud-computing.

Muller R.M. and K. Chung. 2006. Current issues in health care informatics. *Journal of Medical Systems* 30(1):1–2.

National Center for Biotechnology Information (NCBI). 2016. Welcome to NCBI. http://www.ncbi.nlm.nih.gov.

National Center for Biotechnology Information. (NCBI). 2010. U.S. healthcare data today: Current state of play. http://www.ncbi.nlm.nih.gov/books/NBK54296.

Appendix A: Odd-Numbered Answers for Check Your Understanding Sections

Chapter 1

Check Your Understanding 1.1
1. b
3. c
5. d
7. d

Check Your Understanding 1.2
1. a
3. c
5.

  __3__ Knowledge
  __1__ Data
  __5__ Informatics
  __2__ Information
  __4__ Wisdom

Check Your Understanding 1.3
1. False; the policies and procedures must be rewritten to address the new terminology and processes used with the EHR such as screens versus forms, how information is made a part of the record, querying, and so on.
3. d
5. c

Check Your Understanding 1.4
1. c
3. a
5. True

Chapter 2

Check Your Understanding 2.1
1. a
3. d

5. True
7. False; GINA is a comprehensive information nondiscrimination act that defines genetic information to include one's genetic and family genetic information.

Check Your Understanding 2.2
1. d
3. d
5. True
7. True
9. True

Chapter 3

Check Your Understanding 3.1
1. e
3. b
5. c
7. c

Check Your Understanding 3.2
1. b
3. e
5. a
7. a

Chapter 4

Check Your Understanding 4.1
1. a
3. b
5. d

Check Your Understanding 4.2
1. a
3. c

5. d

7. c

9. b

Check Your Understanding 4.3

1. c

3. d

5. b

Check Your Understanding 4.4

1. d

3. b

5. True

Chapter 5
Check Your Understanding 5.1

1. a

3. c

5. d

7. c

9. c

11. c

Check Your Understanding 5.2

1. d

3. c

5. s

7. u

9. u

11. u

Check Your Understanding 5.3

1. d

3. c

5. b

7. c

9. c

Check Your Understanding 5.4

1. g

3. c

5. e

7. j

9. d

11. False; it is an essential and not an optional function.

13. True

15. True

Check Your Understanding 5.5

1. a

3. True

5. True

Chapter 6
Check Your Understanding 6.1

1. b

3. a

Check Your Understanding 6.2

1. b

3. b

5. c

Check Your Understanding 6.3

1. c

3. a

5. c

Chapter 7
Check Your Understanding 7.1

1. a

3. b

5. e

7. c

Check Your Understanding 7.2

1. False; that is the dependent variable.

3. True

5. True

7. c

Check Your Understanding 7.3

1. b
3. c
5. False; that would be MS Excel.
7. True

Check Your Understanding 7.4

1. a
3. d
5. a
7. d

Check Your Understanding 7.5

1. a
3. c
5. True

Check Your Understanding 7.6

1. a
3. b
5. False; it is the SELECT statement.

Chapter 8
Check Your Understanding 8.1

1. True
3. True
5. True
7. False; HIPAA does required the creation of business contingency or disaster plans.
9. True

Check Your Understanding 8.2

1. True
3. True
5. True
7. True
9. d

Check Your Understanding 8.3

1. True
3. False; learnability is an important component of system usability.

5. True
7. True

Chapter 9
Check Your Understanding 9.1

1. True
3. False; they are primarily used by clinicians.
5. False; it is important for organizations to assure interoperability of systems.

Check Your Understanding 9.2

1. False; most electronic patient portals are designed to allow patients to view selected lab results and selected discrete data.
3. False; CAC assists the coder in the coding process, but a human being still makes the critical decisions for final coding.
5. True

Check Your Understanding 9.3

1. False; disparity in healthcare can be improved with DSS use.
3. True
5. True

Chapter 10
Check Your Understanding 10.1

1. e
3. d
5. b
7. True
9. False; at best, some data from some healthcare systems can be uploaded to a PHR, but most cannot due to lack of interoperability.

Chapter 11
Check Your Understanding 11.1

1. d
3. b

5. c

7. a

9. False; Progress notes provide documentation of condition of a patient at specific times throughout the hospitalization. They are in written narrative form without a predefined model and are therefore unstructured data.

Check Your Understanding 11.2

1. a

3. d

5. a

7. False; metadata are needed to provide the details of how the data were created, the data types and allowable values, as well as where they are stored.

9. True

Chapter 12
Check Your Understanding 12.1

1. False; the privacy rule is a part of HIPAA.

3. True

5. True

7. c

9. e

Check Your Understanding 12.2

1. False; the Privacy Rule includes exceptions where authorizations are not required such as for TPO and other specific kinds of requests.

3. True

5. False; that released should only be enough to meet the intended purposes of the request.

7. c

9. a

11. d

Chapter 13
Check Your Understanding 13.1

1. c

3. b

5. d

7. True

9. False; HIPAA Security Rule requires a full evaluation of methods to secure ePHI.

Check Your Understanding 13.2

1. d

3. d

5. c

7. False; encryption is used to allow for a protected transmission but does not alter the information and when decrypted is as the original.

9. True

Chapter 14
Check Your Understanding 14.1

1. False; Each individual facility defines what constitutes the LHR for their facility, therefore the LHR can be different between facilities.

3. False; there has been a significant increase in state laws that provide guidance regarding rules of evidence and civil procedure within each state.

5. False; the record custodian leads activities related to the LHR.

7. False; a designated record set is any set of health records that are maintained with individually

identifiable information or protected health information while the LHR is that defined for disclosure.

Check Your Understanding 14.2

1. False; this is a facility-wide policy for all in the workforce who interact in any way with the LHR.
3. False; it is a best practice for legal council to review to assure the legal aspects are covered completely and appropriately.
5. True
7. False; it is necessary to be able to assess the systems involved.

Check Your Understanding 14.3

1. True
3. False; this response is to describe the processes invoked if the potential for lawsuits or litigation is detected.
5. False; this term applies to any format of evidence.
7. d
9. c

Check Your Understanding 14.4

1. d
3. d
5. True
7. False; it is turning data into documents.

Chapter 15
Check Your Understanding 15.1

1. d
3. True
5. True

Check Your Understanding 15.2

1. d
3. False; an example of other reliable healthcare websites would include associations such as the American Cancer Society and the American Heart Association.
5. False; applications can facilitate the patient maintaining information such as weight, blood pressure, and blood sugar results which can be important to the patient's personal health record.

Chapter 16
Check Your Understanding 16.1

1. d
3. c
5. d
7. d
9. e

Check Your Understanding 16.2

1. False; because there are so many different types of jobs and at all levels, some do not require a degree and some rely more on the skills one has from another degree.
3. False; these are not the general skills required. They are: working knowledge of Microsoft Suite, detail orientation, independent, excellent interpersonal oral and written communication skills, ability to multitask, problem solver and troubleshooter, critical thinking skills, time management, ability to function in a leadership role.

Appendix A: Odd-Numbered Answers for Review Exercises Sections

Chapter 1 Review Exercises

1. d
3. a
5. c
7. d
9. The challenges are primarily due to much of the information being subjective, as seen in physician notes, and the large amount of information.

Chapter 2 Review Exercises

1. a
3. b
5. e
7. True
9. False; this violated the patient's privacy.
11. The manager should meet with the employee and access the Facebook page and the posting. He or she should then discuss the violation with the employee and document the incident. Employees may need a reminder regarding appropriate use of social media.
13. Physician is violating the principles of beneficence and justice because he is not using all data available to recommend the best EHR, instead his decision is based on monetary gain. The potential for harm is that the EHR system does not protect the privacy and security of the patient's PHI and it does not provide the necessary features

to meet the needs of the facility due to security and design flaws. Course of action is to report the physician to your manager and to the Medical Chief of Staff, then form a committee to evaluate the next steps.

Chapter 3 Review Exercises

1. a
3. b
5. a
7. a
9. The EHRs allow for multiple individuals to access a health record at the same time, the records can be accessed from multiple locations, and there is the opportunity to access information in different formats from that of the original document; that is, vital signs over time instead of for each individual recording.

Chapter 4 Review Exercises

1. a
3. c
5. d
7. Two tiered—composed of client and server, fat clients, no business rules or application server, not as scalable due to fat clients.

  Three tiered—composed of client, server, and application server, thin clients, business rules on application server, very scalable.

9. Physical models capture the hardware composition of a system in terms of the computer and other devices. Architectural models as they provide a framework or structure for the flow of data and information within systems.

11. Private cloud—accessible to only one customer and can be operated by the organization, a third party, or a combination of the two, at the customer's location or offsite.

    Community cloud—supported for use by a "community" of users who share some trait, such as security needs, in common.

    Public cloud—open to the general public and owned by an academic institution, the government, or some other organization for the benefit of the public.

    Hybrid cloud—consists of two totally separate cloud infrastructures (private, community, or public) that are unique, but share standardized or proprietary technology facilitating data and application portability.

Chapter 5 Review Exercises

1. b

3. c

5. True

7. True

9. False; this type of data is categorical because the salaries are grouped data.

11. True

13. True

15. Data are raw facts and figures that are processed into information. The types of data are nominal, ordinal, interval, and ratio. Nominal data is categorical data where categories are names, for example, demographic data on a survey. Ordinal or ranked data, are data where the names or labels have an order to them with meaning attached. Interval data is continuous numerical data that has equal intervals of ordered categories. Ratio data is a type of continuous numerical data. In addition to the equal intervals between data points that are found in interval data, ratio data have a true zero point.

17. Unstructured data entry is the use of free text or narrative data in the health record, this can be collected in web forms using free-text boxes, or abstracted from physician's notes in a chart or from recordings. The disadvantage is that is it hard to determine the completeness of the data. Structured data is data where the possible entry fields are constrained, defined, and limited. Structured data are complete and recommended for mandatory government reporting, clinical reporting, and quality measures. The disadvantage is that it cannot capture the clinicians' impressions on a patient, which provide a rich set of data.

Chapter 6 Review Exercises

1. c

3. c

5. a

7. d

9. d

Chapter 7 Review Exercises

1. a
3. c
5. True
7. False; that is the null hypothesis.
9. True
11. The EHR provides structured data for analysis in healthcare research.
    Two examples would include:
    1. Data can be collected from EHRs to determine if patients received prophylactic antibiotics before surgery.
    2. Data could be collected on all diabetic patients to see if diabetic protocols were being utilized correctly.
13. Data visualization tools include MS Excel, SPSS, and R Software.
    This visualization is a single view presenting data from several different sources and joining data from Admission ER tables. Combining these datasets gives idea more clear idea of hospital resource utilization by examining the amount of patients being admitted to the emergency room and the average time these patients spend at the hospital, setting the way for further investigation into peaks, trends, and patterns.

Chapter 8 Review Exercises

1. a
3. d
5. e
7. True
9. True
11. They are needed to bring projects to completion on time, on budget, and with a project the meets the project specification. Roles are project team lead, steering committee lead, implementation team lead, proposal committee member, interface with end users, test team lead, as some examples.
13. The systems development life cycle (SDLC) includes four primary phases: planning and analysis, design, implementation, and support and evaluation. Planning and analysis—defines the goals and scope of the project, organization's business problem, and the resources needed. Design—select project manager, steering committee, hire consultants, develop RFI/RFP, select vendor. Implementation—install system hardware and software, test system, train staff. Support and evaluation—collect data regarding all reported problems, support users.
15. Advantages—can store scanned images and test results, paper part is familiar, advanced directives can be stored online. Disadvantages—requirements of both paper and electronic systems must be addressed, complexity in record location, definition of legal health record, report creation complicated.
17. Disaster planning is defined as a plan for protecting electronic personal health information (ePHI) in the event of a disaster that limits or eliminates access to facilities and ePHI. HIPAA requires that facilities have a disaster recovery plan. Two related issues are the need to

confirm vendors' obligations in a disaster and what control they have over offsite cloud data.

Chapter 9 Review Exercises

1. True
3. True
5. True
7. True
9. False; a human needs to do the critical analysis for appropriate reimbursement.
11. DSSs can be clinical or administrative. CDSSs provide alerts, reminders, and interfaces to assist clinicians with patient care decisions. Administrative CDSSs support administrative decisions using data sources that could include reimbursement, utilization of services, and aggregate patient sociological data.
13. Example answers include graphing data, generating reports, patient portal displays, geospatial mapping of healthcare data, statistical trend analysis.

Chapter 10 Review Exercises

1. True
3. c
5. b
7. Community health management information systems (CHMISs) were first established in 1990, community health information networks followed a few years later, late 1990s and 2000s saw the rise of the regional health information organization (RHIO), and finally the HIEs.

9. a. Advantages: easier to administer; addresses provider concerns about incomplete information; disadvantage: lack of patient control.
   b. Advantage: automatic inclusion of data for more complete data for providers, yet patients can restrict use; disadvantage: procedures for documenting opt-out, so providers know about it, are unclear.
   c. Advantage: much more patient control; disadvantage: very difficult to implement.
   d. Advantages: patient has complete, up front control; provides an opportunity to educate patients; may provide better record matching; disadvantages: obtaining and communicating consent; questions as to how consent can be revoked or withdrawn.
   e. Advantage: patient control up front and very detailed; disadvantage: very, very difficult to manage.
11. Population health is the level and distribution of disease, functional status, and well-being of a defined group of people with specified characteristics. Public health is the study of the health of populations in large areas like states or countries.

Chapter 11 Review Exercises

1. e
3. f
5. b

7. d

9. High-volume, high-velocity, and high-variety information assets. Used for innovative forms of information processing for enhanced insight and decision making. For example, HIE data; Accountable Care Organizations collect the data and use big databases for quality reporting.

Chapter 12 Review Exercises

1. c

3. d

5. c

7. a

9. Use is sharing, employment, application, utilization, examination, or analysis of patient information within the organization. Disclosure refers to release, transfer, provision of access to, or divulging in any other way, the information outside the entity holding the information.

Chapter 13 Review Exercises

1. b

3. b

5. a

7. d

9. To determine potential security risks for a specific facility would involve assessing the vulnerabilities, threats, and risks with appropriate data to provide information on the likelihood of occurrence, potential impact, and level of risk.

Chapter 14 Review Exercises

1. a

3. b

5. c

7. a

9. d

11. False; this concept is of importance to all.

13. False; PE should not be copied and pasted forward from one visit to another because it should be current for the specific stay.

15. The LHR may be completely paper, electronic, or a hybrid combination of both. There are specific requirements for disclosure and e-discovery of electronic and hybrid records in court proceedings as opposed to rules that strictly address requirements of paper records.

17. The LHR policy determines what data and information can or should be released in a response to a request from a third party. Without the LHR policy, a healthcare organization is at risk related to requests for data and information that the organization is not prepared to release.

Chapter 15 Review Exercises

1. a

3. d

5. d

7. Validity is more about accuracy and reliability is more about consistency.

9. A personal health record is a record that is compiled by the patient and remains in possession of the patient.

Chapter 16 Review Exercises

1. b; This is the definition of a genome. Genomics is the branch of biotechnology having to do with applying the techniques of genetics and molecular biology to genetic mapping and DNA sequencing, genetics is the study of heredity and inherited characteristics.

3. a

5. b; This would be CAHIIM, the accrediting association that is associated with AHIMA.

7. c; NIST developed the framework in support of providing greater security; uses activity to achieve their goals for cybersecurity.

9. b; GINA was written to protect this information.

Glossary

Access: The right to inspect and obtain a copy of protected health information about the individual in a designated record set, for as long as the protected health information is maintained in the designated record set

Accountable Care Organization (ACO): An organization of healthcare providers accountable for the quality, cost, and overall care of Medicare beneficiaries who are assigned and enrolled in the traditional fee-for-service program

Accounting of disclosures: A listing of all of the disclosures made outside of the entity holding the protected health information

Accreditation Standards Committee X12 (ASC X12): Committee accredited by ANSI responsible for the development and maintenance of EDI standards for many industries. The ASC "X12N" is the subcommittee of ASC X12 responsible for the EDI health insurance administrative transactions such as 837 Institutional Health Care Claim and 835 Professional Health Care Claim forms (NIST 2011)

Addressable implementation specifications: Standards under the HIPAA Security Rule that should be implemented unless an organization determines that the specification is not reasonable and appropriate. If this is the case, then the organization must document why it is not reasonable and appropriate and adopt an equivalent measure if it is reasonable and appropriate to do so

Ad hoc standards: Standards established by a group of stakeholders without a formal adoption process

Administrative safeguards: Administrative actions such as policies and procedures and documentation retention to manage the selection, development, implementation, and maintenance of security measures to protect electronic protected health information and manage the conduct of the covered entity's or business associate's workforce in relation to the protection of that information

Administrative simplification: The category of provisions in Title II of HIPAA, in addition to the HIPAA Privacy, Security, and Enforcement Rules, Title II or the HIPAA Administrative Simplification Rule also includes rules and standards for transactions and code sets, and identifier standards for employers and providers

Aggregated health information exchange (HIE): Combines all of the data into a centralized repository with a MPI or record locator service. The different HIE participants query, or send a request to, the repository to obtain demographic, clinical, or other information

Alert fatigue: A commonly observed condition among physicians overwhelmed with large numbers to clinically insignificant alerts, thus causing them to "tune out" and potentially miss an important drug–drug or drug allergy alert

Alternate hypothesis: A hypothesis that states that there is an association between independent and dependent variables

AMA Tools for Transactions and Code Set Standards: Provides standards for the electronic exchange of protected health information, for compliance with HIPAA

Ambient intelligence: When numerous objects operate together in harmony

American National Standards Institute (ANSI): The US representative to the International Organization for Standardization (ISO)

American Recovery and Reinvestment Act (ARRA): An economic stimulus bill created to help the United States recover from the downturn of the economy with a total amount of $787 billion allocated to the recovery

American Society for Testing and Materials (ASTM) on Computerized System Standards for HIT: Provides procedures for the development, implementation, utilization, and maintenance of health information systems. Specifies data dictionary definitions to support other standards programs

ANOVA: Test to compare two or more means to determine if they are equal or different

Any and all records: A phrase frequently used by attorneys in the discovery phase of a legal proceeding. Subpoena-based requests containing this phrase may create a situation where the record custodian or provider's legal counsel can work to limit the records disclosed to those defined by a particular healthcare entity's legal health record. Typically, this is only during a subpoena phase, unless the information is legally privileged or similarly protected; the discovery phase of litigation probably can be used to request any and all relevant materials

Application service provider (ASP): A third-party service company that delivers, manages, and remotely hosts standardized applications software via a network through an outsourcing contract based on fixed, monthly usage, or transaction-based pricing

Applied research: Type of research that focuses on the use of scientific theories to improve actual practice, as in medical research applied to the treatment of patients

Architectural models: A framework or structure for the flow of data and information within information

Archival system: A database containing historical copies saved at a particular point in time and used later to recover and restore the information in a database system

Audit log: Chronological record of electronic system(s) activities that enables the reconstruction, review, and examination of the sequence of events surrounding or leading to each event or transaction from its beginning to its end. Includes who performed what event and when it occurred

Authorization: Must be obtained under the HIPAA Privacy Rule for the disclosure of PHI unless the PHI meets an exception stated in the Privacy Rule where an authorization is not required. The authorization must be written in plain language and must contain certain core elements, one of which is a statement that specifies that an authorization is signed

Autonomy: Core ethical principle centered on the individual's right to self-determination that includes respect for the individual; in clinical applications, the patient's right to determine what does or does not happen to him or her in terms of healthcare

Availability: Under the HIPAA Security Rule, the concept of ensuring electronic protected health information can be accessed as needed by authorized users. Encompassed in the concept of availability are many safeguards such as the data backup and storage specification

Backup: The process of maintaining a copy of all software and data for use in the case that the primary source becomes compromised

Basic research: A type of research that focuses on the development and refinement of theories

Beneficence: A legal term that means promoting good for others or providing services that benefit others, such as releasing health information that will help a patient receive care or will ensure payment for services received

Big data: "High-volume, high-velocity and high-variety information assets that demand cost-effective, innovative forms of information processing for enhanced insight and decision making" (Gartner 2016)

Biomedical informatics: Incorporates a core set of methodologies that are applicable for managing data, information, and knowledge across the translational medicine continuum, from bench biology to clinical care and research to public health

Blue Button: A big, virtual button on existing patient portals in order to give patients access to their health information

Breach: The acquisition, access, use, or disclosure of protected health information in a manner not permitted, which compromises the security or privacy of the protected health information

Break the glass: A method that allows users to access data that they may not otherwise be allowed to access. The users are alerted in advance that their actions are being monitored giving them an opportunity to halt their actions, if inappropriate

Broad network access: Any capabilities available over the network can be accessed by a wide variety of interface devices (laptops, smart phones, and so on) using standard mechanisms

Business associate (BA): All entities that are not members of the workforce, but are providing a service or performing a task on behalf of a covered entity with the expectation or possibility that they will have access to protected health information

Business associate agreement (BAA): Clearly documents the requirements of the business associate "to implement administrative, physical, and technical safeguards that reasonably and appropriately protect the confidentiality, integrity, and availability of the PHI that it creates, receives, maintains, or transmits on behalf of the covered entity" (45 CFR 164.308(b)(1) and 164.314)

Business continuity planning (BCP): Includes the recovery and use of the technology as in disaster recovery planning as well as the ability of the organization to continue the processes required for ongoing business operations. Sometimes requires operational procedures in the absence of information technology

Business impact analysis: A method for evaluating and prioritizing the risks that face a business. The goal of the business impact analysis is to identify any gaps in current recovery capability and to develop a strategy for meeting the identified recovery time and recovery point objectives

Cardinality: Describes the relationship between two data tables by referring to the number of elements in each table of a database

Categorical data: Data elements that represent mutually exclusive categories or labels

Cause and effect: Where researcher can state with some confidence that the variable under study caused, or did not cause, the effect under study

Central Authority Platform (CAP): Allows any or all of the classification and terminology coding systems to be used to capture and exchange clinical data

Centralized: A system in which the systems processing functions occur on a single computer

Certification: An evaluation performed to establish the extent to which a particular computer system, network design, or application implementation meets a prespecified set of requirements

Certification Commission for Health Information Technology (CCHIT): An industry-wide initiative engaging a diverse group of stakeholders in a voluntary, consensus-based process that began certifying EHRs in 2006

Characteristics of data quality: Part of the Data Quality Management Model from AHIMA. The 10 characteristics are accessibility, accuracy, consistency, comprehensiveness, currency, definition, granularity, relevancy, precision, and timeliness

Chief clinical information officer (CCIO): Senior manager who provides nursing leadership for nurses, physicians, and other clinicians for leadership in using information systems for the delivery of care, education, and research

Chief information officer (CIO): A senior manager responsible for the overall management of information resources in an organization

Chief knowledge officer (CKO): The person who oversees the entire knowledge acquisition, storage, and dissemination process and identifies subject matter experts to help capture and organize the organization's knowledge assets

Chief medical information officer (CMIO): An emerging position, typically a physician with medical informatics training that provides physician leadership and direction in the deployment of clinical applications in healthcare organizations

Chief nursing informatics officer (CNIO): A position emerging in larger healthcare facilities and organizations. The typical responsibilities in this position are related to the implementation and utilization of HIT systems for clinical care

Civil penalties: Generally fines or money damages used to sanction violators

Classification system: A system that arranges or organizes like or related entities for easy retrieval

Client-server: A network distribution method that involves multiple servers dedicated to different functions with workstations running the application and retrieving data from a server as needed

Clinical analytics: Mining discrete patient healthcare data such as laboratory results, medication, and genetics to make clinical decisions or to aid in translating data for research or further healthcare treatment

Clinical data repository (CDR): A central database that focuses on clinical information

Clinical data warehouse: Snapshots of a variety of clinical databases found throughout a healthcare organization that are combined for the purpose of reporting and analysis

Clinical decision making: The process of utilizing information to formulate a diagnosis

Clinical decision support (CDS): The process in which individual data elements are represented in the computer by a special code to be used in making comparisons, trending results, and supplying clinical reminders and alerts

Clinical decision support system (CDSS): A special subcategory of clinical information systems that is designed to help healthcare providers make knowledge-based clinical decisions

Clinical documentation: The functionality of electronic capture of clinical notes

Clinical informatics: Part of the biomedical continuum. It is focused on information systems to ensure that they support patient care that is safe, efficient, effective, timely, patient-centered, and equitable. Also, the scientific study of patient care, clinical research, and medical education and the effective use of information to support these activities, establish standards, and set policy

Clinical information systems (CIS): Systems designed to facilitate the management of the activities of various clinical departments and to provide electronic charge capture and results reporting

Clinical outcomes assessment: "Measures the actual outcomes of patient care and service against predetermined criteria (expected outcomes), based on the premise that care is delivered to bring about certain results." Also referred to as outcomes analysis (ONC 2012, 19)

Clinical phenotyping: Determining which observable characteristics are applicable for a given subset of patients

Cloud computing: A model for enabling ubiquitous, convenient, on-demand network access to a shared pool of configurable computing resources (such as networks, servers, storage, applications, and services) that can be rapidly provisioned and released with minimal management effort or service provider interaction

Code set: Any set of codes used to encode data elements, such as tables of terms, medical concepts, medical diagnostic codes, or medical procedure codes. A code set includes the codes and the descriptors of the codes

Cold site: A type of data backup facility. Equipment must be brought in, but the site is powered and secure. This is much less expensive than other options, but could take up to a month to operationalize

Column-delimited data: A flat file database format where information is stored in text files as columns of data. The data must be accompanied by documentation that lists the order and position of the variables so that the data may be interpreted

Comma-separated values (CSV): A flat file database format where fields are delimited by a comma. May include the variable names in the first row. If not, then they require documentation to identify the variables in each position

Community cloud: This cloud is supported for use by a community of users who share a trait, such as security needs, in common. One or more of the community may own and operate the cloud, or it may be operated by a third party or a combination of the two. A healthcare example of a community cloud might be the data infrastructure needed for an Accountable Care Organization or that required by a health information exchange

Comparable and consistent: Data that has been normalized or transformed so that they conform to the designated standards

Comparative effectiveness research (CER): Research that generates and synthesizes evidence that compares the benefits and harms of alternative methods to prevent, diagnose, treat, and monitor a clinical condition, or to improve the delivery of care

Computer-aided diagnosis (CAD): The incorporation of computer images with aspects of artificial intelligence to detect and identify potential disease factors

Computer-assisted coding (CAC): Software that extracts and translates transcribed or computer-generated free-text data into diagnosis and procedural codes for billing and coding purposes

Computer-based patient record (CPR): A historical term for an electronic patient record that provides complete and accurate data, alerts, reminders, clinical decision support, links to medical knowledge, and other aids

Computer literate: Having sufficient knowledge and skill to be able to use computers; familiar with the operations of a computer

Computerized provider (physician) order entry (CPOE): Applications that allow providers to write orders for medications or other treatments and transmit them electronically

Computers-on-wheels (COWs): Self-contained rolling carts containing a computer for access to the EHR on each unit

Concept: An idea or unique unit of knowledge or thought created by a unique combination of characteristics

Concept identification: A text processing method that maps the text to standardized concepts using clinical terminologies

Concurrent processes: Processes that run simultaneously and access shared resources such as databases

Confidentiality: A legal and ethical concept that establishes the healthcare provider's responsibility for protecting health records and other personal and private information from unauthorized use or disclosure. In the context of the HIPAA Security Rule, it means that electronic health information is accessible only by authorized people and processes

Consensus standards: Standards are those that are developed through a formal process of comment and feedback by interested stakeholders

Consolidated Health Informatics (CHI): The initiative to adopt existing health information interoperability standards throughout all federal agencies

Consumer: A person who purchases goods and services for personal use

Consumer informatics: The focus is on the interest of the consumer. A goal is to support and inform consumers to facilitate the management of and participation in their own care

Continuous data: Numerical data where there is an equal interval between the data points

Control Authority Platform (CAP): Allows any or all of the classification and terminology coding systems to be used to capture and exchange clinical data

Control group: A comparison study group whose members do not undergo the treatment under study

Correlational research: A design of research that determines the existence and degree of relationships among factors

Cost of ownership: A benefit of cloud computing. Using cloud computing can be more cost effective than maintaining a server on-site. Additional savings may be realized by reducing the number of employees and contractors needed for server maintenance, legacy system conversions, and upgrades

Covered entity (CE): A healthcare provider, health plan, or healthcare clearinghouse that transmits health information in electronic form in connection with healthcare transactions

Criminal penalties: A fine or imprisonment, whether suspended or not

Crosstabs: Serve to highlight any errors where there is an expected or explicit relationship between two data elements

C-suite: Executive management, such as the chief operating officer (COO), chief information officer (CIO), and so on

Dashboard: Reports of process measures to help leaders follow progress to assist with strategic planning

Data: The dates, numbers, images, symbols, letters, and words that represent basic facts and observations about people, processes, measurements, and conditions

Data analysis: The science of examining raw data with the purpose of drawing conclusions about that information. It includes data mining, machine language, development of models, and statistical measurements. Analytics can be descriptive, predictive, or prescriptive

Data cleaning: Sometimes termed data scrubbing, this involves examining the data thoroughly to detect wrong or inconsistent data

Data consolidation: A process for bringing together and summarizing large amounts of data and/or data from multiple sources

Data dictionary: A tool that provides metadata or information about data

Data flow diagram: A method to map out a data model; it maps out the database's boundary and scope

Data governance: Making decisions and exercising authority for data-related matters; establishing a culture where quality data is obtained and valued to drive the business

Data-interchange standards: Establish the means by which a sender transmits or communicates data or information to a receiver (also known as transaction standards)

Data liquidity: The ubiquitous sharing of healthcare data and information

Data mapping: The process of associating concepts or terms from one coding system to concepts or terms in another coding system and defining their equivalence in accordance with a documented rationale and a given purpose

Data mart: Well-organized user-centered searchable databases that contain information drawn from a data warehouse to meet the users needs. It is designed to hold the data that the department requires and is stored according to the users' specific needs

Data mining: The process of extracting and analyzing large volumes of data from a database in order to find patterns in the data

Data model: A representation of the data to be stored in a database and the relationships between the tables and data fields

Data Quality Management Model: A model presented by AHIMA covering the different processes of data handling during which data quality should be addressed. The data handling processes are categorized as application, collection, warehousing, and analysis

Data retrieval: Process of obtaining data from a healthcare database

Data segmentation: Can be used to tag patient information so that selected portions of the record can be shared

Data set standards: Established to assist in the tracking and understanding of important events such as births, deaths, hospital discharges, and so on. Such standards establish the data elements or data variables to be collected and define each data element

Data standards: Standards may be related to the data set, such as the data elements specified for the Uniform Hospital Discharge Data Set, or the allowable data values, such as a selection list being provided for the address data element of State. Standards such as the allowable data elements within a data set, the definitions of the different data elements, or the allowable data values, which constrain the data that can be entered into a field, ensure that the data are as accurate as possible

Data table: Grouping of data organized with records or rows and fields or columns

Data visualization: The representation of data pictorially with graphs and other visual displays

Data warehouse: A database that makes it possible to access data from multiple databases and combine the results into a single query and reporting interface

Database: A collection of data tables

Database management system (DBMS): A system installed locally on each machine that is designed to keep track of data locations and coordinate data modifications; creates and maintains a database. Provides a method for adding or deleting data and also supports methods to extract data for reporting

De facto standards: Standards that have evolved over time to become universally used without a government or other mandate

Decentralized: A system in which the processing functions are split or distributed, among one or more machines in the network system

Decision analysis: A systematic approach to decision making under conditions of imperfect knowledge; a practical application of probability theory that is used to calculate the optimal strategy from among a series of alternative strategies

Decision support database: A common example of a clinical data warehouse. These databases are found in many healthcare entities and may include claims data, financial data, and quality data combined in one database to support both internal and external reporting

Decision support systems (DSS): A computer-based system that gathers data from a variety of sources and assists in providing structure to the data by using various analytical models and visual tools in order to facilitate and improve the ultimate outcome in decision-making tasks associated with nonroutine and nonrepetitive problems

Deidentified health information: Health information that neither identifies nor provides a reasonable basis to identify an individual

Dependability: A benefit of cloud computing. The cloud is up and running 24 hours a day, 7 days a week, every day of the year, which ensures access to much-needed items such as business applications, financial data, and help desk personnel

Dependent variable: A measurable variable in a research study that depends on an independent variable

Descriptive research: A type of research that determines and reports the current status of topics and subjects

Descriptive statistics: A set of statistical techniques used to describe data such as means, frequency distributions, and standard deviations; statistical information that describes the characteristics of a specific group or a population

Designated Record Set: A group of records maintained by or for a covered entity that is (1) the medical records and billing records about individuals maintained by or for a covered health care provider; (2) the enrollment, payment, claims adjudication, and case or medical management record systems maintained by or for a health plan; or (3) used, in whole or in part, by or for the covered entity to make decisions about individuals

Diagram 0: A data flow diagram expanding on the context diagram and adding details regarding the data tables and their relationships

Digital Imaging Communication in Medicine (DICOM): A standard that promotes a digital image communications format and picture archive and communications systems for use with digital images

Digital immigrant: An individual who lived before the advent of the digital age but has adapted more or less to the digital age

Digital native: A person who has only known a world of digital toys and tools

Disaster recovery planning (DRP): Defines the resources, actions, tasks, and data required to manage the business recovery process in the event of a physical disaster

Disclosure: The output and release upon request of appropriate health record documents

Discrete data: Data elements that represent mutually exclusive categories or labels

Disease management: Emphasizes the provider–patient relationship in the development and execution of the plan of care, prevention strategies using evidence-based guidelines to limit complications and exacerbations, and evaluation based on outcomes that support improved overall health

Distributed system: A collection of independent computers connected through a network and managed by system software that enables the computers to coordinate their activities and to share system resources such that the users perceive the system as a single, integrated system

Document and data nonrepudiation: Characteristics that defend against charges questioning the integrity of data or documents. They delineate the methods by which the data are maintained in an accurate form after their creation, free of unauthorized changes, modifications, updates, or similar changes

Double-blind study: A type of clinical trial conducted with strict procedures for randomization in which neither researcher nor subject knows whether the subject is in the control group or the experimental group

e-Discovery: The process of discovering what parts of the patient's records may be used for litigation or further legal proceedings. It is an opportunity for opposing counsel to obtain relevant information. It is named to reflect an emphasis on electronic records; however, paper–electronic hybrids may also be included

e-Health: An emerging field at the intersection of medical informatics, public health, and business, referring to health services and information delivered or enhanced through the Internet and related technologies

e-Health literacy: The ability to seek, find, understand, and appraise health information from electronic sources and apply the knowledge gained to addressing or solving a health problem

Electronic document management system (EDMS): Utilized to manage the plethora of electronically stored images and documents

Electronic media: (1) Electronic storage material on which data is or may be recorded electronically, including, for example, devices in computers (hard drives) and any removable or transportable digital memory medium, such as magnetic tape or disk, optical disk, or digital memory card; (2) transmission media used to exchange information already in electronic storage media. Transmission media include, for example, the Internet, extranet or intranet, leased lines, dial-up lines, private networks, and the physical movement of removable or transportable electronic storage media

Electronic medical record (EMR): An electronic record of health-related information on an individual that can be created, gathered, managed, and consulted by authorized clinicians and staff within a single healthcare organization

Electronic medication administration records (eMAR): Use of technology and bar coding to track medications from when ordered to when given to the patient

Electronic patient portals: Provide access to personal health information from a patient's healthcare organization. These portals provide patients with opportunities to view results of exams and treatment, and also provide alerts for preventive care

Electronic protected health information (ePHI): Individually identifiable health information that is transmitted by electronic media or maintained in electronic media

Encryption: The process of transforming text into an unintelligible string of characters that can be transmitted via communications media with a high degree of security and then decrypted when it reaches a secure destination

Entity relationship diagram (ERD): Displays the relationship between tables in a relational database

Episode of care: The specific instance of a condition or illness with a defined time frame with the beginning and ending times of care identified

e-Prescribing: Allows practitioners to use electronic devices to write and submit prescription orders directly to a participating pharmacy rather than faxing or providing the patient with a written prescription that must then be taken to the pharmacy

Equivalence: In a data mapping, determined by the distribution of map relationships for a given map

Ergonomics: A discipline of functional design associated with the employee in relationship to his or her work environment, including equipment, workstation, and office furniture adaptation to accommodate the employee's unique physical requirements so as to facilitate efficacy of work functions

Ethics: A field of study that deals with moral principles, theories, and values; in healthcare, a formal decision-making process for dealing with the competing perspectives and obligations of the people who have an interest in a common problem

Evidence-based medicine: The use of the current best evidence in making clinical decisions about the care of individual patients by integrating individual clinical expertise with the best available clinical evidence from systematic research

Experimental research: (1) A research design used to establish cause and effect; (2) A controlled investigation in which subjects are assigned randomly to groups that experience carefully controlled interventions that are manipulated by the experimenter according to a strict protocol; *Also called* experimental study

Export: To get the data out of one system

Expressivity: How well a note conveys the patient's and provider's impressions, reasoning, and thought process; level of concern; and uncertainty to those subsequently reviewing the note

Extended or Enhanced Entity Relationship (EER): A "languages" associated with information modeling, began as entity relationship diagramming, it is useful for those who process data better visually

External validity: An attribute of a study's design that allows its findings to be applied to other groups

Extract, transform, and load (ETL): Process of exporting the data from the data source, mapping the data to the data destination and importing the data into the destination data warehouse

Fault tolerant: Systems that are highly available and remain in operation even when hardware, software, or network failures occur

Federal Rules of Civil Procedure (FRCP): The guidelines that govern the procedures for civil trials

Federal Rules of Evidence (FRE): Governs what and how electronic records may be used and the roles of record custodianship for purposes of evidence in a trial

Federated health information exchange (HIE): Designed as provider-to-provider networks using the Internet for connectivity, with no central repository of data. A central entity maintains the master patient index or record locator service, which is used to determine where patients have been treated previously and where their health information might exist

Field: Data elements representing attributes of the information being collected

Field studies: Research done outside the laboratory or place of work

File Server: A distribution method where the system runs entirely on the end user's workstation and transfers entire files

Firewall: Monitors and controls all communication into and out of an intranet. It is implemented by a set of processes that act as a gateway to a network applying the organizational security policy

Flat file: A text file, usually delimited by a comma or tab, with one record found on each row. It has only one table of data

Forecasting: To calculate or predict some future event or condition through study and analysis of available pertinent data

Foreign key: A variable in one table that is a primary key in another table

Forward maps: Those that map from an older source code or data set to a newer target code or data set

Frequency: The number of times that a particular observation or value occurs in a data set

Functional genomics: Studies for genomics include learning the pattern of genes under certain conditions

Functionality: An aspect of an EHR that should be evaluated. It addresses the features of the EHR product, including patient encounter documentation, automating and facilitating office workflow, decision support during patient encounters, and reporting that supports care management and template customization

Future-proofing: A benefit of cloud computing. Computer hardware, software, and networking solutions begin their move toward obsolescence almost as soon as they are implemented, which can be costly. Cloud computing moves the cost of updating certain parts of the technology from the customer to the cloud provider, a substantial benefit given the rapid pace of the growth of the Internet and other technologies

Genetic Information Nondiscrimination Act of 2008 (GINA): This law, which took effect in 2009, provides the legal standard to be followed for the collection, use, and disclosure of genetic information; it was enacted to prohibit discrimination based on genetic information for health coverage and employment

Genetics informatics: Specific to the use of genome sequence data along with computer capabilities and statistical methods to obtain biological information

Genome: All the genetic information present in a given organism

Genomics: A branch of biotechnology concerned with the genetic mapping and DNA sequencing of sets of genes or the complete genomes of selected organisms

Government mandate: Standards that are specified or established by the government for certain purposes

Hacker ethics: Refers to the hackers' beliefs that restrictions on data are objectionable, and that technology is a tool that should be used to perform hands-on actions that make nonhackers' private data publicly accessible while protecting the hacker's personal privacy

Hard disk: The permanent memory of a computer that stores installed application software, files created by the user, and the operating system

Health: The state of being free from illness or injury

Health and Medicine Division (HMD): (Formerly Institute of Medicine) An independent, nonprofit organization that works outside of government to provide unbiased and authoritative advice to decision makers and the public (IOM 2016)

Health informatics: The field of information science concerned with the management of all aspects of health data and information through the application of computers and computer technologies

Health Information and Management Systems Society (HIMSS): A cause-based not-for-profit organization exclusively focused on providing global leadership for the optimal use of IT and management systems for the betterment of healthcare. The HIMSS mission is to lead healthcare transformation through the effective use of health information technology

Health Information Exchange (HIE): As a noun, HIE refers to an organization that supports, oversees, or governs the exchange of health-related information among organizations according to nationally recognized standards. As a verb, health information exchange refers to the actual exchange of health information electronically between providers and others with the same level of interoperability, such as labs and pharmacies

Health information system (HIS): A set of components and procedures organized with the objective of generating information that improves healthcare management decisions at all levels of the health system

Health information technology (HIT): The technical aspects of processing health data and records including classification and coding, abstracting, registry development, and storage

Health Information Technology for Economic and Clinical Health (HITECH) Act: One part of ARRA. Designated funding to modernize the healthcare system by promoting and expanding the adoption of health information technology. HITECH provided $20 billion in Medicare and Medicaid incentive payments to physicians and hospitals for meaningful use of EHRs and $2.6 billion to support ONC initiatives

Health Insurance Portability and Accountability Act (HIPAA): Legislation that addresses standards for transactions and code sets for electronic exchange of health-related information to perform billing or administrative functions; standards for terminologies related to medications including the Food and Drug Administration's names and codes for ingredients, manufactured dosage forms, drug products, and medication packages; and additional standards for privacy and security of patient information

Health IT Standards Committee: An official federal advisory committee established by the Health Information Technology for Economic and Clinical Health (HITECH)

Act enacted as part of the American Recovery and Reinvestment Act (ARRA) of 2009. The committee makes recommendations to the National Coordinator for Health IT on standards, implementation specifications, and certification criteria for the electronic exchange and use of health information

Health Level 7 (HL7): An international organization of healthcare professionals dedicated to creating standards for the exchange, management, and integration of electronic information

Health literacy: The degree to which individuals have the capacity to obtain, process, and understand basic health information and services needed to make appropriate health decisions

Health plan: An individual or group plan that provides, or pays the cost of, medical care

Healthcare clearinghouse: A public or private entity, including a billing service, repricing company, community health management information system, or community health information system, and value-added networks and switches, that do either of the following functions: (1) processes or facilitates the processing of health information received from another entity in a nonstandard format or containing nonstandard data content into standard data elements or a standard transaction; (2) receives a standard transaction from another entity and processes or facilitates the processing of health information into nonstandard format or nonstandard data content for the receiving entity

Healthcare code sets: Any set of codes used for encoding data elements, such as tables of terms, medical concepts, medical diagnostic codes, or medical procedure codes

Healthcare Common Procedure Coding System (HCPCS): Consists of two levels or systems. Level I is CPT, a large, well-curated catalog of clinical and surgical procedures maintained by the American Medical Association as a proprietary and copyrighted resource. Level II of the HCPCS is maintained by CMS. CMS creates and administers the Level II HCPCS codes as alphanumeric identifiers for products, supplies, and services not included in CPT

Healthcare provider: Any person or organization who furnishes, bills, or is paid for healthcare in the normal course of business

HIPAA Enforcement Rule: 45 CFR 160, subparts C, D, and E. This rule spells out the authority of the Office for Civil Rights (OCR) related to the enforcement of the HIPAA Privacy and Security Rules

Historical research: A research design used to investigate past events

HIT Policy Committee: A federal advisory committee established under the HITECH Act

Hot site: A type of data backup facility for critical applications and operations, which can be online within hours. This option is the most expensive

Human Gene Nomenclature (HUGN): A system for exchanging information regarding the role of genes in biomedical research in the federal health sector

Hybrid cloud: This consists of two totally separate cloud infrastructures (private, community, or public) that are unique, but share standardized or proprietary technology facilitating data and application portability

Hybrid (health) record: A type of patient record that is maintained in both paper and electronic formats. It may be part of a mixture of paper and electronic or multiple electronic systems that do not communicate or are not logically architected for record management

Hypertext markup language (HTML): A standardized computer language that allows the electronic transfer of information and communications among many different information systems

Hypothesis: A statement that describes a research question in measurable terms

Imaging informatics: Synonymous with radiology informatics or medical imaging informatics, it utilizes the radiology information gathered from individual patients to enhance patient care by finding ways to efficiently and reliably use the collected data

Import: Brings in data from other systems or databases

Imputation: A process that uses special statistical methods to provide missing values in data records. Imputation methods must be described fully and imputed values clearly labeled

Independent variable: The factors in experimental research that researchers manipulate directly

Inferential statistics: (1) Statistics that are used to make inferences from a smaller group of data to a large one; (2) A set of statistical techniques that allows researchers to make generalizations about a population's characteristics (parameters) on the basis of a sample's characteristics

Informaticist: Individuals in a field of study (informatics) that focuses on the use of technology to improve access to, and utilization of, information

Informatics: Using technology to acquire, manage, maintain, and use information as a basis for the plethora of decisions that must be made in a cost-effective manner. Also, the study of collecting, organizing, storing, and using electronic information

Information governance: The accountability framework and decision rights to achieve enterprise information management (EIM). IG is the responsibility of executive leadership for developing and driving the IG strategy throughout the organization. IG encompasses both data governance (DG) and information technology governance (ITG)

Information infrastructure: Processing, tools, and technologies to support the creation, use, transport, and storage of information

Infrastructure as a service (IaaS): This is the most minimal level of cloud computing where the infrastructure is provided, but the consumer controls the operating systems, storage, and applications. The consumer may also have control over networking components such as the firewall

Institute of Medicine (IOM): An independent, nonprofit organization that works outside of government to provide unbiased and authoritative advice to decision makers and the public

Institutional Review Board (IRB): An administrative body that provides review, oversight, guidance, and approval for research projects carried out by employees serving as researchers, regardless of the location of the research (such as a university or private research agency); responsible for protecting the rights and welfare of the human subjects involved in the research. IRB oversight is mandatory for federally funded research projects

Integrated: Designed to bring together multiple information systems and allow them to communicate in a timely and effective manner and work together as one system

Integrity: Under the HIPAA Security Rule, this means that electronic protected health information is not altered or destroyed in an unauthorized manner

Interfaces: Hardware or software that enable disparate CIS and HIS software systems to communicate with each other

Internal validity: An attribute of a study's design that contributes to the accuracy of its findings

International Classification of Functioning and Disability (ICF): Classification of health and health-related domains that describe the body functions and structures, activities, and participation

International Organization for Standardization (ISO): A worldwide, nongovernmental, internationally recognized standards development body

Internet of Things (IoT): A computing concept where every day physical objects are connected to the Internet and able to identify themselves to other devices

Interoperability: Standards that allow different health information systems to work together within and across organizational boundaries in order to advance the effective delivery of healthcare for individuals and communities

Interval data: A category of continuous data that do not have a true zero and can have negative numbers. An example of interval data is temperature, which can be negative or positive

Join: Combine data from two or more tables in a database

Justice: Treating all people fairly

Knowledge management (KM): The management of information in the facility data repositories, policies and procedures, and other work documents

Laboratory information system (LIS): A system that provides a hub to integrate laboratory information, including orders with results; there may be user access to the information. Other functionality includes scheduling, billing, and other information needed by the lab; rarely is all of this information integrated with an EHR

Legacy data: Existing data, some of which are on paper, and some of which may already be digital. Whatever the current format, they must be converted to a format that is compatible with the new product or system

Legal health records: A concept created to describe the data, documents, reports, and information that comprise the formal business record(s) of any healthcare organization that are to be utilized during legal proceedings

Legal hold: A legal concept that requires special, tracked handling of patient records to ensure no changes can be made to a record involved in litigation. Common in the paper record environment to substantiate the integrity of the record, this is less common in the electronic environment where audit logs are the standard

Limited data set: Protected health information from which certain specified direct identifiers of individuals and their relatives, household members, and employers have been removed

Linearization: A subset of the ICD-11 foundation component, that is fit for a particular purpose (reporting mortality, morbidity, or other uses); jointly exhaustive of the ICD universe (foundation component); composed of entities that are mutually exclusive of each other; and each entity is given a single parent

Litigation response: Typically the term used to describe the processes and procedures invoked if the potential for lawsuits or litigation is detected. It is a set of procedures that, when instituted, protects the relevant records. Litigation response is not only triggered by atypical record disclosure requests but by any sign or action that shows a potential for a lawsuit

Local area network (LAN): A network that connects various devices together via communications within a small geographic area such as a single organization

Logical Observation Identifiers Names and Codes (LOINC): A dictionary of laboratory codes and clinical test descriptors, originated by Regenstrief Institute and funded by federal support grants as a public resource for the common good. It is publicly usable without any fees or license

Meaningful use: The use of a certified EHR in a meaningful manner such as for e-prescribing; clinical decision support; maintenance of a problem list of current and active diagnoses; the exchange of health information; and the submission of quality or other measures. This is evaluated as part of the EHR Incentive Program of CMS

Meaningful use of information: Using systems with certified software to enhance the use of data obtained from health records

Measured service: Use of resources in the cloud can be monitored, controlled, and reported, allowing for better management

Medical identity theft: The assumption of a person's name and sometimes other parts of his or her identity—such as insurance information or Social Security number—without the victim's knowledge or consent to obtain medical services or goods, or when someone uses the person's identity to obtain money by falsifying claims for medical services and falsifying medical records to support those claims

Medical informatics: Both the information and data parts as well as the controlling and automatic nature of data processing itself

Medical scribe: A medical student, nurse practitioner, or physician's assistant who assists the physician with the required documentation in the patient's medical record

Metadata: Data that provide information about another piece of data. Essentially, data about data

Method: A piece of information stored about an object in an object-oriented database. It describes how to use the stored data

mHealth: A form of telehealth where wireless devices and phone technologies are used for the generation, aggregation, and dissemination of health information between patients and providers

Middleware: A bridge between two applications or the software equivalent of an interface

Minimum necessary: Requires covered entities to evaluate their practices and enhance safeguards as needed to limit unnecessary or inappropriate access to and disclosure of protected health information

Mixed methods research: Studies that utilize data collection and data analysis methods from both quantitative and qualitative research in one study

Mobility: A benefit of cloud computing. Data streaming from the clouds allows for greater mobility because the Internet is accessible from multiple mobile devices, such as smart phones and tablets, PDAs, virtual desktops, or traditional laptops or PCs

Moral values: A system of principles by which one guides one's life, usually with regard to right or wrong

Morbidity: Diseases or conditions for which patients seek treatment

Mortality: The cause of death on death certificates. Mortality data are used to present the characteristics of those dying, determine life expectancy, and compare mortality trends with other countries

Narrative-text string: A type of search similar to the find functionality used every day in programs such as Microsoft Word or Adobe Reader

National Council for Prescription Drug Program (NCPDP): A not-for-profit ANSI-accredited standards development organization founded in 1977 that develops standards for exchanging prescription and payment information (NCPDP 2017)

National Drug File–Reference Terminology (NDF-RT): A data set created by the Veterans Administration for specific drug classifications

National Institute of Standards and Technology (NIST): An agency of the US Department of Commerce, founded in 1901 as the nation's first federal physical science research laboratory

Natural experiments: Where researchers have no control over the phenomenon under study. They do have the study planned but are waiting for the event to occur naturally

Natural language processing (NLP): A technology that converts human language (structured or unstructured) into data that can be translated then manipulated by computer systems

Negation: An issue with the widespread use of NLP in the real-time clinical domain. Negation involves the ability of the processor to detect the differences between "no chest pain," meaning it is absent, and "chest pain," meaning it is present

No-consent: A model for HIE that does not require any agreement on the part of the patient to participate in an HIE. HIEs that have adopted this model operate in states that explicitly allow this model via legislation

Nominal data: Those data where the categories are simply names. For example, a data element often collected for healthcare consumers is gender

Nonexperimental research: Where there is no random selection of participants nor is there any random assignment of participants to study groups

Nonmaleficence: A legal principle that means "first do no harm"

Notice of Privacy Practices (NPP): An essential document regarding an individual's right to receive adequate notice of how a covered entity may use and disclose his or her PHI. The notice also must describe the individual's rights and the covered entity's legal duties with respect to that information

Null hypothesis: A hypothesis that states there is no association between the independent and dependent variables in a research study

Numerical (computational) literacy: The ability to calculate or reason numerically. An example of the need for this can be found in an understanding of body mass index calculations or if drug dosing may call for calculations

Nursing informatics: Where the practice of nursing intersects with computers and information science. At the basic level it is using technology to improve patient care. The more advanced level is with the nurse scholar conducting research to validate practice and identify means of improving nursing practice to achieve enhanced outcomes and greater patient satisfaction

Object-oriented databases: Designed to handle data types beyond text and numbers. An object-oriented database stores two types of information about the object, the data itself and the method

Object-Role Modeling (ORM): A language associated with information modeling, sometimes called fact-oriented modeling. It uses graphical and textual languages to model and query information, as well as a procedural language for designing conceptual models

Office for Civil Rights (OCR): The enforcement agency for the HIPAA Privacy and Security Rule. Since April 14, 2003, the Privacy Rule has been enforced by the OCR. The OCR has enforced the Security Rule since July 26, 2009

Office of the National Coordinator for Health Information Technology (ONC): Principal adviser to the secretary of the Department of Health and Human Services on the development, application, and use of health information technology

ONC-Authorized Testing and Certification Bodies (ATCBs): Empowered to perform complete EHR or EHR module testing and certification. They utilize conformance testing requirements, test cases, and test tools developed by the NIST to determine whether the software complies with the EHR Incentive Program requirements for establishing meaningful use of an EHR

On-demand self-service: Anyone with the appropriate permissions can make use of the resources without additional intervention

Online diagnosers: Individuals who use the Internet to determine a diagnosis or identify a medical condition

Ontology: A system of categories used as a method for combining data; a common vocabulary organized by meaning that allows for an understanding of the structure of descriptive information that facilitates a specific topic or domain

Open System Interconnection Model (OSI): Seven-layer model presenting the protocol layers that a typical data packet traverses beginning with the electronic signal that starts the source data transmission, and ending with the application layer in the destination application on a PC or server that receives the transmitted data packet and translates it into meaningful data for display (ISO 2016)

Openness: Flexibility to extend and improve the existing system with minimal impact

Operations: In the context of HIPAA, any of the following activities: (1) quality assessment and improvement activities, including outcomes evaluation, patient safety activities, population-based activities, protocol development, and case management and care coordination; (2) competency assurance activities, including provider or health plan performance evaluation, credentialing, and accreditation; (3) conducting or arranging for medical reviews, audits, or legal services, including fraud and abuse detection and compliance programs; (4) specified insurance functions, such as underwriting, enrollment, premium rating, related to the creation, renewal, or replacement of health insurance or benefits, along with risk rating and reinsuring risk relating to healthcare claims; (5) business planning, development, management, and administration; and (6) business management and general administrative activities of the entity, including but not limited to deidentifying protected health information, creating a limited data set, and certain fundraising for the benefit of the covered entity

Opt-in: A model for HIE that requires patients to specifically affirm their desire to have their data made available for exchange within an HIE. This option provides up-front control for patients since because data cannot be included unless they have agreed

Opt-in with restrictions: A model for HIE that allows patients to make all or some defined amount of their data available for electronic exchange. Patients may restrict how their data is used by allowing access only to specific providers, by allowing only specific data elements to be included, or by allowing data to be accessed only for specific purposes

Opt-out: A model for HIE that allows for a predetermined set of data to be automatically included in an HIE, but a patient may still deny access to information in the exchange. This model allows the consumer to prevent their data and information from inclusion in the HIE

Opt-out with exceptions: A model for HIE that makes the patient's information available in the exchange, but enables the patient to selectively exclude data from an HIE, limit information to specific providers, or limit exchange of information to exchange for specific purposes

Ordinal data: Data where the names or labels have an order to them with meaning attached. For example, a patient may be diagnosed with cancer, which is often represented as Stage I, Stage II, Stage III, or Stage IV

Patient-centered medical home: Also referred to as medical home, this is a program to provide comprehensive primary care that partners physicians with the patient and their family to allow better access to healthcare and improved outcomes

Patient portal: A secure method of communication between the healthcare provider and the patient

Payment: Encompasses activities of a health plan to obtain premiums or to determine or fulfill its responsibility for coverage and provision of benefits under the health plan, and furnish or obtain reimbursement for healthcare delivered to an individual and activities of a healthcare provider to obtain payment or be reimbursed for the provision of healthcare to an individual

Personal health record (PHR): An example of consumer informatics. It is an electronic or paper health record maintained and updated by an individual for himself or herself, a tool that individuals can use to collect, track, and share past and current information about their health or the health of someone in their care

Physical models: Capture the hardware composition of a system in terms of the computer and other devices. The model is a pictorial representation of the arrangement of the different pieces and connection points

Physical safeguards: Physical measures, policies, and procedures to protect a covered entity's electronic information systems and related buildings and equipment, from natural and environmental hazards, and unauthorized intrusion

Physician champion: A physician tasked with the responsibility of representing the views of the physician users

Physician Consortium for Performance Improvement (PCPI): Develops, evaluates, uses, and disseminates best practices based on evidence-based measures

Picture archiving and communication systems (PACS): Provides storage of electronic images and reports

Placebo: Does not contain the study medication/intervention

Platform as a service (PaaS): At this intermediate level of capability consumers create or acquire applications using programming languages and tools supported by the cloud computing service provider. Although the consumer does not control the underlying infrastructure they do exercise more control over the applications

Point-of-care testing (POCT): Where the diagnostic tests are performed at or near where the patient care is taking place

Population (as related to research): The universe of phenomena, objects, people, or data under investigation from which a sample is taken

Population health: The capture and reporting of healthcare data that are used for public health purposes. It allows the healthcare providers to report infection diseases, immunizations, cancer, and other reportable conditions to public health officials

Post hoc text processing: Using algorithms after the data is entered to structure the data for processing

Practicality: An aspect of an EHR that should be evaluated. It addresses costs including goals about price, internal resources to maintain the EHR, whether the EHR is integrated or interfaced with the practice management systems, and interfaces with labs

Practice management system (PMS): Supports scheduling, financial, and billing activities. PMSs generally include patient registration, scheduling, eligibility verification, charge capture, electronic claims processing, billing, and collections

Precision medicine: Tailoring medical treatments to the individual characteristics of each patient through the ability to identify and classify subpopulations that differ in their susceptibility to a specific disease, and in the biology and prognosis of conditions they may acquire, and their response to specific treatments

Predictive analysis: Predicts future outcomes and is often used for simulating future scenarios that help managers optimize their outcomes

Predictive modeling: Where multiple data points are analyzed utilizing sophisticated software programs to identify the one characteristic that results in a problem or provides the solution

Pre-empt: In law, the principle that a statute at one level supersedes or is applied over the same or similar statute at a lower level

Primary data use: Use of healthcare data for direct patient care

Primary key: Uniquely identifies the row in a database

Privacy: The quality or state of being hidden from, or undisturbed by, the observation or activities of other persons, or freedom from unauthorized intrusion; in healthcare-related contexts, the right of a patient to control disclosure of protected health information

Private cloud: Accessible to only one customer and can be operated by the organization, a third party, or a combination of the two, at the customer's location or off-site. Healthcare organizations, especially larger ones, may choose this option due to the need for patient information security or if sensitive research is being conducted

Probability: Using patient-related data to determine the likelihood of various occurrences in the disease process and modes of treatment

Protected health information (PHI): Individually identifiable health information that is transmitted by electronic media, maintained in electronic media, or transmitted or maintained in any other form or medium

Public cloud: This cloud is open to the general public and owned by an academic institution, the government, or some other organization for the benefit of the public. The owner or a third party or some combination thereof can operate it, at any location

Public health: The level and distribution of disease, functional status, and well-being of all of the inhabitants of a given neighborhood, city, region, state, country, or the world

Public health informatics: The systematic application of information and utilization of computer technology to support public health initiatives as related to research, education, and delivery of public health services

Qualitative research: A philosophy of research that assumes that multiple contextual truths exist and bias is always present

Quality improvement (QI): A set of activities that measures the quality of a service or product through systems or process evaluation and then implements revised processes that result in better healthcare outcomes for patients, based on standards of care

Quantitative research: A philosophy of research that assumes that there is a single truth across time and place and that researchers are able to adopt a neutral, unbiased stance and establish causation

Quasi-experimental: A research design that resembles experimental research but lacks random assignment to a group and manipulation of treatment

Random access memory (RAM): Temporary memory used when a software application is in use or when the computer starts up

Random sample: An unbiased selection of subjects that includes methods such as simple random sampling, stratified random sampling, systematic sampling, and cluster sampling

Rapid elasticity: Service is provided on demand, meaning that more can quickly be provided when needed and reduced just as fast, so the consumer only pays for what they need and use

Ratio data: In addition to the equal intervals between data points seen in continuous data, ratio data have a true zero (0) point. An example of ratio data in healthcare would be "patient weight"

Read only memory (ROM): Permanent memory that can be read from but not changed by any applications' or users' actions

Record: In database terminology, a collection of fields that are related in a database

Record custodians: Also known as record stewards, they are commonly charged with leading multidisciplinary definition projects for both the HIPAA-required Designated Record Set and the legal health record. They are also expected to develop proper organization, management, guidelines, and processes related to the use of business records as a protective legal defense tool

Recovery point objective (RPO): The length of time that you can operate without a particular application

Recovery time objective (RTO): The maximum amount of time tolerable for data loss and capture

Red flags: Suspicious documents, information, or behaviors that indicate the possibility of identity theft. Examples of red flags include inconsistencies in documents (driver's license and insurance card), documents that appear to be altered, and not having more than one form of ID (insurance card but no other form of ID)

Regional Extension Centers (RECs): Established by the ONC to assist primary care providers in quickly becoming adept and meaningful users of EHRs. RECs provide training and support services to assist doctors and other providers in adopting EHRs, share information and guidance to help with EHR implementation, and give technical assistance as needed

Relational database: In such a database, data with a common purpose, concept, or source are arranged into tables. The relationship between the tables is displayed in an entity relationship diagram (ERD)

Reliability: A measure of consistency of data items based on their reproducibility and an estimation of their error of measurement

Rendition: The act of rendering data into documents, usually in report form. Report writers are the most common form of rendering, but there are others such as the creation of documents for continuity of care based on preprogrammed routines as required by meaningful use

Reputation: The reputation of the vendor should also be evaluated when purchasing an EHR, including how established the vendor is, references from other clients, and confirmation that their software is certified

Request for information (RFI): The RFI is used to ask vendors for information about their products and services. It is often used to obtain information from a large number of vendors to narrow the field of vendors to whom a request for proposals will be issued

Request for proposal (RFP): The RFP is a formal request to vendors to provide specific information about how they can meet the organization's specific requirements. In the RFP, the organization should describe the goals and priorities for the IT acquisition including technical and functional requirements

Required implementation specifications: Standards under the HIPAA Security Rule that are not optional, but must be implemented in conformance with the regulation

Research: (1) An inquiry process aimed at discovering new information about a subject or revising old information. Investigation or experimentation aimed at the discovery and interpretation of facts, revision of accepted theories or laws in the light of new facts, or practical application of such new or revised theories or laws; the collecting of information about a particular subject; (2) As amended by HITECH, a systemic investigation, including research development, testing, and evaluation, designed to develop or contribute to generalized knowledge (45 CFR 164.501 2013)

Research question: Research questions restate the research problem, name the independent and dependent variables, participants, and research site, but with a narrowed focus

Resource pooling: The cloud computing provider resources serve multiple consumers, usually independent of location, though these can be specified by the consumer

Resource sharing: Being able to use the hardware, software, or data anywhere in the system

Retrospective research: A type of research conducted by reviewing records from the past (for example, birth and death certificates or health records) or by obtaining information about past events through surveys or interviews

Reverse map: Goes from a newer source code or data set to an older target code or data set

Risk: The probability of incurring injury or loss, the probable amount of loss foreseen by an insurer in issuing a contract, or a formal insurance term denoting liability to compensate individuals for injuries sustained in a healthcare facility

RxNORM: A system created by the National Library of Medicine, for describing clinical drugs. RxNorm is the meaningful use specification for pharmaceutical names and codes in the United States

Sample: A set of units selected for study that represents a population

Sanctions policy: Under the HIPAA Security Rules, this must outline how cases of noncompliance will be addressed within the organization knowing that even with a strong risk management plan, the potential for noncompliance (either intentional or nonintentional) still exists

Scalability: The ability to support growth while maintaining the same level of service

Scatterplot: A visual representation of data points on an interval or ratio level used to depict relationships between two variables

Seamless care: Consistent, coherent, logical, without discontinuities or disparities, and of uniform quality care

Secondary data use: The nondirect care use of personal health information and other healthcare data

Secondary release of information: When the authorized recipient will be distributing the information to other individuals or agencies

Security: A benefit of cloud computing. The security of the cloud application is paramount for healthcare providers to be able to ensure the privacy of individually identifiable healthcare data. Cloud computing service companies working with providers and others would be subject to all aspects of the HIPAA Privacy and Security Rules

Security incident: The attempted or successful unauthorized access, use, disclosure, modification, or destruction of information or interference with system operations in an information system

Security Risk Analysis: Provides covered entities and business associates with the structural framework upon which to build their HIPAA Security Plan. Covered entities and business associates are required to conduct a Security Risk Analysis to evaluate risks and vulnerabilities in their environment and to implement reasonable and appropriate measures to protect against reasonably anticipated threats or hazards to the security or integrity of electronic protected health information

Select query: The purpose of a select query in SQL is to pull records that meet a certain criteria from a particular table or combination of tables

Semantic interoperability: The ability to exchange data and information with its original meaning intact and understood by all receivers

Social media: Websites and applications that enable users to create and share content or to participate in social networking

Software as a service (SaaS): The highest level of cloud computing service models, SaaS enables access to the cloud computing provider's applications via a variety of devices, usually through an interface such as a web browser

Source: The code or data set from which the data map originates

Spoliation: The malicious alteration, concealment, or destruction of evidence

Standards development organizations (SDOs): An organization involved, in the healthcare context, in creating and maintaining healthcare standards. In order to promulgate a recognized standard, SDOs must be accredited by ANSI and, if applicable, the ISO

State Rules of Civil Procedure: State laws adopted by the state from the US Federal Rules of Civil Procedure that provide guidance regarding civil procedure within each state (US Courts 2016)

State Rules of Evidence: State laws adapted by the state from the US Federal Rules of Civil Procedure that provide guidance regarding rules of evidence and civil procedure within each state (US Courts 2016)

Structured data: Binary, machine-readable data in discrete fields, with limitations on what can be entered into the field. The structured entry of healthcare data involves the use of templates and on-screen forms with the possible entry fields and the potential entries in those fields controlled, defined, and limited. Structured data can have many benefits including completeness, quality, and accessibility of the data for a variety of purposes

Structured Query Language (SQL): A fourth-generation computer language that includes both DDL and DML components and is used to create and manipulate relational databases

Systematized Nomenclature of Medicine Clinical Terms (SNOMED CT): A processable collection of medical terminology covering most areas of clinical information such as lab results, nonlab interventions and procedures, anatomy, diagnosis and problems, and nursing. It is a logically organized and massive terminology, mostly ordered by a formal description logic, which permits SNOMED CT to benefit from the classifying reasons developed by computer science and the fields of formal ontology and logic

Target: The code or data set in which one is attempting to find a code or data representation with an equivalent meaning

Technical safeguards: The technology and the policy and procedures for its use that protect electronic protected health information and control access to it

Technology literacy: Entails having some basic knowledge about technology, some basic technical capabilities, and the ability to think critically about technological issues and act accordingly

Telehealth: A telecommunications system that links healthcare organizations and patients from diverse geographic locations and transmits text and images for (medical) consultation and treatment

Telemedicine: The remote delivery of healthcare services over a telecommunications network

Temporal: An issue with the widespread use of NLP in the real-time clinical domain. Temporal means the computer can detect any time frames included when the concept is identified. For example, "past history of cancer" is very different from simply "cancer"

Terminal emulation software: Used on a personal computer to allow a user to connect to a host as if the user is on a dumb terminal

Terminal-to-host: The application and any data stay on a host computer with the user connecting either via a dumb terminal or using terminal emulation software on a personal computer to connect as if the user is on a dumb terminal. Sometimes this arrangement is also termed a thin client, with most of the actual processing taking place on a central computer

Terminology: A set of terms representing the system of concepts of a particular subject field

Threat: The potential for exploitation of a vulnerability or potential danger to a computer, network, or data

Three-tiered architecture: Expands on the two-tier system with the addition of an application server that contains the software applications and the business rules. Clients in this architecture are called "thin clients" because most of the processing is done on the server, and the client has very little software installed on it

Topology: The network's physical layout. Types of cabled network topologies include point-to-point, star, bus, tree, or ring

Transaction: The transmission of information between two parties to carry out financial or administrative activities related to healthcare

Transaction set: The data required to complete a specified communication

Transaction standards: Establish the means by which a sender transmits or communicates data or information to a receiver (also known as data-interchange standards)

Translational medicine: Taking the scientific knowledge gained from basic advances in research to the bedside by developing new procedures and modes of treatment to improve healthcare

Transparency: The end user sees the distributed system as a single machine

Treatment: The provision, coordination, or management of healthcare and related services for an individual by one or more healthcare providers, including consultation between providers regarding a patient and referral of a patient by one provider to another

T-test: Used to compare current data to a company benchmark

Two-tiered model: A model composed of several client computers that are used to capture and process the data. The servers in this configuration are powerful machines that have application software installed on them and in turn store the data captured by client machines

Unified Modeling Language (UML): A common data-modeling notation used in conjunction with object-oriented database design

Uniform Rules for e-Discovery: Amendments to the FRCP specifically designed for electronically stored information

Unintended consequences: Unanticipated and undesirable issues or problems

Unstructured data: Unstructured data entry is the use of free text or string data in the health record. This does not mean that there is no organization to the data, just that it is not structured with specific data elements, allowable values, and so on. In the paper record a large amount of the data, especially the day-to-day progress notes, were unstructured

Usability: An aspect of an EHR that should be evaluated. It addresses the speed and ease of use, including goals about tasks that must be done fast, computer literacy of the practice staff, and the methods by which data will be entered

Use case: A technique that develops scenarios based on how users will use information to assist in developing information systems that support the information requirements

Valid authorization: Under HIPAA, a valid authorization under section 164.508 must contain at least the following elements: (i) A description of the information to be used or disclosed that identifies the information in a specific and meaningful fashion; (ii) The name or other specific identification of the person(s), or class of persons, authorized to make the requested use or disclosure; (iii) The name or other specific identification of the person(s), or the class of persons, to whom the covered entity may make the requested use or disclosure; (iv) A description of each purpose of the requested use or disclosure; (v) An expiration date or an expiration event that relates to the individual or the purpose of the use or disclose; (vi) Signature of the individual and the date. If the authorization is signed by a personal representative of the individual, a description of such representative's authority to act for the individual must also be provided (45 CFR 164.508 2013)

Validity: (1) The extent to which data correspond to the actual state of affairs or that an instrument measures what it purports to measure; (2) A term referring to a test's ability to accurately and consistently measure what it purports to measure

Values: What ethics and morals are based on; the beliefs or standards, on which we base our judgment

Variable: A characteristic or property that may take on different values

Virtual private networks (VPNs): Extend the firewall protection boundary beyond the local intranet by the use of cryptographically protected secure channels at the IP level. A VPN is a private network that uses a public network (usually the Internet) to connect remote sites or users together privately

Visual literacy: The ability to understand graphs or other visual information. For example, the consumer may need to understand a graph trend line of laboratory results

Vital statistics: Statistics on events such as birth and death; important enough that a government collects information on them through certain registration procedures

Vocabulary: A dictionary of terms; that is, words and phrases with their meanings

Vulnerability: An inherent weakness or absence of a safeguard that could be exploited by a threat

Vulnerable subjects: In the context of research studies are children, pregnant women, human fetuses, neonates, mentally disabled individuals, educationally or economically disadvantaged, prisoners or persons with incurable or fatal diseases. The study participants in these categories require additional consideration and/or protection

Warm site: A type of data backup facility. IT provides basic infrastructure, but takes time, possibly a week, to activate. This is less expensive than a hot site

Whistle-blower: One who reports a wrongdoing

Wide area network (WAN): A computer network that connects devices across a large geographic area

Workforce: Employees, volunteers, trainees, and other persons whose conduct, in the performance of work for a covered entity or business associate, is under the direct control of such covered entity or business associate, whether or not they are paid by the covered entity or business associate

World Wide Web (WWW): A global network of networks offering services to users with web browsers

References

Gartner. 2016. IT Glossary. http://blogs.gartner.com/it-glossary/big-data/.

Institute of Medicine of the National Academies. 2016. Advising the nation/Improving health. https://www.nationalacademies.org/hmd/~/media/Files/About%20the%20 IOM/IOM-brochure-website.pdf.

International Standards Organization. 2016. ISO 9000- Quality Management. http://www.iso.org/iso/home/standards/management-standards/iso_9000.htm.

National Institute of Standards and Technology (NIST). 2011. Accredited Standards Committee (ASC) X12. Response to the National Institute of Standards and Technology, Federal Agency Participation. https://www.nist.gov/sites/default/files/documents /standardsgov/ASC-X12-Consolidated-NIST-NFI-Response-2-16-11.pdf.

ONC. 2012. Component 5: History or Health Information Technology in the US. (Spring):19. https://www.healthit.gov/sites/default/files/Comp-05-Instructor-Manual .pdf.

US Courts. 2016. Current Rules of Practice and Procedure. http://www.uscourts.gov /rules-policies/current-rules-practice-procedure.

National Council for Prescription Drug Programs (NCPDP). 2017. About Us. http://www.ncpdp.org/About-Us.

Index